Endoscopic Spine Surgery and Instrumentation

Percutaneous Procedures

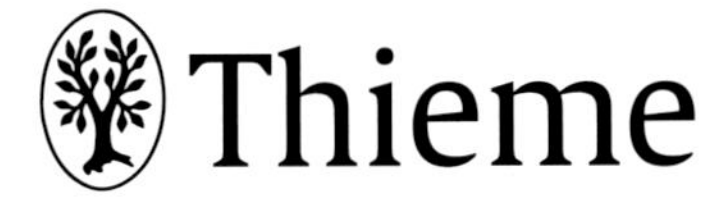

Endoscopic Spine Surgery and Instrumentation

Percutaneous Procedures

Daniel H. Kim, M.D., F.A.C.S.
Director, Spinal Neurosurgery and Reconstructive Peripheral Nerve Surgery
Department of Neurosurgery
Stanford University Medical Center
Stanford, CA

Richard G. Fessler, M.D., Ph.D.
Professor of Surgery
Chief, Section of Neurosurgery
University of Chicago Hospitals
Chicago, IL

John J. Regan, M.D.
Co-Director
Institute for Spinal Disorders
Cedars-Sinai Medical Center
Los Angeles, CA

Thieme
New York • Stuttgart

Thieme Medical Publishers, Inc.
333 Seventh Ave.
New York, NY 10001

Editor: Timothy Hiscock
Assistant Editor: Jennifer Berger
Vice President, Production and Electronic Publishing: Anne T. Vinnicombe
Production Editor: Print Matters, Inc.
Marketing Director: Phyllis Gold
Director of Sales: Ross Lumpkin
Chief Financial Officer: Peter van Woerden
President: Brian D. Scanlan
Compositor: Compset, Inc.
Printer: Everbest Printing Co.

Library of Congress Cataloging-in-Publication Data

Endoscopic spine surgery and instrumentation: percutaneous procedures. / [edited by] Daniel H. Kim, Richard G. Fessler, John J. Regan.
p. ; cm.
Includes bibliographical references and index.
ISBN 1-58890-225-0
1. Spine—Endoscopic surgery. 2. Surgical instruments and apparatus. I. Kim, Daniel H. II. Fessler, Richard G. III. Regan, John J., 1952–
[DNLM: 1. Endoscopy—methods. 2. Spine—surgery. WE 725 E56 2004]
RD533E537 2004
617.5′60597—dc22 2004048082

Important note: Medical knowledge is ever-changing. As new research and clinical experience broaden our knowledge, changes in treatment and drug therapy may be required. The authors and editors of the material herein have consulted sources believed to be reliable in their efforts to provide information that is complete and in accord with the standards accepted at the time of publication. However, in view of the possibility of human error by the authors, editors, or publisher of the work herein or changes in medical knowledge, neither the authors, editors, or publisher, nor any other party who has been involved in the preparation of this work, warrants that the information contained herein is in every respect accurate or complete, and they are not responsible for any errors or omissions or for the results obtained from use of such information. Readers are encouraged to confirm the information contained herein with other sources. For example, readers are advised to check the product information sheet included in the package of each drug they plan to administer to be certain that the information contained in this publication is accurate and that changes have not been made in the recommended dose or in the contraindications for administration. This recommendation is of particular importance in connection with new or infrequently used drugs.

Some of the product names, patents, and registered designs referred to in this book are in fact registered trademarks or proprietary names even though specific reference to this fact is not always made in the text. Therefore, the appearance of a name without designation as proprietary is not to be construed as a representation by the publisher that it is in the public domain.

Printed in China

5 4 3 2 1

TNY ISBN 1-58890-225-0
GTV ISBN 3-13-136651-6

To David G. Kline, M.D., the greatest mentor and teacher of all time.

Daniel H. Kim

To the many fellows, residents, medical students, nurses, and technicians who contributed to our work in so many meaningful ways.

Richard G. Fessler

To my father, Leo J. Regan, for teaching me honesty, perseverance, and the pursuit of a better life for all.

John J. Regan

Contents

Foreword

Spinal surgery became an important part of neurosurgery even while the specialty was being developed. One of Victor Horsley's early triumphs was the removal of a thoracic spinal cord tumor. There were no imaging studies, and clinical localization proved to be imprecise. But Horsley persisted in spite of initial negative exploration, extending the surgery to eventually find and remove the tumor. Walter Dandy recognized and removed herniated lumbar disks in the 1920s. Charles Elsberg was probably the first neurosurgeon to specialize in the spine. Mixter and Barr thoroughly described herniation of the intervertebral disk and its surgical treatment. By the 1940s operations on herniated lumbar and cervical disks via posterior approaches were widely described and discussed in the neurosurgical literature. By the 1960s the anterior approach to the cervical spine was firmly established.

Throughout the second half of the twentieth century, most neurosurgeons in the United States spent a majority of their time dealing with spinal diseases. Operations for the herniated disk, some spinal deformities, and to a lesser extent, spinal stenosis represented the majority of neurosurgical operations. Intracranial procedures were perceived as more glamorous, but spinal operations dominated the neurosurgical practice. At the same time, spine surgery in orthopedics grew in a somewhat different way with a great emphasis upon scoliosis and the repair of spinal deformity. By the 1980s the lines between orthopedic spine practice and neurosurgical spine practice had begun to blur, and by the 1990s there were few distinguishing features unique to one specialty or the other.

The introduction of the operating microscope in the 1970s revolutionized many aspects of intracranial surgery. But the microscope had no such decisive effect upon most spinal surgery. Although some surgeons utilized high magnification for spinal surgery, the majority did not. Obliteration of arterial venous malformations and removal of spinal cord tumors were both greatly enhanced by microtechniques, however, high magnification microsurgery had a much greater impact on intracranial surgery than spinal surgery.

Most spinal surgery has required large exposures with much soft tissue and bony disruption. Even so, a few surgeons began to work with limited exposures early in the development of spinal surgery. Pool introduced myeloscopy in 1938 for direct visualization of intraspinal contents. Collis demonstrated successful keyhole surgery for disk herniation through a speculum in the 1960s. The advent of better endoscopes, high resolution videoscopy, the operating microscope, and high quality perioperative imaging have set the stage for advances in minimally invasive spinal surgery.

As these procedures proliferate, there has developed a simultaneous need for an authoritative reference for both educational and clinical uses. The editors of this volume have created such a text. The offerings in this book begin with fundamental considerations of what equipment is needed and how that equipment should be deployed to greatest advantage. Practical topics range from simple disk excision and nerve root decompression (a procedure done for many years in a variety of ways) to complex spinal fixator implantations. We can expect that the repertoire of the minimally invasive surgeon is going to expand dramatically. For most procedures, minimally invasive only speaks to the skin incision and exposure required; complex surgeries can be accomplished with these limited exposures. Concepts of spinal surgery haven't changed with reduced exposure.

There is another area of minimally invasive surgery that is just now being developed. Vertebroplasty is a simple way to reinforce the weakened collapsed spine that is both safe and enormously successful in well selected patients. This is only a first step in percutaneous procedures. CT is already used to provide precise placement for diagnostic and therapeutic injections of all kinds. I think it will not be long before we are injecting materials to induce regrowth of cartilage, ligament, and bone. Induction of bone growth through the injection of a variety of growth factors is likely to supplant many open fusion procedures. Direct injection of specific neurolytic materials to deactivate nociceptors is feasible. It is not a serious stretch of the imagination to think that substances to reduce the bulk of ligaments, absorb bony spurs, or shrink protruding disks will become a reality. Many of the chapters in this book are on the cutting edge of such advances. At present minimally invasive surgery is valued for reducing tissue trauma and thus the risk and discomfort for patients. I predict, however, that these approaches will soon expand into regenerative techniques that sound like science fiction today.

There is another aspect of minimally invasive surgery that is very important: high quality perioperative imaging. This kind of imaging carries with it the promise of verifying the success of any given procedure at the time it is being done. Thus every patient should have the desired effect proven by imaging before they leave the interventional suite or operating room. Because at least one-third of the spine surgery failures that I see relate to failure of the original surgeon to meet the desired goals of surgery, I believe this added perioperative imaging will be an important change in practice as well.

Neuronavigation and robotics are also important aspects of this field. Robotics are particularly appropriate for spinal surgery, and I believe that the development of robots for automatic placement of fixators will be an important application in this area. Only a short time ago these minimally invasive procedures were appearing on our meeting programs as "look what I can do " oddities. In a very brief period of time they have become a standard part of the neurosurgical armamentarium and should be learned by everyone performing spine surgery. The concept of minimally invasive surgery is rapidly becoming as revolutionary a force in spinal surgery as the introduction of the operating microscope was to intracranial surgery.

The character of spinal surgery is changing. Subspecialization in the spine is now common and subspecialization in minimally invasive spine surgery will soon become common as well. As these techniques are developed, the number of diseases and abnormalities that can be treated will expand. With these techniques we can help an increasing number of patients achieve relief from the consequences of spinal deformities and disease. Because back and neck pain are among the most common complaints of patients throughout the world, the impact of expanding our armamentarium to both understand and treat them will be enormous. The editors and their authors are to be congratulated for this pioneering work that so dramatically expands the horizons of spinal surgery and equally expands our ability to help our patients.

Donlin M. Long, M.D., Ph.D.

Preface

Spinal surgery has evolved dramatically within the last twenty years. Innovative techniques, from the use of the operating microscope to image guidance, have changed the approach to surgical problems. In addition, improved instrumentation, from odontoid screws and lateral mass screws to sacropelvic fixation, has improved the surgical management of countless patients. It is these changes that have collectively led to the advancement of spinal surgery and subsequent improved outcomes.

One of the major advancements in this arena within the last decade has been in the development of minimally invasive spinal surgery. Since its inception, progress within this area has been dramatic. From percutaneous procedures to multilevel fusions, the advancement in this field has been unparalleled.

This book summarizes the enormous progress made in every aspect of minimally invasive spinal surgery. The text is divided anatomically, starting from the occipital cervical junction and moving down to the lumbosacral region. In this journey, everything from percutaneous procedures to multilevel endoscopic thoracic fusions is reviewed. This is a yeoman's review of minimal access surgery, reviewing its history as well as the latest in technology.

This book is meant for those who specialize in minimally invasive spinal surgery. Subdivided into cervical, thoracic, and lumbar surgery, the text and images are easily referenced. From decompressive procedures to instrumentation, details of surgical techniques are outlined. In addition, indications, contraindications, and outcomes are also discussed.

Endoscopic Spine Surgery was also written for every spine surgeon. As minimal access technology has grown, its use has spread to all aspects of spine surgery. Thus, even critics will agree that every spine surgeon should understand these procedures and utilize them as part of their armamentarium.

Lastly, this text was written for the vast array of people affiliated with spinal surgery. Addressing the broader audience from those in industry to the nurses in the operating room, we hope to promote the advancement of minimal access surgery by increasing the research and development in this subspecialty. We also hope to educate all of those involved in this area, decreasing anxiety and increase comfort level for all within the operating room.

Minimally invasive spine surgery is here to stay. Since its inception, it has led to improvement in patient care. This has been demonstrated through decreased postoperative pain and length of hospitalization with good neurological outcomes. We hope to further decrease the stigma behind endoscopic surgery by familiarizing readers with this area of specialty.

Acknowledgments

I would like to acknowledge the following individuals whose hard work made this book possible: Hoang Le, Raju S.V. Balabhadra, Max Lee, David W. Schaal, Michelle Mitchell, T.J. Hwang, Jessica Dillon, Karen M. Shibata, and all of the neurosurgery residents at Stanford University Medical Center.

Daniel H. Kim, M.D.

I would like to acknowledge my co-authors, Anthony K. Frempong-Boadu, Faheem Sandhu, Paul Santiago, and Daniel Refai, and my associates, Laurie Rice, Lacey Bresnahan, and Melody Hrubes, for the generous contributions.

Richard G. Fessler, M.D., Ph.D.

I would like to acknowledge Edgar Dawson, M.D., for his support through my career.

John J. Regan, M.D.

Contributors

Yong Ahn, M.D.
Chief, Department of Neurosurgery
Wooridul Spine Hospital
Seoul, Korea

John L. Andreshak, M.D.
Spine Surgery
Orthopaedic Associates
Warrenville, IL

Anthony Altimari, M.D.
Central DuPage Health Physician Staff
Central DuPage Hospital
Wheaton, IL

Calvin L. Au, M.D.
Attending Anesthesiologist
Department of Anesthesia
University of British Columbia
Vancouver General Hospital
Vancouver, British Columbia, Canada

Raju S.V. Balabhadra, M.D.
Department of Neurosurgery
Stanford University Medical Center
Stanford, CA

John Beiner, M.D.
Orthopaedic Surgeon
Connecticut Orthopaedic Specialists
Hamden, CT

Rudolf Beisse, M.D.
Vice Chairman and Head Trauma Surgeon
Department for Surgery and Traumasurgery
Trauma Center Murnau
Murnau, Germany

Darren Bergey, M.D.
Department of Orthopedics
Loma Linda University
Loma Linda, CA

Randal Betz, M.D.
Chief of Staff
Shriners Hospital
Philadelphia, PA

Sarjoo M. Bhagia, M.D.
Miller Orthopedic Clinic
Charlotte, NC

Christopher M. Bono, M.D.
Department of Orthopaedic Surgery
Boston University Medical Center
Boston, MA

John C. Chiu, M.D., F.R.C.S.
Chairman and Director
Neurospine Division
Department of Neurosurgery
California Spine Institute
Thousand Oaks, CA

David Clements, M.D.
Director, Spine Surgery
Cooper Hospital/University Medical Plaza
Camden, NJ
Co-Director of the Spinal Surgery Fellowship
Temple University Hospital
Philadelphia, PA

Alvin Crawford, M.D.
Director
Division of Pediatric Orthopaedic Surgery
Cincinnati Children's Hospital Medical Center
Cincinnati, OH

Jean Destandau, M.D.
Neurosurgeon
Bordeaux, France

Huy M. Do, M.D.
Stanford University Medical Center
Department of Radiology
Stanford, CA

Richard G. Fessler, M.D., Ph.D.
Professor of Surgery
Chief, Section of Neurosurgery
University of Chicago Hospitals
Chicago, IL

Kevin T. Foley, M.D.
Image Guided Research Center
Memphis, TN

Anthony K. Frempong-Boadu, M.D.
Assistant Professor
Department of Neurosurgery
New York University School of Medicine
New York, NY

Steven R. Garfin, M.D.
Professor and Chair
Department of Orthopaedics
University of California at San Diego
University of California at San Diego Medical Center
San Diego, CA

Russell V. Gilchrist, M.D.
Department of Neurological Surgery
University of Pittsburgh
School of Medicine
UPMC-Health System
Presbyterian University Hospital
Pittsburgh, PA

James M. Giuffre, M.D.
Director of Research
International Spinal Development and Research Foundation
Las Vegas, NV

Jonathan N. Grauer, M.D.
Assistant Professor and Co-Director
Orthopaedic Spine Service
Yale Orthopaedics
New Haven, CT

Tooraj Gravori, M.D.
Department of Neurosurgery
University of California at Los Angeles
Los Angeles, CA

Mark W. Hawk, M.D.
Spine Fellow
Department of Neurological Surgery
University of California at Davis
Sacramento, CA

Stephen E. Heim, M.D., F.A.C.S.
Co-Medical Director
Neuro-Spine Center
Director
Spine Surgical Training Center
Central DuPage Hospital
Carol Stream, IL

Langston T. Holly, M.D.
Assistant Professor
Division of Neurosurgery
University of California at Los Angeles
Los Angeles, CA

Zacharia Isaac, M.D.
Director, Interventional Physiatry
Division of Physical Medicine and Rehabilitation
Brigham and Women's Hospital
Boston, MA

David H. Jho, B.A.
Jho Institute for Minimally Invasive Neurosurgery
Department of Neurological Surgery
Allegheny General Hospital
Pittsburgh, PA

Hae-Dong Jho, M.D., Ph.D.
Jho Institute for Minimally Invasive Neurosurgery
Department of Neurosurgery
Allegheny General Hospital
Pittsburgh, PA

J. Patrick Johnson, M.D.
Director, Cedars-Sinai Institute for Spinal Disorders
University of California at Los Angeles
Los Angeles, CA

Larry T. Khoo, M.D.
Assistant Professor
Neurological and Orthopedic Spinal Surgery
Co-Director, UCLA Comprehensive Spine Center
UCLA Medical Center
Los Angeles, CA

Brian S. Kim, B.S.
Palo Alto, CA

Daniel H. Kim, M.D., F.A.C.S.
Director, Spinal Neurosurgery and Reconstructive Peripheral Nerve Surgery
Department of Neurosurgery
Stanford University Medical Center
Stanford, CA

David H. Kim, M.D.
The Boston Spine Group,
Boston, MA

Kee D. Kim, M.D.
Assistant Professor of Neurological Surgery
Department of Neurosurgery
University of California at Davis
Sacramento, CA

Brian K. Kwon, M.D.
Department of Orthopaedics
Thomas Jefferson University
Philadelphia, PA

David Le, M.D.
Stanford University Medical Center
Department of Neurosurgery
Stanford, CA

Sang-Ho Lee, M.D., Ph.D.
Wooridul Spine Hospital
Seoul, Korea

Michael A. Lefkowitz, M.D.
Long Island Neurological Associates
New Hyde Park, NY

Isador H. Lieberman, M.D., M.B.A., F.R.C.S.(C.)
Section of Spinal Surgery
Department of Orthopaedic Surgery
The Cleveland Clinic Foundation
Cleveland, OH

John M. Luce, M.D.
Professor of Medicine
Department of Medicine
Division of Pulmonary and Critical Care Medicine
University of California at San Francisco
San Francisco General Hospital
San Francisco, CA

Calvin R. Maurer Jr., Ph.D.
Senior Research Scientist
Co-Director, Image Guidance Laboratories
Department of Neurosurgery
Stanford University
Stanford, CA

Peter O. Newton, M.D.
Children's Hospital and Health Center
San Diego, CA

Mick J. Perez-Cruet, M.S., M.D.
Director, Minimally Invasive Spine Surgery and Spine Program, Michigan Head and Spine Institute
Providence Medical Center
Southfield, MI

George D. Picetti III, M.D.
Associate Clinical Professor
Department of Orthopaedics
Chief of Spine Surgery
Kaiser Sacramento
University of California at San Francisco
San Francisco, CA

Michael Potulski, M.D.
Head of Department
Spinal Cord Injuries
Trauma Center Murnau
Murnau, Germany

Y. Raja Rampersaud, M.D.
Toronto Western Hospital
Toronto, Ontario, Canada

Daniel Refai, M.D.
Resident
Department of Neurosurgery
Washington University in St. Louis
St. Louis, MO

John J. Regan, M.D.
Co-Director
Institute for Spinal Disorders
Cedars-Sinai Medical Center
Los Angeles, CA

Crystal D. Rogers
Georgetown University
Washington, D.C.

Daniel Rosenthal, M.D.
Neurosurgical Associate
Hamburg, Germany

Dino Samartzis, B.S., P.C. E.H.H.C., Dip. E.B.H.C., M.A.(C.), M.S.(C.)
Graduate Division
Harvard University
Cambridge, MA
Division of Health Sciences
The University of Oxford
Oxford, England
London School of Economics and Political Science
University of London
London, England

Faheem A. Sandu, M.D., Ph.D.
Fort Worth Brain and Spine Institute
Fort Worth, TX

James A. Sanfilippo
Medical Student
The University of Medicine and Dentistry of New Jersey
Newark, NJ

Paul Santiago, M.D.
Spine Fellow
Section of Neurological Surgery
University of Chicago Hospitals
Chicago, IL

Ramin Shahidi, Ph.D.
Assistant Professor
Director, Image Guidance Laboratories
Department of Neurosurgery
Stanford University
Stanford, CA

Adnan Siddiqui, M.D., Ph.D.
Resident
Department of Neurosurgery
SUNY Upstate Medical University Hospital
Syracuse, NY

Curtis W. Slipman, M.D.
Associate Professor
Department of Physical Medicine & Rehabilitation
University of Pennsylvania Health System
Philadelphia, PA

John S. Thalgott, M.D.
International Spinal Development and Research Foundation
Las Vegas, NV

Alexander R. Vaccaro, M.D.
Professor of Orthopaedic Surgery
Thomas Jefferson University and the Rothman Institute
Co-Director
The Delaware Valley Regional Spinal Cord Injury Center
Thomas Jefferson University
Philadelphia, PA

Anthony Virella, M.D.
Department of Neurosurgery
UCLA Medical Center
Los Angeles, CA

Michael Y. Wang, M.D.
University of Southern California
Los Angeles, CA

Jay B. West, Ph.D.
Imaging Scientist
Accuray, Inc.
Sunnyvale, CA

Russell Woo, M.D.
General Surgery Resident
Stanford University Medical Center
Stanford, CA

Michael Yee, F.N.P.
Kaiser Sacramento Spine Center
Roseville, CA

Anthony T. Yeung, M.D.
Arizona Institute for Minimally Invasive Spine Care
Arizona Orthopedic Surgeons
Phoenix, AZ

Christopher A. Yeung, M.D.
Arizona Institute for Minimally Invasive Spine Care
Arizona Orthopedic Surgeons
Phoenix, AZ

Kenneth S. Yonemura, M.D.
Assistant Professor
Department of Neurosurgery
SUNY Upstate Medical University Hospital
Syracuse, NY

■ SECTION ONE ■

Minimally Invasive Spine Surgery

1

Historical Background of Minimally Invasive Spine Surgery

MICK J. PEREZ-CRUET, RAJU S. V. BALABHADRA, DINO SAMARTZIS, AND DANIEL H. KIM

Demands from health insurance organizations and hospitals to remain competitive in the health care market, as well as the impact of cost, patient satisfaction, and a quicker return to normal daily function, have pressured physicians and biotechnology manufacturers to address the needs of an evolving work-oriented society. Stemming from the initial experiences of successful early ambulation following surgery and the advantages of outpatient surgery to the patient, hospital, and physician, a trend toward more minimally invasive procedures ensued.[1] Thus, to reduce operative time and complications, minimize intraoperative tissue trauma, diminish the length of hospital stays, lessen postoperative use of narcotics, and enhance postoperative outcomes, minimally invasive techniques have been developed to address morbidities associated with more open surgical procedures of the spine.

The earliest indication of spine pathology was found in Egyptian mummies dated 2900 BC and further elucidated in the Edwin Smith papyrus written circa 1550 BC. In fact, the first description of the spinal column was offered by the Egyptians in the djet symbol used for the god Osiris to represent stability, duration, and durability.[2] Emerging from the age of antiquity, Hippocrates has been credited as the father of spine surgery, as evidenced by his seminal teachings and writings, underlined by his principles of sound reasoning and accurate observation[3]; however, the first concrete delineation of operative treatment of the spinal column was proposed by Paulus of Aegina in the seventh century.[4] He advocated and conducted direct removal of osseous tissue at the site of pathology. Since then, various approaches and techniques for operative treatment of the spine have been developed and evolved to address numerous conditions. In this chapter, we will review the evolution of minimally invasive techniques in the spine.

Cervical Spine

Endoscopic-Assisted Transoral Surgery

Fang and Ong[5] published the first series of patients to undergo transoral decompression for irreducible atlantoaxial abnormalities in 1962; however, undue morbidity and mortality caused poor acceptance of this approach. Advancements in imaging techniques and the availability of the operative microscope improved the safety and efficacy of the approach. This approach, though, requires such wide exposures as soft/hard palate splitting and extended maxillotomies for decompressing clival abnormalities, resulting in increased operating time, complexity, prolonged recovery, and patient morbidity.[6] Frempong-Boadu et al[6] demonstrated the efficacy of endoscopic-assisted transoral surgery in limiting these extended approaches in a series of seven patients. One of the disadvantages of using the microscope is that the optics are located at a distance from the location of the abnormality. With the endoscope, the optics and illumination are in the field of the abnormality. With the use of the 30-degree angled endoscope, one can clearly visualize the clivus abnormality, obviating the need for extensive palatal splitting.[6]

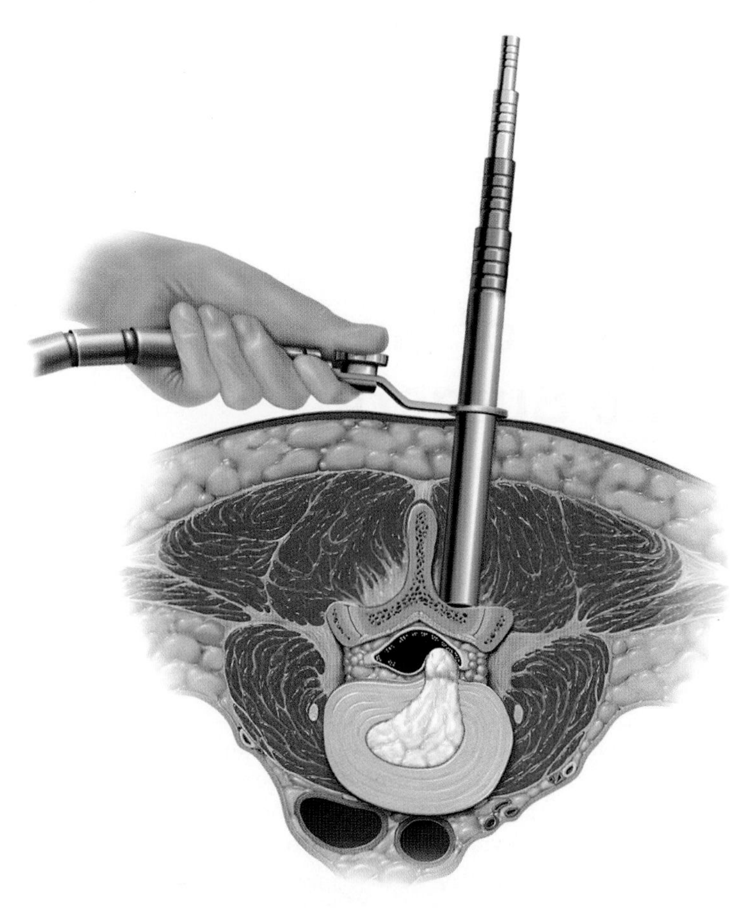

FIGURE 1–1 The microendoscopic diskectomy system comprising tubular dilators and retractor system can be used for cervical as well as lumbar surgeries.

Cervical Microendoscopic Laminectomy/Diskectomy

Scoville and Whitcomb[7] introduced the concept of posterior cervical disk surgery. Although the anterior approach to the cervical spine has become more popular, the posterior approach is an effective procedure in selected cases. It is indicated in cases with laterally herniated disk fragments, isolated foraminal narrowing, multilevel foraminal narrowing without central stenosis, continued root symptoms after anterior cervical diskectomy and fusion, and patients for whom anterior approaches are contraindicated; however, it is usually necessary to use moderate-size incisions and to perform significant paraspinous muscle dissection in these operations. Postoperative wound pain and muscle spasms can therefore be significant, and postoperative recovery is often relatively slow.

The microendoscopic diskectomy (MED) system was developed to minimize the tissue trauma and postoperative discomfort seen with open procedures (Fig. 1–1). It enables posterior cervical and lumbar diskectomy through a tubular retractor, with endoscopic observation. A guidewire is inserted through the posterior cervical musculature, with the tip being fluoroscopically directed to the operative disk space. Dilators are sequentially inserted through the posterior neck musculature, at the junction of the lamina and the lateral mass (Fig. 1–2). A 16 mm tubular retractor is then inserted over the largest dilator and fixed to the flexible arm assembly on the table. The endoscope is fixed inside the

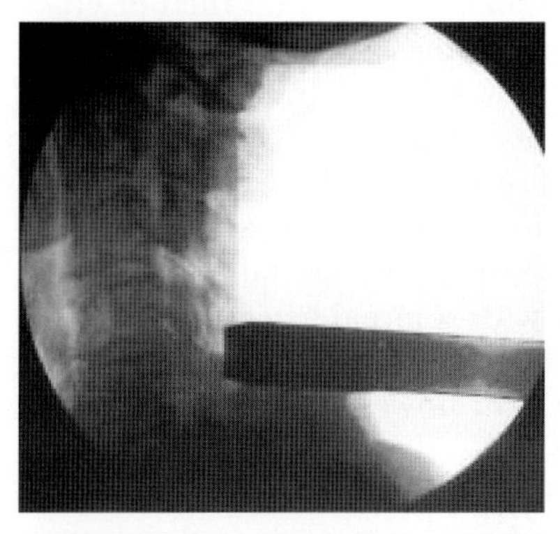

FIGURE 1–2 Intraoperative lateral fluoroscopic scan confirming the position of the working channel of the microendoscopic diskectomy system for a C4–C5 foraminotomy and diskectomy.

tubular retractor. The tubular retractor tip is positioned to expose the lateral portion of the superior and inferior laminae and the medial portion of the corresponding facet joint. After exposure has been achieved, a small curved curette is used to define the edge of the superior lamina and the lateral mass. Bone removal begins on the inferolateral portion of the superior lamina and proceeds to the superolateral portion of the inferior lamina. After palpation of the medial edge of the superior and inferior pedicles with a microprobe, bone removal is extended into the medial facet joint to expose the nerve root. Bone removal is performed with a small Kerrison punch or a high-speed drill as in open procedures. The MED system provides equally good exposure of the involved segment and decompression compared with open microdiskectomy.

In cadaveric studies, Roh et al[8] performed posterior cervical foraminotomies using either the MED system or conventional open techniques. Their results demonstrated that the average vertical diameter of decompression and percentage of facet removed were greater for the MED technique. The transverse diameter of the laminotomy area and the average length of decompressed root were not significantly different. Transmuscular dilation with an endoscopic tubular working channel can minimize postsurgical pain and provide rapid postoperative recovery.

Thoracic Spine

Thoracoscopic Spine Surgery

Jacobaeus, a professor of internal medicine in Stockholm, Sweden, is credited with performing the first thoracoscopic procedure in 1910.[9] As an internist, he was involved in the diagnosis and treatment of pulmonary tuberculosis, and he thought that the ability to observe the pleural space was crucial. After his initial diagnostic procedures, Jacobaeus described the technique of lysis of tuberculous pleural adhesions, which was performed with a cystoscope and a heated platinum loop.[10] In 1990, with the introduction of video imaging to standard endoscopy, the modern era of thoracoscopy began. Mack et al[11] in the United States and Rosenthal et al[12] in Europe first reported the technique of video-assisted thoracic surgery (VATS) in 1993. Thoracoscopic spine procedures were initially implemented to treat disk herniations, pathologies of the vertebral body, and drainage of abscesses, as well as for tumor biopsies. In the ensuing years it was used in cases of scoliosis, anterior interbody fusions, osteotomies and bone grafting, corpectomies, and vertebral instrumentation for tumors and fractures.

Thoracoscopic access is achieved by temporarily deflating the lung on the ipsilateral side of the spinal exposure using a double-lumen endotracheal tube. Narrow portals are introduced through small incisions in the intercostal spaces. The endoscope is then introduced through one of the portals, with the other portals serving as working channels and being used interchangeably.

Thoracoscopy can be used to access the entire thoracic spine and thoracolumbar junction (to L2), providing visualization of the disks, vertebral bodies, and ipsilateral pedicle (Fig. 1–3). It offers several advantages over conventional open thoracotomy to treat spinal disorders. VATS allows visualization of the procedure to the entire operating team, and two surgeons may work side by side. VATS uses small incisions and a minimal amount of rib resection, and there is no spreading of the ribs, thus minimizing postoperative discomfort, reducing incisional pain, creating fewer respiratory and shoulder girdle problems, and decreasing blood loss. It has also shortened hospitalization time and length of rehabilitation after surgery.

Like most endoscopic techniques, the successful application of VATS has a steep learning curve that requires the operator to acquire the technical skills needed to use the long working arms of the endoscopic equipment. Bony dissection requires stable and precise manipulation of standard open equipment with modified longer working arms. Thus, it is crucial to use both hands to stabilize and achieve precise control over the drill, curettes, or bone rongeurs used to avoid devastating neural or vascular injuries.

Thoracoscopic sympathectomy has also been used with success for treatment of anhydrosis in an ambulatory setting. Furthermore, thoracoscopic sympathectomies have been performed with multiportal and biportal systems; even uniportal approaches are now being used.

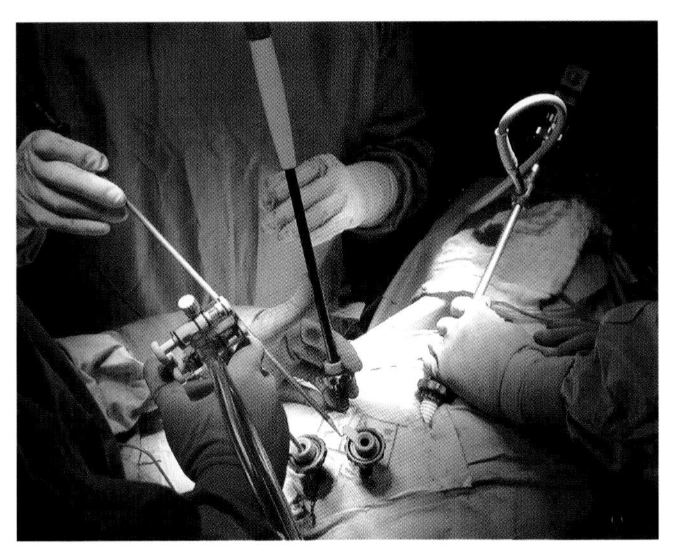

FIGURE 1–3 Thoracoscopic surgery. The image illustrates thoracoscopic techniques to obtain thoracolumbar decompression and stabilization for a severe TIZ burst fracture.

Posterior/Posterolateral Endoscopic Diskectomy

In a further attempt to reduce tissue trauma and enhance postoperative outcome, a thoracic microendoscopic diskectomy instrumentation and approach have been developed and employed with preliminary success to treat thoracic disk herniations from a direct posterior or posterolateral endoscopic approach. Jho[13] described the technique of endoscopic transpedicular thoracic diskectomy with a 0- and 70-degree 4 mm endoscope requiring relatively small 1.5 to 2 mm incisions and minimal tissue dissection. This approach avoids the need for separate skin incisions in the chest wall (required for thoracoscopic approaches) and the need for postoperative chest drainage. Chiu and Clifford[14] demonstrated the safety and efficacy of posterolateral endoscopic thoracic diskectomy followed by low-energy nonablative laser for shrinkage and tightening of the disk (laser thermodiskoplasty) using a 4 mm 0-degree endoscope.

Lumbar Spine

Chemonucleolysis

In 1941, Eugene Jansen and Arnold Balls[15] first isolated chymopapain, a proteolytic enzyme extracted from papaya latex. In 1956, Lewis Thomas[16] administered intravenous injections of crude papain to rabbits and noticed that their ears drooped. Intrigued by Thomas's article, Lyman Smith postulated the therapeutic use of papain to treat chondroblastic tumors. In 1963, Smith et al[17] were the first to inject chymopapain into a herniated nucleus pulposus for the treatment of sciatica. This process, aptly called chemonucleolysis, alters the characteristics of the nucleus pulposus by liberation of chondroitin sulfate and keratin sulfate by hydrolysis of noncollagenous proteins of mucopolysaccharide involvement and leading to polymerization of the nucleus pulposus. It has been used safely to treat disk disease in the spine for the past three decades. Despite the extensive use of chymopapain, chemonucleolysis still provokes controversy. After more than 30 years of clinical experience, research, double-blind trials, and Food and Drug Administration (FDA) approval, differing views persist. Nordby and Javid[18] published the results of a 14-year study of 3000 patients, with an 82% success rate for the first 1000 patients and an overall success rate of 87.2%; however, others have questioned the safety and indications for the use of chymopapain to treat disk disease.

Some 75 investigators in the United States and Canada administered injections to nearly 17,000 patients in phase III chemonucleolysis trials, which ended in July 1975. The results of the phase III trials were mixed, with several enthusiastic reports and several others that questioned the safety and efficacy of chymopapain.[19,20] To date, there is no consensus in the neurosurgical and orthopedic communities regarding the use of chymopapain. Proper patient selection is crucial for any intervention, and this is especially true for percutaneous chemonucleolysis. Chemonucleolysis should be reserved for patients presenting with radicular symptoms, with radiological studies [magnetic resonance imaging (MRI), computed tomographic (CT), and/or myelographic scans] confirming a herniated soft disk, and who have experienced failure of conservative nonsurgical treatment. The size and shape of the disk are not factors for safe chemonucleolysis. The proponents of chymopapain claim that lack of familiarity, training, and indications could explain some of the complications. Age can be a factor because patients over 60 years of age may lack sufficient mucoprotein for hydrolysis of the herniated disk. For patients younger than 20 years of age, 80 to 90% success rates have been reported.[21]

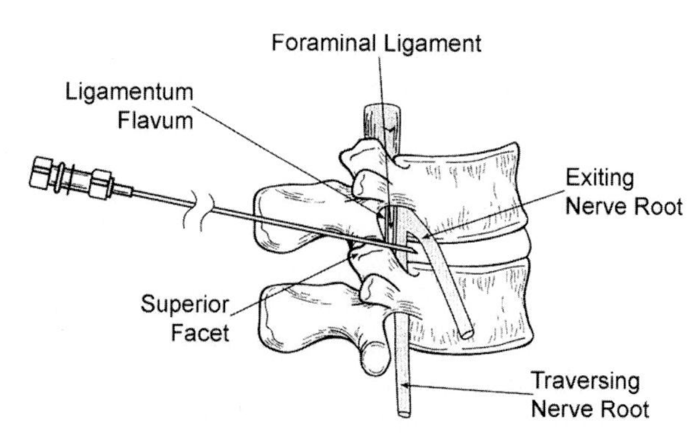

FIGURE 1–4 Diagram showing anatomic features of the relevant structures close to the path of the needle.

Chemonucleolysis is performed with the patient placed in either a lateral or a prone position; the needle is positioned in the center of the offending disk, with fluoroscopic guidance (Fig. 1–4). The currently recommended dose is 1000 to 2000 units/disk space. With chymopapain sensitivity testing and administration of antihistamine agents before chymopapain injection, anaphylaxis has been reduced to 0.25% of total allergic reactions. The vast majority (87%) of the reported complications occurred before 1984, and no major anaphylactic complications have been reported in the United States since July 1987.[22]

There is significant cost effectiveness in the use of chemonucleolysis for the treatment of intervertebral disk disease. As noted by Ramirez and David,[23] the cost of chemonucleolysis is, on average, 23% lower than that of surgical treatment of disk herniation.

Percutaneous Diskectomy

In 1975, Hijikata et al[24] demonstrated a percutaneous nucleotomy by utilizing arthroscopic techniques for disk removal via intradiscal access for the treatment of posterior or posterolateral lumbar disk herniations under local anesthesia. After diskography using Evans blue dye, specially designed instruments were placed in a 5 mm cannula and inserted against the lateral anulus. A circular incision was made in the anulus, and the blue-stained nucleus pulposus was removed with pituitary forceps. In 1983, Kambin and Gellman[25] performed a diskectomy by inserting a Craig cannula and a small forceps into the disk space after an open laminectomy to evacuate the nucleus pulposus. In 1985, Onik et al[26] reported the development of a 2 mm blunt-tipped suction cutting probe for automated percutaneous diskectomy at L4–L5 or higher levels.

The selection criteria for patients undergoing percutaneous diskectomy are similar to those for patients undergoing chymopapain treatment. Patients are selected on the basis of clinical symptoms and radiological evidence that removal of the nucleus pulposus would decompress the affected nerve root. It is also important to identify the presence or absence of extruded fragments. On T2-weighted MRI scans, extruded disks appear brighter than contained disks, which exhibit dark coloration similar to that of degenerated disks. CT diskograms can demonstrate the presence or absence of extruded disk fragments. The size of the protrusion is an important factor in obtaining successful outcomes with percutaneous diskectomy. If the disk herniation is >50% of the anteroposterior diameter of the thecal sac, then there is a >90% chance that the patient will experience a poor outcome after percutaneous diskectomy. Patients with narrowed disk spaces are also poor candidates for percutaneous diskectomy.

Kambin and Sampson[27] initiated the use of fluoroscopy before the procedure for confirmation of the appropriate disk level. The anteroposterior view is used to confirm that the patient is in line without rotation. The lateral view should indicate that the end plates are parallel. Preoperative CT or MRI scans of the entire abdomen through the involved disk space should be obtained to avoid damaging crucial structures in a far lateral approach.

Suction diskectomy is performed with the patient in either a prone or a lateral position. Flexion of the hips reduces lumbar lordosis and allows for a larger entry zone posteriorly. The procedure is performed using mild sedation and local anesthesia. An 18-gauge, 25 cm, hubless, stainless steel trocar is inserted and advanced obliquely, with fluoroscopic guidance, toward the posterior margin of the intervertebral disk to reach the appropriate level. The starting point on the skin is usually 10 cm from the midline. When the trocar is in the appropriate position, a 2.8 mm cannula with an internal, blunt-end, tapered dilator is placed over the hubless trocar. When the cannula and dilator are in the correct position, the dilator is removed. The cannula is pressed against the anulus, and a 2 mm, open-ended, circular cutting tool is inserted through the cannula to cut a hole in the anulus. The nucleotome is advanced into the disk space. The nucleotome is 20 cm in length, with a rounded tip. The reciprocating action of the cutting tool and aspiration occur simultaneously. Saline solution is delivered to the disk space by flowing between the inner and outer cannulas, producing a suspension of macerated disk material as the inner cannula reciprocates at 180 cycles/min, permitting rapid cutting. The slurry of saline solution and disk material is aspirated through the inner cannula into a collection bottle. After the disk space has been accessed, the diskectomy can be completed in 15 to 20 min.

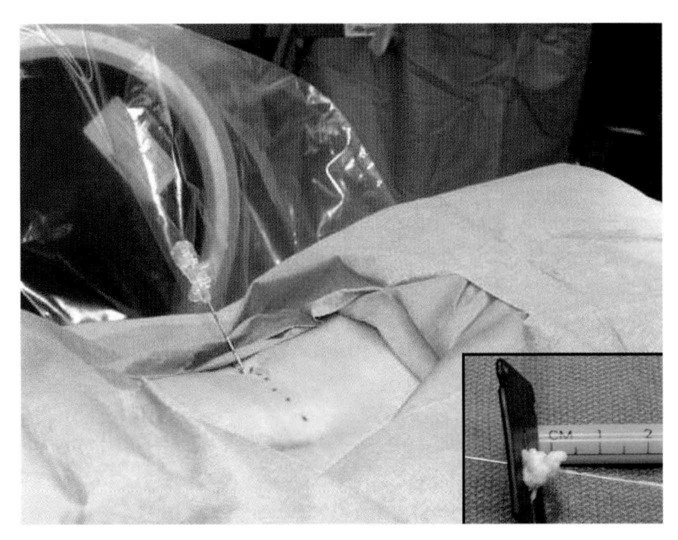

FIGURE 1–5 Result of using an automated percutaneous lumbar diskectomy system for a single-level disk herniation.

Minimally invasive lumbar surgery can be performed successfully using percutaneous techniques. The outcomes of more than 4500 automated or manual percutaneous lumbar diskectomies (PLDs) have been reported. The reported outcomes indicate an overall success rate of 75%, with a complication rate of 1%. Automated PLD is appropriate for patients with single-level disk disease (Fig. 1–5). It is not considered an option for patients with a history of previous chymopapain or surgical treatment for disk disease, progressive neurologic deficits, bowel or bladder problems, sequestered disk fragments, or evidence of vertebral disease (e.g., spinal stenosis or spondylolisthesis).

The role of PLD remains investigational until prospective, randomized, controlled studies reliably validate outcomes. In the future, spinal endoscopy may facilitate observation of the area of nucleotomy and increase the amount of disk removal.

Percutaneous Laser Diskectomy

Ascher and Heppner[28] were the first to use the technique of percutaneous laser diskectomy to treat lumbar disk disease. Their technique involved measuring the intradiscal pressure before and after laser diskectomy, using a saline manometer. They postulated that the removal of even a small volume of tissue from the disk caused a corresponding decrease in intradiscal pressure.[28] This procedure is not indicated for patients with uncontained disk extrusions or disk fragments outside the disk space. The combined results of Ascher,[29] Choy et al,[30] and others demonstrated 70 to 80% rates of long-lasting pain relief for more than 1000 patients. In 1990, Yonezawa et al[31] used a neodymium:yttrium-aluminum-garnet (Nd:YAG) laser through a double-lumen needle with a fiberoptic, quartz-fiber tip to measure pressure before and after the procedure.

Percutaneous laser diskectomy is an outpatient procedure that requires percutaneous placement of a single needle in the disk space. With fluoroscopic verification of the level and placement of the needle and with coupling via a fiber, laser energy is passed into the disk space. The laser energy is transmitted in short bursts to avoid excessive heating of the adjacent tissue. The consensus is that percutaneous laser diskectomy should demonstrate indications and successes similar to those of other percutaneous modalities.

In 1992, Davis[32] used a potassium-titanal-phosphate (KTP) laser for lumbar disk ablation, achieving a success rate of 80%. Producing a light that is lime green at 531 nm, the KTP laser can be coupled to a fiberoptic cable and can be easily directed into the intervertebral disk space through a spinal needle. The procedure is appropriate for patients with contained disk herniations associated with radicular symptoms. The KTP laser has also been approved for percutaneous laser diskectomy. Advances have allowed the development of side-firing probes, which provide better directional control and allow better observation. The side-firing laser probe reduces the risk of injury to such anterior structures as the vena cava, aorta, and iliac vessels. Yeung[33] recommended injecting the disks with indocyanine green (to act as a chromophore), thus maximizing delivery and minimizing the chance of injury to adjacent structures.

The holmium:YAG laser has a 2.1 μm wavelength (in the midinfrared region), which can easily be delivered to the intervertebral disk space. In contrast to the continuous-wave lasers of other systems, the holmium: YAG system has a unique pulsed laser, which enables adjustment of the pulse width and frequency, to reduce damage to adjacent tissue. In bench testing with a pulse width of 250 msec at 10 Hz and 1.6 J/pulse, no temperature increase was noted in adjacent tissues. The disk cavitation caused by the laser results in a reduction in intradiscal pressure, decreasing the force driving the herniated fragments posteriorly. The only reported complication was a case of diskitis in a series of 333 procedures described by Choy et al.[34] The possible complications theoretically include perforation of the aorta, vena cava, iliac vessels, or abdominal contents and cauda equina syndrome.

The results of percutaneous laser disk decompression in cases involving back and leg pain with disk protrusions are still unclear. No controlled prospective studies have been performed to evaluate the results of percutaneous laser diskectomy. The largest experience in the literature was reported by Choy et al.[34] They found excellent results in 87.4% in a study of 333 patients, with a mean follow-up of 26 months. Early experience with the KTP/532 device was reported by Davis,[35] who achieved an 85% success rate. Yeung[33] reported good to excellent results in 84% with the KTP/532 device.

Percutaneous laser diskectomy is one step in the development of safer techniques for disk removal. Various laser wavelengths have been used for this purpose, but no consensus exists regarding success with this form of treatment. Published results demonstrated 70 to 80% success rates for selected groups; unfortunately, laser diskectomy as a stand-alone procedure adds controversy to the field of percutaneous treatment of lumbar disk disease. Current techniques, however, involve manual removal of disk material with laser modulation under endoscopic control. The use of lasers under direct observation can be performed safely and effectively.

Arthoscopic Microdiskectomy

Ottolenghi and Argentina[36] in 1955 and Craig[37] in 1956 described posterolateral biopsy of the spine. In 1983 and 1986, Kambin[25,27] and co-workers combined open laminectomy with nucleotomy, via Craig instrumentation, to observe the effects of nucleus pulposus removal on the surrounding anatomic features. In 1975, Hijikata et al[24] developed mechanical tools for nucleotomy using similar principles. Refinements to the technique involved the use of an automated system.

Subsequent developments led to the design of a 2.7 mm glass arthroscope combined with a videodiscoscope with a single working portal.[38] This development enabled observation of periannular structures, including the foramina and the spinal nerve. Arthroscopic disk surgery allows removal of herniated disks via a posterolateral approach. This is accomplished with biportal access via triangulation into the intervertebral disk, with adequate irrigation and suction.[38]

The mechanism of pain relief after arthroscopic microdiskectomy and central nucleotomy is believed to involve reduced intradiscal pressure, removal of inflammatory agents, reductions in intervertebral disk height, and lower tension on the nerve. The dramatic cessation of radicular pain after extraction of a herniated nuclear fragment in the course of an open surgical procedure proves that removing tension and irritation from the nerve root helps provide pain relief.

Small rigid arthroscopes allow inspection of the anulus, spinal nerve, and foramina. Intradiscal arthroscopic observation is not required for simple nucleotomy or disk debulking. Localization and removal of posteriorly herniated disk fragments require good arthroscopic illumination and observation. There are currently 0-, 30-, and 70-degree angled arthroscopes and flexible arthroscopes are available.

Patients with herniated lumbar disks who are selected for arthroscopic microdiskectomies should demonstrate symptoms of nerve root irritation and present correlative radiological evidence. All intra-annular, subligamentous, and extraligamentous herniations are accessible with arthroscopic microdiskectomy; however, extraligamentous disk fragments that have migrated in caudal or cephalad directions cannot safely be removed using arthroscopic microdiskectomy.

The triangular working zone has been defined as a safe zone in the posterolateral anulus, allowing safe passage of instruments with minimal risk to the exiting nerve.[25,27] As the nerve exits the foramen, it extends laterally and distally, forming the anterior borders of the triangular working zone. The inferior border of this safe zone is the vertebral end plate of the lower body. It is bordered posteriorly by the articular process and superior articulating facet of the lower vertebrae and medially by the traversing root and dura (Fig. 1–6).

Uniportal access is achieved with a 5 mm internal diameter cannula, which provides access for central and posterior extraction of herniated intra-annular fragments. The instruments required for arthroscopic microdiskectomy include 18-gauge needles, guidewires, a cannulated obturator, a 6.4 mm (outer diameter) access cannula, a suction irrigation valve and cannula stopper, trephines, flexible-tip forceps, a videodiscoscope, suction forceps, and a variety of powered resecting instruments (Fig. 1–7). With uniportal access, resecting

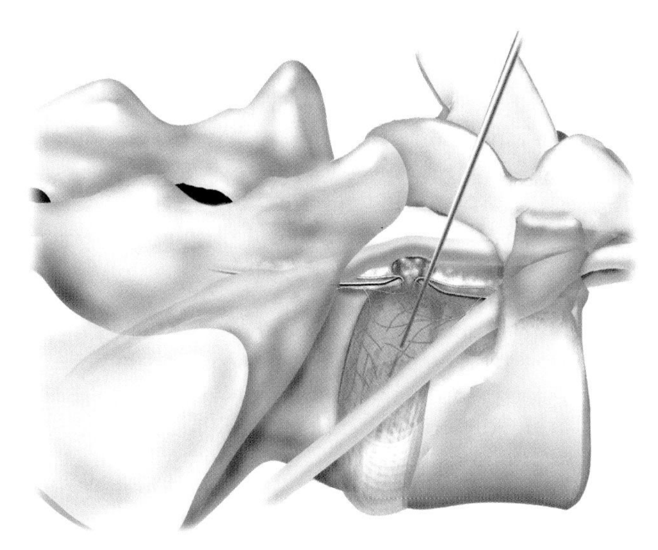

FIGURE 1–6 Red shaded area represents the triangular working zone (Kambin's triangle) defined as the "safe zone" at the posterolateral anulus, allowing safe passage of endoscopic instruments to the disk space with minimal risk to the exiting nerve roots.

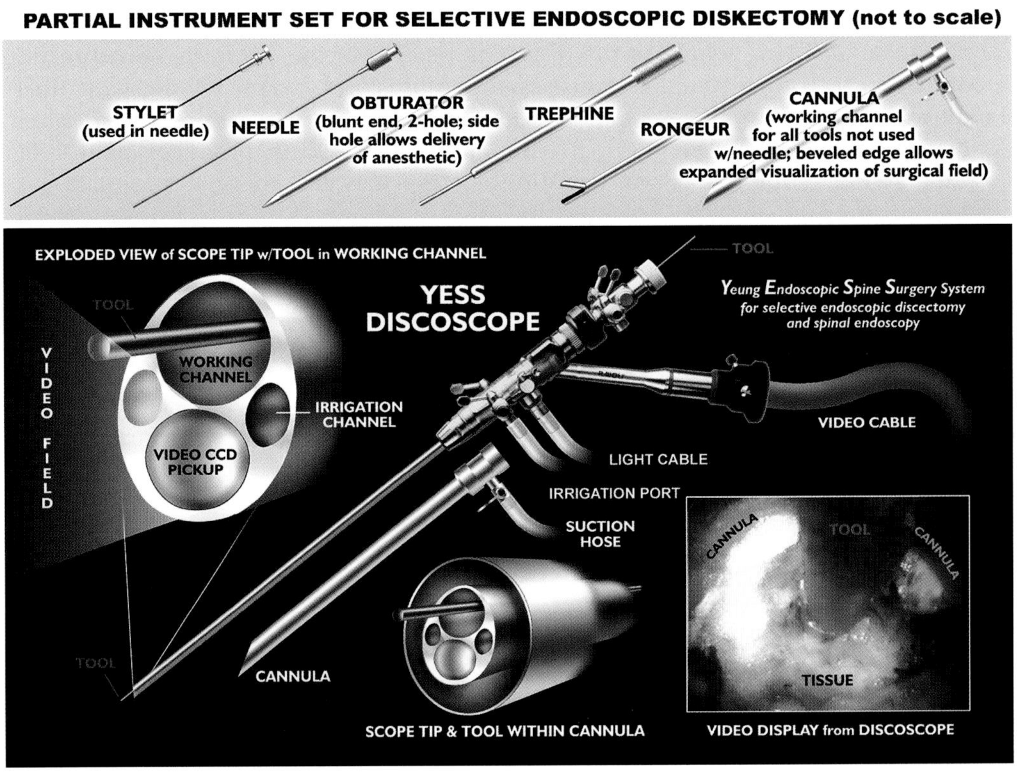

PARTIAL INSTRUMENT SET FOR SELECTIVE ENDOSCOPIC DISKECTOMY (not to scale)

STYLET (used in needle)
NEEDLE
OBTURATOR (blunt end, 2-hole; side hole allows delivery of anesthetic)
TREPHINE
RONGEUR
CANNULA (working channel for all tools not used w/needle; beveled edge allows expanded visualization of surgical field)

EXPLODED VIEW of SCOPE TIP w/TOOL in WORKING CHANNEL
YESS DISCOSCOPE
Yeung Endoscopic Spine Surgery System for selective endoscopic discectomy and spinal endoscopy
TOOL
WORKING CHANNEL
IRRIGATION CHANNEL
VIDEO CCD PICKUP
VIDEO FIELD
VIDEO CABLE
LIGHT CABLE
IRRIGATION PORT
SUCTION HOSE
CANNULA
TISSUE
SCOPE TIP & TOOL WITHIN CANNULA
VIDEO DISPLAY from DISCOSCOPE

FIGURE 1–7 The YESS (Yeung Endoscopic Spine Surgery) system used for posterolateral diskectomy consists of multichannel endoscopes, working cannulas, and specialized instruments.

instruments and the videoscope are inserted alternately for observation and safe resection. On the other hand, an access cannula with an outer diameter of 12 to 14 mm can be used, permitting exploration of the exiting nerve and foraminal decompression. The lateral recess can be accessed through this cannula, with partial resection of the pars and facet joints. The cannula is also used to perform a mini-laminotomy and extraction of the free fragments. This device has a side fenestration that permits introduction of the videoscope; simultaneous observation and resection can thus be performed.

The patient is conscious, minimally sedated, and positioned prone on a radiolucent frame. The C-arm is positioned to obtain a lateral view of the spine. An entry site 10 cm from the midline is made, and the needle is advanced in a horizontal plane. The facet joint is often palpated with the tip of the needle, which is then reinserted in a more vertical direction in the safe triangular working zone. Resistance is felt as the needle makes contact with the anulus. In the anteroposterior plane, the needle is in the midpedicular line. At this point, the stylet is removed and a guidewire is passed through it. A small incision is made, and the cannulated obturator is placed over the guidewire and advanced toward the anulus. The access cannula is passed over the cannulated obturator and advanced until it reaches the anulus. Arthroscopic observation of the periannular structures around the annulotomy is performed, with the adipose tissue and superficial veins often requiring coagulation.

After observation of the anulus, cottonoid pads soaked in local anesthetic are placed over the anulus. This helps control the pain because the annular surface has a rich supply of sensory fibers. The anulus is penetrated with a 3 mm trephine using a slow rotary motion. A 4.9 mm trephine is then introduced to enlarge the annulotomy. Use of an upbiting forceps further enlarges the annulotomy. The access cannula is advanced until it is engaged in the annular fibers. A suction punch or trimmer blade is used for posterior nucleotomy.

Numerous studies on the efficacy of arthroscopic disk surgery have been published. Kambin and colleagues[25,27] reported an 87% successful outcome rate with arthroscopic microdiskectomy, and others have reported similar success. In a prospective randomized study evaluating the efficacy of microscopic disk surgery compared with endoscopic disk extraction, Mayer and Brock[39] achieved favorable outcomes, with minimal complications, with the percutaneous arthroscopic technique. The reported complications include diskitis, instrument breakage, and psoas hematomas; no neurovascular complications arising from posterolateral access to the intervertebral disks of the lumbar spine have been encountered. Proper patient selection makes this an attractive option, with same-day surgery, negligible blood loss, avoidance of general anesthesia, and minimization of scar tissue all contributing to satisfactory outcomes.

Percutaneous Intradiscal Radio-Frequency Thermocoagulation

Percutaneous intradiscal nucleotomy using lasers was first performed by Ascher and co-workers in 1987.[28,29] The laser energy causes vaporization of the nucleus pulposus, thus reducing the intradiscal pressure and symptoms related to the herniated disk. Radio-frequency lesioning has gained wider acceptance and is used to treat trigeminal neuralgia and create pallidotomy and thalamotomy lesions. The size of the lesion can be well controlled, and the lesion is usually placed around the tip of the electrode. A high-frequency alternating current flows from the tip of the electrode into the tissue. Most radio-frequency lesions are produced at probe temperatures of 60 to 80°C (Fig. 1–8).

Intradiscal electrothermal coagulation is a therapeutic innovation specifically designed to treat internal disk disruption. This is a condition in which the disk is rendered painful because of the development of radial fissures extending into the outer one third of the anulus fibrosus. The diagnosis of this condition is based on history and radiological findings, in the form of diskograms and/or postdiskography CT scans. Intradiscal electrothermal coagulation involves percutaneously threading a flexible heating electrode into the disk so that the electrode passes circumferentially around the inner surface of the disk. The heating of the electrode denatures the collagen of the anulus and coagulates the pain fibers supplying the anulus. Direct application of thermal energy to the intervertebral disk produces pain relief via two different mechanisms, thermal coagulation of

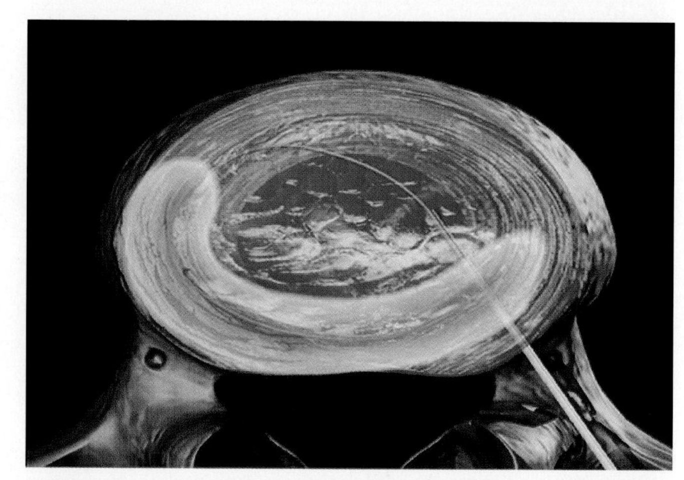

FIGURE 1–8 Drawing demonstrating intradiscal electrothermal coagulation, performed by percutaneously threading a flexible heating electrode into the disk.

nociceptors and increased disk stability due to contraction of collagen type I fibers.

A common method of achieving temperatures of 60 to 80°C involves using a needle powered by a radiofrequency generator in the center of the nucleus. Saal and Saal[40] developed a novel resistive heating catheter that can be introduced into the anulus and navigated through the nucleus and around the inner wall of the anulus. Oratec Interventions Inc. (Menlo Park, CA) has conducted several clinical trials of intradiscal electrothermal treatment for internal disk disruption. Their study included 140 patients who presented with chronic lower back pain between February 1998 and October 1998. To be eligible for that study, patients were required to satisfy the International Association for the Study of Pain criteria for internal disk disruption: reproducibility of pain with stimulation of the affected disk and CT evidence of a grade III annular tear. Fifty-three patients satisfied the diagnostic criteria and were invited to participate in the study. Of those patients, 36 consented to undergoing intradiscal electrothermal coagulation. The control treatment consisted of an established physical therapy and rehabilitation program. The results of that study indicated that 60% of the selected patients experienced profound reductions in pain.[40] All of these studies indicate that, for carefully selected patients, intradiscal electrothermal annuloplasty seems promising, both as a technique to reduce chronic pain of discogenic origin and as an alternative to invasive spine surgery.

Spinal Endoscopy

In 1931, Burman[41] introduced the concept of myeloscopy for direct spinal cord observation. In 1934, Mixter and Barr[42] reported an open hemilaminectomy with intraoperative discotomy for treatment of intervertebral disk rupture into the spinal canal. In 1938, Pool[43] expanded on Burman's work and reported myeloscopic inspection of the dorsal nerve roots of the cauda equina. In 1942, Pool[44] introduced the concept of intrathecal endoscopy and reported the results of more than 400 myeloscopic procedures.

Myeloscopy fell out of favor for a time because of the morbidity associated with insertion of a large-bore scope into the neural cavity. The state of spinal endoscopy remained essentially the same until Ooi et al[45] used an endoscope to examine the intrathecal space before surgery. Using improved technology, Ooi et al[46] were able to describe pathological features in greater detail, including chronic arachnoiditis and nerve root excursion during claudication associated with lumbar spinal stenosis.

Current FDA-approved indications for spinal endoscopy are documentation of pathological features and decompression of structures, direct nerve inspection, inspection of internal fixation, and delivery of therapeutic agents. The current uses of spinal endoscopy have been expanded to include closed decompression of spinal roots, use with lasers, epidural biopsies, percutaneous interbody fusion, and decompression of thoracic disk herniations. Spinal endoscopy has been used to perform thoracoscopy-assisted diskectomies, correction of kyphosis, biopsies, drainage of epidural abscesses, and disk space fusion. In addition, the uses of spinal endoscopy have been expanded to include laparoscopic techniques to treat such lumbar spine pathological conditions as lumbar diskectomy and fusion (anterior vs. posterior).

Lumbar Microendoscopic Diskectomy

MED to treat nerve root compression is a relatively new procedure that provides minimally invasive access to the spinal column. Medtronic Sofamor Danek (Memphis, TN) developed the instruments and technology (Figs. 1–9 and 1–10).

MED combines standard lumbar microsurgical techniques with endoscopy, enabling surgeons successfully to address free-fragment disk pathological factors and lateral recess stenosis. The endoscopic approach allows smaller incisions and less tissue trauma, compared with standard open microdiskectomy. Routine outpatient

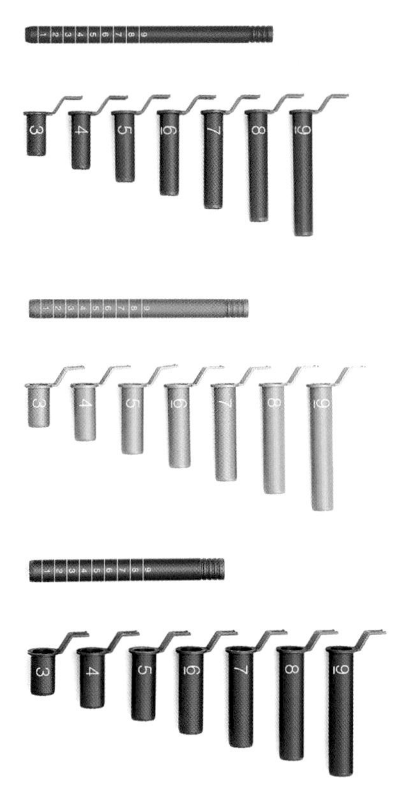

FIGURE 1–9 Photograph of the microendoscopic diskectomy (MED) system: the set of dilators of incremental sizes, and the working channel used for MED.

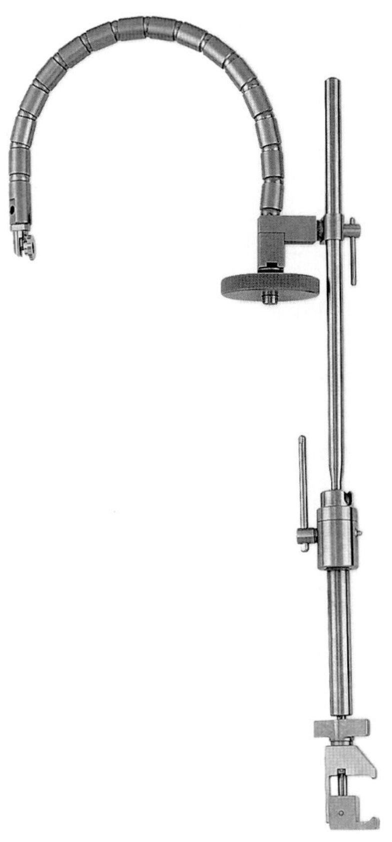

FIGURE 1–10 Photograph of the articulated clamp used to secure the working channel and the endoscope of the microendoscopic diskectomy system.

application and the avoidance of general anesthesia reduce hospital stays and costs.

Muramatsu et al[47] reported on their series of 70 patients who underwent MED and 15 patients for whom Love's method was used to treat lumbar disk disease. MED resulted in less blood loss (mean = 12.1 ml) than Love's method (mean = 59.1 ml); analgesics (suppositories) were required by 52.0% of the MED-treated patients after surgery, whereas all of the patients treated with Love's procedure required analgesics; and MED reduced the mean number of days before the patients became ambulatory (MED, 1.0 day; Love's method, 4.9 days).

MED has the same indications as open microdiskectomy procedures. Muramatsu et al[47] did not use MED to treat patients with herniation associated with segmental instability and lower back pain, patients with combined lumbar canal stenosis and herniation, or patients who had previously undergone back surgery. Guiot et al[48] have shown the technical feasibility of percutaneous microendoscopic bilateral decompression of lumbar stenosis via a unilateral approach in a human cadaveric study.

Endoscopic Pedicle Screw Fixation of Lumbar Spine

The video-assisted posterolateral approach was developed by Boden and associates.[49] Posterior keyhole approaches for endoscopic placement of pedicle screws has been done using multiple portals or a single portal between the two pedicles. Muller et al[50] described the use of multiple portals in a cadaveric study to identify bony landmarks and to test the feasibility of performing endoscopic pedicle screw fixation. Endius (Plainville, MA) developed a system for a single portal approach for posterolateral transpedicular screw fixation and posterolateral lumbar arthrodesis (Fig. 1–11).

In both techniques, a transmuscular approach is performed to place the endoscope over the working area. A needle probe is positioned at the desired level, with biplanar fluoroscopic confirmation. Making a small skin

A

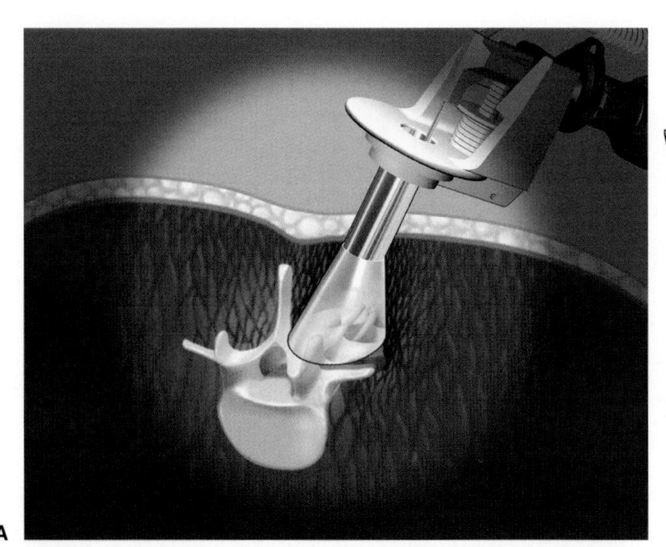

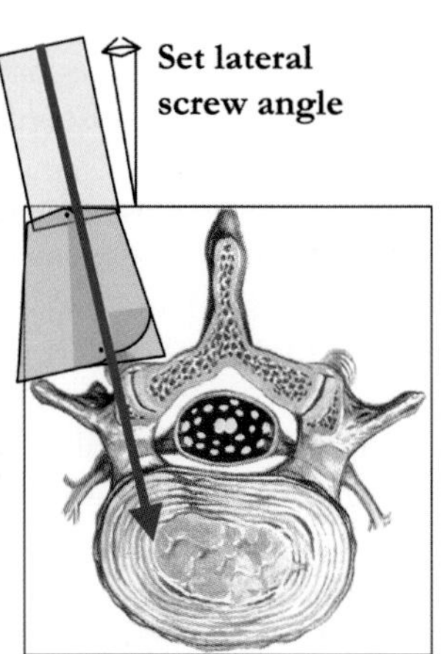

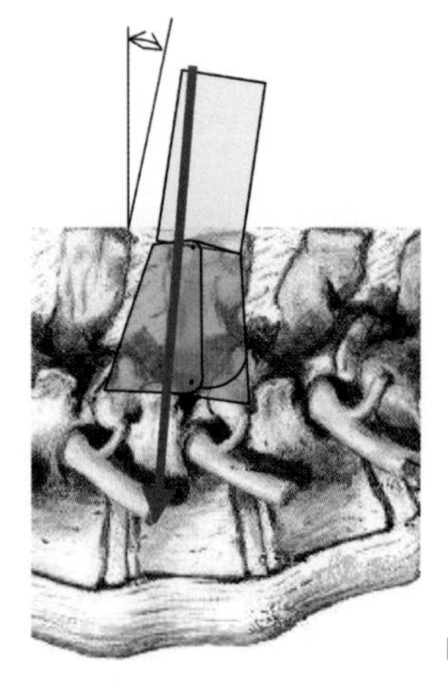

B

FIGURE 1–11 (A) The Endius system used in percutaneous transpedicular screw insertion. **(B)** Lateral and axial schematic representation of the Endius system used in transpedicular screw placement. The retractor system can be repositioned using the same entry point to obtain exposure for the adjacent pedicle.

incision around the probe, dilators of incremental size are passed over the probe until the desired blunt-tipped obdurator can be placed.

Muller et al[50] performed a transmuscular insertion of a pedicle screw-rod fixation device using a rigid operating sheath. This sheath (Thoracoport, AutoSuture Co., Norwalk, CT) measured 1.5 cm in diameter and 5 cm in length, and was used with a disposable trocar system consisting of a blunt-tipped obdurator, a threaded sleeve, and a shroud to secure the system. The surgical field was illuminated by an endoscope (Hopkins 11, Karl Storz GmbH & Co., Tuttlingen, Germany) with a diameter of 4 mm, a length of 18 cm, and angles of 0, 30, and 70 degrees. The Diapason pedicle probe (Stryker Instruments, Kalamazoo, MI) with a blunt tip was used to discover whether the pedicle walls were intact. The system has pedicle screws that have a U-shaped screw head.[50] The connecting rods are fixed in the screw heads via a ball-ring interface and are locked with locking screws. The pedicle screws are placed using an inclinometer, which provides the surgeon with instant feedback during the placement of pedicle screws.

The Endius system consists of similar dilators and probes. In addition, the Endius system has a fan apparatus that allows the surgeon to use blunt dissection techniques to visualize both pedicles and the interspace between them. Thus, this system accomplishes pedicle screw fixation of one motion segment with a single portal in each side. The visualization afforded is large enough to place pedicle screw constructs using rods/plates at the desired levels (Fig. 1–11).

Laparoscopic Lumbar Spine Surgery

The modern era of laparoscopy began in the 1980s, when Kurt Semm performed the first appendectomy in Germany. Semm, a physician and an engineer, developed many tools that are still in use. The first human laparoscopic cholecystectomy was performed in 1987 by DuBois et al.[51] With the advantages of laparoscopic exposures being championed by urological, gynecological, and general surgeons, it is natural that spine surgeons would consider extending the advantages of laparoscopic exposures to the anterior lumbar spine. The significant advantages of transperitoneal laparoscopic surgical treatment include improved observation of surgical anatomic features, marked reductions in postoperative pain, early hospital discharges, and reduced incidence of postoperative ileus. In 1991, Obenchain[52] reported the first use of a laparoscopic approach to the lumbar spine for a diskectomy (Fig. 1–12). Regan et al[53] described the technique and reported preliminary results for laparoscopic anterior lumbar fusion.

Gaur[54] was the first to describe an endoscopic retroperitoneal approach for urological procedures, which was later applied to treatment of the lumbar spine. Retroperitoneal, minimally invasive, endoscopic spine surgery has the advantage of not requiring carbon dioxide insufflation or entrance into the peritoneal cavity, and it avoids dissection near the large vessels and the hypogastric plexus. Advances in interbody fusion cage technology have generated a great deal of interest in

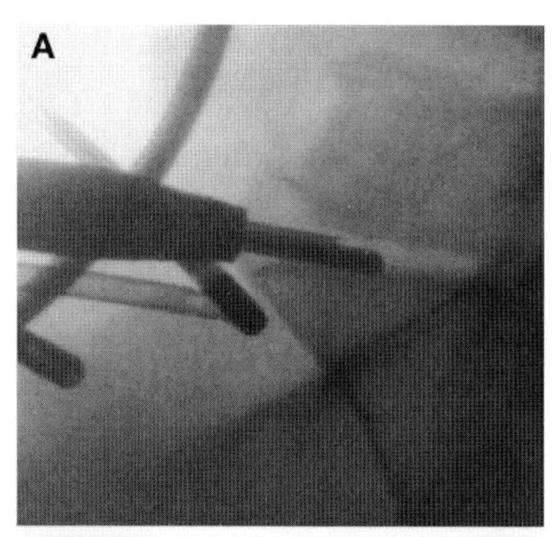

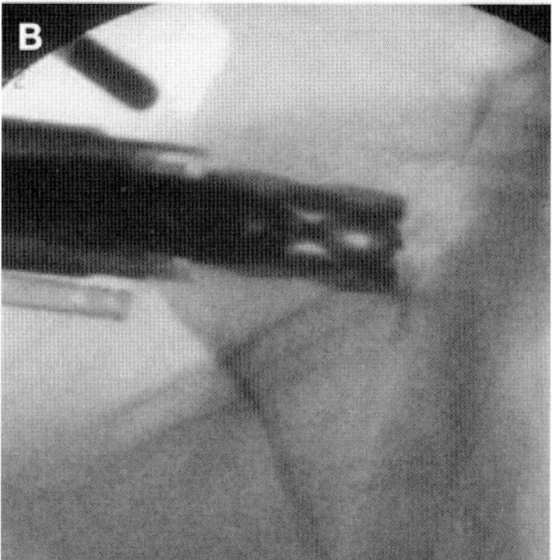

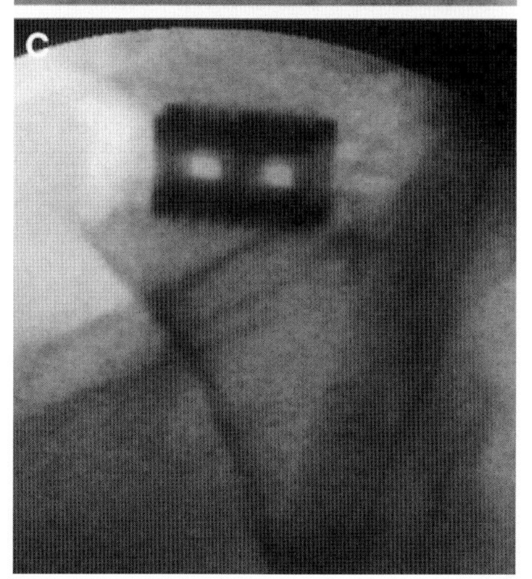

FIGURE 1–12 **(A)** Lateral radiographs showing fluoroscopic guidance of L5–S1 disk space with positioning of working channel/dilator for performing diskectomy. **(B)** Preparation of the disk space with drill and tap. **(C)** Lateral radiographs after laparoscopic insertion of the BAK cage.

laparoscopic techniques. Spinal fusion systems inserted with laparoscopic techniques maintain posterior load-bearing elements and reduce postoperative pain.

Additional Minimally Invasive Developments

Application of Image-Guidance Systems in the Spine

Since its introduction, transpedicular screw fixation has significantly changed the scope of spine surgery.[55] Several complex spinal abnormalities, including neoplasms, degenerative diseases, trauma, and infections, are commonly treated with instrumentation to promote fusion via stabilization. The anatomic features of the diseased motion segments and the adjacent neural structures may be distorted and are often difficult to appreciate. Serious complications resulting from screw misplacement or pedicle cortex perforation can lead to devastating neurologic or vascular damage. Pedicle screw fixation provides the most stable construct. To increase the safety of the procedure, various methods have been used to target the pedicle better with respect to the trajectory and depth of screw placement. Most surgeons use assessments of anatomical landmarks, supplemented by fluoroscopy, to identify the anatomical features of the pedicles before placement of the pedicle screws. Weinstein et al[56] reported pedicle cortex violation in nearly 20% of cases.

Image guidance systems are widely used in intracranial surgery and have been adapted to assist with screw placement since the mid-1990s. The use of image guidance systems for pedicle screw placement has improved the accuracy of placement. The system relies on precise localization of the pedicles with CT. In addition, the transverse width, longitudinal depth, and trajectory angle can be measured (Fig. 1–13).

Nolte et al[57] described the principles of computer-assisted pedicle screw fixation. The overall accuracy of their system was 1.74 mm, using CT scans with 2 mm image increments. Intraoperative surgical exposure of the posterior vertebral elements was performed using standard surgical techniques. An infrared camera (Optotrak; Northern Digital, Waterloo, Ontario, Canada) tracked specific instruments (i.e., pedicle probe, awl, and space pointer) equipped with light-emitting diodes. The dynamic reference was fixed to the spinous process of the vertebra to be instrumented. Normal bony landmarks and their correlations with the images confirmed the calibration accuracy. Using that computerized system, they reported a pedicle screw misplacement rate of 4.3% under clinical conditions.

Choi et al[58] reported the use of computer-assisted fluoroscopic targeting for pedicle screw fixation. They described a system in which the pedicle entry site and the depth of insertion were determined by intraoperative

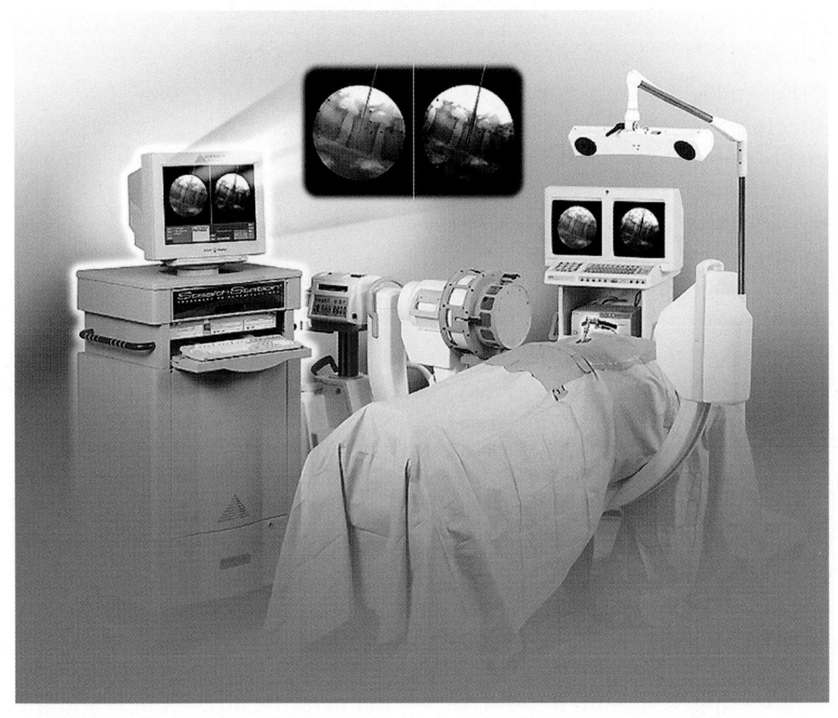

FIGURE 1–13 The virtual fluoroscopy system used for image-guided spinal surgery.

anteroposterior and lateral fluoroscopic scans. Those authors compared the accuracy of placement with the fluoroscopy-guided system versus the image guidance system and observed no significant differences.

Improved accuracy and ease of use with image guidance spine systems will facilitate localization of anatomical bony landmarks and expedite fixation for cervical, thoracic, and lumbar stabilization. With improvements in endoscopic and image-based guidance, the use of a combination of endoscopic and image guidance systems for thoracoscopic or laparoscopic stabilization procedures can be envisioned.

Vertebroplasty

The spine is composed of a rich trabecular lattice of cancellous bone encased in a hard cortical shell. Moreover, the spine is exposed to degrees of compressive loads and tensile stresses that are in symbiotic biomechanical play with the inner and outer matrixes of the vertebral bodies. Osteoporotic and neoplastic invasion of the vertebral bodies results in erosion of the cancellous network and development of vertebral compression fractures (VCFs), which can contribute to neurologic deficit, gross spinal instability, and ensuing deformity. Surgical management involves significant risks because all of these patients have significant comorbid conditions. It involves internal fixation using screws, plates, wires, cages, or rods and requires extensive surgical exposure. The time required for recuperation from open fixation procedures can be long. Obtaining satisfactory fixation in osteoporotic bone can be technically difficult, and the failure rate for spinal arthrodesis is significant.

Open procedures with the implementation of instrumentation were utilized in an attempt to establish pain control and address neurologic compromise. In an attempt to reduce such invasive operative treatment, percutaneous vertebroplasty (PVP) was developed in 1984 by Galibert and Deramond[59] in France as a minimally invasive outpatient procedure to offer immediate pain relief by the injection of polymethylmethacrylate (PMMA) bone cement into the vertebral body through a transpedicular percutaneous approach. Although a popular procedure in Europe, PVP was not performed in the United States until 1994.[60] This is currently used in the treatment of vertebral fractures involving osteoporosis, primary or secondary tumors of the spine, and spinal trauma.

Kyphoplasty

In an effort to reduce the high incidence of cement extravasation and detrimental sequelae, infection, cement toxicity, and adjacent fracture development due to an altered sagittal balance, kyphoplasty was developed in the mid-1990s by Dr. Mark Reiley. Kyphoplasty implements inflatable bone tamps inserted by a bilateral transpedicular approach that decreases intravertebral pressure and inserts PMMA into the cavity to elevate the vertebral end plates and restore vertebral height.[61] The injection of highly viscous PMMA under lower pressures into a preformed cavity formed by the bone tamps greatly reduces the risk of extravertebral extravasation of the PMMA. Furthermore, kyphoplasty offers immediate pain relief, restores sagittal balance, enhances biomechanical regional milieu, improves vital capacity, thereby increasing mobility, and eradicates the detrimental psychological cascade that often affects patients with VCFs and an altered spinal alignment. In addition, the risk of subsequent vertebral fractures is decreased due to the restoration of the sagittal balance. Although PMMA has been successful in a slue of orthopedic and spine-related procedures, various bioactive substrates possessing osteoconductive and osteoinductive potential have been under investigation as alternatives to PMMA.

Endoscopic/Percutaneous Applications of Biological Agents

One of the many bioactive substrates under heated investigation are bone morphogenetic proteins (BMPs). These proteins, initially identified in 1965 by Urist,[62] are multifunctional cytokines that function as osteoinductive agents in the formation of visceral development, cell proliferation and differentiation, and chondroblast and osteoblast formation. Recombinant BMPs promote and enhance solid fusion, obviate the need for autograft harvest and its associated morbidities, diminish the need for internal instrumentation, avoid reoperation rates associated with nonunions or implant failure, decrease hospital costs, and improve postoperative outcome. Early results, especially with BMP-2 and BMP-7, in animal models and in human subjects have been promising.[63,64] Furthermore, heated investigation of the vast potential of gene therapy is ongoing and motivated by the ability of direct application as well as prolonged and desired osteoinduction signaling.[65,66] Preliminary results have indicated the promotion of bone and intervertebral disk formation, as well as the encoding of various desired factors. The availability of these bone growth factors and gene therapy opens newer avenues for bone fusion by endoscopic or percutaneous methods to avoid the morbidity and risks associated with fusion by open methods.

The field of spine surgery has been witness to immeasurable growth in the past four decades. The evolution of surgical techniques and treatment methodologies is testament to the optimal quality of care each physician seeks to offer the patient. Although there has been an inclination toward more minimally invasive techniques in spine surgery, indications and proper patient selection are essential pragmatic dogmas that must be employed in consideration of an operative treatment modality to obtain optimal clinical outcome and patient satisfaction.

REFERENCES

1. Detmer DE, Buchanan-Davidson DJ. Ambulatory surgery. In: Rutknow IM, ed. *Socioeconomics of Surgery*. St. Louis: CV Mosby; 1989:30–50.
2. Lang JK, Kolenda H. First appearance and sense of the term "spinal column" in ancient Egypt. *J Neurosurg*. 2002;97:152–155.
3. Marketos SG, Skiadas P. Hippocrates: the father of spine surgery. *Spine*. 1999;24:1381–1387.
4. Knoeller SM, Seifried C. History of spine surgery. *Spine*. 2000;25:2838–2843.
5. Fang HSY, Ong GB. Direct anterior approach to the upper cervical spine. *J Bone Joint Surg Am*. 1962;44A:1588–1604.
6. Frempong-Boadu AK, Faunce WA, Fessler RG. Endoscopically assisted transoral-transpharyngeal approach to the craniovertebral junction. *Neurosurgery*. 2002;51:60–66.
7. Scoville WB, Whitcomb BB. Lateral rupture of cervical intervertebral discs. *Postgrad Med*. 1966;39:174–180.
8. Roh SW, Kim DH, Cardoso AC, Fessler RG. Endoscopic foraminotomy using MED system in cadaveric specimens. *Spine*. 2000;25:260–264.
9. Jacobaeus HC. Possibility of the use of cystoscope for investigation of serious cavities. *Munch Med Wochenschr*. 1910;57:2090–2092.
10. Jacobaeus HC. The practical importance of thoracoscopy in surgery of the chest. *Surg Gynecol Obstet*. 1921;32:493–500.
11. Mack MJ, Regan JJ, Bobechko WP, et al. Application of thorascopy for diseases of the spine. *Ann Thorac Surg*. 1993;56:736–738.
12. Rosenthal DJ, Rosenthal DR, Simone A. Removal of a protruded thoracic disc using microsurgical endoscopy: a new technique. *Spine*. 1994;19:1087–1091.
13. Jho HD. Endoscopic microscopic transpedicular thoracic discectomy: technical note. *J Neurosurg*. 1997;87:125–129.
14. Chiu J, Clifford T. Microdecompressive percutaneous discectomy: spinal discectomy with new laser thermodiskoplasty for nonextruded herniated nucleus pulposus. *Surg Technol Int*. 1999;8:343–351.
15. Jansen EF, Balls AK. Chymopapain: a new crystalline proteinase from papaya latex. *J Biol Chem*. 1941;137:459–460.
16. Thomas L. Reversible collapse of rabbit ears after intravenous papain and prevention of recovery by cortisone. *J Exp Med*. 1956;104:245–252.
17. Smith L, Garvin PJ, Jennings RB, Gesler RM. Enzvme dissolution of the nucleus pulposus. *Nature*. 1963;198:1311–1312.
18. Nordby EJ, Javid MJ. Continuing experience with chemonucleolysis. *Mt Sinai J Med*. 2000;67:311–313.
19. Nordbv EJ, Brown MD. Present status of chymopapain and chemonucleolysis. *Clin Orthop*. 1977;129:79–83.
20. Nordby EJ, Lucas GL. A comparative analysis of lumbar disk disease treated by laminectomy or chemonucleolysis. *Clin Orthop*. 1973;90:119–129.
21. Lorenz M, McCulloch J. Chemonucleolysis for herniated nucleus pulposus in adolescents. *J Bone Joint Surg Am*. 1985;67A:1402–1404.
22. Nordby EJ, Wright PH, Schofield SR. Safety of chemonucleolysis: adverse effects reported in the United States, 1982–1991. *Clin Orthop*. 1993;293:122–134.
23. Ramirez LF, David MJ. Cost effectiveness of chemonucleolysis versus laminectomy in the treatment of herniated nucleus pulposus. *Spine*. 1985;10:363–367.
24. Hijikata S, Yamagishi M, Nakayama T, Oomori K. Percutaneous diskectomy: a new treatment method for lumbar disc herniation. *J Toden Hosp*. 1975;39:5–13.
25. Kambin P, Gellman H. Percutaneous lateral discectomy of the lumbar spine: a preliminary report. *Clin Orthop*. 1983;174:127–132.
26. Onik G, Helms CA, Ginsberg L, Hoagland FT, Morris J. Percutaneous lumbar diskectomy using a new aspiration probe: porcine and cadaver model. *Radiology*. 1985;155:251–252.
27. Kambin P, Sampson S. Posterolateral percutaneous suction-excision of herniated lumbar intervertebral discs: report of interim results. *Clin Orthop*. 1986;207:37–43.
28. Ascher PW, Heppner F. CO_2-laser in neurosurgery. *Neurosurg Rev*. 1984;7:123–133.
29. Ascher PW. Status quo and new horizons of laser therapy in neurosurgery. *Lasers Surg Med*. 1985;5:499–506.
30. Choy DS, Case RB, Fielding W, Hughes J, Liebler W, Ascher P. Percutaneous laser nucleolysis of lumbar disks. *N Engl J Med*. 1987;317:771–772.
31. Yonezawa T, Onomura T, Kosaka R, et al. The system and procedures of percutaneous intradiscal laser nucleotomy. *Spine*. 1990;15:1175–1185.
32. Davis JK. Percutaneous discectomy improved with KTP laser. *Clin Laser Mon*. 1990;8:105–106.
33. Yeung AT. Consideration for the use of the KTP laser for disc decompression and ablation. In: Sherk HIT, ed. *Spine: State of the Art Reviews—Laser Discectomy*. Philadelphia: Hanley & Belfus;1993:67–93.
34. Choy DS, Ascher PW, Saddekni S. Percutaneous laser disc decompression. *Spine*. 1992;17:949–956.
35. Davis JK. Early experience with laser disc decompression: a percutaneous method. *J Fla Med Assoc*. 1992;79:37–39.
36. Ottolenghi CE, Argentina PA. Diagnosis of orthopaedic lesions by aspiration biopsy: results of 1061 punctures. *J Bone Joint Surg Am*. 1955;37A:443–464.
37. Craig FS. Vertebral body biopsy. *J Bone Joint Surg Am*. 1956;38A:93–102.
38. Kambin P. Arthroscopic microdiscectomy. *Arthroscopy*. 1992;8:287–295.
39. Mayer HM, Brock M. Percutaneous endoscopic discectomy: surgical technique and preliminary results compared to microsurgical discectomy. *J Neurosurg*. 1993;78:216–225.
40. Saal JA, Saal JS. Intradiscal electrothermal treatment for chronic discogenic low back pain: a prospective outcome study with minimum 1-year follow-up. *Spine*. 2000;25:2622–2627.
41. Burman MS. Myeloscopy or the direct visualization of the spinal cord and its contents. *J Bone Joint Surg*. 1931;13:695–696.
42. Mixter WJ, Barr JS. Rupture of intervertebral disc with involvement of spinal canal. *N Engl J Med*. 1934;211:210–215.
43. Pool JL. Direct visualization of dorsal nerve roots of the cauda equina by means of a myeloscope. *Arch Neurol Psychiatr*. 1938;39:1308–1312.
44. Pool JL. Myeloscopy: intraspinal endoscopy. *Surgery*. 1942;11:169–182.
45. Ooi Y, Sato Y, Mikanagi K, Morisaki N. [Myeloscopy.] *No To Shinkei*. 1977;29:569–574.
46. Ooi Y, Sato Y, Morisaki N. Myeloscopy: the possibility of observing the lumbar intrathecal space by use of an endoscope. *Endoscopy*. 1973;5:901–906.
47. Muramatsu K, Hachiya Y, Morita C. Postoperative magnetic resonance imaging of lumbar disc herniation: comparison of microendoscopic discectomy and Love's method. *Spine*. 2001;26:1599–1605.
48. Guiot BH, Khoo LT, Fessler RG. A minimally invasive technique for decompression of the lumbar spine. *Spine*. 2002;27:432–438.
49. Boden SD, Moskovitz PA, Morone MA, Torihitake Y. Video-assisted lateral intertransverse process arthrodesis: validation of a new minimally invasive lumbar spinal fusion technique in the rabbit and nonhuman primate (*Rhesus*) models. *Spine*. 1996;21:2689–2697.
50. Muller A, Gall C, Marz U, Reulen HJ. A keyhole approach for endoscopically assisted pedicle screw fixation in lumbar spine instability. *Neurosurgery*. 2000;47:85–96.

51. Dubois F, Icard P, Berthelot G, Levard H. Coelioscopic cholecystectomy: preliminary report of 36 cases. *Ann Surg.* 1990;211:60–62.
52. Obenchain TG. Laparoscopic lumbar discectomy. *J Laparoendosc Surg.* 1991;1:145–149.
53. Regan JJ, McAfee PC, Guyer RD, Aronoff RJ. Laparoscopic fusion of the lumbar spine in a multicenter series of the first 34 consecutive patients. *Surg Laparosc Endosc.* 1996;6:459–468.
54. Gaur DD. Laparoscopic operative retroperitoneoscopy: use of a new device. *J Urol.* 1992;148:1137–1139.
55. Roy-Camille R, Saillant G, Berteaux D, Marie-Anne S, Mamoudy P. Vertebral osteosynthesis using metal plates: its different uses. *Chirurgie.* 1979;105:597–603.
56. Weinstein JN, Spratt KF, Spengler D, Brick C, Reid S. Spinal pedicle fixation: reliability and validity of roentgenogram-based assessment and surgical factors on successful screw placement. *Spine.* 1988;13:1012–1018.
57. Nolte LP, Zamorano LJ, Jiang Z, Wang Q, Langlotz F, Berlemann L. Image-guided insertion of transpedicular screws: a laboratory set-up. *Spine.* 1995;20:497–500.
58. Choi WW, Green BA, Levi AD. Computer-assisted fluoroscopic targeting system for pedicle screw insertion. *Neurosurgery.* 2000;47:872–878.
59. Galibert P, Deramond H. La vertebroplastie percutanée comme traitement des angiomas vertebraux et des affections dolorigenes et fragilisantes du rachis. *Chirurgie.* 1990;116:326–335.
60. Barr JD, Barr MS, Lemley TJ, McCann RM. Percutaneous vertebroplasty for pain relief and spinal stabilization. *Spine.* 2000;25:923–928.
61. Dudeney S, Lieberman IH, Reinhardt MK, Hussein M. Kyphoplasty in the treatment of osteolytic vertebral compression fractures as a result of multiple myeloma. *J Clin Oncol.* 2002;20:2382–2387.
62. Urist M. Bone formation by autoinduction. *Science.* 1965;150:893–899.
63. Boden SD, Martin GJ Jr, Horton WC, et al. Laparoscopic anterior spinal arthrodesis with rhBMP-2 in a titanium interbody threaded cage. *J Spinal Disord.* 1998;11:95–101.
64. Boden SD, Hair GA, Viggeswarapu M, Liu Y, Titus L. Gene therapy for spine fusion. *Clin Orthop.* 2000;379(suppl):S225–S233.
65. Cha CW, Boden SD. Gene therapy applications for spine fusion. *Spine.* 2003;28(suppl):S74–84
66. Alden TD, Pittman DD, Beres EJ, Hankins GR, Kallmes DF, Wisotsky BM, Kerns KM, Helm GA. Percutaneous spinal fusion using bone morphogenetic protein-2 gene therapy. *J Neurosurg.* 1999;90(suppl):109–114

2

Endoscopic Surgical Equipment

LARRY T. KHOO AND ANTHONY VIRELLA

The concept of percutaneous access via small tubular or cylindrical portals is fundamental to the concept of minimally invasive and endoscopic spinal surgery.[1] The tubular configuration of these access cannulas allows for the use of progressive, tissue-sparing dilation, as well as for a minimal amount of retraction pressure on adjacent vital tissues during the surgical procedure. Extensive literature has documented the less-invasive nature of portal access for a variety of spinal procedures with significant improvements in the degree of postoperative pain and disability.[2–5] These portals come in a variety of shapes and sizes, and they can range from metallic to plastic and from rigid to flexible. As a principle, these tubular cannulas require some type of trocar device for insertion through the outer musculoligamentous wall to provide access and visualization of the target pathology and spinal column. Whereas standard retraction systems can often induce regional ischemia within the adjacent soft tissues, tubular retractors, by definition, exert minimal pressures on the tissue, thereby significantly improving tissue perfusion during prolonged procedures.[6]

Endoscopic Surgical Access

Selection of the appropriate access portals will vary according to the specific nature and location of the operative procedure. For thoracoscopic procedures, simple small-diameter working portals are all that are required to provide access sheaths for the long-working instruments required for the procedure. In general, thoracoscopic portals are designed to accommodate only one instrument at a time, with subsequent ports placed for visualization and additional working instruments (Fig. 2–1A).[4,7] As such, soft, flexible portals can be used during thoracoscopy because maintenance of a corridor of direct visualization through the port is not essential. This offers the benefit of less pressure on the intercostal neurovascular bundle at the edge of the rib and thus a decreased incidence of postoperative intercostal neuralgia.[8,9]

Like all portals, flexible thoracoscopic portals are available in a variety of working diameters, with the length being customizable by simply cutting off the excess. The presence of screw-type ridges on the portal walls helps to facilitate placement, stabilize it in the soft tissue, and decrease minor run-down-type venous bleeding that can often obscure intraoperative visualization. All thoracoscopic and laparoscopic portals typically have a widened cuff base to maintain their position on the chest or abdominal wall. This cuff can be sutured or stapled to the skin surface to further secure them during the procedure. Rigid portals used for laparoscopic procedures generally have a valve mechanism incorporated to seal the cannula, thereby allowing for carbon dioxide (CO_2) insufflation that is typically integral to these abdominal procedures. Insufflation is usually not used, however, for the majority of thoracic procedures where simple deflation of the ipsilateral lung provides more than an adequate working space.

Similar to the variety of portals available, the trocars used for their introduction are also available in a wide range of designs. For thoracoscopic procedures, initial blunt dissection with a tonsil into the intercostal space is typically followed by introduction of a simple rigid plastic trocar integral within the working portal.[8–10] After

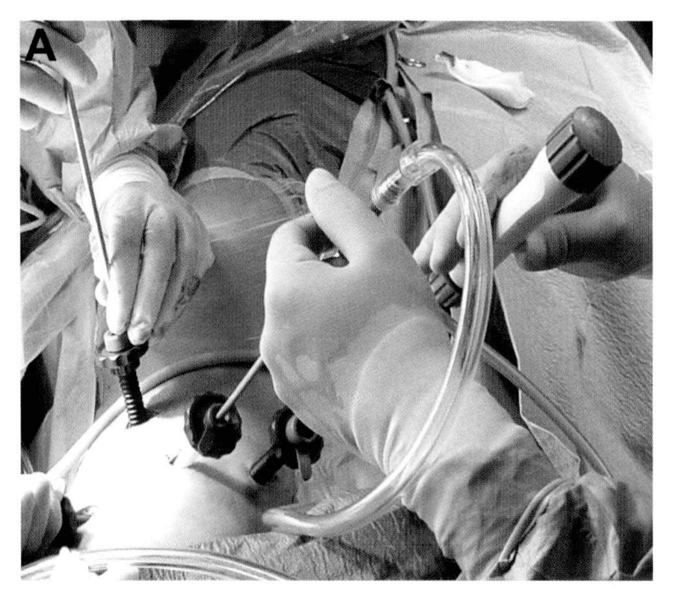

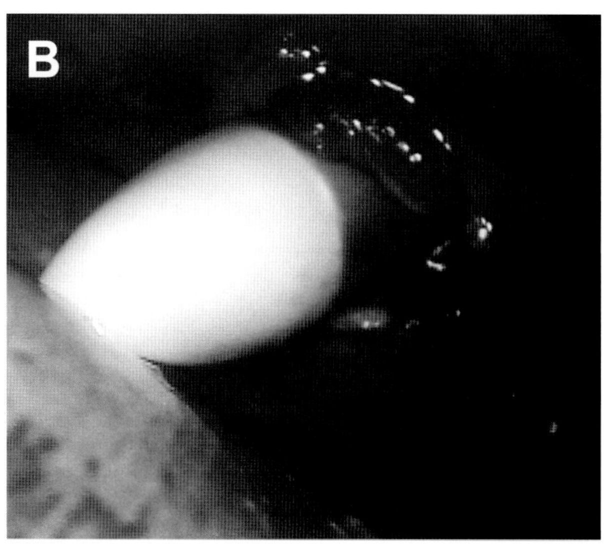

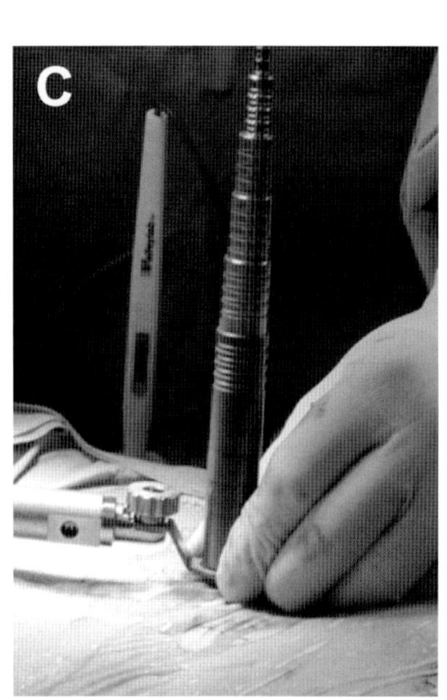

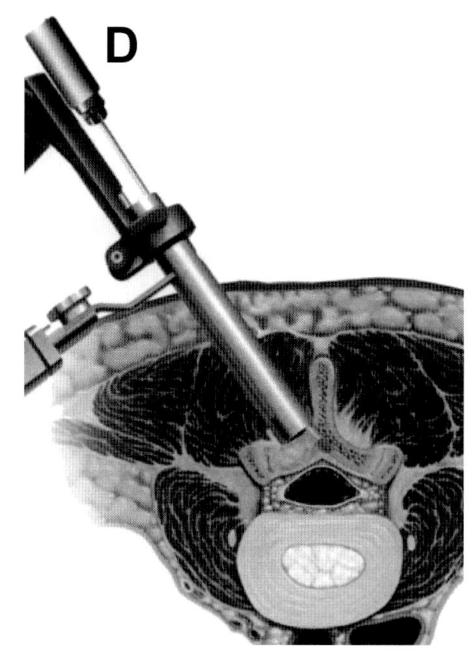

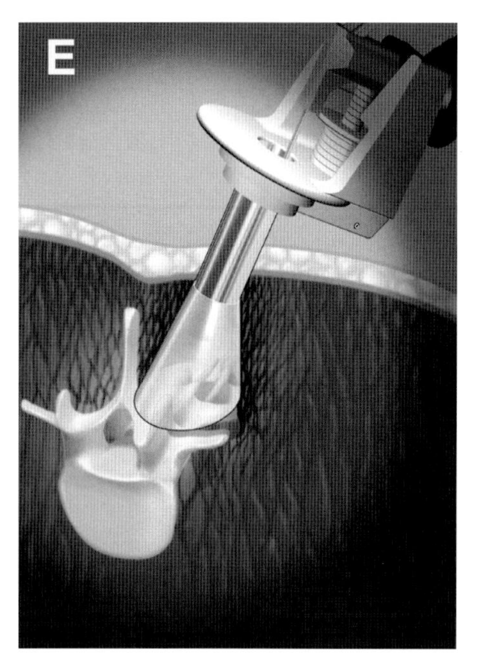

FIGURE 2–1 (A) Multiple access portals are typically placed during anterior thoracoscopic or laparoscopic procedures. Separate channels are used for the working instruments, suction, and camera, allowing for triangulation at the working target area. **(B)** Blunt plastic trocars are needed to introduce thoracoscopic portals into the thorax and to avoid inadvertent injury to the underlying parenchyma. **(C)** Serial tubular dilators are sequentially introduced through a dorsal approach to displace the posterior musculoligamentous complex gradually with a minimum of neurovascular and direct cautery injury. **(D)** Coaxial endoscopic-assisted visualization is employed during small diameter approaches to the dorsal spine because the direct line of sight is greatly impaired through the small working portal. **(E)** Whereas rigid tubular portals are often adequate for simple decompressive procedures, such expandable cannulas as the Endius Flexposure portal (Plainville, MA) allow for wide surgical exposures at depth through a small dorsal incision.

proper placement within the intercostal space, the trocar is removed with the portal, then secured at the chest wall (Fig. 2–1B). Optical portals optionally allow for direct illuminated, endoscopic visualization during passage of the trocar tip to prevent inadvertent injury to the subjacent organs during initial placement of the working portals. These optical portals are of particular value in laparoscopic access because the abdominal contents are easily perforated during percutaneous cannulation. Once placed, these optical trocars can also be used to insufflate the working space, thereby pushing the visceral contents away from the abdominal wall and facilitating safe placement of subsequent working portals. When CO_2-positive pressure insufflation is used, it is critical that the portals be vented intermittently and that a surveillance system is present to monitor intra-abdominal pressures. Self-venting, integrated laparoscopic control systems are critical in such procedures to prevent accidental vascular embolism and visceral injury. Careful attention to technique during portal placement will similarly help to maintain the seal required within the abdominal cavity for laparoscopic procedures. Specialized optical portals with integrated balloon-dilating mechanisms for preperitoneal and retroperitoneal exposures are available to facilitate entrance and dissection of these potential anatomic spaces.[11]

For endoscopic posterior spinal procedures, a series of metallic sequential tubular dilators is often substituted for a single introductory trocar. This allows for targeted placement of a small Steinmann pin or Kirschner wire to the region of interest and subsequent confirmation with fluoroscopy or image guidance. Progressive dilation with integral dilators gradually creates a working channel by splitting the muscular fibers along their natural orientation, thereby minimizing the amount of iatrogenic injury. After dilation to the desired diameter, a final working portal is placed, then secured to a bed-mounted retractor (Fig. 2–1C). Unlike thoracoscopic or laparoscopic procedures, where the optical camera is placed through a separate portal, posterior spinal endoscopic procedures typically utilize a coaxial endoscopic camera to provide illumination and magnification of the working cannula (Fig. 2–1D). Surgical instruments and fixation are all applied directly through this same port. Examples of commercial access systems include the Access Port (Spinal Concepts; Austin, TX), the METRx Minimal Access System (Medtronic Sofamor Danek; Memphis, TN), the Nuvasive system (Nuvasive; San Diego, CA), and the ATAVI system (Endius; Plainville, MA). The central mechanism of each of these systems is still fundamentally that of tubular dilation and a cylindrical working portal. For more multilevel decompressive or fusion procedures, more extensile percutaneous exposure is provided by specialized cannulas that can be expanded after standard progressive tubular dilation. These include the Xpand system (Medtronic Sofamor Danek) and the ATAVI Flexposure cannula (Endius). With expansion, ultimate working diameters of up to 40 to 60 mm can be achieved with these systems (Fig. 2–1E).

Operative Guidance

During endoscopic spinal procedures, working within a confined space with a limited number of anatomical landmarks often leads to significant intraoperative disorientation. This leads to problems with localization, adequate decompression, complete lesion resection, proper correction of the preoperative deformity, and proper placement of spinal instrumentation. For example, correct localization of a thoracic herniated disk is often a daunting intraoperative task without clear anatomical landmarks within the thoracic cavity (Fig. 2–2A). As such, intraoperative fluoroscopy is essential to confirm the working level prior to decompression (Fig. 2–2B). Fluoroscopic confirmation of Steinmann pin placement is similarly essential during initial targeting for endoscopic posterior spinal procedures (Fig. 2–2C). To facilitate spinal fixation through very constrained working portals, significant improvements in implant design and materials over the last decade have resulted in improved strength, ergonomics, ease of use, and performance. Despite these advances, the safety and efficacy of screw-based spinal instrumentation continue to be limited by anatomical constraints. Whereas the lumbar spine pedicles are typically capacious, other fixation corridors (e.g., the high thoracic pedicles and the C1–C2 transarticular pathway) are often diminutive in caliber. Image guidance thus plays an essential role in improving the accuracy of screw placement in such anatomically challenging areas. Plain radiographs, fluoroscopy, and virtual multiplanar fluoroscopy have all been used for guidance during decompression and instrumentation for endoscopic spinal surgery. Although each modality provides significant operative value, none has been able to provide completely accurate axial or three-dimensional information to the surgeon (Fig. 2–2D). Although classic stereotactic volumetric image guidance systems such as these are able to provide some of this information, their use has been limited by the need for intraoperative coregistration of the preoperative dataset to the operative field (Fig. 2–2E).

With the introduction of three-dimensional fluoroscopy, rapid acquisition of an intraoperative computed tomographic (CT) scan of the bony vertebral column is now possible (SireMobile Iso-C Fluoroscopic System; Siemens, Munich, Germany). This imaging technology represents a significant stride in the quest for an ideal image guidance modality for spinal instrumentation. Such intraoperative CT data provide for accurate,

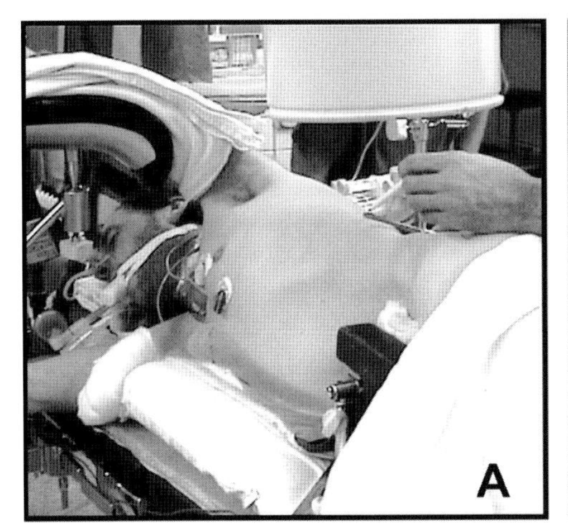

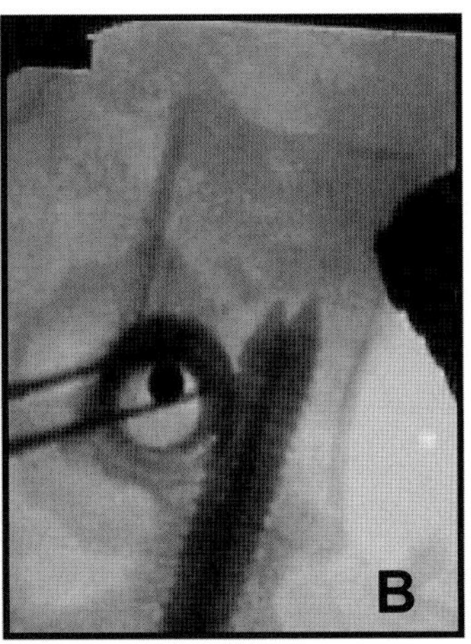

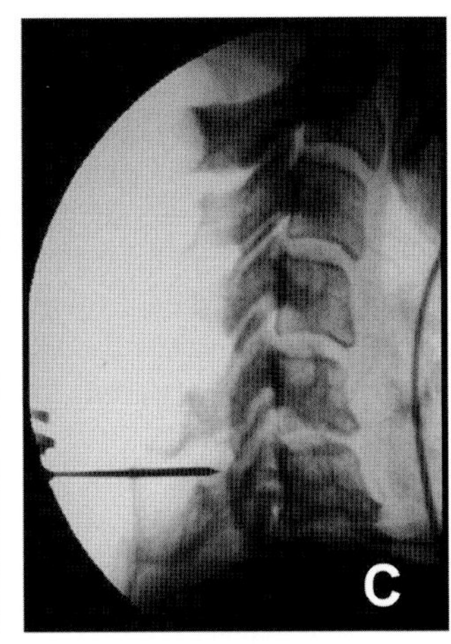

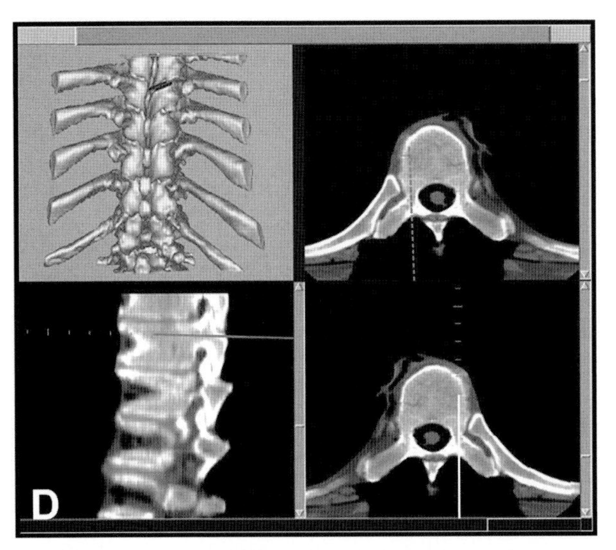

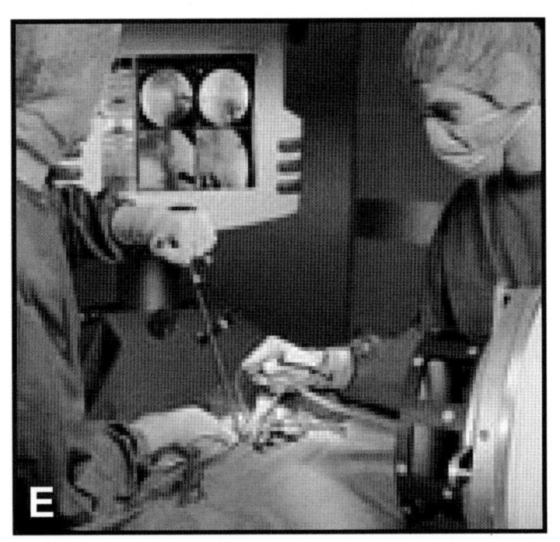

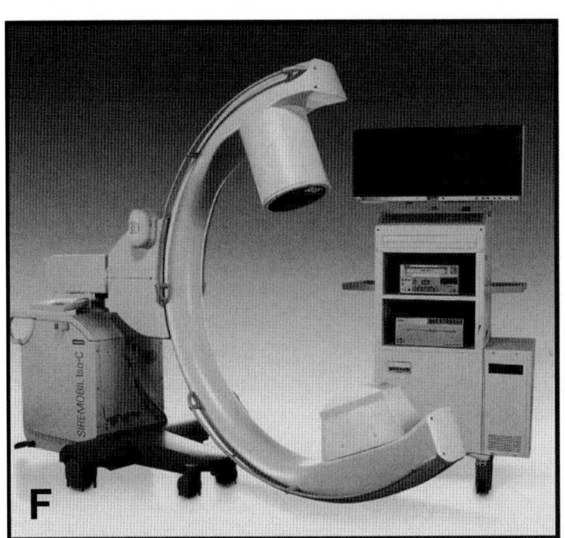

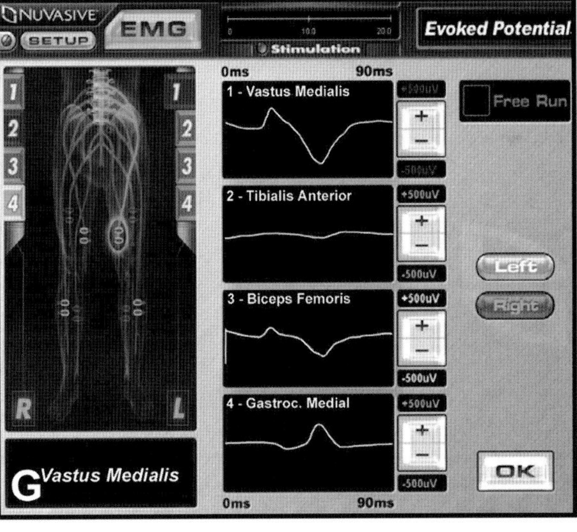

FIGURE 2–2 Operative surgical access. **(A)** Frequent preoperative and **(B)** intraoperative localization of the target level and pathology is critical in planning and execution of minimally invasive portal-type approaches because there is little leeway for "cheating" up or down during the procedure. **(C)** During dorsal tubular approaches, the surgical approach is typically defined, to a large extent, by the trajectory of the initial Steinmann pin placement. As such, careful fluoroscopic confirmation of the initial location of the pin will greatly facilitate the overall success and ease of the procedure. **(D)** Stereotactic three-dimensional image guidance systems allow for real-time axial information, which helps the surgeon facilitate safe decompression and placement of instrumentation. In addition, 3-D "virtual" views can be provided, thereby helping the surgeon compensate for the narrow minimally invasive access portals and their constrained field of view. **(E)** Intraoperative registration and the need for direct line-of-sight tracking of the working tools, however, greatly constrain the ergonomic facility of these technologies. **(F)** Use of intraoperative CT scans as provided by the Siemens Iso-C unit, which serves a dual function as a standard fluoroscopic arm and a simple motorized CT scan unit, can provide real-time intraoperative 3-D information and also avoid registration-type problems. **(G)** Real-time electromyography stimulation of pedicle screws with such systems as Neurovision (Nuvasive; San Diego, CA) helps to facilitate safe placement by detecting cortical breaches and potential injury to adjacent neural structures.

up-to-date anatomical information that can be reformatted in numerous projection planes (Fig. 2–2F). Thus, the need for coregistration to preoperative volumes is eliminated, thereby increasing the speed and cost effectiveness of operative cases. When merged with a frameless stereotactic image guidance system, targeting, decompression, and screw insertion can be planned, visualized, and tracked virtually according to the patient's unique anatomy, thereby greatly improving the surgical efficacy of each component of the endoscopic procedure.

In addition to these visual image guidance systems, neurologic surveillance and guidance are a potentially important aspect of endoscopic and minimally invasive spinal procedures. Because endoscopic procedures are often two-dimensional in their view, additional surveillance with somatosensory evoked potentials (SSEP) and stimulated electromyography (EMG) can provide useful adjuncts to prevent inadvertent neurologic injury during decompression and instrumentation. Whereas an abnormal SSEP is sometimes correlative with neurologic injury, a negative elicited EMG during pedicle cannulation strongly indicates intraosseous placement.[12,13] Such commercial systems as Neurovision (Nuvasive; San Diego, CA) provide such intraoperative EMG thresholds to facilitate accurate pedicle screw placement during minimally invasive spinal instrumentation (Fig. 2–2G).

Endoscopic Visualization

Endoscope Considerations

The operating endoscopes and cameras used during endoscopic and minimally invasive spinal procedures are used in a similar fashion to that of a standard operating microscope. Like microscopes, they provide illumination and magnification. Furthermore, they provide illumination at depth and can be steered directly over the working area to provide an unobstructed, clear visualization of the surgical field far superior to the long line of sight afforded by a microscope. For laparoscopic and thoracoscopic procedures, the surgical endoscopes used are typically rigid, glass-rod-type, 1 cm diameter endoscopes that provide a clear, high-resolution picture. For such procedures, there usually are no working ports in the endoscope because the surgical instruments are introduced through separate, additional working portals in the chest and abdominal wall. The surgeon works through a process of triangulating these operative instruments with the optic or endoscope positioned between them directly over the operating site (Fig. 2–3A). Endoscopes give the surgeon a view that is free from the obstruction that surgical instruments would cause in a standard line of sight viewed with loupes or a microscope. In posterior endoscopic-assisted procedures, the endoscope is mounted on a ring on the working portal that keeps it coaxial with the surgeon's view and the trajectory of the operative instruments (see Fig. 2–1D, 2–1E). By steering the endoscope downward, the surgeon is able to "see around" his or her own hands, thereby gaining an unobstructed field of view.

Whereas the aforementioned procedures are endoscopically assisted, some spinal procedures truly work "through" the endoscope. The most common of these are the posterolateral lumbar diskectomy techniques popularized by Kambin, Yeung, and Tsou.[14–16] With these techniques, dissection, decompression, cautery, and disk removal are often achieved directly through the endoscope, thereby necessitating a working channel of appropriate caliber that the surgical instruments can pass through (Fig. 2–3B). In addition, irrigating ports are needed in combination with appropriate valves on the endoscopes to manage the flow of fluid.

Most hospitals today carry high-quality surgical endoscopes in their inventory for a variety of procedures, including cardiac, thoracic, esophageal, gastric, hepatic, urological, and gynecological procedures. The necessary system components of a digital camera, light cable, illumination source, signal processor, video monitor, image capture, video recorder, and image printer are also usually readily available as well. The spinal surgeon fundamentally should ensure that the telescope used will be a large (1 cm) diameter scope that can provide a broad field with variable illumination, zoom ability, adjustable focus, high-definition image and resolution, accurate color reproduction, and multiple offset angle choices. The advent of three-dimensional (3-D) dual-chamber endoscopes can provide the surgeon the additional benefits of depth perception during particularly complex or microsurgical-type tasks.

The majority of surgical telescopes used today are still based on the time-proven rigid Hopkins lens system that couples air and multiple quartz rod lenses to provide a bright accurate image with minimal distortion. Flexible, low-resolution, or small-diameter endoscopes (e.g., ventriculoscopes) should be avoided for spinal procedures. A distal objective, a relay, and a proximal eyepiece lens are typically used in combination. For most telescopes, a working field of view subtends an 80- to 90-degree arc. Telescopes with varying angles of views or offsets ranging from 0 to 60 degrees are available (Fig. 2–3C). Whereas 0-degree endoscopes afford the least disorientation by providing a direct ahead view, off-axis telescopes provide the surgeon the ability to look around corners or edges at the depths of the operative field. The surgeon can also look around the entire thorax or abdomen by simply spinning the scope around its long axis. Finally, off-axis scopes can be placed well away from the working surgical instruments to avoid collision in the cavity.[2,7,9,10,17] Disadvantages of offset telescopes include

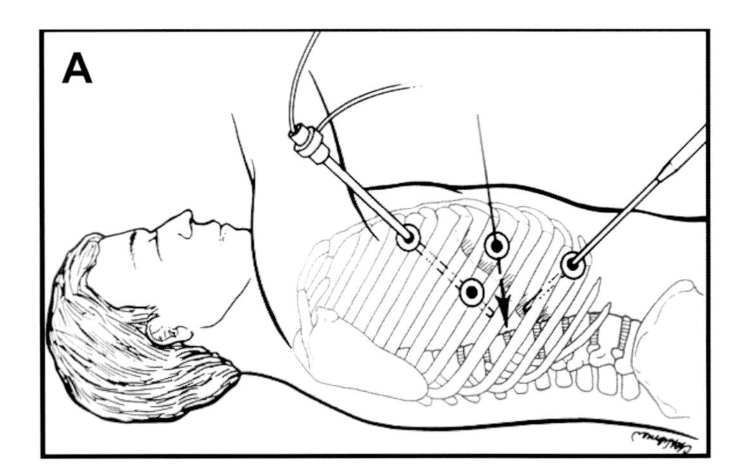

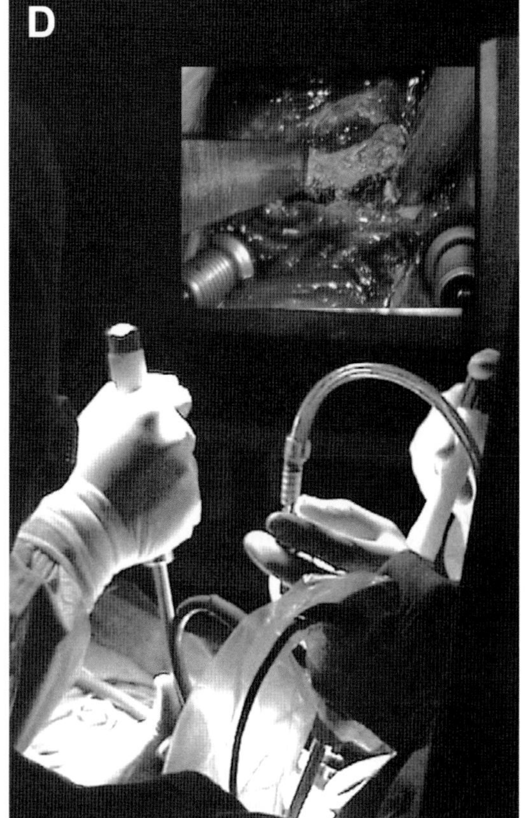

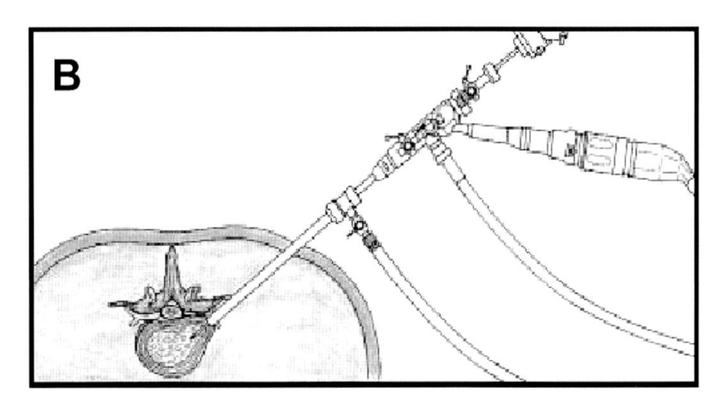

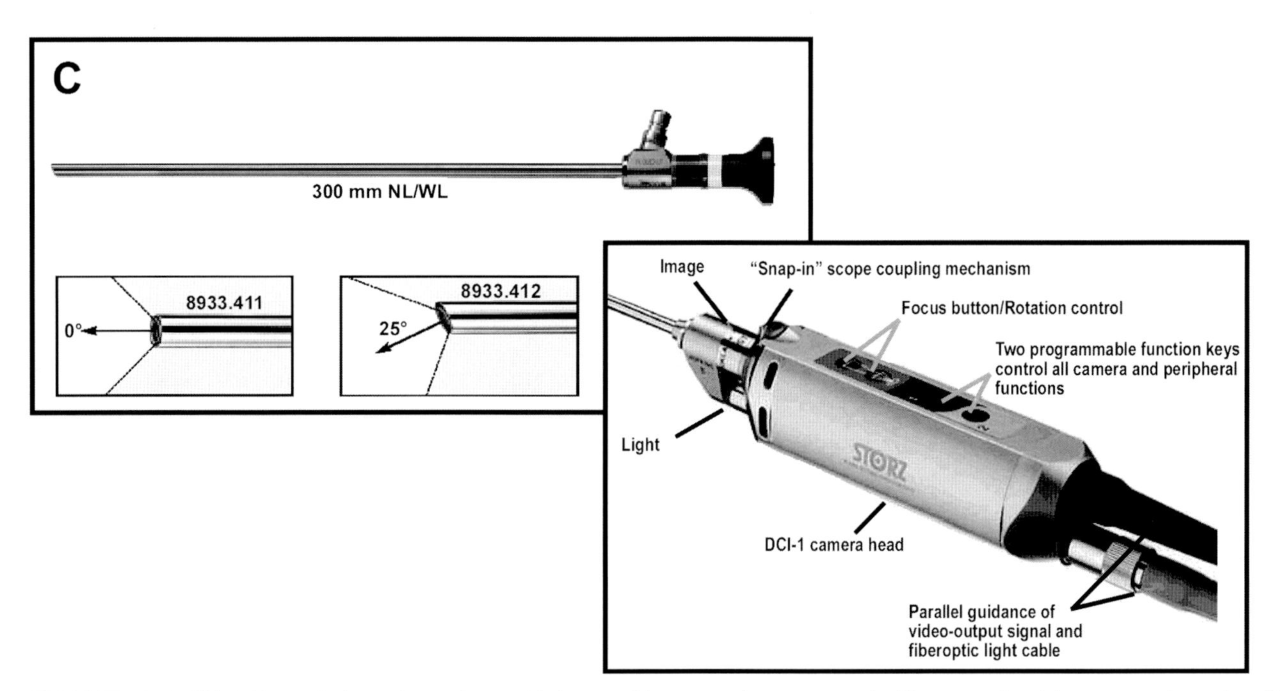

FIGURE 2–3 (A) Triangulation through multiple working portals allows for improved ergonomics and visualization during anterior thoracoscopic and laparoscopic procedures. Such triangulation is not possible during uniportal dorsal approaches. **(B)** Multiple working channels are required through the single portal to allow for simultaneous passage of the instruments, suction, and optic. **(C)** Multiple choices are available with regard to the working angle of the surgical endoscope to facilitate optimal intraoperative visualization. **(D)** The majority of endoscopic procedures are accomplished by the surgeon watching the procedure on large video monitors mounted throughout the operative suite visible to the entire surgical team. Transformation of the analog optical signal seen at the tip of the endoscope to a digital, transmissible image is accomplished through the use of a charged coupling device.

slightly less intense illumination and mild disorientation on the assistant's behalf. We have found that 30-degree endoscopes are particularly versatile for spinal endoscopic-assisted procedures.[4] Facility with both straight and offset telescopes is ultimately desirable.

Digital Imaging

Whereas the original surgical endoscopes used an eyepiece for direct viewing and required that the surgeon place his or her face on or near the end of the sterile telescope, modern endoscopic spinal surgery uses lightweight digital cameras connected to video monitors for large, bright, magnified intraoperative visualization (Fig. 2–3D). The images can also be routed to other devices, including multiple video monitors for the rest of the surgical team and anesthesiology, video recording devices, still image digital capture devices, and photo printers. All this equipment is typically modular and can be mixed and matched for integration into a single ergonomic cart (Fig. 2–4A).

A significant advance in surgical endoscopy was made with the advent of the charged coupling device (CCD), which made possible the conversion of an analog optical image into a clear, accurate, high-resolution digital signal via silicon optical chips. These specialized silicon chips contain a grid of thousands of photosensitive detectors, or pixels, that emit an electronic signal when struck by a photon. These signals are integrated and reconstructed by an in-line digital image processor. The CCD chip can be located either directly at the tip of the endoscope (i.e., "chip on a stick") or, more commonly, on the extracavitary proximal end of the telescope. The processor then uses a series of analog transformations to reassemble the images into a television-type image that can be transmitted out to the operative viewing monitors. With advances in signal processing and color encoding, the images provided by such CCD telescopes far exceed those afforded by classical optical or fiberoptic methods. Furthermore, high-resolution flexible and three-dimensional endoscopes are now available thanks to breakthroughs in CCD technology.

A brief overview of CCD technology is needed to understand the options available. CCD-type cameras originally employed a single chip with a single detector grid whose pixels differentially sensed red, green, or blue light. Although efficient, the color reproduction and resultant clarity of these images were not optimal, especially in the often reddish environs of the operative field. This led to the advent of the alternating single-chip CCD that utilized a 30-Hz strobe light to allow the sensing grid to cycle between sensing green, red, and blue light in 1⁄30 sec intervals. This color separation allowed for significantly improved clarity and color reproduction in the final reintegrated video image. The highest-quality images come from those cameras that simply use three-chip CCD to detect each color spectrum separately. Although the three-chip devices clearly provide the best images, they are also substantially more expensive than the single-chip alternating CCD-type cameras. Finally, it is crucial that the digital processor/integrator unit that is used to couple the camera to the monitor also be up-to-date to ensure the highest quality image processing and reconstruction.

For the novice, one of the most dreaded hurdles of endoscopic spinal surgery is the lack of three-dimensional information. With advances, true 3-D endoscopic visualization is now possible by incorporating two separate optical channels into a single telescope. Much like real-life human binocular vision, such systems use two separate cameras that then transmit their respective images to the digital processor. Other techniques include a single lens with two full-color CCD images at slightly different angles in a single shaft and a splitting lens that separates a left and right image from a single main objective lens. All these techniques ultimately result in separate binocular images being sent to the digital video processor. Viewing of these separate images typically requires either a head-mounted visor display that yields two separate images to the respective eyes or special viewing glasses that flicker as the left and right images are alternately projected on a single-monitor screen (Fig. 2–4B). There is a special infrared emitter located at the top of the video screen that alternately "blacks out" either the right or left eyepiece of the glasses, depending on which image is being presented on the screen. Because of the discomfort, headache, and ergonomic limitations presented by both systems, popularity of 3-D visualization systems has been limited.[2]

Illumination

The type and source of illumination available during the procedure are as important as the camera in many respects. Most modern operating rooms use either xenon or halogen illumination sources mounted via either liquid-filled or fiberoptic cables. Whereas liquid-filled cables are more durable, they conduct and heat up more rapidly, thereby requiring early connection to the endoscope. By contrast, fiberoptic cables remain cooler, but they are much more susceptible to breaking, with a gradual decrease in intensity as more fibers become damaged. The light sources typically range from 250 to 400 W and must be viewed with caution. The intensity of the light can be varied via automated or manual controls. Whereas xenon provides brighter illumination, halogen is often more useful operatively because the light is not as hot as that provided by the xenon source. Particular caution must be paid to not placing the tip of the endoscope or the light cable on the operative field

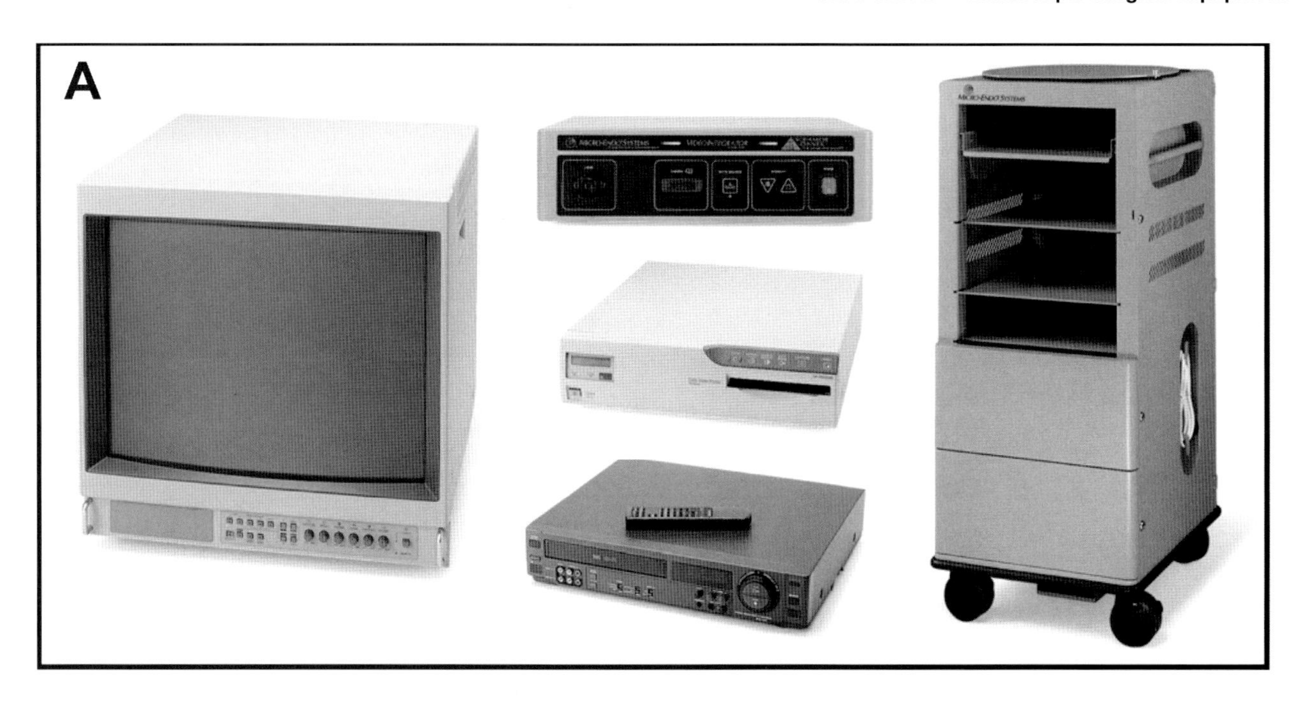

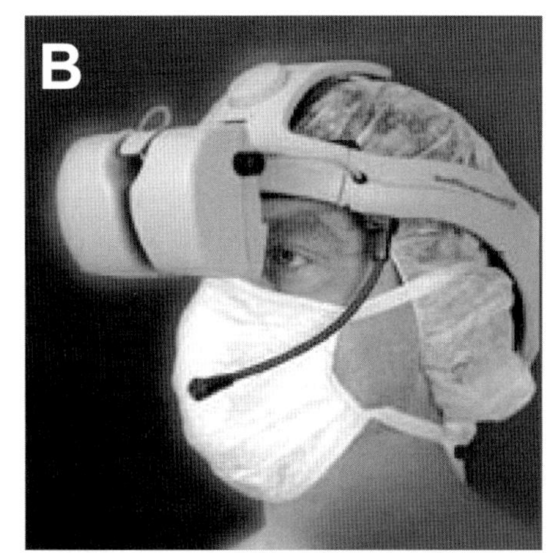

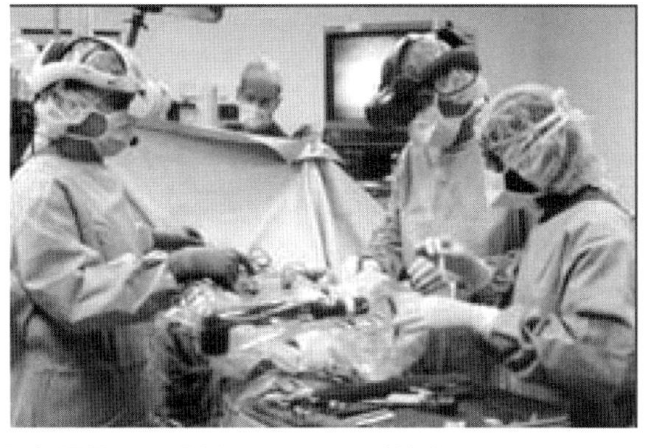

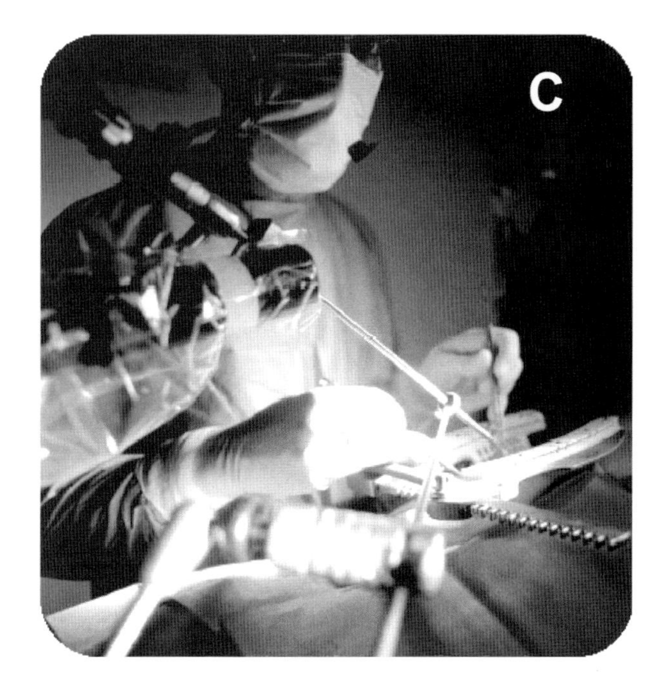

FIGURE 2–4 Digital imaging. **(A)** Because endoscopic procedures are digital-image based, numerous additional equipment options are available for archival and visualization purposes. The surgeon may choose to combine the monitors, camera, CCDs, printers, and recorders into a single cart to conserve space. **(B)** To provide true 3-D visualization from appropriate dual-chamber endoscopes, special heads-up binocular liquid crystal display projection systems are available (Vista; Salt Lake City, UT). **(C)** Robotic holding and endoscopic platforms provide additional ergonomic assistance, if so desired.

because there have been documented cases of intraoperative ignition of paper drapes.[2,9,10] Although brief contact with the patient's tissues is associated with minimal risk of thermal injury, the surgeon and team should be cautious to avoid directly touching the tip of the endoscope upon removal from the body, except with a moist gauze to clean the lens.

Intraoperative Considerations

Regardless of the offset angle of the endoscope, it is crucial that the surgeon rotate the camera at the end of the telescope to the proper orientation prior to beginning the operation. A surgical team typically should establish a convention (i.e., a standard view) such that every member of the surgical team should be oriented the same way. As such, the assistant holding the telescope and camera should know to keep the view so that the surgeon is oriented at all times.

Because the endoscope and camera are significantly cooler and less humid than the body's environment, intraoperative fogging of the lens is a primary concern during endoscopic spinal procedures. Prewarming the endoscope in a bucket or warm body-temperature saline for several minutes prior to introduction within the working cavity or portal can cut down on this fogging. In addition, sterile defogging solution, or FRED (Fog Reduction and Elimination Device; U.S. Surgical, Norwalk, CT), should be applied to the endoscope tip on the lens as a surfactant to reduce fogging. FRED can also be reapplied by soaking a small sponge stick and wiping the tip of the endoscope while it is still in the wound to reduce time needed for removing and reintroducing the optic each time it needs to be cleaned. Several proprietary systems exist for intracavitary cleaning of the endoscope as well. Some telescopes have an integrated washing and cleaning mechanism available for additional cost.

A stable but adjustable view of the surgical field is critical for facilitating endoscopic spinal surgery. During the initial phases of the operation, when the orientation of the images is changed frequently, a surgical assistant can be devoted to holding the endoscope to maintain a relatively stable perspective; however, an assistant usually fatigues easily and poorly stabilizes images for long procedures. A moving image is difficult to follow and unnecessarily distracts the surgeon; therefore, mechanical endoscope holders are extremely useful for reliable fixation of the position of the endoscope in relation to the patient's chest and spine. These devices use mechanical or pneumatic arms that are mounted onto the operating table (see Fig. 2–1E). Robotic, voice-activated computerized endoscope holders are also available (Fig. 2–4C). Endoscope holders simplify the operation, provide stable images, and free the assistant's hands for other tasks.

Image Capture and Recording

Numerous options exist with regard to the capture and storage of intraoperative images during spinal endoscopic procedures. Images can be captured as still shots, brief video motion sequences, or continuous video recording. Archival format options include standard photographic images, digital images (JPEG, TIFF), S-VHS analog, 8 mm digital, regular or minidigital video (DV), and DVD digital disc. In the case of standard still-photo film photographs, a regular high-quality camera must be integrated into the telescope or camera prior to digital processing. Such capture devices are limited in their ease of use. With the advent of digital cameras, however, this process has been greatly simplified, and images can simply be fed from the digital video integrator and processor to a printer. Such devices can provide extremely high-resolution capture of 3 to 5 megapixels in size. More limited, however, is the ability to print these images because most high-quality photo printers still produce images at or under 1200 × 1200 resolution. For video capture, most hospitals still routinely use S-VHS or 8 mm digital formats that are actually beneath the resolution of newer CCDs and processors. For maximal clarity, it is recommended that routine capture of video be accomplished through such true digital formats as that of the mini-DV tape or DVD disc recorders. These formats provide exceptionally crisp playback on standard home and office player units. Furthermore, they provide the ability for postproduction enhancement and editing on most computer laptops and workstations with only a minimal amount of additional equipment. Expensive proprietary archival systems available for image and video capture provide elegant in-line mechanisms to acquire, date, log, and store images in conjunction with demographic data, the operative timeline, and the surgeon's annotations.

Endoscopic Surgical Instruments

On first glance, the operative instruments used during endoscopic spinal procedures are familiar to most spine surgeons; however, careful inspection soon reveals several significant differences. During thoracoscopic and laparoscopic procedures, the working length is substantially longer than that of standard open transcavitary surgery. The working distance can range from 14 to 30 cm, thereby necessitating modification of standard instruments. Endoscopic instruments used for these anterior spinal procedures are thus much longer and also have etched depth markings to facilitate visualization and orientation during two-dimensional dissection of the regional anatomy (Fig. 2–5A). Because of the long lever arm between the portal and the tip of the tools, the surgeon's hand movements are often amplified.

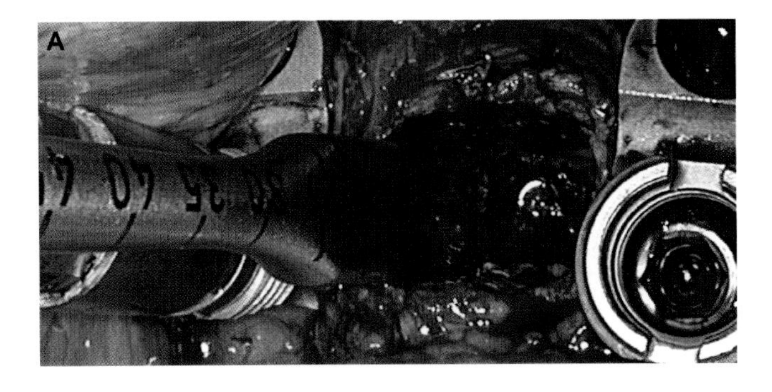

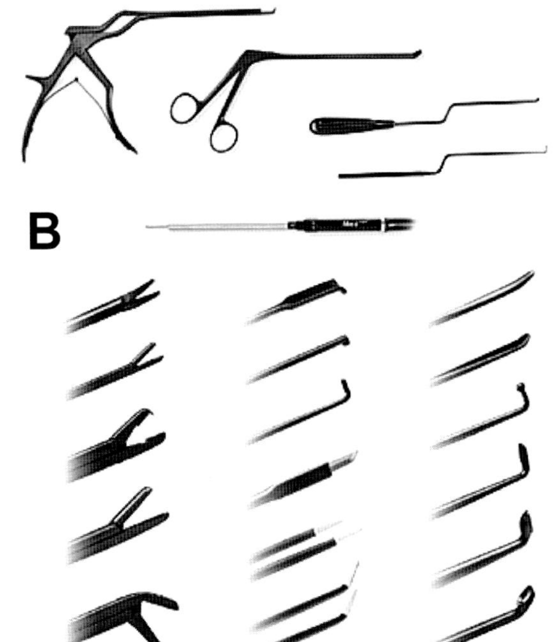

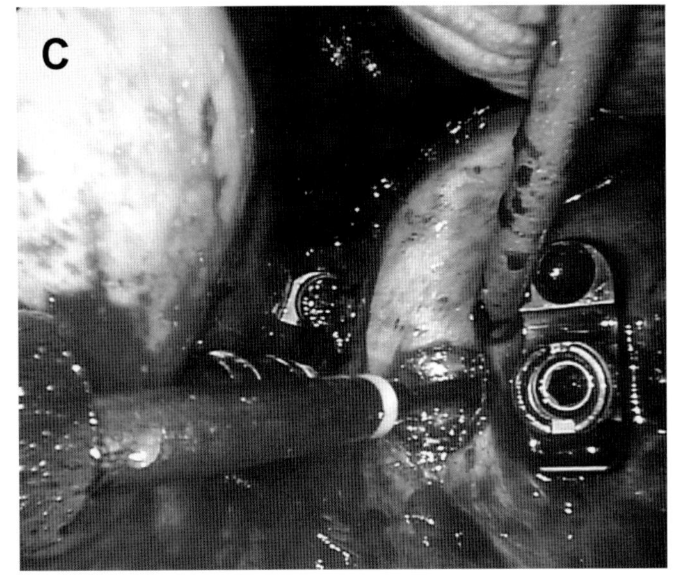

FIGURE 2–5 Endoscopic surgical instruments. **(A)** For endoscopic procedures, modifications of standard surgical instruments are needed to improve the ergonomics and ease of use. Graduation with depth markings is invaluable to avoid accidental plunging and appropriate assessment of depth during such procedures. **(B)** For single-portal access procedures where line-of-sight considerations are limiting, bayoneting of the instruments and changes in their working angle and length are needed. **(C)** Integration of cautery into the surgical instruments helps reduce the number of objects placed into the portal at one time as well as the number of exchanges needed to accomplish a given surgical maneuver.

Surgeons must therefore adopt new strategies for manipulating tools precisely. The surgeon must often use both hands to anchor and guide the handle and shaft of the tools. The tool may also need to be steadied by stabilizing the shaft against the endoscopic portal within the chest wall. Lightweight tools (e.g., suctions, bipolar cauterization devices, endoscopic scissors, and forceps) can usually be controlled adequately with one hand. The surgeon can then work simultaneously with tools in both hands for dissection; however, to gain precise control of heavier tools (e.g., Kerrison rongeurs and curettes) or tools used close to the dura, the surgeon often must use both hands.

Dissection Tools

In their design, the majority of endoscopic spinal tools are very similar to open instruments. As mentioned earlier, they are typically much longer, with mechanisms that allow for shaft rotation to facilitate dissection at depth. Furthermore, beveling or angling of the working tip slightly off the main axis is frequently seen in endoscopic spinal instruments to allow for improved visualization of the working tip during surgery. These curved-tip instruments and dissectors are particularly useful to incise and dissect the fascia, pleura, or peritoneum away from the segmental vessels, spine, and chest wall. The working angle allows for such dissection with simple turns of the surgeon's wrist during these long-distance manipulations. Some instrument systems (e.g., METRx; Medtronic Sofamor Danek) provide bayoneted instruments that are useful to keep the hands away from the central working corridor of a single working portal as well as to improve line-of-sight issues when direct vision (e.g., loupes or microscopes) is used (Fig. 2–5B). The hand grip interfaces are at first unfamiliar to spinal surgeons because they are often ring forceps or pistol grips or have some type of locking mechanism. Because placement of multiple instruments is often limited by only one access portal, many endoscopic spinal instruments have integrated irrigation, suction, and cautery mechanisms to obviate the need for placement of additional instruments through an often-constrained working corridor. Of particular use during thoracoscopic and laparoscopic procedures are integrated dissecting scissors (straight and curved), Debakey-type tissue forceps, right-angled clamps (e.g., Maryland clamp), pleural dissectors, and bipolars. Thus, dissection and cautery can be achieved with maximal ergonomic efficiency (Fig. 2–5C). Nerve root retractors with integrated suction are especially useful during endoscopic-assisted posterior spinal procedures. Many of these multipurpose instruments are available in disposable form for single use.

Retractors

During endoscopic procedures, retraction of adjacent structures is often challenging because of limited access afforded by the portals. As such, thoracoscopic and laparoscopic procedures routinely employ tissue-friendly forceps (e.g., lung forceps, Allis clamps, and Babcock clamps) to hold and move important structures away from the operative field. The fan-bladed retractors that are used to mobilize both lung and visceral structures away from the spine are especially important. These are available in a variety of designs, but all incorporate blunt-tipped, broad-surfaced blades that "fan" out after placement through the portal to allow for a broad, gentle retraction surface (Fig. 2–6A). These retractors frequently have an additional joint that allows for angling and towing in without additional manipulation of the working shaft angle, which is constrained by the access portal. With proper patient positioning and rotation of the patient, the atelectatic lung often can be encouraged to fall away from the spine, thereby minimizing excessive retraction of the lung and viscera to avoid inadvertent injury.

Irrigation and Suction

Like retraction issues, suction and irrigation during endoscopic procedures are also both critical and technically challenging to accomplish. Because the tools are often long, strong suction can be difficult to maintain. Excessive blood, cautery burn, and clot tend to absorb light, thus decreasing the illumination provided by the endoscope. To clear these undesirable elements, long Frazier-tipped or trumpet-type suction tools with integrated suction, irrigation, and cautery are needed. These specialized suction devices require an integrated means of delivering forceful irrigation to dislodge blood and clots from tissue surfaces (Fig. 2–6A-C). Pressurized bags of saline or intravenous fluid are typically mounted in-line with the suction tip to accomplish this goal. A cheaper alternative to such commercially available devices is a simple 50 cc syringe with a long central venous introducer sheath attached to it for irrigating within the thoracic or abdominal cavity.

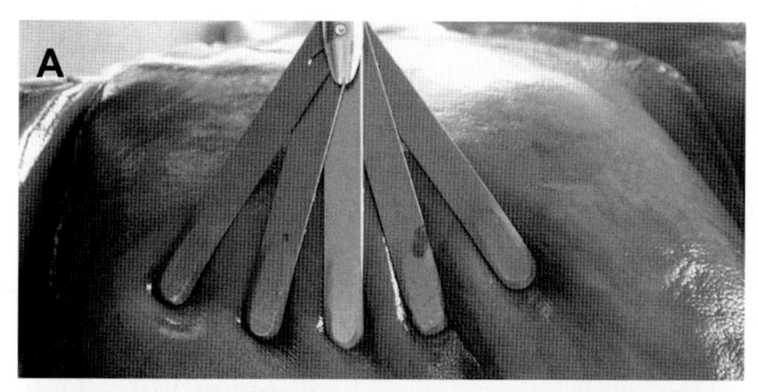

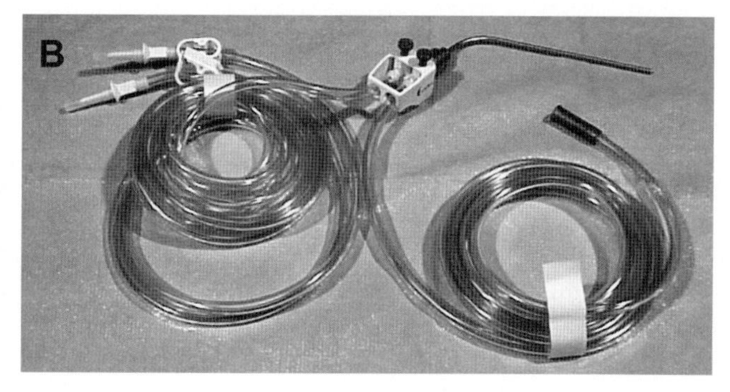

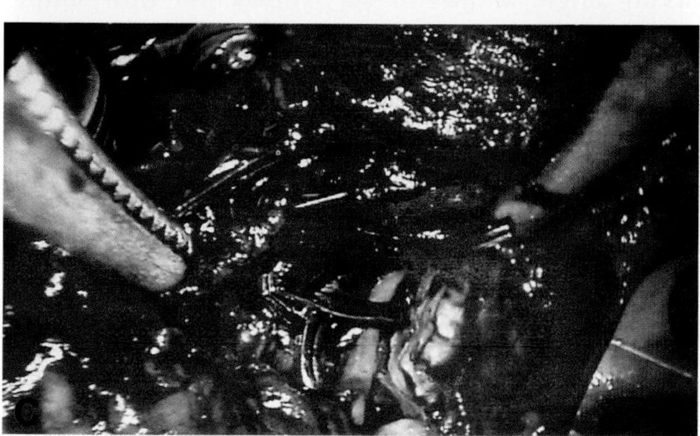

FIGURE 2–6 **(A)** Such specialized tools as the fan-bladed design for thoracoscopic surgery are required to retract visceral structures during these procedures. **(B)** Integration of suction and cautery into an ergonomically friendly device is necessary to provide a clear operative field during endoscopic procedures. **(C)** Subtle changes in the working length and angle of endovascular clip appliers are needed to provide proper ligation and hemostasis during minimally invasive surgeries.

Hemostasis and Cautery

Whereas the fundamental techniques of endoscopic hemostasis are the same as that of conventional open spinal surgery, the tools used, as with all instruments, require modification. As mentioned earlier, cautery is commonly integrated into many of the dissection, suction, and irrigation tools for ergonomic reasons. Both monopolar and bipolar cautery options are typically available, depending on the type of instrument being used. Dedicated cautery devices are also available in thoracoscopic, laparoscopic, and posterior endoscopic instrument sets. Because normal bipolars are useless in these procedures, longer, pistol-grip shafts are used. In addition, beveled bipolar tips are often helpful to reach underneath structures or beyond the immediate field of view. Ultrasonic or harmonic scalpels (Ethicon Endosurgery; Somerville, NJ) can be used as a combined cutting and cautery tool that allows for a shallow depth of penetration with a minimum of thermal damage, smoke, and adjacent tissue injury. With its blade that oscillates at 55 kHz and amplitude of 60 to 80 μ, it is able to denature collagen and effectively seal vessels smaller than 1 mm in diameter; however, it is not effective for hemostasis of larger vessels.

In a similar fashion, hemoclip appliers must be modified for use in endoscopic procedures. Automated, disposable, multiuse clip appliers with rotating shafts allow for variable angle of placement or several clips without having to reload each time. These endoscopic clip appliers are available in a variety of working angles to facilitate dissection and placement underneath vascular structures. Because secure hemostasis of large-caliber segmental vessels often necessitates multiple clip placements, such rapid-fire devices are invaluable.

With regard to hemostatic agents, such standard surgical agents as Gelfoam (Upjohn, Kalamazoo, MI),

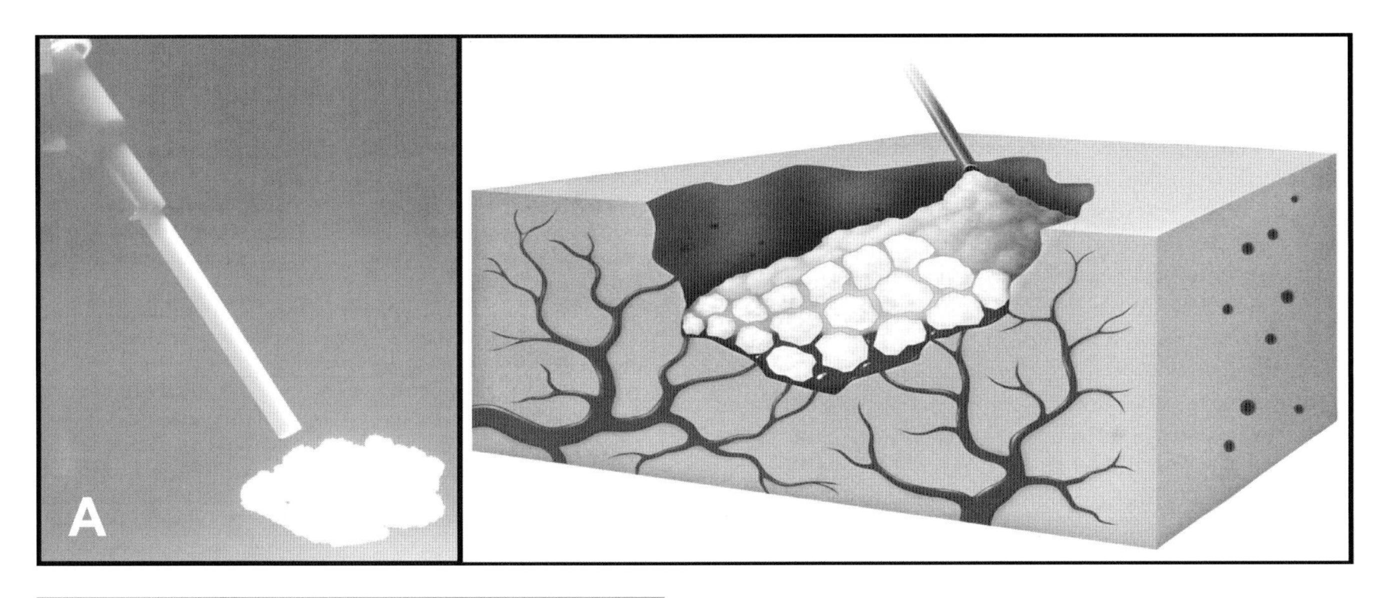

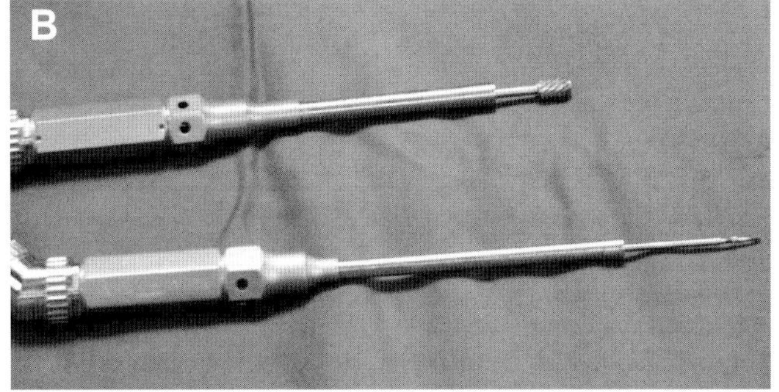

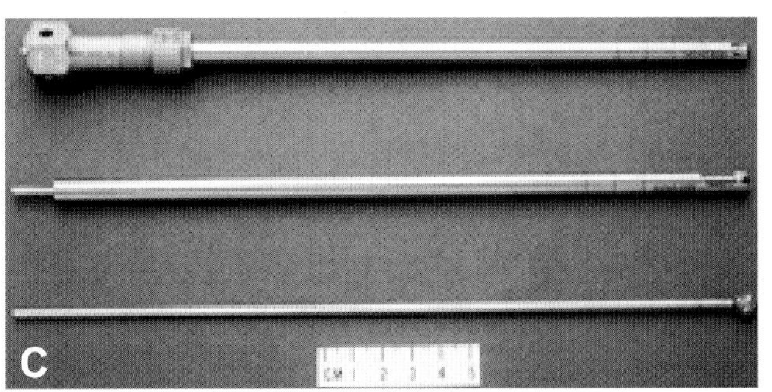

FIGURE 2–7 Endoscopic hemostatic and drills. **(A)** In addition to modified surgical instruments, modification of hemostatic agents with regard to form and shape help to facilitate hemostasis during minimally invasive procedures. Floseal (BaxterHealthcare) allows for local hemostasis through enlarging thrombin-soaked gelatin granules that allow for local tamponade and are not washed off during gentle irrigation as compared with standard pieces of thrombin-soaked Gelfoam. **(B)** For endoscopic procedures, additional length and smaller spin diameters are required in the drills used. **(C)** Because of the two-dimensional view and the inability to see proximal to the working area, shielded drill bits allow for additional safety during thoracoscopic and laparoscopic procedures.

Avitene (C. R. Bard, Inc., Murray Hill, NJ), and Nu-Knit (Johnson & Johnson, Arlington, TX) can be used via specialized delivery systems. Bone wax applied on the long end of cherry cotton dissectors or endoscopic peanuts can be used in a standard fashion. Delivery of Gelfoam with thrombin or Avitene can be accomplished via long delivery cylinders with central plungers. The roll of Avitene is then expressed in the working field and delivered to the bleeding site via manipulation with a small cottonoid or dissector. The advent of powdered or gelatin granules of Gelfoam impregnated with thrombin (e.g., Floseal; Baxter Healthcare, Deerfield, IL) allows for delivery through a syringe and a long endoscopic tip directly into such bleeding sites as the epidural gutters. As the granules swell, local hemostasis is readily achieved. After a few minutes, moderate irrigation removes loose granules, leaving the clot in place (Fig. 2–7A). In our experience, the use of such agents has resulted in significant decrements in our operative blood loss. This experience echoes that of the cardiothoracic endoscopic experience as well.

Endoscopic Drills

As with standard open spinal procedures, the use of a modern, low-torque, high-speed drill is essential for the majority of endoscopic spinal procedures. High-speed pneumatic devices were preferred for most endoscopic bone dissection applications; however, such newer high-speed electric drills as the TPS system (Stryker, Kalamazoo, MI) are now able to deliver similar power and efficiency to that of pneumatic devices. The long bits and guiding shafts of endoscopic drills require additional stabilizing elements such as a pistol grip. This allows the operative surgeon stable, three-point control of the drill by bracing the pistol grip along the chest wall, thereby allowing for more precise control of the distal working tip. The Midas Rex drill system (Midas Rex Pneumatic Tools, Inc., Fort Worth, TX) has bits that are 25 cm (R- or L-attachments) or 40 cm long (Rx attachment), both of which are useful for thoracoscopic spine work (Fig. 2–7B). These attachments have a long, protective sheath that prevents injury to the lung and paraspinal soft tissue. A telescoping, adjustable sheath allows the surgeon to carry the length of the exposed drill tip to protect the soft tissues of the thorax. Various drill bits are available for endoscopic use (Fig. 2–7C). Coarse diamond burrs are useful for endoscopic drilling of the vertebral body but do create significant heat around neural structures. The coarse diamond burrs create bone dust slurry that fills the interstices of the cancellous bone and reduces bone bleeding without generating excessive debris within the chest cavity.

Technological advances in endoscopic equipment and instrumentation have greatly expanded the indications for minimally invasive spine surgical procedures. Developments in imaging technology with better resolution of endoscopic images, greater use of working channels, and improved 3-D imaging will allow for improved surgical outcomes. Integration of endoscopic equipment with image-guidance and robotic systems presents an exciting promise for further refinement of endoscopic procedures.

REFERENCES

1. Kim DH, Jaikumar S, Kam AC. Minimally invasive spine instrumentation. *Neurosurgery.* 2002;51:15–25.
2. Dickman CA, Perin NI. Instrumentation and equipment for thoracoscopic spine surgery. In: Dickman CA, Rosenthal DJ, Perin NI, eds. *Thoracoscopic Spine Surgery.* New York: Thieme Medical Publishers;1999:37–48.
3. Fessler RG, Khoo L. Minimally invasive cervical microendoscopic foraminotomy (MEF): an initial clinical experience. *Neurosurgery.* 2002;51:37–45.
4. Khoo L, Beisse R, Potulski M. Minimally invasive endoscopic repair of thoracolumbar burst fractures. *Neurosurgery.* 2002;51:104–117.
5. Khoo L, Fessler RG. Microendoscopic decompressive laminotomy for lumbar stenosis. *Neurosurgery.* 2002;51:146–154.
6. Styf JR, Willen J. The effects of external compression by three different retractors on pressure in the erector spine muscles during and after posterior lumbar spine surgery in humans. *Spine.* 1998;23:354–358.
7. Aronoff RJ, Mack MJ. Equipment and instrumentation for thoracoscopy and laparoscopy. In: Regan JJ, McAfee PC, Mack MJ, eds. *Atlas of Endoscopic Spine Surgery.* St. Louis: Quality Medical Publishing; 1995:35–38.
8. Krasna MJ, Mack MJ. Equipment and instrumentation. In: Krasna MJ, Mack MJ, eds. *Atlas of Thoracoscopic Surgery.* St Louis: Quality Medical Publishing; 1994:19–34.
9. Regan JJ. Equipment and instrumentation for endoscopic spine surgery. In: Regan JJ, McAfee PC, Mack MJ, eds. *Atlas of Endoscopic Spine Surgery.* St. Louis: Quality Medical Publishing; 1995:69–82.
10. Landreneau RJ, Mack MJ, Hazelrigg SR, et al. Video-assisted thoracic surgery: basic technical concepts and intercostal approach strategies. *Ann Thorac Surg.* 1992;54:800–807.
11. Allen MS, Trastek VF, Daly RC, et al. Equipment for thoracoscopy. *Ann Thorac Surg.* 1993;56:620–623.
12. Glassman SD, Dimar JR, Puno RM, Johnson JR, Shields CB, Linden RD. A prospective analysis of intraoperative electromyographic monitoring of pedicle screw placement with computed tomographic scan confirmation. *Spine.* 1995;20:1375–1379.
13. Manninen RH. Clinical measurement-monitoring evoked potentials during spinal surgery in one institution. *Can J Anesth.* 1998;45: 460–465.
14. Kambin P. Posterolateral percutaneous lumbar discectomy and decompression. In: Kambin P, ed. *Arthroscopic Microdiscectomy: Minimal Intervention in Spinal Surgery.* Baltimore: Williams & Wilkins; 1991:67–100.
15. Kambin P, Casey K, O'Brien E, et al. Transforaminal arthroscopic decompression of lateral recess stenosis. *J Neurosurg.* 1996;84: 462–467.
16. Yeung AT, Tsou PM. Posterolateral endoscopic excision for lumbar disc herniation. *Spine.* 2002;27:722–731.
17. Talamini MA, Gadacz TR. Laparoscopic equipment and instrumentation. In: Zucker KA, Bailey RW, Reddick EJ, eds. *Surgical Laparoscopy Update.* St. Louis: Quality Medical Publishing; 1995: 69–81.

3

Anesthetic Considerations and Operating Room Setup for Minimally Invasive Endoscopic Spine Surgery

BRIAN K. KWON, CALVIN L. AU, JOHN BEINER, JONATHAN N. GRAUER, JAMES A. SANFILIPPO, DAVID H. KIM, AND ALEXANDER R. VACCARO

The spinal community has witnessed increasing interest in endoscopic, minimally invasive surgical techniques. Spine surgeons have been encouraged by the prospect of emulating the reduced perioperative morbidity achieved by the general and cardiothoracic surgeons who have championed laparoscopic and thoracoscopic technologies. Endoscopic procedures present anesthetic challenges that are distinct from traditional open procedures. A fairly substantial assembly of specialized equipment is necessary to navigate the spine successfully in a minimally invasive manner. The initial presurgical preparations necessitate careful planning with regard to the operating room setup, patient positioning, and surrounding configuration of all surgical personnel and required equipment.

Anesthetic Considerations for Thoracoscopy

Although thoracoscopic access to the spine obviates the need for a large thoracotomy incision, it does require retraction or collapse of the nondependent lung for adequate visualization. This and the resultant single-lung ventilation of the dependent side can have significant cardiopulmonary implications, which are important to recognize when undertaking a minimally invasive thoracic procedure. Signs and symptoms of preexisting cardiac and pulmonary disease must be identified and carefully evaluated preoperatively by the appropriate medical consultants. Although the patient may have an adequate baseline level of functioning, he or she will be largely dependent on the pulmonary function of a single lung during a potentially prolonged thoracoscopic procedure. Pulmonary function tests may be warranted in patients with chronic obstructive pulmonary disease (COPD) or other respiratory disorders. The spine patients being managed thoracoscopically for anterior release to correct deformity or for symptomatic thoracic disk herniation fortunately are typically younger and can therefore tolerate single-lung ventilation for the often-prolonged duration of these surgical procedures. Smoking is unfortunately relatively common in patients with spinal disorders. Such patients should be implored to stop smoking at least 6 to 8 weeks prior to surgery because a decrease in sputum production and improvement in ciliary activity will lessen the chance of postoperative respiratory complications.[1,2] Of course, beyond the pulmonary implications of smoking that are inherently relevant to the thoracoscopy procedure itself, the adverse effects of smoking on bone fusion and tissue healing are well recognized.[3]

Perioperative Monitoring

Perioperative monitoring of patients undergoing thoracoscopy includes such routine measures as electrocardiogram (ECG), pulse oximetry, blood pressure, temperature, and capnography. Pulse oximetry and capnography provide important information with regard to oxygenation and ventilatory status, and it can provide early warnings for a variety of ventilation problems. Most anesthesiologists place an arterial line for cases involving trespass of the thoracic cavity and single-lung ventilation. Periodic arterial blood gas measurements may also be warranted, especially in patients with preexisting pulmonary disease whose end-tidal CO_2 can be misleading. Large-bore peripheral intravenous lines should be established at the onset of the procedure, and consideration should be given to the placement of a central venous catheter, depending on the nature of the procedure. A surgical misadventure leading to a large vessel injury in the thoracic cavity may quickly turn the procedure into a life-threatening hemorrhagic emergency. Central venous access is invaluable for the rapid infusion of resuscitative fluids and pharmacologic agents and for the central monitoring of their effects. A surgical suite setup incapable of rapidly converting to an open thoracotomy and lacking in the necessary blood product resources for urgent hemodynamic resuscitation is suboptimal for minimally invasive thoracoscopic surgery. These deficiencies arguably should be corrected prior to undertaking such procedures. A Swan-Ganz catheter is also useful in settings of large blood loss or in patients with severe preexisting cardiopulmonary disease, although it should be recognized that pulmonary blood-flow alterations associated with single-lung ventilation may invalidate the assumption of uniform pulmonary capillary resistance upon which cardiac output and left-ventricular end-diastolic volume are calculated.[4]

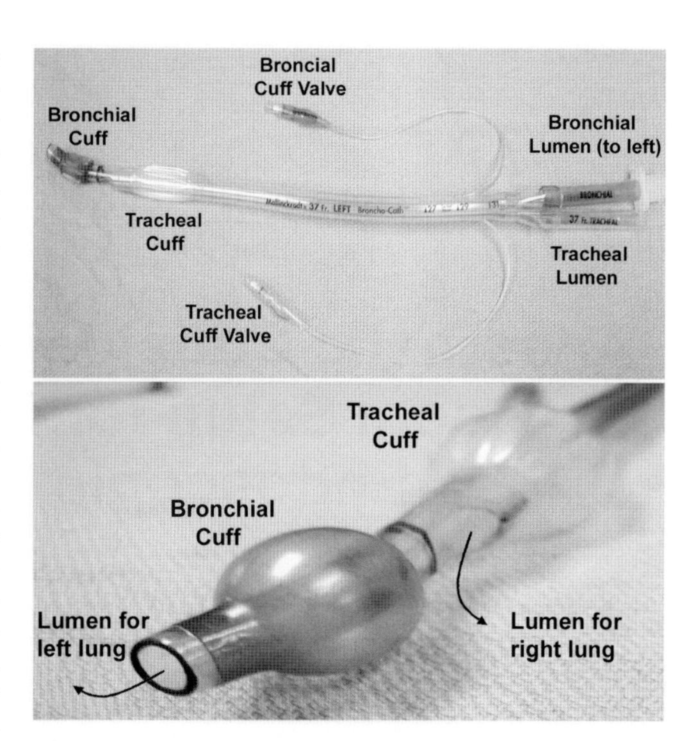

FIGURE 3–1 Double lumen endotracheal tube. Note that the tube has two cuffs that can be inflated independently, with the bronchial cuff inflated within the left mainstem bronchus. Such a tube can be used for single-lung ventilation of either right or left lung. For left-lung ventilation, gas exchange occurs through the lumen to the left lung, with the tracheal lumen occluded. For right-lung ventilation, gas exchange occurs through the tracheal lumen, with the left lumen occluded.

Single-Lung Ventilation

The effects of single-lung ventilation of the dependent lung are arguably the most significant anesthetic consideration for thoracoscopy. Collapse of the nondependent lung is important for visualization of the spine and for minimizing iatrogenic lung injury from various thoracoscopic instruments. Deflation of the nondependent lung is accomplished using a double-lumen endotracheal tube or any one of a variety of specially designed single-lumen tubes with built-in bronchial blockers. In general, complete deflation of the lung takes ~15 to 20 minutes. If collapse of the lung is not sufficient to provide adequate visualization of the thoracic spine, CO_2 can be insufflated into the pleural cavity to provide pressure retraction of the mobile lung tissues. Elevating the intrathoracic pressure unfortunately can cause significant hemodynamic alterations, including a tension pneumothorax. It is recommended that insufflation pressures not exceed 10 mm Hg, below which cardiovascular consequences are minimized.[5]

For the induction of single-lung ventilation, double-lumen tubes are currently favored because of their relative ease of placement, although single-lumen tubes are used most commonly in pediatric patients due to their more compact dimensions. Double-lumen endotracheal tubes have two lumens and two occlusive balloons (Fig. 3–1). The proximal balloon is inflated in the trachea, and the distal balloon is inflated at the entrance to the mainstem bronchus. Many anesthesiologists use a left-sided double-lumen tube regardless of the intended operative side because a right-sided double-lumen tube is more difficult to place without inadvertently occluding the right upper lobe. Single-lung ventilation is then accomplished by ventilating only the dependent lung and opening the nondependent lung to atmospheric pressure, allowing it to collapse naturally. Double-lumen tubes are larger in caliber than are single-lumen tubes; thus, they are more likely to cause tracheobronchial injury. Great care must also be taken to position the two occlusive balloons precisely within the tracheobronchial tree to ensure proper function. Problems with positioning are the most common cause of ventilatory difficulties during single-lung ventilation. Although the presence of breath sounds and ventilation or oxygenation parameters are indicative of accurate tube positioning, direct visualization and confirmation of the tube position are advisable with fiberoptic bronchoscopy.[6]

Several physiologic alterations occur when the nondependent lung is deflated. Ventilation and pulmonary perfusion are normally well matched. This means that areas of lung that receive the most blood also receive the most ventilation. When the nondependent lung is deflated, blood passes through the atelectatic lung, and a ventilation-perfusion (V/Q) mismatch, or shunt, occurs, resulting in suboptimal blood oxygenation. At first, this is compensated by hypoxic pulmonary vasoconstriction (HPV), an autoregulatory mechanism that increases pulmonary vascular resistance in the face of low PaO_2 and PvO_2. This redirects blood flow to areas of the lung that are well ventilated. HPV ceases to function, however, when ~70% of the lung has collapsed due to a lack of normoxic regions in the lung to which blood can be redirected.[7] When full collapse is finally achieved, therefore, significant hypoxia may occur due to both the reduction in pulmonary surface area for gas exchange and the significant V/P mismatch. With the patient in a lateral decubitus position, further deterioration in PaO_2 can occur from impaired ventilation within the dependent, "down" lung.[8] These physiologic alterations highlight the need to evaluate the cardiopulmonary status of the patient carefully before undertaking a minimally invasive thoracoscopic procedure.

Anesthetic Considerations for Laparoscopy

Laparoscopic procedures do not directly affect the cardiopulmonary system to the extent of thoracoscopic procedures, but they do have their own systemic influences, which are largely related to the frequent use of intraperitoneal CO_2 insufflation and to patient positioning. Pneumoperitoneum with CO_2 remains the most common and reliable method of achieving laparoscopic visualization of the lumbar spine. The peritoneal cavity is entered initially with a periumbilical trocar or Veress needle, through which CO_2 is introduced to expand the abdomen and to allow for the introduction of other instruments and for exposure to the spine. A peak intraperitoneal pressure no greater than 15 mm Hg is recommended because the hemodynamic consequences at or below this level are relatively modest and well tolerated. In general, the greater the intraperitoneal pressure applied, the greater the compression of the abdominal aorta and inferior vena cava, and hence enhanced potential for hemodynamic disturbance.[9] Compression of the aorta increases systemic vascular resistance and afterload, whereas compression of the vena cava decreases venous return and preload. These factors, in association with the hemodynamic effects of anesthetic induction and patient positioning, may transiently reduce cardiac output by as much as 50% of normal.[10] These changes tend to normalize within the first 10 to 30 min, but nevertheless represent important considerations in the patient with limited cardiac reserve.

Insufflated CO_2 itself may have a direct and indirect effect on systemic circulation. The diffusion of CO_2 into the systemic circulation results in slightly increased end-tidal CO_2. The direct effects of this (beyond the mechanical effects of insufflation) are not entirely clear, although it may contribute to acidemia, hypercapnea, and reduced stroke volume,[11] particularly in patients with severe pulmonary disease and the impaired ventilatory function to eliminate CO_2 (e.g., COPD).

Laparoscopy systems that rely on specialized retractor systems to lift abdominal wall contents instead of CO_2 insufflation have been described.[12] Although this minimizes the potential adverse hemodynamic effects of CO_2 insufflation, the advantages of such gasless techniques may be offset somewhat by inferior surgical visualization.[13]

Endoscopic spine procedures typically require Trendelenburg positioning of the patient to move the abdominal contents superiorly and facilitate access to the L4–L5 and L5–S1 disk spaces. It appears that the establishment of pneumoperitoneum in either the Trendelenburg or reverse Trendelenburg position significantly worsens the hemodynamic abnormalities associated with CO_2 insufflation. Both positions affect venous return to the heart, albeit in opposite manners. The reverse Trendelenburg position is associated with significant venous pooling in the lower extremities, leading to decreased preload and a reduction in cardiac output. Trendelenburg positioning results in an opposite physiologic phenomenon (i.e., an increase in venous return to the heart and increased cardiac output).[14] In addition to altering hemodynamic function, intraperitoneal insufflation and the Trendelenburg position both push the diaphragm superiorly, thus reducing diaphragmatic excursion, functional residual capacity, and pulmonary compliance. Although these changes may be well tolerated by the young, healthy individual, they may have significant adverse effects on patients with preexisting pulmonary disease. Trendelenburg positioning may also cause the carina to move superiorly and alter the relative position of the endotracheal tube. Sudden intraoperative changes in ventilatory status of the patient during such procedures therefore warrant an immediate evaluation of endotracheal tube position.

Although both thoracoscopy and laparoscopy involve several anesthetic considerations that warrant cautious attention, one should not overlook the potential for these minimally invasive procedures to reduce overall morbidity and improve patient care in comparison to open procedures that necessitate larger incisions. The increasing interest in endoscopic surgery as an alternative to large-incision open exposures is a testimony to this. Nevertheless, unique anesthetic issues exist for thoracoscopic and laparoscopic surgery, which need to be acknowledged, particularly in patients with preexisting medical conditions.

Operating Room Setup for Endoscopic Spine Surgery

Endoscopic spinal procedures are quite resource-intensive in terms of operating room personnel and equipment needs. In addition to the obligatory surgical and anesthetic teams (including assistants and nurses), these procedures may require two or more circulating nurses, a neuromonitoring team, and a dedicated x-ray technician. A thoracic, cardiovascular, or general surgeon proficient in endoscopy is often beneficial as a cosurgeon or assistant to the spine surgeon to assist in the exposure and to provide urgent open access should the need arise. For example, it is estimated that conversion from thoracoscopy to open thoracotomy occurs in 6 to 20% of cases, most often because of the need to gain better access to the surgical pathology.[15] A physically large operating room is helpful to accommodate the required personnel and equipment necessary for such minimally invasive procedures as a fluoroscopy machine, multiple video monitors (these need to be positioned on either side of the patient in a direct line of sight for the surgeon and assistant), and, possibly, image guidance systems. The myriad of specialized endoscopic spinal instruments requires a well-familiarized surgical team of assistants and nurses, a substantial amount of sterile table space, and a cogent strategy to maintain all of the equipment in an orderly fashion within the operative field. The scrub nurse should have the Mayo stand arranged toward the foot of the bed in such a way that such commonly used equipment as the electrocautery and suction are easily delivered to surgeons on either side of the table.

In thoracoscopy procedures, the patient is positioned in the lateral decubitus position with the lung and side of the spine to be accessed lying superiorly. Ensuring an exact lateral position is helpful for orientation both visually with the thoracoscope and radiographically with fluoroscopy. A radiolucent table is helpful for achieving both anterior and lateral fluoroscopic images of the spine. The operating table should be capable of rotating in a side-to-side manner and tilting in a head up or down manner to allow the atelectatic lung to fall away from the region of the spine being accessed (Fig. 3–2). An axillary roll is placed as padding under the dependent axilla, and all other bony prominences are padded with foam or pillows. Given the possibility that the

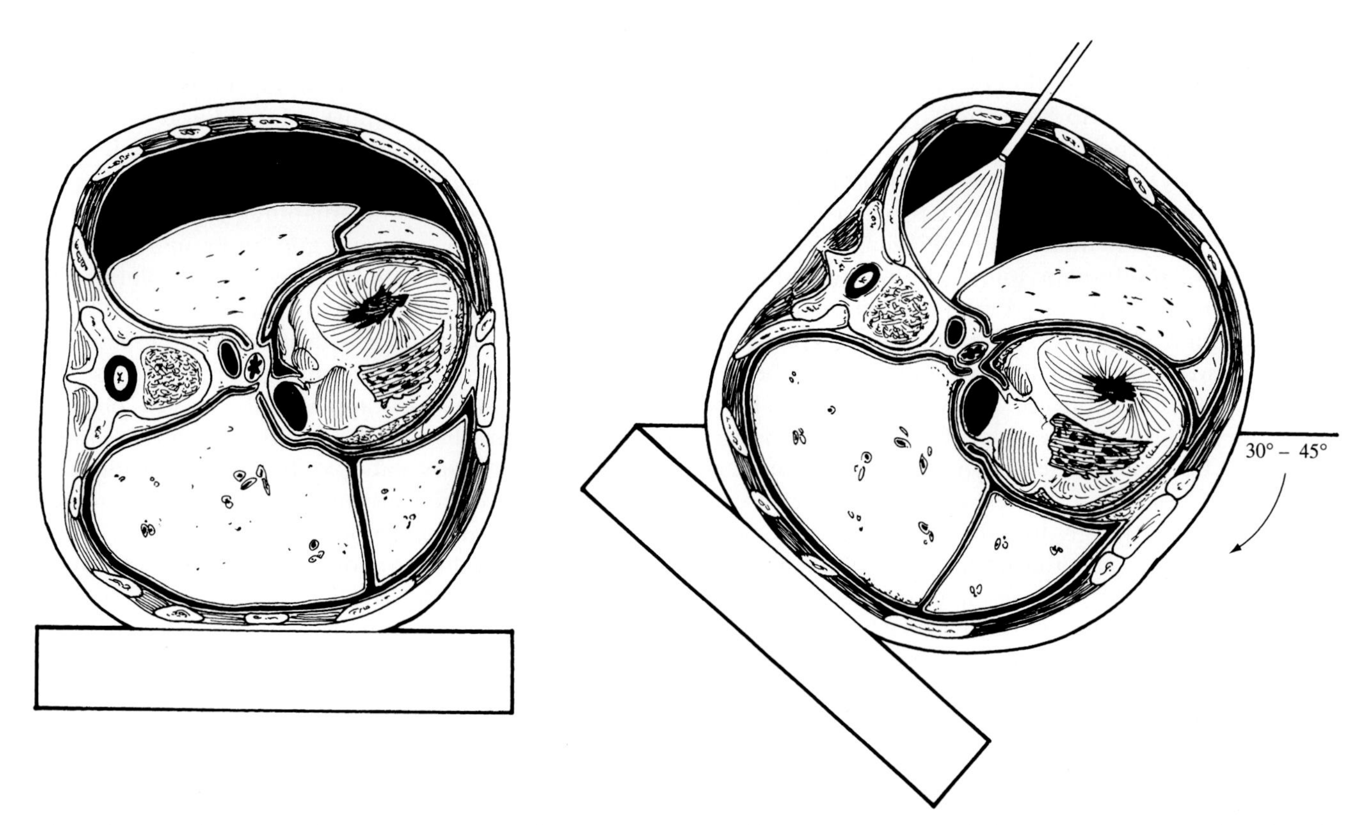

FIGURE 3–2 Tilting the patient forward during thoracoscopic procedures will use gravity to move the lung away from the spine and thus facilitate visualization. (With permission from Rosenthal DJ, Dickman CA. Operating room setup and patient positioning. In: Dickman C, Rosenthal DJ, Perin NI, eds. *Thoracoscopic Spine Surgery.* New York: Thieme Medical Publishers; 1999:104.)

thoracoscopic procedure may be quite prolonged, careful attention must be paid to ensuring adequate padding and protection during the case. A sling or elevated armboard attachment can be used to keep the ipsilateral arm flexed at the shoulder and out of the way for access to the upper thoracic spine (Fig. 3–3). Adhesive tape, belts, or clamps should be used to secure the patient to the table and prevent motion when changing the table inclination. The thoracic region should be draped completely so that the procedure can be converted to an open thoracotomy if necessary.

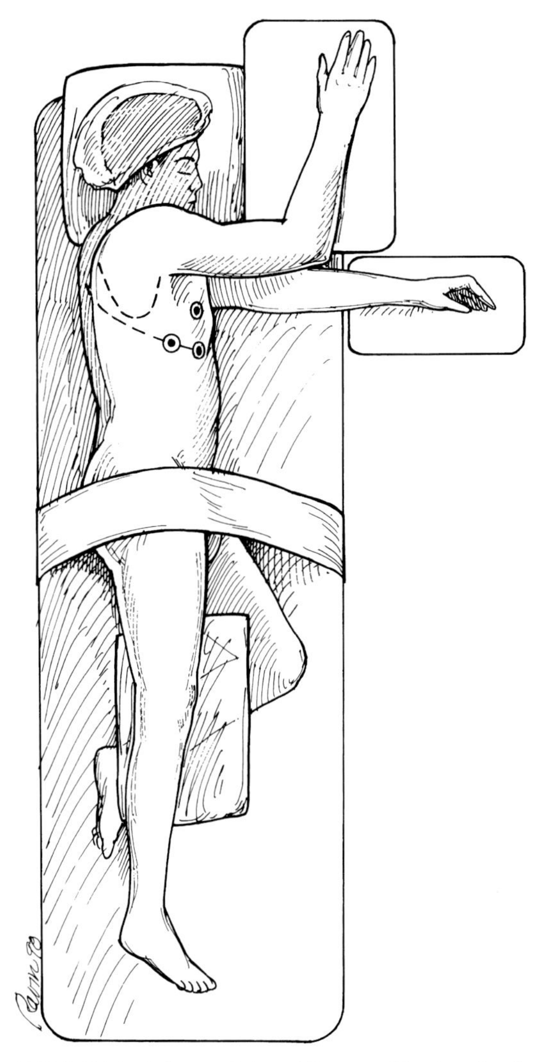

FIGURE 3–3 Lateral decubitus positioning for the patient undergoing thoracoscopy. Ensuring that the patient is in the direct lateral position will aid in fluoroscopic visualization. Attention should be paid to padding the arms, axilla, and bony prominences of the hip/pelvis and lower extremities adequately. To access the upper thoracic spine, the right arm can be abducted up and out of the way so that the portals can be inserted in a sufficiently cephalic position. (With permission from Rosenthal DJ, Dickman CA. Operating room setup and patient positioning. In: Dickman C, Rosenthal DJ, Perin NI, eds. *Thoracoscopic Spine Surgery.* New York: Thieme Medical Publishers; 1999:103.)

In laparoscopy procedures, the patient is placed supine on a radiolucent table that can be tilted into a fairly steep reverse Trendelenburg position to allow for the abdominal contents to fall away from the lower lumbar spine. The arms may be tucked at the patient's side. If this results in obstruction of fluoroscopic visualization, the shoulders may be abducted 90 degrees to move them up and away from the axial spine. When performing an anterior interbody procedure, the table can be extended if possible, or a large gel-pad can be placed under the lumbosacral junction in order to extend the lumbar spine focally. This will provide maximal access to the anterior disk space and will facilitate the restoration of normal sagittal alignment. Again, the patient should be secured to the table to prevent sliding when placed in the Trendelenburg position.

Efficient staff and equipment positioning around the patient undergoing a minimally invasive procedure are absolute prerequisites prior to commencing surgery. In practice, the exact arrangement of the surgical personnel and equipment will be influenced by the actual procedure and the equipment availability. In thoracoscopy, a commonly used positioning arrangement is to have the spine surgeon and the first assistant standing in front of the patient, who is lying in the lateral decubitus position, with an additional assistant or scrub nurse standing behind the patient (Fig. 3–4). The primary surgeon controls the primary operating instruments (e.g., the rongeurs, burrs, and dissecting tools). The first assistant often operates the camera and helps with visualization, and the second assistant across the table often helps to retract the lung and provide suction. One video monitor should be placed toward the head of the bed, directly across the table from the primary surgeon so that the surgeon's eyes and hands can be kept in a frontal position, obviating the need to turn his or her head while operating. A second monitor is placed toward the head of the bed on the surgeon's side to be viewed by the assistant from the other side of the table. Surgical members committed to working an endoscopic instrument should have a video monitor placed as directly in front of them as possible.

Similar principles exist for the arrangement of equipment and personnel for laparoscopic surgery. With the patient lying supine, the primary surgeon can choose to stand on either the right or left side of the patient based on familiarity, hand dominance, and side of pathology. The laparoscope camera is usually inserted into the superior aspect of the abdomen. The surgical assistant who holds the scope generally stands above the primary surgeon toward the head of the bed. The fluoroscopic unit is introduced from the side of the patient at the level of surgical pathology when needed. Video

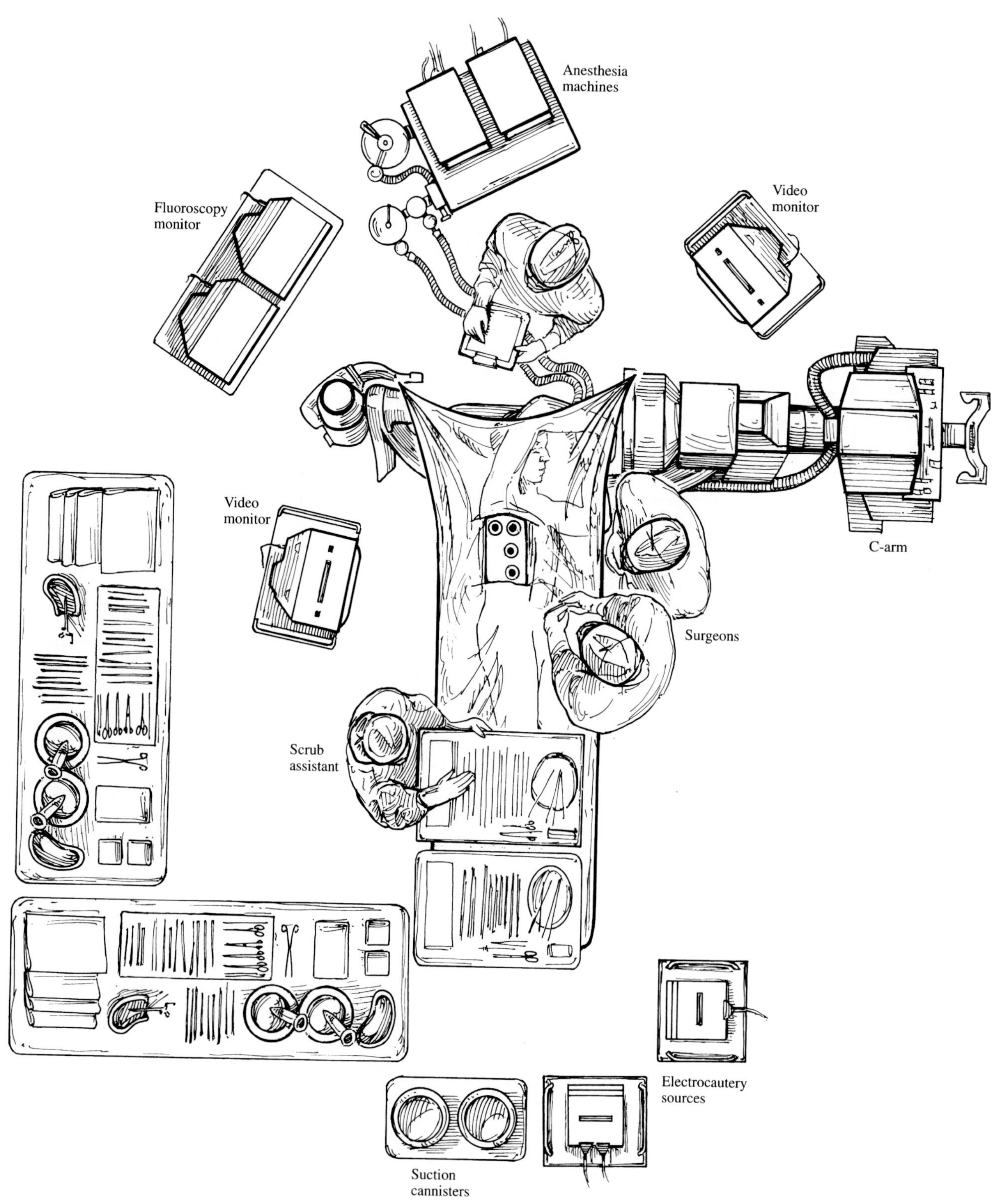

FIGURE 3–4 Commonly used arrangement for thoracoscopy. Note that the video monitors are in the direct line of sight for the surgeon and assistant. The video monitor at the head of the bed may be used by the scrub assistant opposite the surgeon. In this configuration, the C-arm is brought in from the head of the bed, but alternatively it can come up from the foot. (With permission from Rosenthal DJ, Dickman CA. Operating room setup and patient positioning. In: Dickman C, Rosenthal DJ, Perin NI, eds. *Thoracoscopic Spine* Surgery. New York: Thieme Medical Publishers; 1999:96.)

monitors should be positioned in a comfortable line of sight for the surgeon and the assistants. One monitor is usually positioned to the right or left of the patient in front of the primary surgeon's line of sight. Another monitor is usually placed at the foot of the bed for efficient visualization by the assistants.

Endoscopic techniques to address spinal pathology will likely increase in popularity in the future. The anesthetic considerations of thoracoscopy and laparoscopy (e.g., the effects of single-lung ventilation and pneumoperitoneum) should be clearly appreciated by the spinal surgeon. Whereas the expectation of lowered morbidity will encourage surgeons to develop skills in endoscopic procedures, it should be recognized that the learning curve for these techniques is steep. Prior to undertaking such procedures, a sufficient degree of training must be obtained, and one must have a strong appreciation for the need to develop thoughtful strategies with regard to operating room setup and equipment requirements.

REFERENCES

1. Buist AS, Sexton GJ, Nagy JM, Ross BB. The effect of smoking cessation and modification on lung function. *Am Rev Respir Dis.* 1976;114:115–122.
2. Pearce AC, Jones RM. Smoking and anesthesia: preoperative abstinence and perioperative morbidity. *Anesthesiology.* 1984;61:576–584.
3. Hadley MN, Reddy SV. Smoking and the human vertebral column: a review of the impact of cigarette use on vertebral bone metabolism and spinal fusion. *Neurosurgery.* 1997;41:116–124.
4. Tuman KJ, Carroll GC, Ivankovich AD. Pitfalls in interpretation of pulmonary artery catheter data. *J Cardiothorac Anesth.* 1989;3:625–641.
5. Fredman B. Physiologic changes during thoracoscopy. *Anesthesiol Clin North Am.* 2001;19:141–152.
6. Shah JS, Bready LL. Anesthesia for thoracoscopy. *Anesthesiol Clin North Am.* 2001;19:153–171.
7. Marshall BE, Marshall C. Continuity of response to hypoxic pulmonary vasoconstriction. *J Appl Physiol.* 1980;49:189–196.
8. Dieter RA Jr, Kuzycz GB. Complications and contraindications of thoracoscopy. *Int Surg.* 1997;82:232–239.
9. Dexter SP, Vucevic M, Gibson J, McMahon MJ. Hemodynamic consequences of high and low-pressure capnoperitoneum during laparoscopic cholecystectomy. *Surg Endosc.* 1999;13:376–381.
10. Joris JL, Noirot DP, Legrand MJ, Jacquet NJ, Lamy ML. Hemodynamic changes during laparoscopic cholecystectomy. *Anesth Analg.* 1993;76:1067–1071.
11. Ho HS, Saunders CJ, Gunther RA, Wolfe BM. Effector of hemodynamics during laparoscopy: CO_2 absorption or intra-abdominal pressure? *J Surg Res.* 1995;59:497–503.
12. Transfeldt EE, Schultz L. Approach to the lumbar spine without insufflation. In: Regan JJ, McAfee PC, Mack MJ, eds. *Atlas of Endoscopic Spine Surgery.* St. Louis: Quality Medical Publishing; 1995:137–150.
13. Goldberg JM, Maurer WG. A randomized comparison of gasless laparoscopy and CO_2 pneumoperitoneum. *Obstet Gynecol.* 1997;90:416–420.
14. Cunningham AJ, Brull SJ. Laparoscopic cholecystectomy: anesthetic implications. *Anesth Analg.* 1993;76:1120–1133.
15. Latham P, Dullye KK. Complications of thoracoscopy. *Anesthesiol Clin North Am.* 2001;19:187–200.

SECTION TWO

Cervical Spine

4

Endoscopic-Assisted Transoral Odontoidectomy

DANIEL REFAI, FAHEEM A. SANDHU, ANTHONY K. FREMPONG-BOADU, AND RICHARD G. FESSLER

The transoral approach is commonly used to treat anterior pathological lesions in the lower clivus, foramen magnum, and upper cervical spine. It provides excellent visualization of extradural lesions that extend from the mid-clivus to the level of the C2 vertebral body. The standard microsurgical transoral technique has permitted a safe and direct approach to anterior pathology of the upper cervical spine and lower clivus with reduced mortality and morbidity.[1–3] Refinements using neuronavigation have further optimized this procedure.[4,5]

Despite advances in microneurosurgical techniques, the standard transoral approach does have limitations. The narrow working space can limit rostral and caudal exposure. Hard palate resection and extensive maxillotomies are used to enhance cephalad visualization. Splitting the mandible and glossectomy can improve caudal exposure. In an effort to reduce morbidities associated with additional surgical exposure, surgeons have begun to explore adjuvant intraoperative techniques and equipment.

In this chapter, we will describe the use of a magnifying endoscope in the transoral approach for anterior cervicomedullary junction decompression. The endoscopically assisted transoral (EATO) approach offers superior visualization and illumination compared with the standard anterior microsurgical approach to the caudal clivus and upper cervical spine. In our experience, use of the endoscope, which has a 30-degree angle, has obviated the need for extensive soft palate splitting, hard palate resection, and extended maxillotomy except in cases of very high clival pathology.[6] Thus, the EATO approach represents a less-invasive means of achieving transoral decompression of the upper cervical spine and lower clivus.

Indications

Indications for the endoscopic-assisted and standard transoral approaches are essentially the same. Numerous anterior pathologies (e.g., extradural tumor, translocation of the odontoid process in rheumatoid arthritis, basilar impression, congenital atlantoaxial subluxation, fracture-dislocation at the craniocervical junction, vertebrobasilar aneurysm, and anterior compression of the neural structures) can be approached by the transoral route. For lesions that may require extensive additional surgical exposure to visualize rostral or caudal disease, EATO is especially indicated because additional surgical exposure may be avoided altogether. Although some authors have successfully used the transoral approach for intradural lesions, the transoral approach is not generally recommended for intradural lesions because of the risk of complications related with dural opening (e.g. cerebrospinal fluid, CSF, leak and meningitis).[7] In addition, the transoral procedure is contraindicated in patients with ectatic vertebral or basilar artery located in the operative field, or if an active infectious process is present in the nasopharyngeal cavity.[3]

Preoperative Procedures

Preoperative Assessment

Preoperative evaluation of the oral cavity is extremely important before doing the transoral procedure. An interdental length of 2.5 cm is the minimum distance required for adequate exposure using the transoral route;

therefore, in any patient with less than 2.5 cm of interdental space, splitting the mandible and glossectomy usually provides the additional room necessary for performing surgery. A culture of the nasal and oropharyngeal cavities is obtained preoperatively to identify unusual organisms and guides perioperative antibiotic selection. On the other hand, triple antibiosis can be used routinely.

Patient Positioning

The patient is positioned supine on the operating table, with the head slightly extended and fixated rigidly with a head holder (Fig. 4–1A). Rigid fixation of the head, however, is not used in some institutions to avoid potential injury during the procedure that may result from distal segment movement away from a fixed craniocervical junction.[3,8] A halo brace can be used if the patient had preoperative spinal instability. Awake, fiberoptic oral intubation is indicated for patients with instability. Tracheostomy is generally reserved for cases with severe respiratory disturbance or lower cranial deficits that require prolonged postoperative ventilatory support.

OR Setup and Equipment

Several items of equipment are needed to perform an endoscopic transoral procedure safely. First, C-arm fluoroscopy is essential for verifying correct patient positioning and localization during surgery. The C-arm should be draped into the field (Fig. 4–1B). Some authors have further advocated the use of neuronavigation software in standard transoral approaches to reduce postoperative morbidity.[4,5] At this time, it is not

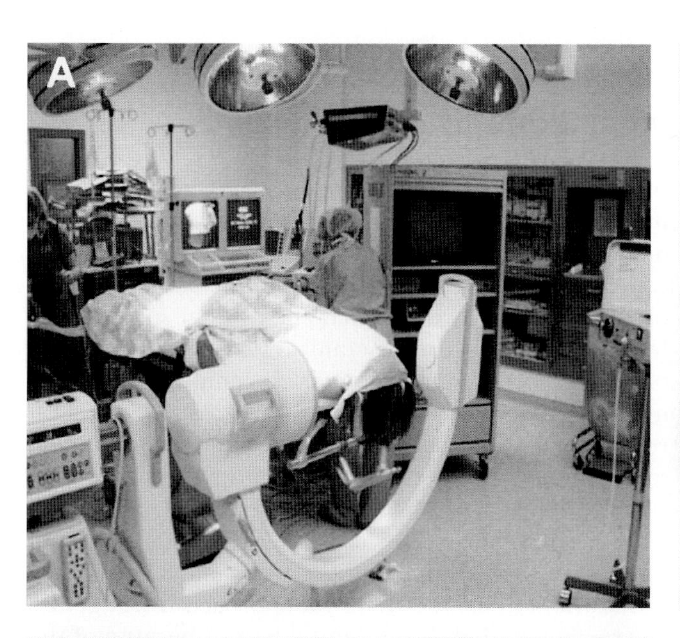

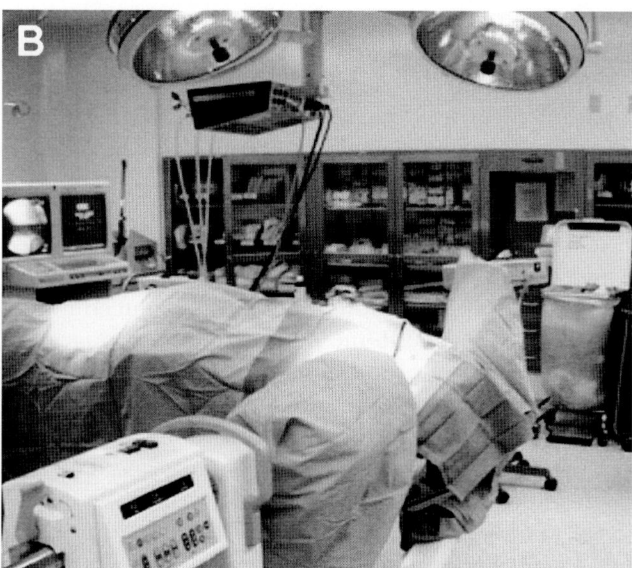

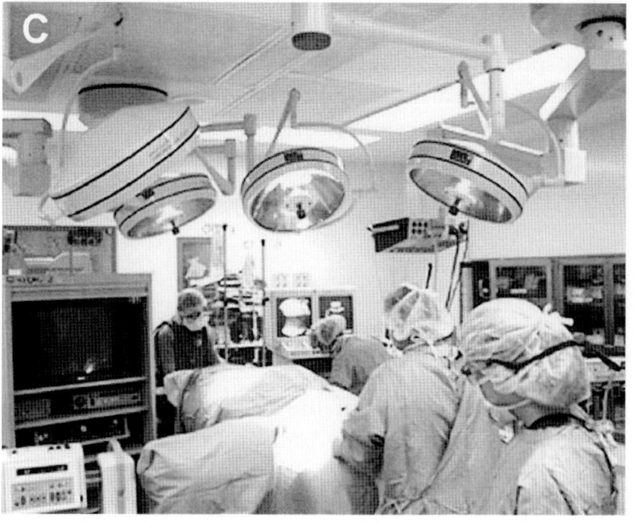

FIGURE 4–1 Operating room setup. **(A)** The patient is placed supine, in three-point head fixation, in mild extension. **(B)** The patient is draped to include the fluoroscopy and to allow access to the nasal-pharyngeal cavity. **(C)** For convenience, anesthesia is located at the foot of the bed. The video tower is placed opposite the surgeon, and the fluoroscopy monitor is placed at the foot of the bed. (With permission from Frempong-Boadu AK, Faunce WA, Fessler RG. Endoscopically assisted transoral-transpharyngeal approach to the craniovertebral junction. *Neurosurgery.* 2002;51:60–66.)

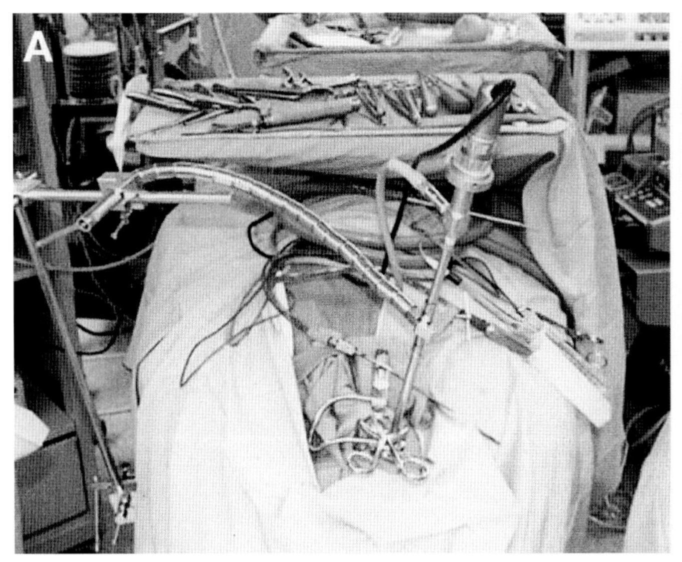

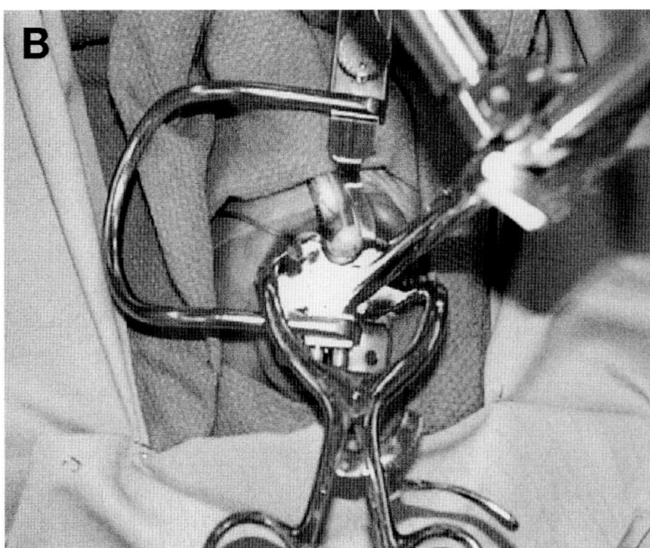

FIGURE 4–2 The endoscopic position. **(A)** The endoscope is held in place via a flexible arm that is secured to the operating table. **(B)** The endoscope is placed in the operative field and provides illumination and magnification. (With permission from Frempong-Boadu AK, Faunce WA, Fessler RG. Endoscopically assisted transoral-transpharyngeal approach to the craniovertebral junction. *Neurosurgery.* 2002;51:60–66.)

our practice to use image guidance for the EATO procedure. Next, a Dingman retractor with rubber guards is used to keep the tongue depressed and the mouth open and to protect the airway. The choice of endoscopes is important, and we currently use the 10- and 30-degree angled 10 mm Karl Storz endoscopes (Karl Storz Endoscopy-America, Inc., Culver City, CA). The basic surgical setup is similar to the standard transoral approach (see Fig. 4–1C). A high-speed drill (Midas Rex, Ft. Worth, TX) is required to remove bone, as well as pituitary rongeurs and curettes.

Surgical Technique

Following induction and intubation, gauze throat packs are placed to occlude the larynx and the esophagus to limit accumulation of blood in the stomach. The oropharyngeal cavity is sterilized with 10% providine iodine solution and hydrogen peroxide. The patient is then draped to allow access to the mouth and the nasal cavity (see Fig. 4–1B). A Dingman retractor is placed over the teeth and used to keep the mouth open. Self-retaining retractors are fastened to the Dingman to keep the tongue depressed. It is a good practice to release tongue retraction every 30 min to prevent lingual congestion from venous and lymphatic compression.

Next, the soft palate is injected with 1% lidocaine with 1/100,000 epinephrine. With the aid of loupe magnification, a midline incision is made in the soft palate to the base of the uvula deviating to one side of it. Crockard self-retaining retractors are inserted to retract the leaves of the soft palate, allowing exposure of the high nasopharynx. The posterior pharyngeal wall is anesthetized with 1% lidocaine with 1/100,000 epinephrine. Ten- and 30-degree 10 mm Karl Storz endoscopes are used for illumination and visualization of the operative field (Fig. 4–2). A midline posterior pharyngeal incision is made that extends from the base of the clivus to the upper border of the third cervical vertebra as guided by lateral fluoroscopy. The pharyngeal flaps are elevated and retracted using a Crockard self-retaining retractor exposing the prevertebral and retropharyngeal muscles. The incision is carried down to the bone using an insulated electrocautery, and a subperiosteal dissection of the longus coli and longus capitis muscles is then done. It is important to limit the lateral exposure to 15 mm from the midline bilaterally to prevent injury to the hypoglossal nerves, eustachian tubes, and vertebral arteries at the C1–C2 interspace.[6] Self-retaining retractors are placed to expose the lower clivus, C1, and C2.

Using a high-speed drill under endoscopic and lateral fluoroscopic guidance, the anterior arch of C1 and the mid- to caudal clivus are removed as needed to expose the dens completely (Fig. 4–3). A large amount of pannus is frequently present between the anterior arch of C1 and the dens, especially in rheumatoid patients. This can be removed using the cautery, curettes, and pituitary rongeurs, remembering to expose no more than 15 mm lateral to the midline. The apical ligament is then incised and removed. In cases of severe odontoid invagination, the caudal clivus is resected using the

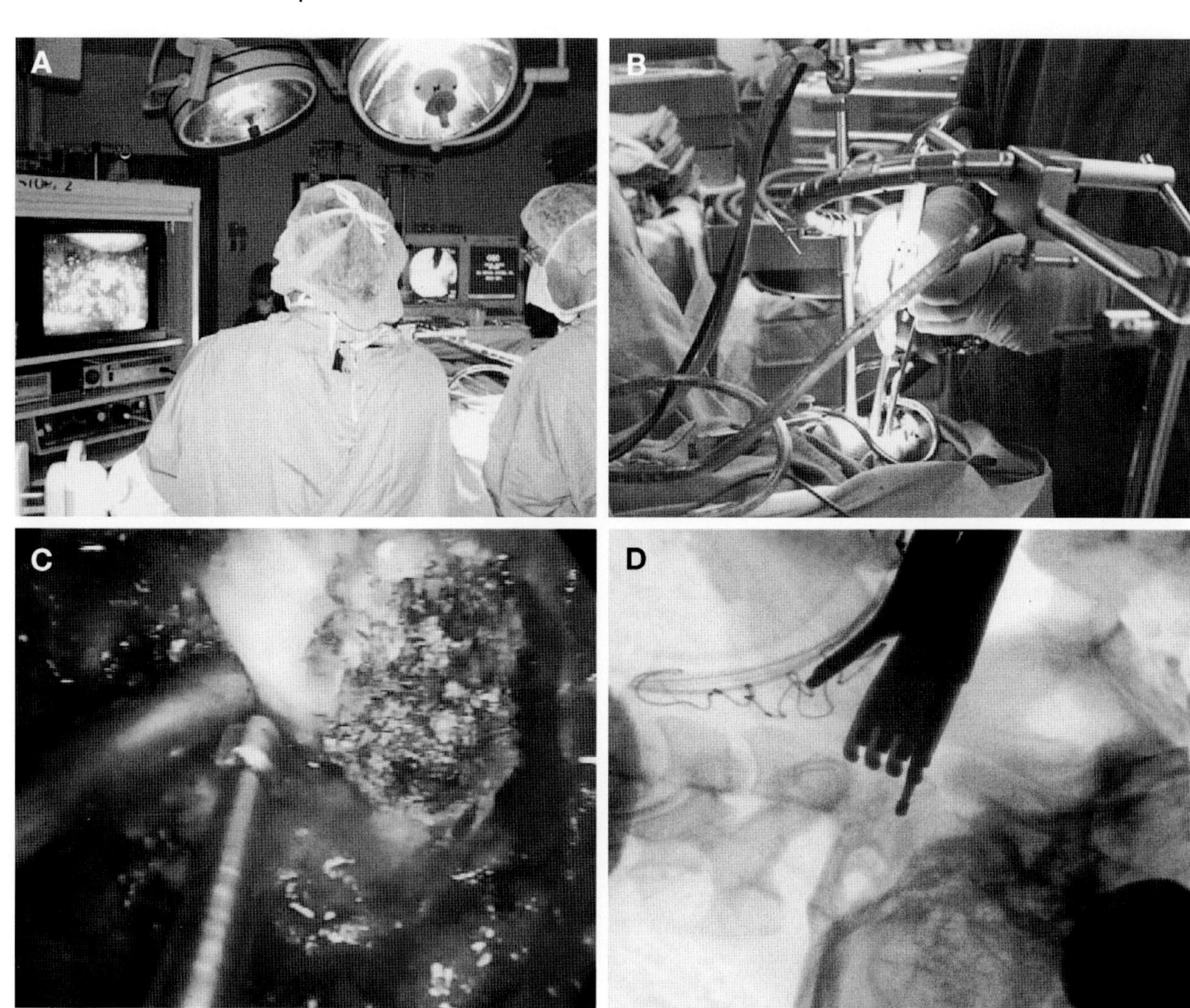

FIGURE 4–3 The anatomic exposure **(A)** The surgeon views the decompression on the video monitor. **(B)** A closer view of the surgeon working in the operative field. **(C)** An endoscopic view of the transoral decompression. **(D)** Fluoroscopy of C2 decompression in progress. (With permission from Frempong-Boadu AK, Faunce WA, Fessler RG. Endoscopically assisted transoral-transpharyngeal approach to the craniovertebral junction. *Neurosurgery.* 2002;51:60–66.)

high-speed drill under endoscopic and lateral fluoroscopic guidance. Care must be taken because the tissue posterior to the clivus is often adherent to the dura. Bleeding can occur if the marginal sinus is violated at the level of the foramen magnum, but this is easily controlled using Gelfoam and the bipolar cautery.

Removal of the dens is then accomplished in a rostral-caudal direction using a high-speed drill. Complete removal of the dens requires sectioning of the rostral alar and apical ligaments, which are often adherent to the dura. Sectioning of these ligaments is easier if the base of the dens is still intact and the tip is not floating.[1] After bony removal, the pannus is resected. This is also accomplished in a rostral to caudal direction after identification of the dura/ligamentous plane rostrally. Decompression should be extensive, including the fibrous capsule around the odontoid and the overlying synovial tissue. Cervicomedullary decompression is judged to be complete when dural pulsations are observed at the decompression site. Adequacy of decompression is then confirmed using lateral fluoroscopy and locally applied iodinated contrast agent.

Hemostasis is achieved after the decompression is completed, and a Valsalva maneuver is performed to rule out cerebrospinal fluid (CSF) leak. If the dura is opened, primary closure of the dura with a fascial graft and fat pad should be attempted. Fibrin glue can also be used to reinforce dural closure. A lumbar drain and intravenous antibiotics are maintained for 7 to 10 days following the procedure to prevent further CSF leak and fistula formation.

The pharyngeal musculature and aponeurosis should be closed in two layers using interrupted 3–0 Vicryl suture. The soft palate, if opened, is approximated in three layers, first bringing together the nasal mucosa with interrupted 3-0 Vicryl and subsequently the muscularis and the oral mucosa with interrupted 3–0 Vicryl suture. The Dingman retractor is removed, a weighted feeding tube is placed, and triamcinolone acetonide cream (0.025%) (E. Fougera, Mellville, NY) is applied to the tongue to help reduce postoperative lingual swelling.

Complications and Their Avoidance

Several potential complications can be precluded by careful attention during the intraoperative and postoperative periods. These include complications of dural tears, postoperative nutritional support, and spinal stability.

Dural tears ideally will be prevented by meticulous surgical dissection; however, in the event of a durotomy, optimal treatment is aimed at primary closure with a fascial graft, fat pad, or fibrin glue. Dural tears that are not recognized and corrected intraoperatively should be suspected if the patient complains of headache, nuchal tenderness, or a sensation of mucous discharge along the pharynx. A lumbar drain for 7 to 10 days with intravenous antibiotics is considered appropriate initial therapy.

During the immediate postoperative period, the patient should remain intubated for 1 to 3 days while tongue swelling subsides. Topical steroid may help reduce soft tissue swelling of the oral cavity. Nutritional support is important during the immediate postoperative period and starts with feeding through a nasogastric tube. The

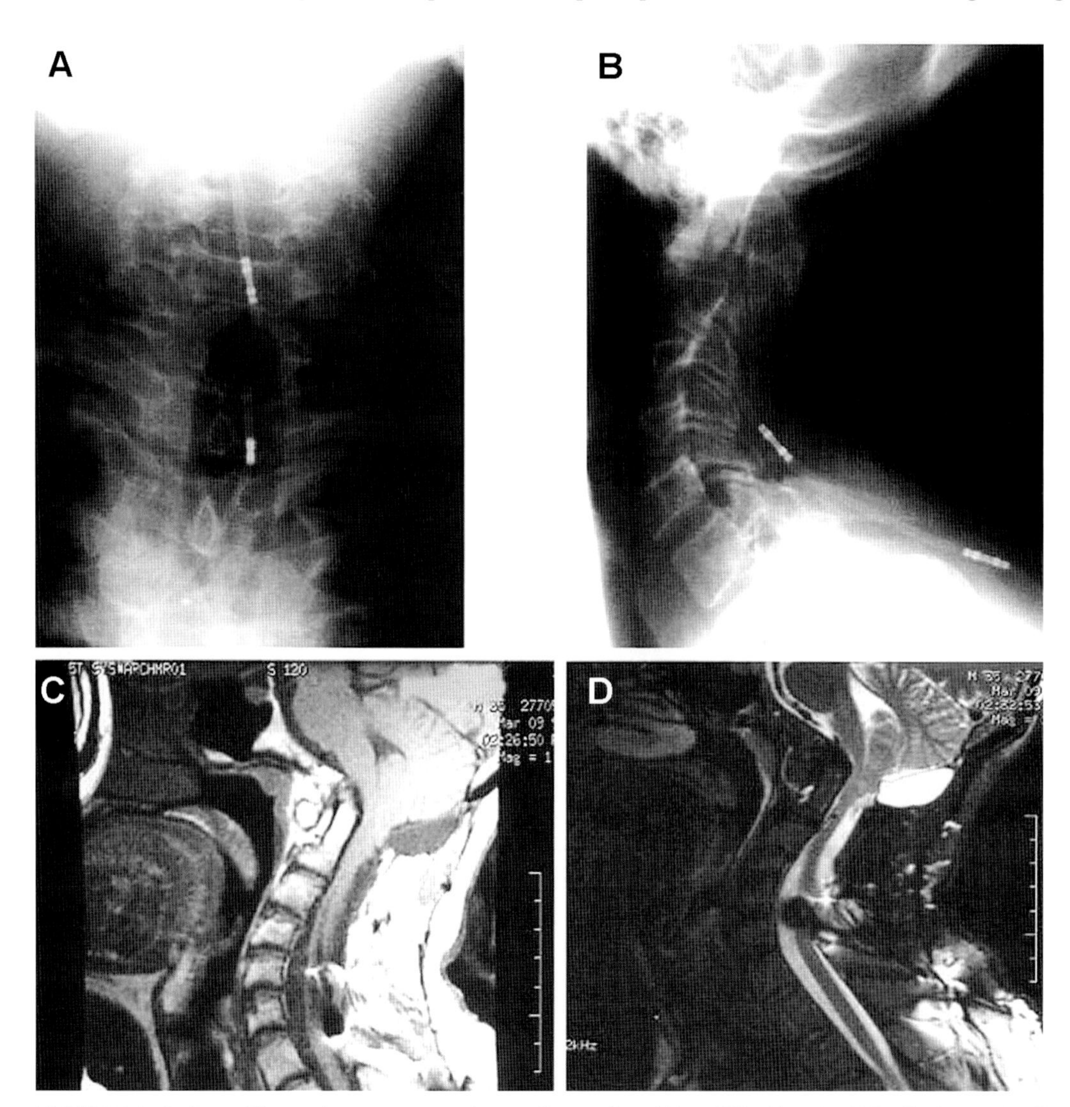

FIGURE 4–4 Case illustration, preoperative radiographs. **(A)** Anteroposterior x-rays. **(B)** Lateral x-ray. **(C)**. T1-weighted sagittal magnetic resonance imaging (MRI). **(D)** T2-weighted MRI. (With permission from Frempong-Boadu AK, Faunce WA, Fessler RG. Endoscopically assisted transoral-transpharyngeal approach to the craniovertebral junction. *Neurosurgery.* 2002;51:60–66.)

diet can be advanced to clear liquids at the end of postoperative week 1 and then to a soft diet the following week.

Postoperative spinal stability should also be evaluated carefully because the odontoidectomy may create instability at the craniocervical junction. Menezes and Van Gilder[3] consider all patients with rheumatoid arthritis who undergo transoral odontoidectomy as unstable. If the craniocervical junction is unstable, patients must be immobilized with a cervical orthosis, and an occipitocervical fusion needs to be performed. Some surgeons advocate doing the odontoidectomy and posterior fusion on the same day.[7,9] Tuite et al[10] have demonstrated successful fusion in pediatric patients who underwent perioperative posterior fusion following transoral decompression.

Case Illustration

A 36-year-old man with a history of type I Chiari malformation with syringomyelia presented to an outside institution complaining of neck pain and progressive difficulty with upper extremity fine motor control. He was initially treated with cervical laminectomy and syrinx-to-peritoneal shunt placement. He did well initially, but he noted a gradual return of his symptoms during the course of the next year, which prompted a revision of his syrinx-to-peritoneal shunt. When this failed to improve his symptoms, he underwent posterior fossa decompression with duroplasty. He again did well but noted an 8-month history of progressive numbness extending from his head to his fingertips, with difficulty walking with frequent falls, and an inability to have or maintain

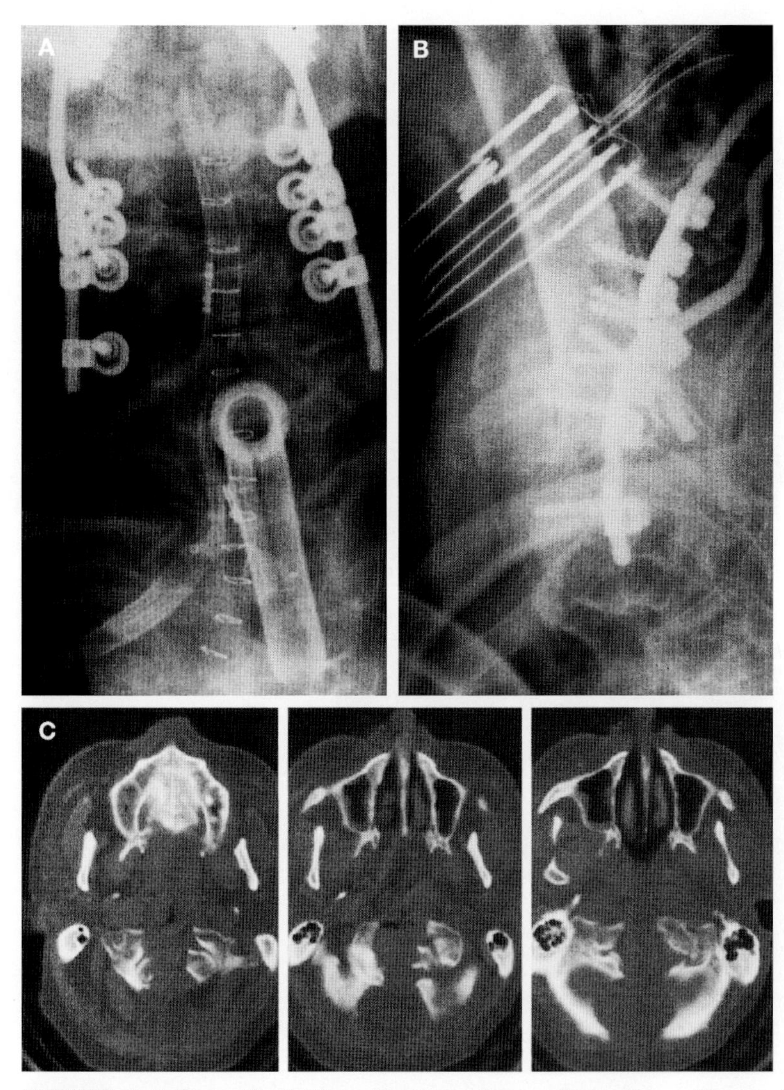

FIGURE 4–5 Case illustration. Postoperative radiographs: **(A)** Anteroposterior x-ray. **(B)** Lateral x-ray. **(C)** Computed tomographic scan of C1 and C2 showing extent of decompression. (With permission from Frempong-Boadu AK, Faunce WA, Fessler RG. Endoscopically assisted transoral-transpharyngeal approach to the craniovertebral junction. *Neurosurgery.* 2002;51:60–66.)

erections. He also reported changes in the tone and quality of his voice and severe difficulty swallowing, prompting placement of a gastrostomy tube.

On examination, he had down-beating nystagmus, hypophonia, and diminished gag reflex. On motor testing he was 5/5 in all muscle groups. He had diffuse hyperreflexia at 4+ throughout with sustained clonus, bilateral Hoffmann's, and Babinski's reflexes. He was in a wheelchair secondary to his severe spasticity.

CT and magnetic resonance imaging (MRI) revealed severe compression of his cervicomedullary junction caused by a posteriorly migrated dens with platybasia of the clivus, cranial settling, and occipitalization of C1. He had adequate posterior fossa decompression and a multilevel cervical laminectomy with placement of a shunt (Fig. 4–4).

The patient underwent placement of a tracheostomy, followed by an EATO decompression of his posteriorly migrated dens and caudal clivus and by an occipitocervical fusion performed under a separate anesthesia (Fig. 4–5). He was decannulated at 3 weeks postoperatively and had complete resolution of his erectile dysfunction as well as an improvement in his swallowing function with removal of his G-tube. By his 6-month follow-up visit, he was ambulatory with a quad cane.

The endoscopic-assisted transoral approach presents a viable alternative to the standard microsurgical transoral approach for treating anterior compressive lesions at the craniovertebral junction. The ability with endoscopic-assisted surgery to look superoinferiorly, laterally, and around the corners often obviates the need for extensive soft palate splitting, hard palate resection, or extended exposures.

REFERENCES

1. Menezes AH, VanGilder JC, Graf CJ, et al. Craniocervical abnormalities: a comprehensive surgical approach. *J Neurosurg*. 1980;53: 444–455.
2. Piper JG, Menezes AH. Management strategies for tumors of the axis vertebra. *J Neurosurg*. 1996;84:543–551.
3. Menezes AH, Van Gilder JC. Transoral-transpharyngeal approach to the anterior craniocervical junction: ten year experience with 72 patients. *J Neurosurg*. 1988;69:895–903.
4. Veres R, Bago A, Fedorcsak I. Early experiences with image-guided transoral surgery for the pathologies of the upper cervical spine. *Spine*. 2001;26:1385–1388.
5. Vougioukas VI, Hubbe U, Schipper J, et al. Navigated transoral approach to the cranial base and the craniocervical junction: technical note. *Neurosurgery*. 2003;52:247–250.
6. Frempong-Boadu AK, Faunce WA, Fessler RG. Endoscopically assisted transoral-transpharyngeal approach to the craniovertebral junction. *Neurosurgery*. 2002;51:60–66.
7. James D, Crockard HA. Surgical access to the base of the skull and upper cervical spine by extended maxillotomy. *Neurosurgery*. 1991; 29:411–416.
8. Menezes AH, Traynelis VC. Tumors of the craniovertebral junction. In: Youmans JR, ed. *Neurological Surgery*. Philadelphia: WB Saunders; 1996:3041–3072.
9. Dickman CA, Locantro J, Fessler RG. The influence of transoral odontoid resection on stability of the craniovertebral junction. *J Neurosurg*. 1992;77:525–530.
10. Tuite GF, Veres R, Crockard HA, et al. Pediatric transoral surgery: indications, complications, and long-term outcome. *J Neurosurg*. 1996;84:573–583.

5

Anterior Endoscopic Cervical Microdiskectomy

JOHN C. CHIU

Anterior cervical diskectomy with or without bony fusion has been the standard treatment for cervical disk protrusions since the 1950s[1–4]; however, these operations are associated with significant local morbidity[5,6] (e.g., graft collapse, graft extrusion, hardware failure, nonfusion with resultant instability, infections, esophageal perforation with infection, and permanent pain, peripheral nerve injury, or infection at the graft donor site). In contrast, anterior endoscopic cervical microdiskectomy (AECM)[7,8] is a minimally invasive, outpatient procedure with much less morbidity, no graft donor site to cause secondary problems, and a significant decrease in the period of convalescence and costs.

The evolution of spinal surgery is trending toward less-invasive techniques, with clever procedures not thought possible a few years ago.[9–14] Advancements in microinstrumentation, fiberoptics, improved fluoroscopic imaging, and high-resolution digital video imaging endoscopy, along with the accumulation of experience in percutaneous lumbar diskectomy[15–18] and spinal laser applications,[18–20] have facilitated the development of AECM.[7]

In 1995, the use of a Holmium laser at low, nonablative levels of energy to cause contraction of the disk tissue, further reducing the size of the protrusion and hardening the disk (laser thermodiskoplasty) to prevent recurrence, was added to our standard protocol for percutaneous AECM. Anterior cervical fusion (ACF) is associated with a 15% or greater chance of junctional disk herniation at interspaces adjacent to fused levels, presumably because fusion places additional stress on adjacent vertebral segments. Minimally invasive endoscopic diskectomy does not affect the stability of adjacent vertebral segments.

Multiple levels of symptomatic cervical disk disease do occur. ACF is often an unattractive treatment in the presence of multiple symptomatic disk levels in a patient, but AECM, a minimally invasive outpatient spinal surgery, can be safely utilized for these cases.

This chapter will describe the surgical technique of AECM step by step, using current endoscopic equipment, instrumentation, surgical tools, potential surgical complications, and complication avoidance in the treatment of symptomatic herniated cervical disks.

Indications

The AECM approach is indicated in the following clinical situations[7]:

- Neck pain with radiation down the arm (radicular pain)
- Symptoms of tingling and numbness, as well as signs of sensory loss, muscle weakness, and/or decreased reflexes in the upper extremities, correlated with the level of involvement
- Severe intractable cervicogenic headache associated with neck pain
- No improvement of symptoms after a minimum of 12 weeks of conservative therapy
- Magnetic resonance imaging (MRI) or computed tomographic (CT) scan positive for disk herniation, consistent with dermatome of clinical symptoms (MRI is the imaging study of choice)

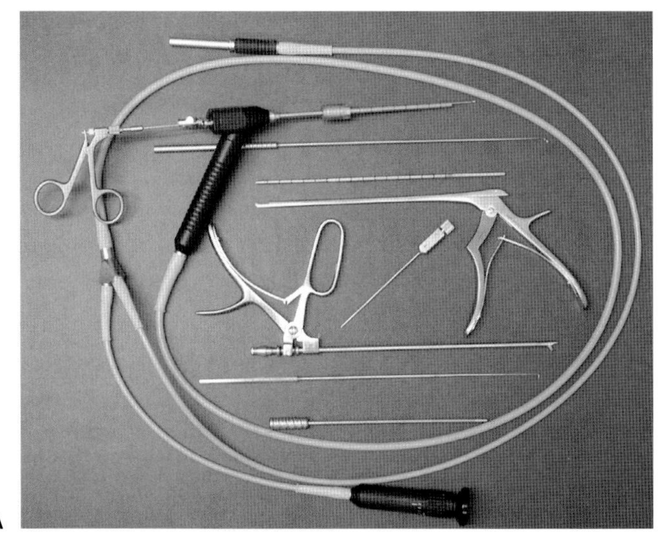

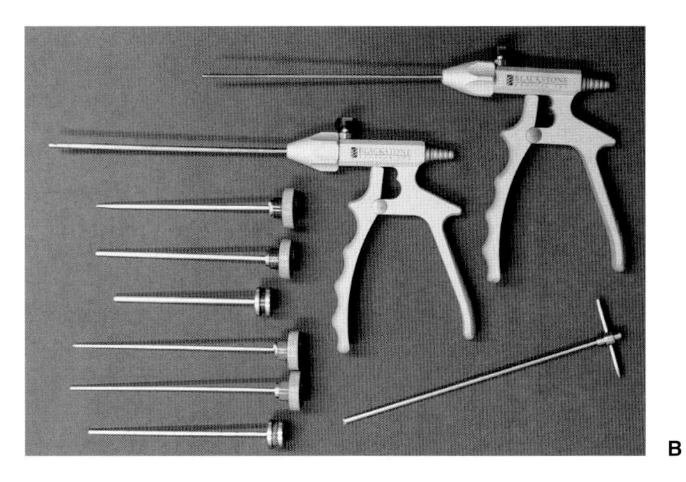

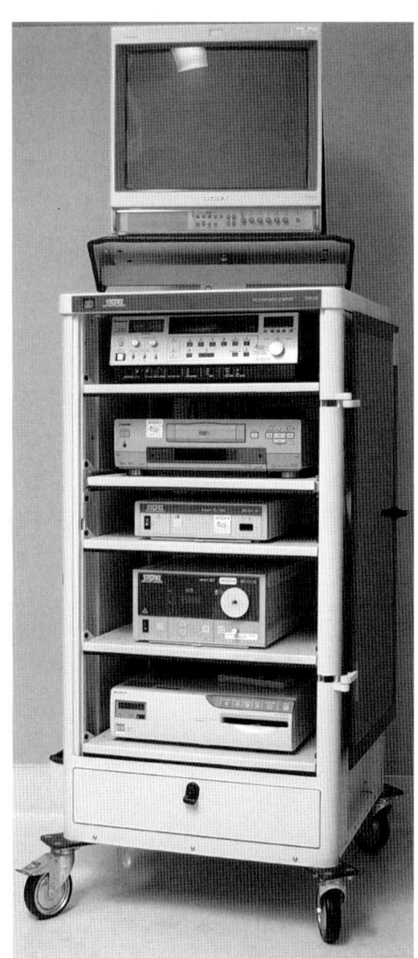

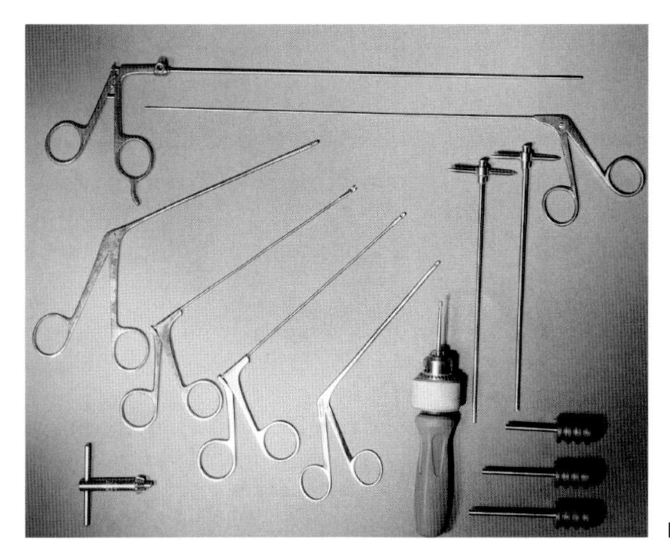

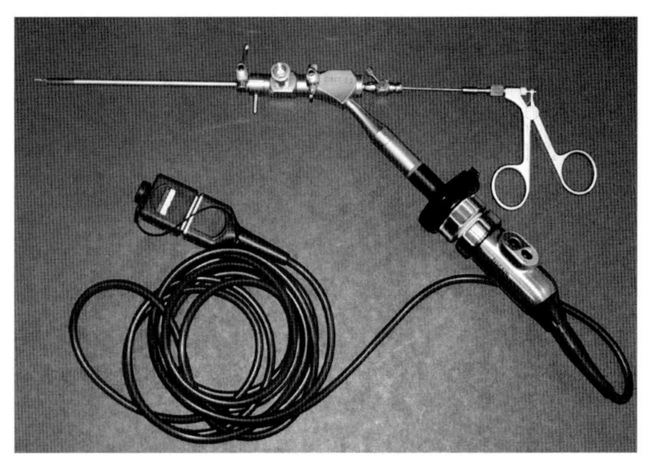

FIGURE 5–1 Video digital endoscopy tower and anterior cervical endoscopic instruments. **(A)** Cervical 0-degree endoscopes and endoscopic instruments. **(B)** Diskectomes, working channel sets. **(D)** Diskectomy set, forceps, trephines, and burr. **(E)** Trichip digital camera with cervical 6-degree endoscope and forceps. **(C)** Video digital endoscopic tower.

- Junctional cervical disk herniation syndrome in postcervical fusion
- Positive pre- or intraoperative diskogram and pain provocation test
- Positive electromyography is considered helpful
- Multiple cervical disks can be treated at one sitting

Contraindications

- Severe cervical spinal canal stenosis
- A significant migrated-free disk fragment, not located at disk level
- Advanced spondylosis (significant bone spurs) with severe disk space narrowing and with osteophytes blocking entry into the disk space
- Significant ossification of posterior longitudinal ligament

Surgical Equipment and Instruments

The following surgical equipment and instruments are necessary to perform AECM:

- Cervical endoscopic diskectomy set (Karl Storz, Tuttlingen, Germany), including 4 mm, 0-degree endoscope (Fig. 5–1A)
- Cervical diskectomy sets (2.5 and 3.5 mm) (Blackstone Medical, Inc., Springfield, MA) with short cervical diskectomes (Fig. 5–1B).
- Endoscopic tower equipped with digital video monitor, DVT/VHS recorder, light source, and photo printer, with trichip digital camera system (Fig. 5–1C)
- Endoscopic grasping and cutting forceps (Fig. 5–1D)
- Endoscopic probe, knife, rasp, and burr (Fig. 5–1D)
- More aggressively toothed trephines used for spurs and spondylitic ridges at the anterior and posterior disk space (Fig. 5–1D)
- 3.5 mm, 6-degree cervical operating endoscope (Fig. 5–1E)
- Holmium:YAG laser generator (Trimedyne, Irvine, CA) with right-angle (side-firing) probe (Fig. 5–2A,B)
- Digital fluoroscopy equipment (C-arm) and monitor

Anesthesia

This procedure is done under local anesthesia with monitored conscious sedation or occasionally, if indicated, general anesthesia. Two grams of Ancef (cefazolin) and 8.0 mg of Decadron (dexamethasone) are routinely given intravenously at the start of anesthesia. The esophagus is made more palpable by inserting an esophageal or nasogastric tube. The pulse of the carotid artery may be augmented with use of sympathomimetics (e.g., ephedrine) to raise systolic blood pressure to a minimum of 130 mm Hg. Surface electroencephalogram (EEG) (SNAP, Nicolet Biomedical, Madison, WI) provides added precision for anesthesia.

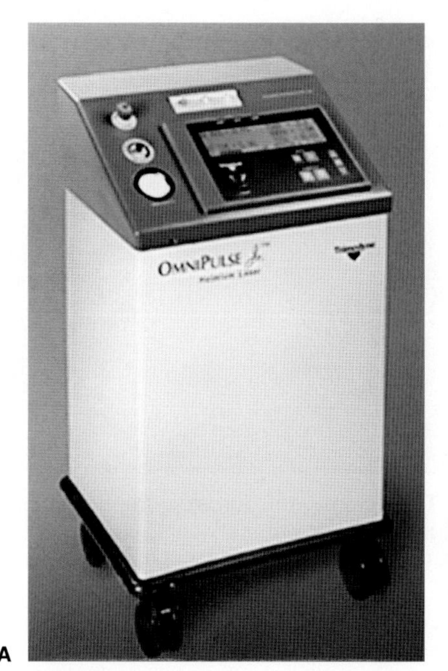

A

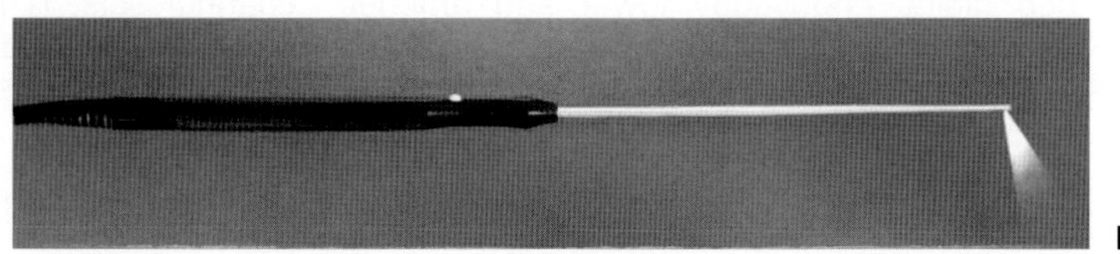

B

FIGURE 5–2 Holmium: yttrium-aluminum-garnet (YAG) laser equipment for laser thermodiskoplasty. **(A)** Holmium:YAG laser generator. **(B)** Right-angle (side-firing) laser probe.

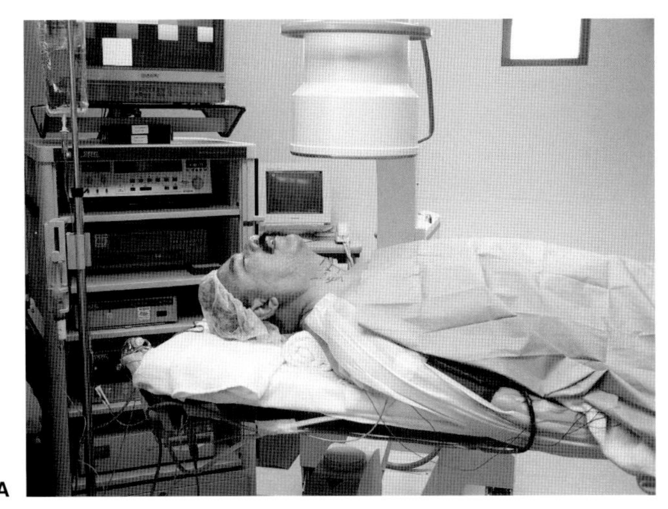
A

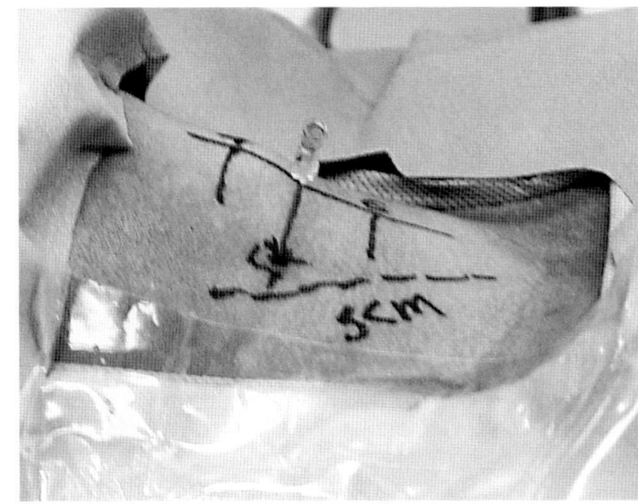

B

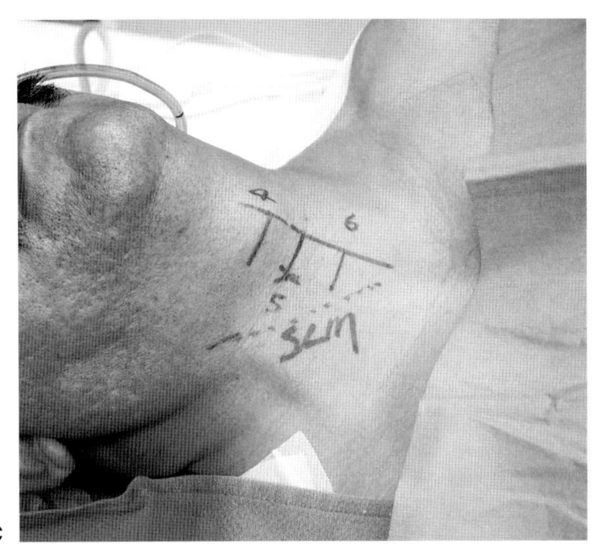

C

FIGURE 5–3 Patient positioning and localization. **(A)** Patient positioning. **(B)** Localization: skin marking. **(C)** Placement of needle.

Patient Positioning

The patient is placed in a supine position, with the neck extended over a rolled towel under the shoulders, on an adjustable radiolucent surgical table.[7] A soft strap is placed over the forehead to stabilize it. The shoulders are distracted gently downward with tape (Fig. 5–3A). Digital C-arm fluoroscopy is used in anteroposterior (AP) and lateral planes to control the placement of all instruments throughout the operation. Electromysgraphy (EMG) needles are placed in areas of distribution of the nerve roots from the spinal levels being operated on to provide continuous neurophysiologic-neuromuscular monitoring throughout the procedure for added safety.

Localization

Initial localizing AP fluoroscopic x-rays are made with Allis clamps attached to the drapes and crossing the neck horizontally at the expected level. The midline, the levels, and the point of entry (operating portal) for surgery are marked on the skin with a marking pen (Fig. 5–3B,C). On the other hand, using sterile technique, the level of the disk can be accurately identified by inserting an 18-gauge needle into a disk under fluoroscopy (Fig. 5–4A–D), as described under Surgical Techniques.

Surgical Techniques

The initial point of entry (operating portal) is adjacent to the medial border of the right sternocleidomastoid muscle, where firm pressure is applied digitally in the space between that muscle and the trachea, pointing toward the vertebral surface (see Fig. 5–4A,B). The larynx and trachea are displaced medially and the carotid artery laterally (see Fig. 5–4A,B). The anterior cervical spine is palpated with the fingertips. An 18-gauge spinal

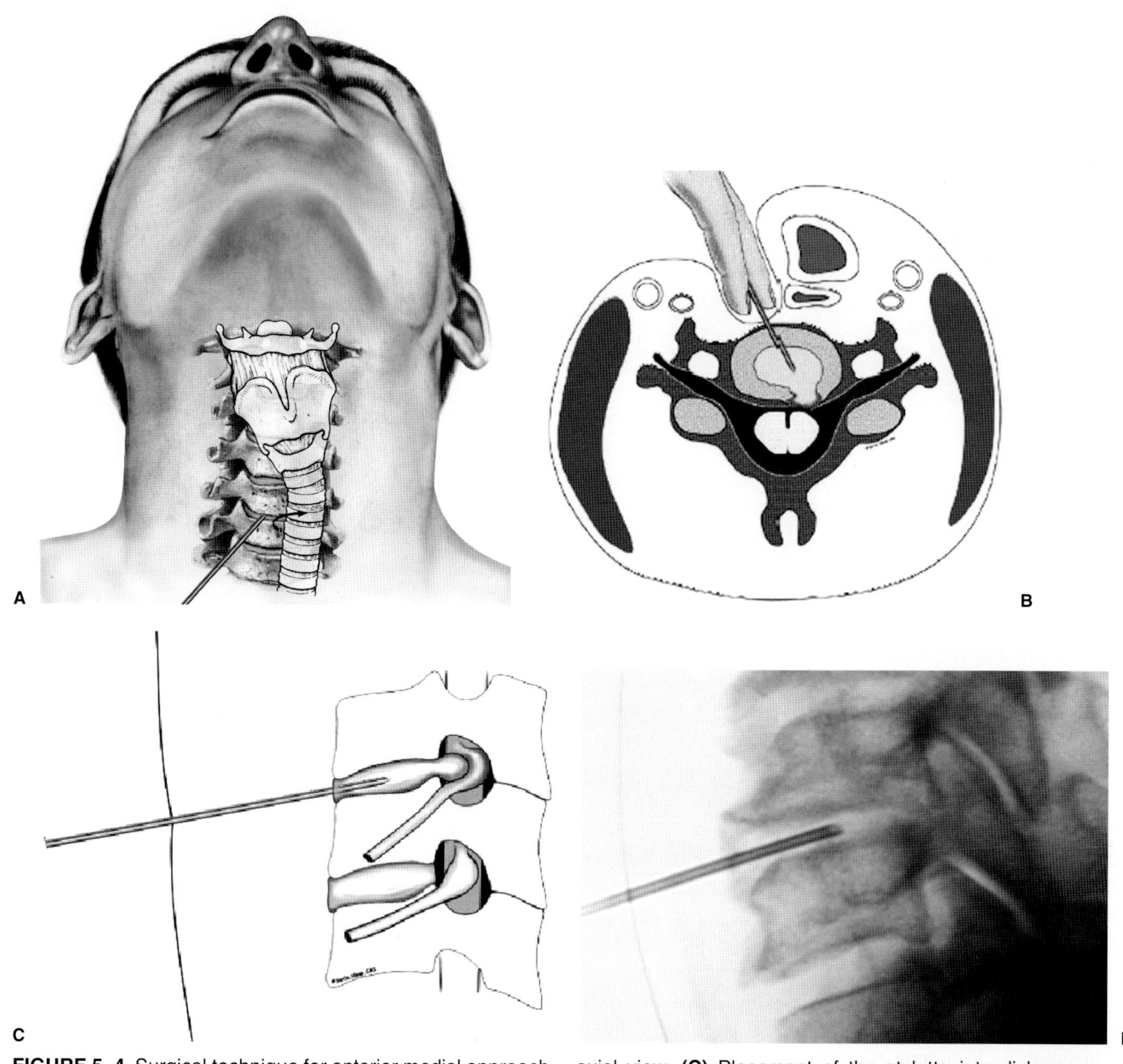

FIGURE 5–4 Surgical technique for anterior medial approach for needle and stylette placement into the disk. **(A)** Retraction of trachea/esophagus for needle placement—frontal view. **(B)** Retraction of trachea/esophagus for needle placement—axial view. **(C)** Placement of the stylette into disk space—lateral view. **(D)** Placement of the stylette—fluoroscopic lateral view.

stylette is passed transdermally into the disk space, and its position is confirmed fluoroscopically (see Fig. 5–4C,D). If a pain provocation test and diskogram have not been done preoperatively, they are done now. If results are confirmatory, the operation is performed. A 3 mm skin incision is made, and a narrow guidewire stylette is passed through the needle, which is then removed. A 2.5 mm or 3.5 mm internal diameter cannula/dilator is introduced over the stylette and into the disk interspace.

A standard number 18 guidewire replaces the narrow one. A trephine replaces the dilator and incises the anulus. Under fluoroscopic and endoscopic visualization, minicurettes and forceps (Figs. 5–5A, 5–6) loosen and remove disk fragments prior to introducing the diskectome through the cannula to remove the disk. The diskectome employs a high-pressure irrigation-suction system and a guillotine-cutting blade (Figs. 5–5B, 5–7A). The instruments removing the disk material are

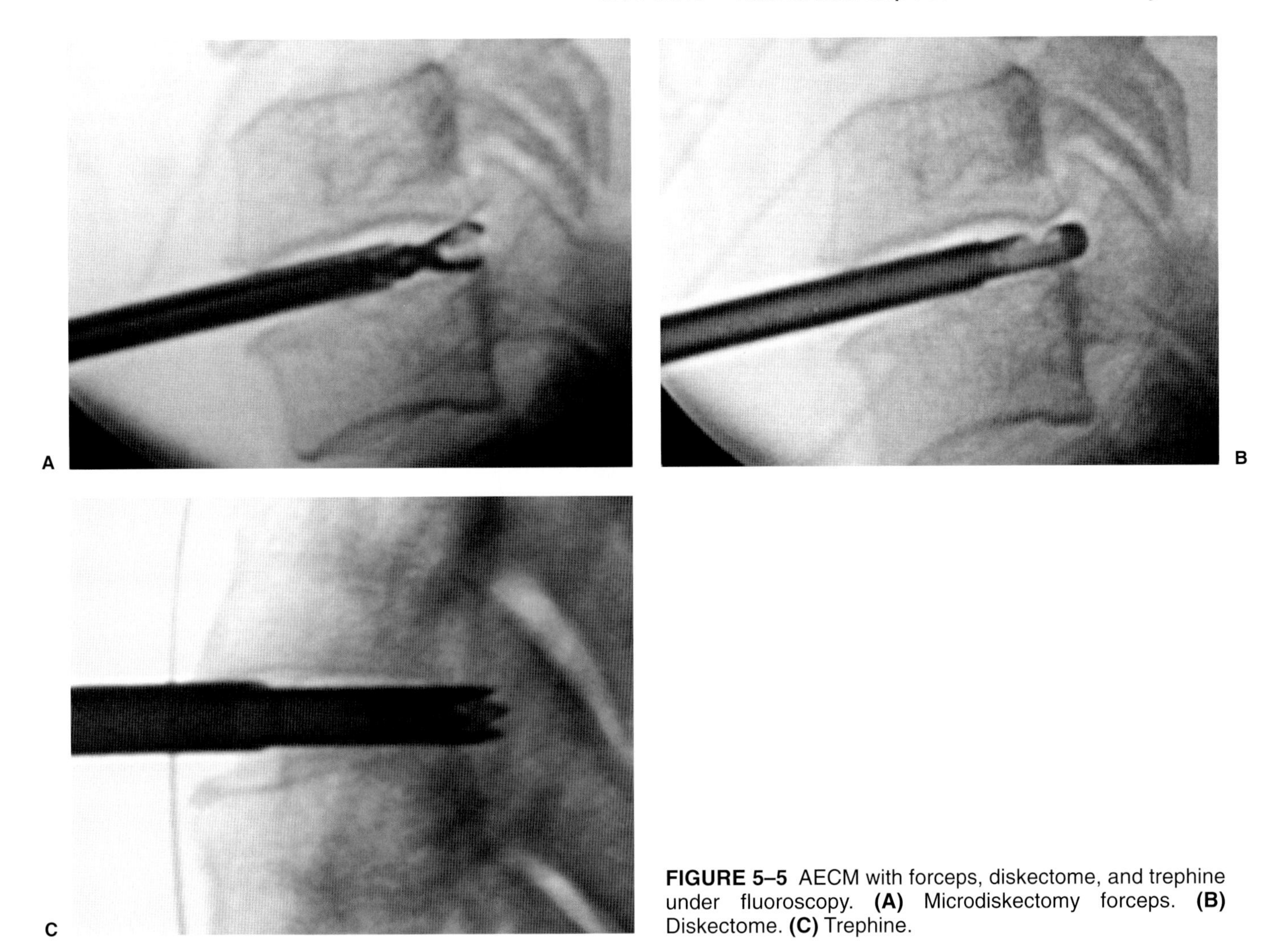

FIGURE 5–5 AECM with forceps, diskectome, and trephine under fluoroscopy. **(A)** Microdiskectomy forceps. **(B)** Diskectome. **(C)** Trephine.

FIGURE 5–6 (A,B) Endoscopic views of anterior endoscopic cervical microdiskectomy with forceps removing disk material.

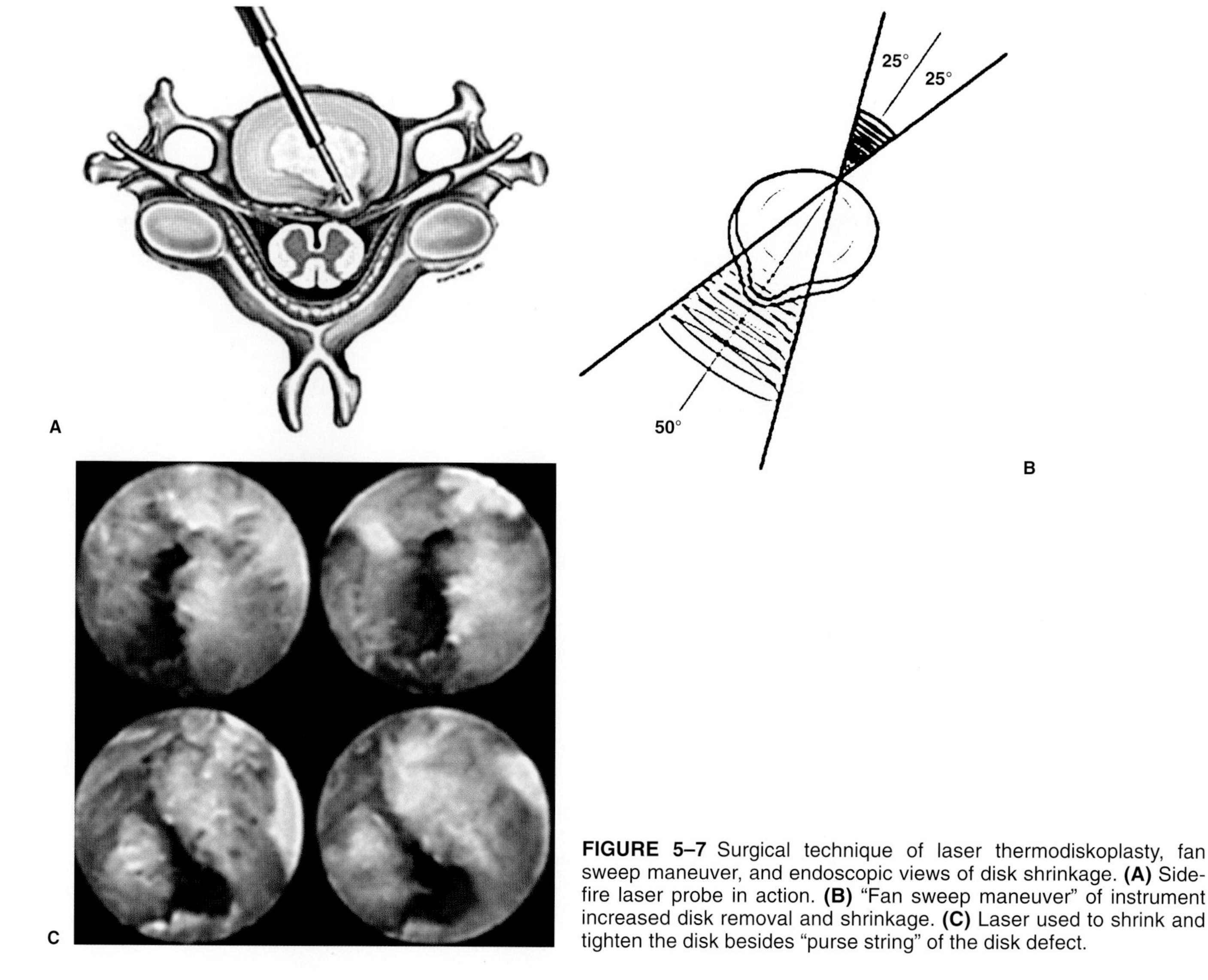

FIGURE 5–7 Surgical technique of laser thermodiskoplasty, fan sweep maneuver, and endoscopic views of disk shrinkage. **(A)** Side-fire laser probe in action. **(B)** "Fan sweep maneuver" of instrument increased disk removal and shrinkage. **(C)** Laser used to shrink and tighten the disk besides "purse string" of the disk defect.

moved in a "critical fan sweep maneuver" with a 25-degree "rocking" excursion of the cannula hub from side to side to increase the area of total disk removed up to approximately a 50-degree inverted cone-shaped area within the disk space (Fig. 5–7B).[7] All maneuvers are closely monitored with fluoroscopy and by endoscopy. Trephines with more aggressive teeth are used to remove bone spurs or osteophytes. Very large bone spurs can be removed with a short cannula system with a burr (Fig. 5–8). The holmium: yttrium-aluminum-garnet (YAG) laser with right-angle (side-firing) probe facilitates removal of disk material further. In addition, it is used at nonablative levels of laser energy (Table 5–1) for laser thermodiskoplasty [i.e., collagen and disk shrinking (Fig. 5–7C) and tightening effect to further decompress and to harden the disk]. Endoscopy is used for direct visualization (Fig. 5–9A,B) and for confirmation of diskectomy and laser thermodiskoplasty. Again, after using the diskectome for laser disk debris removal in the disk space, the probe and cannula are removed. Marcaine (0.25%) is infiltrated subcutaneously around the wound. The tiny incisional wound is closed with a bandage.

Postoperative Care

Patients are ambulatory within 1 hour postoperatively and discharged subsequently. They may shower the following day. A soft cervical collar is used for 2 to 3 days, or as needed. An ice pack is helpful. Mild analgesics and muscle relaxants are required at times. Progressive neck exercise begins on the second postoperative day. Patients are allowed to return to work in 1 to 2 weeks, provided heavy labor and prolonged sitting are not

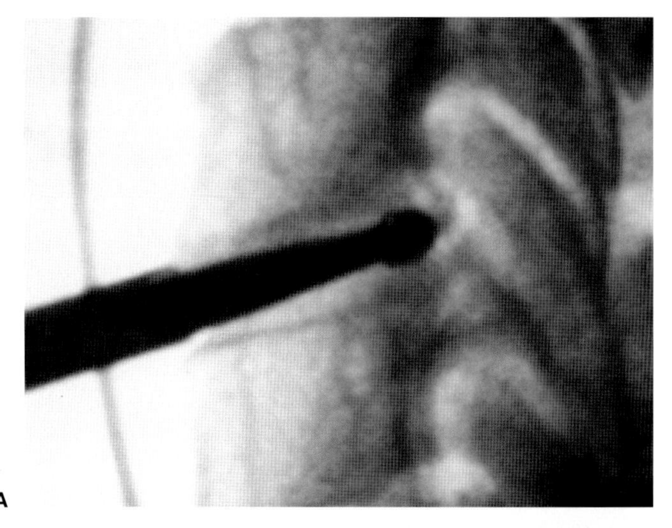

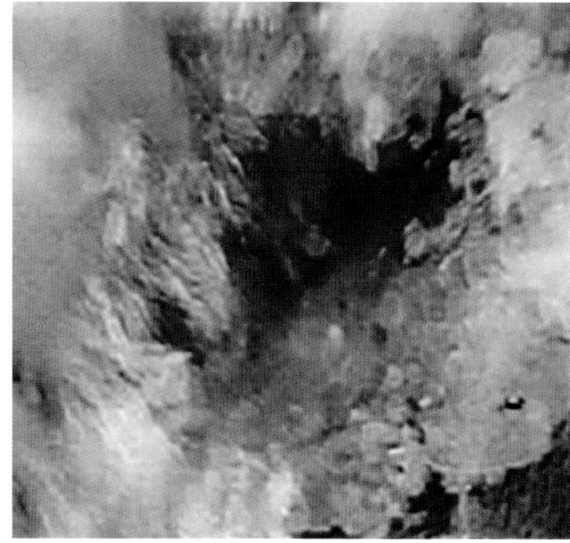

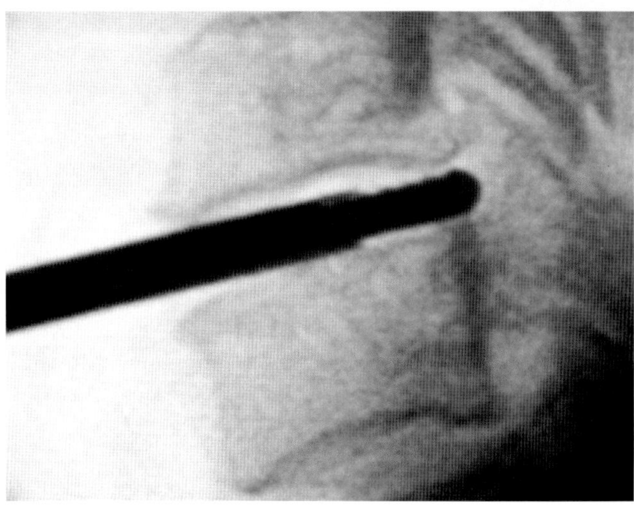

FIGURE 5–8 Rasp and burr used to remove osteophyte. **(A)** Burr to remove osteophyte. **(B)** Endoscopic view of disk space after osteophyte removal. **(C)** Rasp in action.

involved. This procedure can be extremely gratifying for patients.

Outcome

Ninety-four percent of surgical patients with single disk problems have good-to-excellent relief of symptoms postoperatively,[7,19] resuming usual activity in a few days and full active lives in 3 to 7 weeks.

TABLE 5–1 Lumen laser setting for cervical laser thermodiskoplasty Nonablative levels of laser energy at 10 Hz 5 sec on and 5 sec off

	Stage	*Watts*	*Joules*
Cervical	First stage	8	300
Cervical	Second stage	5	200

Complications and Avoidance

A thorough knowledge of the AECM procedure and surgical anatomy of the neck, careful selection of patients, and preoperative surgical planning with appropriate diagnostic evaluations facilitate the AECM and prevent potential complications. All potential complications of open anterior disk surgery are possible, but they are rare or much less frequent in AECM.

Infection

Infection can be avoided by careful sterile technique, using prophylactic antibiotics IV intraoperatively and the much smaller incisional area. Infection and complications secondary to a donor graft site are obviated. Aseptic diskitis can be prevented by aiming the laser beam in a "bowtie" fashion to avoid damaging the end plates (at 6 and 12 o'clock).

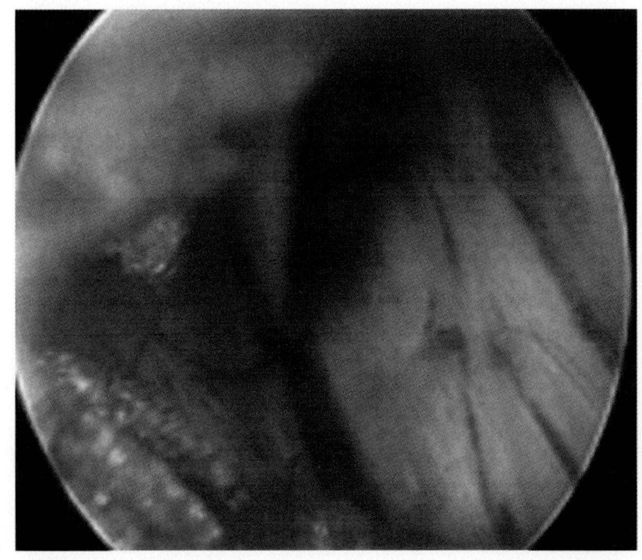

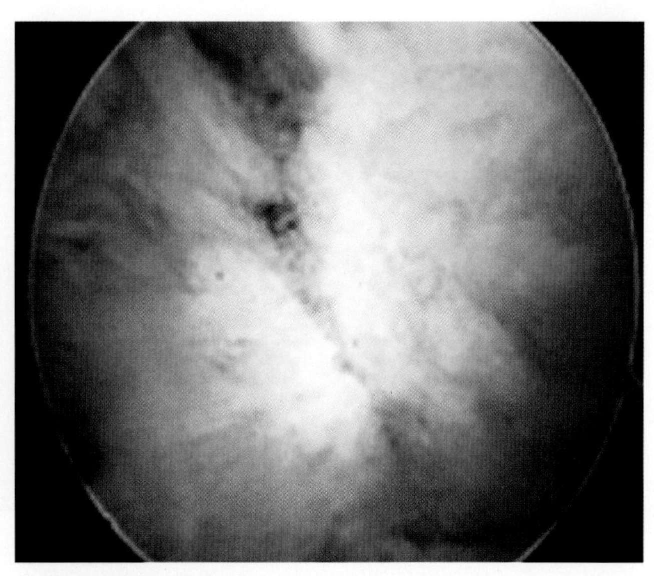

FIGURE 5–9 Endoscopic views of uncinate joint and nerve root after decompression, and fissure in cervical disk. **(A)** Uncinate joint and nerve root after endoscopic microdecompression. **(B)** Intraoperative endoscopic view of fissure in cervical disk.

Hematoma (Subcutaneous and Deep)

Hematoma occurs post-ACF and may occur with minimally invasive spinal surgery, but is minimized by careful technique, by not prescribing aspirin or nonsteroidal anti-inflammatory drugs (NSAIDs) within 1 week prior to surgery, by application of gentle digital pressure, or by placing an IV bag over the operative site for the first 5 minutes after surgery and application of an ice bag thereafter.

Vascular Injuries

Vascular injuries are extremely rare when care is taken to locate and protect the carotid artery, jugular vein, and other vascular structures, including the vertebral artery in the foramen transversarium laterally and the inferior and superior thyroid arteries. No carotid artery injury has been reported in the United States. The carotid sheath should be identified and protected under the surgeon's fingers. If carotid arterial pulsation is hard to palpate, it can be augmented by IV ephedrine. No prolonged retraction of the carotid sheath and artery is required because it is in anterior cervical fusion; hence, direct trauma and embolic complications involving carotid vessels are unlikely.

Neural Injuries

Neural injuries are extremely rare with minimally invasive approaches. No spinal cord injuries have been reported. Nerve root and spinal cord injury, although possible, can be avoided with continuous intraoperative neurophysiologic monitoring [EMG/nerve conduction velocity (NCV)] and direct endoscopic visualization. Neural complications of ACF, including hypoglossal, spinal accessory, and phrenic, auricular, and cutaneous nerves, can be prevented by careful technique. Recurrent laryngeal nerve injury, although a recognized complication of ACF, is extremely rare with AECM. One case with hiccough and one with hoarseness have postoperatively occurred transiently out of 1200 cases of AECM.

Sympathetic Nerve Injuries

Sympathetic nerve injuries are extremely rare, but they can occur from injury to cervical sympathetic and stellate ganglia. One incidental transient Horner's syndrome or oculosympathetic dysfunction lasting 1 day following AECM was noted.

Excessive Sedation

Excessive sedation can be avoided by surface EEG monitoring, providing more precise estimation of the depth of anesthesia, reducing the amount of anesthetics, and preventing excessive or insufficient sedation.

Operation on the Wrong Level

A major complication of ACF or AECM is operating at the wrong level and with improper instrumentation. Proper utilization of digital C-arm fluoroscopy for anatomical localization avoids complications caused by poor placement of instruments or operating at the wrong disk level.

Dural Tears

Dural tears have not been reported in AECM.

Soft Tissue Injuries

Although soft tissue injuries may occur due to prolonged forceful retraction, as occurs in ACF operations, they are not an issue with AECM. Failure of fusion, collapse of the bone plug, migration of the bone plug, and hardware failure similarly cannot occur.

Dysphasia and Postoperative Airway Obstructions Due to Edema

Airway obstructions may occur, but they can be avoided by careful surgical procedures and identification of these organs. Esophageal and tracheal injury due to edema or perforation can be avoided by careful palpation and digital retraction at the site of needle insertion. Having the anesthesiologist place a nasogastric tube into the esophagus aids in identifying and retracting that structure by palpation.

Inadequate Decompression of Disk Material

Inadequate decompression of disk material is minimized by using multiple modalities and instruments (e.g., forceps, trephining the posterior ligament, diskectome, burr and rasp, and laser application to both vaporize tissue and perform thermodiskoplasty).

Thyroid Gland Injury

Injury to the thyroid can be avoided by approaching the glands posteriorly and not encountering the parenchyma. A large goiter requires special care because of its vascularity.

Advantages of AECM

The advantages of AECM are those of minimally invasive spinal surgery[7]:

- Same-day outpatient procedure (less traumatic, both physically and psychologically)
- Small incision and less scarring of the neck
- No dissection of muscle, bone, or ligaments, or manipulation of the dural sac or nerve roots
- Little or no epidural bleeding
- Does not promote further instability of spinal segments or postcervical fusion junctional disk herniation
- Early return to activities of daily living
- Commonly done under local anesthesia
- Costs less than conventional diskectomy
- Multiple-level diskectomy feasible and well tolerated
- Least challenging to medically high-risk patients (e.g., those with cardiopulmonary problems and the morbidly obese)
- Exercise programs begun same day as surgery
- Direct endoscopic visualization and confirmation of the efficacy of surgery

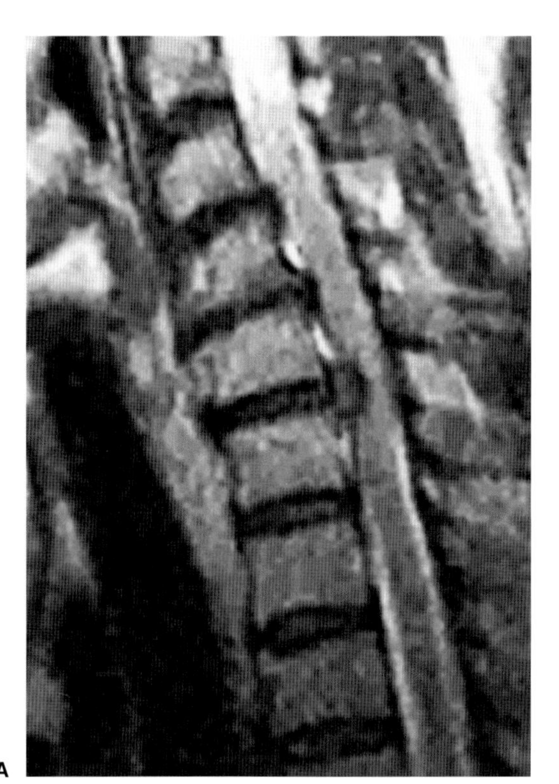
A

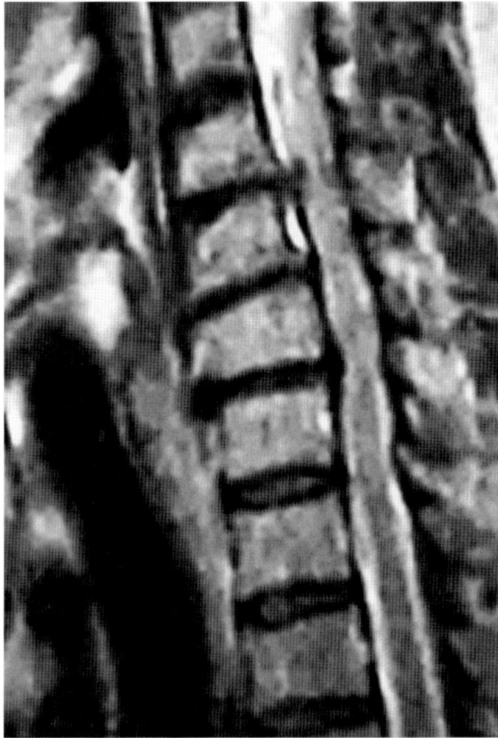
B

FIGURE 5–10 Large 8 mm herniated C6–C7 disk compressing spinal cord. **(A)** Pre- and **(B)** postoperative magnetic resonance imaging scans.

Case Illustration

A 62-year-old female patient complained of progressive neck, shoulder, and bilateral arm pain for 3 years, with increasing stiffness of the legs, along with stool and urinary incontinence for 3 months. The left biceps reflex was reduced, and knee and ankle reflexes were 2+. Hypoalgesia was present in the left middle and ring fingers. Babinski's reflex was equivocal on the right. Mild spastic gait was evident. EMG was abnormal in a left C6–C7 distribution. MRI (Fig. 5–10A) confirmed a large 8 mm herniated C6–C7 disk causing spinal cord compression, a 2 mm disk protrusion at C4–C5, and a 2 to 3 mm protrusion at C5–C6. Provocative diskogram and anterior endoscopic microdecompressive diskectomy with laser thermodiskoplasty were performed. Very brief transient worsening of gait was followed postoperatively by rapid improvement of all symptoms and disappearance of incontinence by the third postoperative day. She was asymptomatic and free of pain at follow-up 1 year later. She had resumed all her normal activities. Comparative pre- and postoperative MRI scans showed complete removal of the large herniated C6–C7 disk (Fig. 5–10B).

Conclusion

Anterior endoscopic cervical microdiskectomy, which represents a new procedure for treating symptomatic herniated cervical disks anteriorly through an endoscope, aims to reduce tissue trauma from conventional open cervical surgery. Low-energy nonablative laser is applied for shrinkage and tightening of the disk (laser thermodiskoplasty). With appropriate endoscopic spinal surgical training, thorough knowledge of the AECM procedure, and surgical experience, AECM is a safe and efficacious procedure. This minimally invasive and less traumatic outpatient procedure results in less morbidity, more rapid recovery, and significant economic savings.

REFERENCES

1. Bailey RW, Badgely CE. Stabilization of the cervical spine by anterior fusion. *Bone Joint Surg.* 1958;40A:607–624.
2. Cloward RB. The anterior approach for removal of ruptured cervical discs. *J Neurosurg.* 1958;15:602–617.
3. Robinson RA, Smith GW. Anterolateral cervical disc removal and interbody fusion for cervical disc syndrome. *Bull Johns Hopkins Hosp.* 1955;96:223–224.
4. Robertson JT. Anterior removal of cervical disc without fusion. *Clin Neurosurg.* 1973;20:259–261.
5. McCulloch J, Young P. Complications of cervical spine microsurgery. In: McCuloch JA, ed. *Essentials of Spinal Microsurgery.* Philadelphia: Lippincott-Raven; 1998;209–215.
6. Shea M, Takeuchi TY, Wittenberg RH, White AA III, Hayes WC. A comparison of the effects of automated percutaneous diskectomy and conventional diskectomy on intradiscal pressure, disc geometry, and stiffness. *J Spinal Disord.* 1994;7:317–325.
7. Chiu J, Clifford T. Cervical endoscopic discectomy with laser thermodiskoplasty. In: Savitz MH, Chiu JC, Yeung AT, eds. *The Practice of Minimally Invasive Spinal Technique.* Richmond: AAMISMS Education; 2000:141–148.
8. Lee SH. Comparison of percutaneous endoscopic discectomy to open anterior discectomy for cervical herniations. *J Min Inv Spinal Tech.* 2001;1:17–19.
9. Hijikata S. Percutaneous nucleotomy: a new concept of technique and 12 years experience. *Clin Orthop.* 1989;238:9–23.
10. Davis GW, Onik, Helms O. Automated percutaneous discectomy. *Spine.* 1991;16:359–363.
11. Onik G, Mooney G, Maroon JC, et al. Automated percutaneous discectomy: a prospective multi-institutional study. *Neurosurgery.* 1990;26:228–233.
12. Ascher PW. Application of the laser in neurosurgery. *Laser Surg Med.* 1986;2:91–97.
13. Krause D, Drape JL, Jambon F, et al. Cervical nucleolysis: indications, technique, results. *J Neuroradiol.* 1993;20:42–59.
14. Kambin P. Posterolateral percutaneous lumbar discectomy and decompression: arthroscopic microdiscectomy. In: Kambin P, ed. *Arthroscopic Microdiscectomy: Minimal Intervention in Spinal Surgery.* Baltimore: Urban & Schwarzenberg; 1991:67–100.
15. Mayer HM, Brock M. Percutaneous endoscopic discectomy: surgical technique and preliminary results compared to microsurgical discectomy. *J Neurosurg.* 1993;78:216–225.
16. Schreiber A, Suezawa Y, Leu HJ. Does percutaneous nucleotomy with discoscopy replace conventional discectomy? Eight years of experience and results in treatment of herniated lumbar disc. *Clin Orthop.* 1989;238:35–42.
17. Fukishima T, Ishijima B, Hirakawa K, et al. Ventriculofiberscope: a new technique for endoscopic diagnosis and operation. *J Neurosurg.* 1973;38:251–256.
18. Yonezawa T, Onomura T, Kosaka R, et al. The system and procedures of percutaneous intradiscal laser nucleotomy. *Spine.* 1990; 15:1175–1185.
19. Chiu J, Clifford T, Greenspan M. Percutaneous microdecompressive endoscopic cervical discectomy with laser thermodiskoplasty. *Mt Sinai J Med.* 2000;67:278–282.
20. Chiu J, Clifford T. Multiple herniated discs at single and multiple spinal segments treated with endoscopic microdecompressive surgery. *J Minim Invasive Spinal Tech.* 2001;1:15–19.

6

Percutaneous Endoscopic Cervical Diskectomy and Stabilization

SANG-HO LEE AND YONG AHN

Percutaneous endoscopic cervical diskectomy (PECD) is a new surgical method for treating soft cervical disk herniations. The goal of the procedure is decompression of the spinal nerve root by percutaneous removal of the herniated mass and shrinkage of the nucleus pulposus under local anesthesia. The anterior interbody fusion, achieved by removing the intervertebral disk and inserting a bone graft under general anesthesia, remains the mainstay of surgical treatment for cervical disk herniation. The open anteromedial diskectomy with fusion, however, usually requires entrance into the spinal canal, with the accompanying risk of such complications as epidural bleeding, perineural fibrosis, transient or permanent myelopathy, graft-related problems (e.g., donor site morbidity, painful pseudarthrosis, graft extrusion or angular collapse, kyphotic deformity, graft impaction into the body), dysphasia, and hoarseness (e.g., temporary or permanent vocal cord paresis).[1–7] The minimally invasive PECD under local anesthesia can avoid these complications and offers an alternative to open therapeutic methods in cervicobrachial neuralgia or radiculopathy due to soft cervical disk herniation. It has already undergone successful biomechanical tests and cadaveric studies. In cases of failure, PECD does not impede conventional surgical approaches, and it offers such numerous advantages as the absence of risk of epidural bleeding and periradicular fibrosis, maintenance of stability of the intervertebral mobile segment, and reduced risk for recurrence after performing an anterior diskal window. The procedure provides an excellent cosmetic effect, and the reduced operation time and hospital stay allow the patient to recover to normal daily activity more rapidly.

Although PECD provides an effective and attractive alternative to open diskectomy and fusion, it has limitations. For example, PECD is ineffective in the presence of segmental instability or cervical discogenic pain syndromes. Spinal stabilization performed by conventional open procedures, however, often requires an extended pathway through the neck to insert the fusion/spacer devices into the disk space. Specially designed expandable holders can be used as interbody spacers to achieve stability without open diskectomy fusion, thus avoiding many approach-related complications seen with open techniques.

History

Since its first description of cervical percutaneous diskectomy by Tajima et al., there has been a remarkable evolution of various minimally invasive techniques for cervical disk disease. These include such percutaneous cervical diskotomy (PCD) as chemonucleolysis using chymopapain,[9] automated percutaneous cervical diskectomy (APCD),[10–12] the combination of chymopapain injection followed by APCD,[13] and laser percutaneous cervical decompression (LPCD),[14–17] all of which are well established. We have performed PECD with cervical laser-assisted spinal endoscopy (LASE) since 1993.

Indications

Most patients with cervicobrachial neuralgia due to disk herniation respond well to medical treatment; however, symptoms related to perineural cicatricial fibrosis due to a prolonged pressure on the nerve root can become irreversible. The occurrence or aggravation of a neurologica deficit even after an adequate period of conservative treatment therefore requires one to consider surgical decompression. PECD is indicated in the surgical treatment of soft cervical disk herniation contained by the posterior longitudinal ligament (subligamentous protrusion) and confirmed by magnetic resonance imaging. If the radicular symptoms are aggravated with neck extension and reduced by flexion of the neck, and if rotating the head toward the affected extremity and compressing the vertex of the head reproduce symptoms, whereas abduction of the shoulder and elevation of the head bring relief of symptoms, it is a good indication for PECD. Cervicoencephalic symptoms (e.g., headache and dizziness lasting for more than 1 year due to soft cervical disk herniation) diagnosed by diskography are also a good indication for PECD. A very bulky hernia is not a contraindication as long as the patient has no myelopathic symptoms and signs. Stabilization after diskectomy is considered in all patients with cervical instability and cervical discogenic syndromes.

Contraindications

PECD is contraindicated in patients presenting a severe neurologic deficit, segmental instability, acute pyramidal syndrome, progressive myelopathy, and other pathological conditions (e.g., fracture, tumor, pregnancy, and active infection).

Instruments and Equipment

The oldest working tube Tajima et al. made in 1981 was 2 mm in diameter and 8 cm in length. He added two dilators, one guide needle for diskography, and three disk forceps (i.e., small, medium, and large). The small forceps (disk rongeur) was principally utilized for excision of osteophytes. Using medium and large forceps, Tajima et al. performed diskectomy of the posterior disk. These instruments might be broken inside the disk.[8] The revised instruments required for PECD include an 18-gauge spinal needle, a thin guidewire, dilating obturators, working cannulas, an anulus trephine, and various forceps with or without an irrigation hole (Fig. 6–1). Visual control of percutaneous diskectomy is possible intermittently with a small, rigid endoscope and continuously with a flexible endoscopic holmium: yttrium-aluminum-garnet (YAG) laser kit or working endoscope (cervical LASE) (Fig. 6–2). The procedure should be performed only after a clear view of the entire operative disk under lateral and anteroposterior (AP) fluoroscopic projection has been obtained. The operating table must

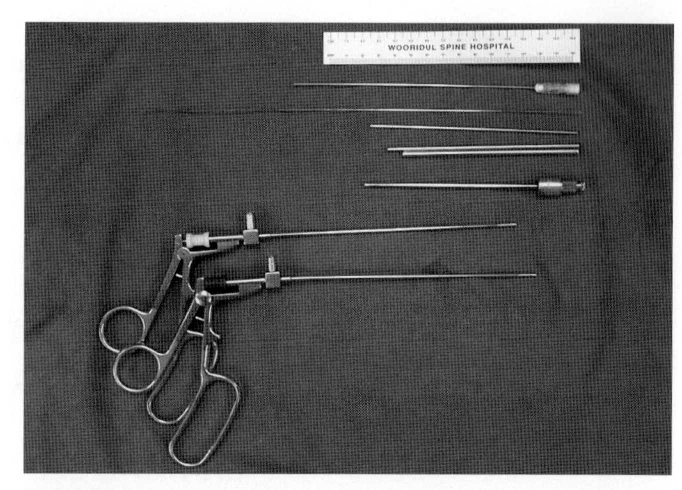

FIGURE 6–1 Instruments for percutaneous endoscopic cervical diskectomy WSA: 1 and 2 mm dilators; 3, 4, and 5 mm working tubes; forceps; and an annular trephine.

be radiolucent. Equipment for general anesthesia and instruments for open anterior cervical diskectomy with fusion should be prepared in case of a need for conversion to an open procedure or for the rare occasion of airway obstruction due to hematoma.

Preparation and Anesthesia

Preoperative antibiotics (i.e., usually cefazolin 1.0 g) should be given to decrease the risk of infection. Preoperative sedatives are recommended. PECD must be performed in an operating room with strict asepsis. The patient is placed in a supine position, with the neck mildly extended on a radiolucent table. The forehead must be fixed with plaster. A pillow is put under the shoulder and

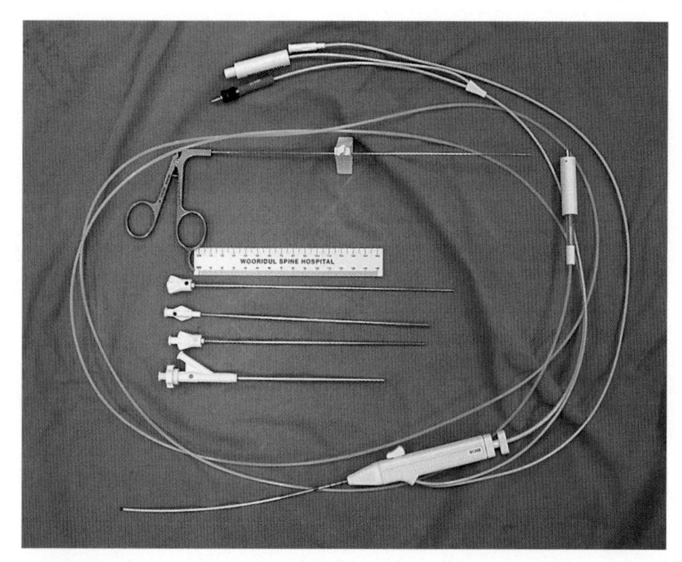

FIGURE 6–2 WSH cervical LASE (laser-assisted spinal endoscopy) system for percutaneous endoscopic cervical diskectomy.

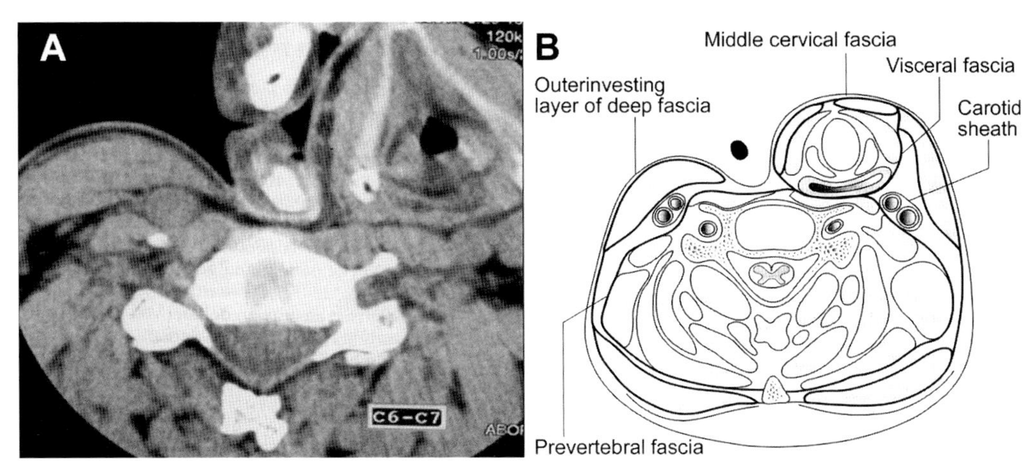

FIGURE 6–3 (A,B) Axial MRI and drawing after pushing trachea with a finger showing a clear way toward cervical disks.

neck. The shoulders are sloped down with a plaster fixed on the table. The C-arm of the fluoroscope is put in front, then in profile, and the area of the operation is carefully marked on the skin with a felt pen using a metal instrument on the front and profile. The lesion is marked by counting the cervical vertebrae downward, then up from the bottom. For better visualization of the C6–C7 level, a slight slope of the fluoroscope may be necessary. The felt pen marks the internal edge of the sternocleidomastoid muscle, the median axis of the neck, and the upper edge of the sternum. The skin is distempered with an antiseptic. The fluoroscope is covered with a sterile field, then the face is surrounded with a plastic field that is held up over the patient's head in order for an anesthesiologist to observe and speak with the patient. Communication between the operator and the patient is necessary during the procedure. The operation is typically conducted under local anesthesia and analgesia by neuroleptics so the surgeon may know immediately any changes in symptoms and signs of the patient. General anesthesia may be used in a few patients who want it or cannot tolerate the position. If the cervical diskography or other procedures aggravate the spinal cord compression, patients can recognize and comment on the development of extremity weakness only under local anesthesia. Under general anesthesia, the urgent need for conversion to open surgery may not be detected early. A solution of 1% lidocaine is usually used to infiltrate the skin and subcutaneous tissue. To minimize the thickening of underlying tissues and to allow a minute palpation of the spinal axis, we prefer not to infiltrate more deeply with lidocaine.

Surgical Technique

Needle Insertion

The surgeon gently pushes the trachea or larynx toward the opposite side with the index and middle finger, then applies a firm pressure in the space between the muscle and trachea and pointed toward the vertebral surface (Fig. 6–3 A,B). The trachea and larynx are displaced medially and the carotid artery laterally. The puncture needle is then inserted through the space between the tracheoesophagus and the carotid artery (Fig. 6–4). The tip of the needle should be positioned on the center of the anterior anulus. The position is confirmed fluoroscopically, and the needle is advanced ~5 mm into the disk. Intraoperative diskography is performed to identify the herniation type or annular tear. Up to 0.5 ml of contrast media is injected to specify the posterior part of the disk. A guidewire is then inserted to replace the puncture needle. A small skin incision (>5 mm) is made.

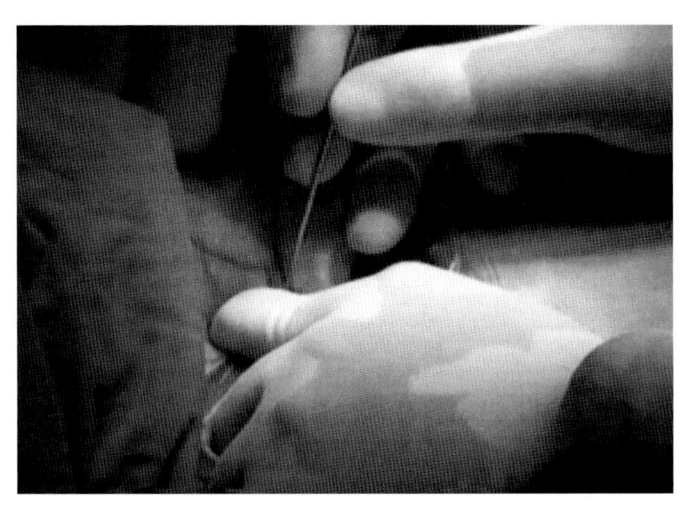

FIGURE 6–4 An 18-gauge needle is shown between the operator's and the assistant's index fingers. The operator's and/or the assistant's index finger pulls the trachea to allow the other finger to touch the anterior surface of the cervical spine.

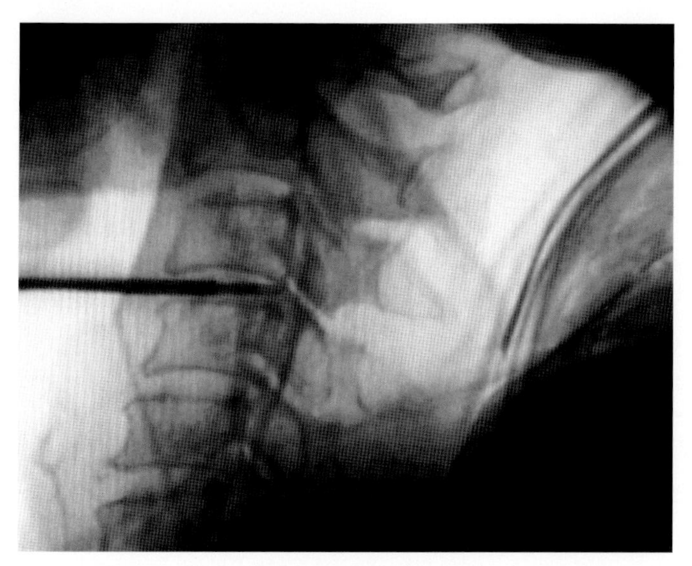

FIGURE 6–5 The position of the forceps tip.

Working Cannula Insertion

After skin incision, the surgeon inserts 1 to 5 mm dilation cannulas sequentially along the guidewire. It is safer to dilate the insertion site gradually. Before insertion of the final working cannula, the anterior anulus is cut by an annulotomy trephine. The final working cannula is then inserted into the disk space, and its position is confirmed by C-arm fluoroscopy. Depending on the disk space height, working cannulas of diameters from 3.0 to 5.0 mm are useful.

Manual Diskectomy

The next step is manual diskectomy under C-arm guidance. The surgeon cuts the anterior anulus as a small hole using the annulotomy trephine, then decompresses the posterior disk widely. The surgeon can thus preserve most of the anterior structures (unlike in the open diskectomy). The forceps are used to remove the nucleus. It should be reached at the end of the posterior margin to remove the herniated mass effectively, with care taken not to injure the spinal cord (Fig. 6–5). The medial nucleus is removed first, then the lateral side according to the position of the lesion. Extraction of the tail of the hernia mass, which is more fibrotic and collagenous, is attempted. The anterior part of the disk should not be removed to avoid postoperative kyphosis. The intradiskal space is rinsed continuously with cefazolin-mixed fluid through an irrigation channel in the forceps.

Endoscopic Laser Diskectomy

After removal of the hernia mass by forceps, a sophisticated laser decompression is performed using the holmium:YAG laser. The endoscopic holmium:YAG laser works precisely with a 0.3 to 0.5 mm cutting depth for direct ablation and shrinkage of the disk (Fig. 6–6A). Continuous saline irrigation is performed to protect the spinal cord or nerve root from energy transmission. To ablate the tissue near or inside the hernia mass, the surgeon should see inside the disk with a small endoscope (Fig. 6–6B).

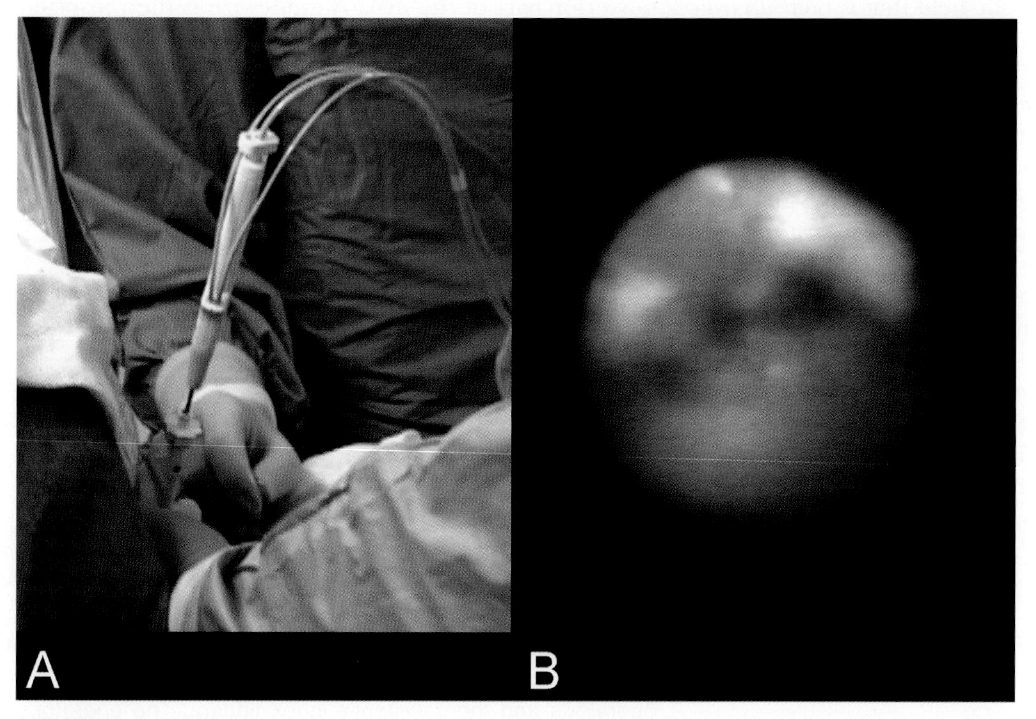

FIGURE 6–6 **(A)** The endoscopic holmium: yttrium-aluminum-garnet laser. **(B)** Endoscopic view of disk ablation by laser.

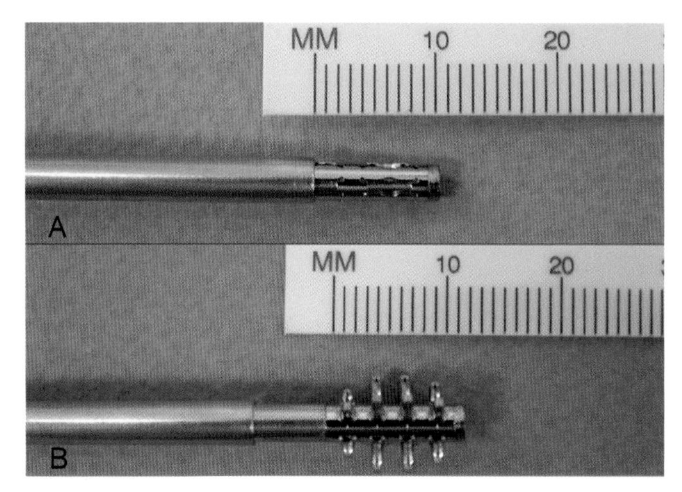

FIGURE 6–7 (A) Initially narrowed form of cervical expandable holder (3.3 mm). **(B)** Expanded form (5/7/7/6 mm).

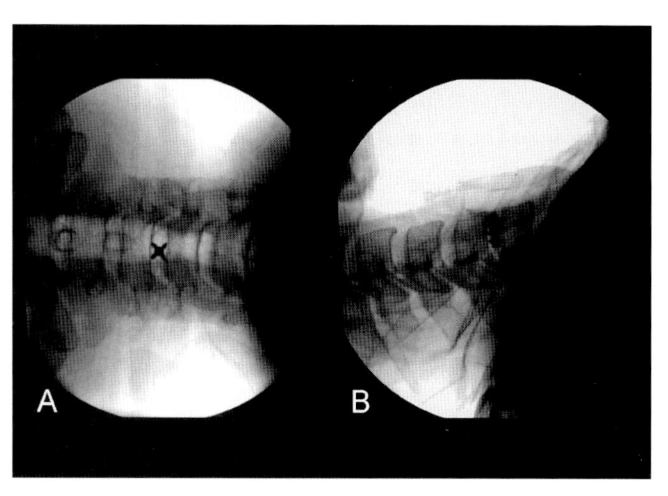

FIGURE 6–8 (A,B) Intraoperative C-arm view of fixed cervical expandable holder at C5–C6.

Furthermore, pumping irrigation with saline during the operation has an antibacterial effect; we have observed no diskitis at all so far.

Stabilization with Expandable Holder

The expandable spinal fusion system, which can be applied by this less invasive technique, allows for spinal stability with minimal tissue dissection. The implant is introduced into the intervertebral space in a narrowed form (Fig. 6–8A). It requires an opening less than 5 mm at the skin entry site. Following the insertion of the implant into the disk space, the implant is expanded to its final form segment by segment by rotating the expander rotational handle (Fig. 6–8B). It is then fixed to the disk space to maintain the disk height (Fig. 6–9).

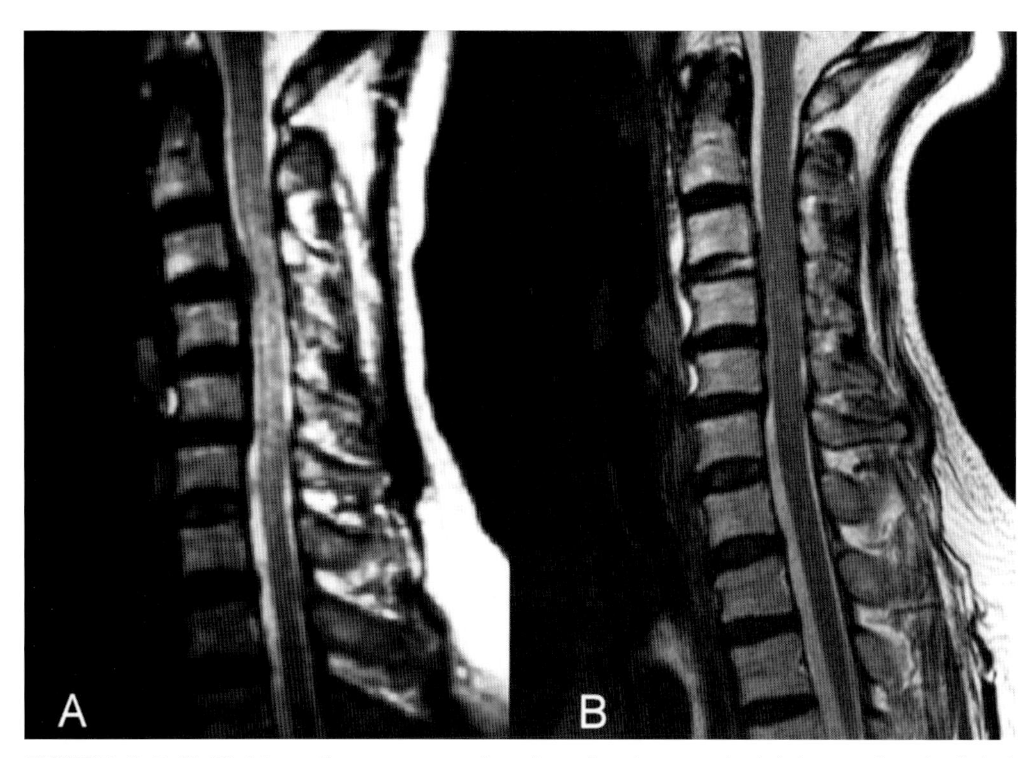

FIGURE 6–9 (A,B) Magnetic resonance imaging showing good shrinkage of soft disk herniation after percutaneous endoscopic cervical diskectomy.

Complications and Avoidance

The surgeon should recognize and manually feel the pulsation of the carotid artery to insert the needle and cannula away from the carotid artery. The surgeon should confirm the position of a needle or a cannula on the AP fluoroscopic view to prevent penetration of the vertebral artery. The fingertips of the operator or the assistant should touch the anterior surface of the vertebral body to avoid perforating the trachea or esophagus. The surgeon should confirm the tip of the guidewire, the annular trephine, the pituitary forceps, and the laser fiber on the lateral fluoroscopic view, so that the ends of the instruments do not pass more than 2 mm beyond the posterior vertebral body line to protect the spinal cord. The disk space should be irrigated frequently with 1000 ml saline mixed with antibiotics to reduce the chance of diskitis or epidural abscess.

Postoperative Management

The patient should be observed for 3 hours to detect possible complications. All patients are permitted to go home on the day of surgery (it is an outpatient surgery). The patient does not need bed rest for more than 1 night. Postoperative oral antibiotics and analgesics are recommended for 3 to 10 days. A cervical collar is recommended for 3 to 14 days, depending on the patient's condition. Mild physical therapy may be helpful for fast recovery within 2 weeks postoperatively if cervicobrachialgia does not disappear completely. Should pain and discomfort remain, complementary epidural injection of steroids with lidocaine may be added so that no further open procedure is necessary. This is a combined therapeutic logic of mechanical decompression with PECD and the reduction of inflammatory components by steroids.[9] Rehabilitation exercises for neck muscle strengthening and improvement of range of motion are recommended twice a week for 3 months after 4 to 6 weeks postoperatively.

Clinical Results

Between 1993 and 2002, a total of 1127 patients were treated by PECD at Wooridul Spine Hospital (Seoul, Korea). Most patients experienced immediate improvement of their pain during the procedure. Immediate postoperative magnetic resonance imaging (MRI) demonstrates that the disk herniation is removed completely (Fig. 6–9). We conducted a retrospective study with 113 patients selected randomly at 3 years after PECD. All of the 113 patients were followed by MRI and computed tomographic (CT) scans. Ninety-eight patients (86.7%) presented radiculopathies. Neck pains were noticed in 67 patients (59%), headache and dizziness in 13 (12%), and mild myelopathy in 5 (4.4%). The mean duration of symptoms was 24 months (range: from 1 to 300 months). The locations of herniation were paramedial in 48 patients (42%), central in 31 (27%), foraminal and lateral in 22 (19%), and diffuse in 13 (12%). Excellent or good results were shown in 94 patients (83%), fair in 13 patients (11%), and poor in 6 (5%) according to Macnab criteria.[18] Two cases (1.8%) needed open diskectomy; one had worsened neck pain after PECD and underwent anterior cervical diskectomy with fusion, and the other had worsened shoulder and arm

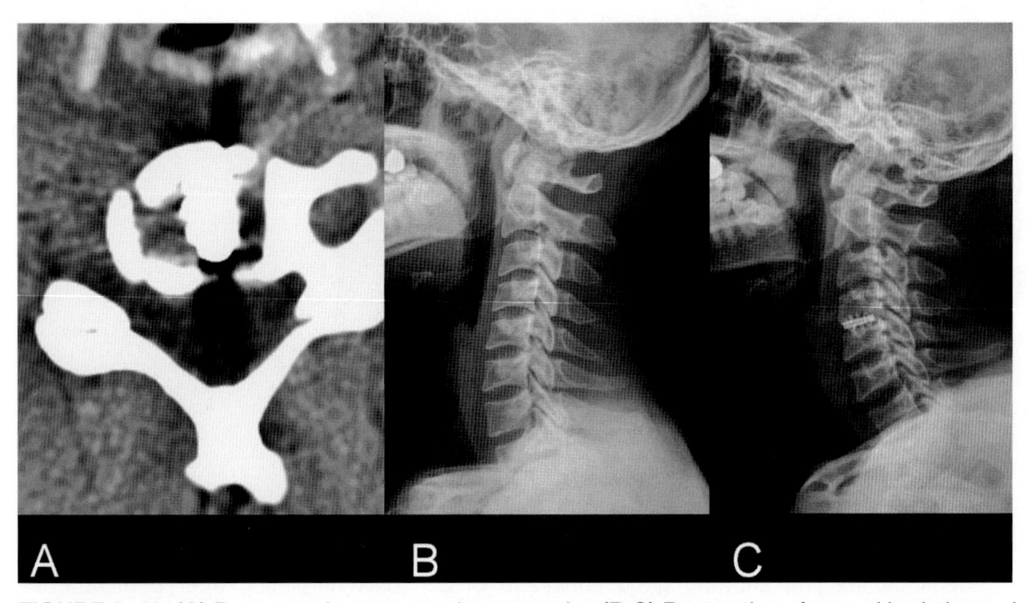

FIGURE 6–10 **(A)** Postoperative computed tomography. **(B,C)** Restoration of normal lordotic cervical alignment after surgery.

pain and underwent anterior cervical foraminotomy. There were no complications (e.g., esophageal, vascular, or nerve injuries), infection, or cerebrospinal fluid leakage.

Since 2001, seven patients underwent the PECD and stabilization with an expandable holder. All patients had remarkable relief of pain after the procedure. Postoperative CT scans showed satisfactory positioning of the implant (Fig. 6–10A). Preoperative kyphotic alignment improved postoperatively (Fig. 6–10B and C). There were no procedure-related complications.

Minimally invasive techniques combining the percutaneous C-arm-guided manual diskectomy and endoscopic holmium:YAG laser diskectomy to treat soft cervical disk herniations with radiculopathy have proven to be conservative and not destructive. The clinical results were comparable to those obtained with open diskectomy and fusion. The PECD is an outpatient surgery and can be as safe and efficacious as open anteromedial cervical diskectomy in select patients. Stabilization following PECD can be performed safely and effectively in cases of soft cervical disk herniations with segmental instability or discogenic neck pain.

REFERENCES

1. Brodke DS. Zdeblick TA. Modified Smith-Robinson procedure for anterior cervical diskectomy and fusion. *Spine.* 1992;17 (10 suppl.):427–430.
2. Bulger RF, Rejowski JE, Beatty RA. Vocal cord paralysis associated with anterior cervical fusion: considerations for prevention and treatment. *J Neurosurg.* 1985;62:657–661.
3. Clements DH, O'Leary PF. Anterior cervical diskectomy and fusion. *Spine.* 1990;15:1023–1025.
4. Flynn TB. Neurologic complications of anterior cervical interbody fusion. *Spine.* 1982;7:536–539.
5. Kadoya S, Nakamura T, Kwak R. Microsurgical anterior osteophytectomy of cervical spondylotic myelopathy. *Spine.* 1984;9:437–441.
6. Lunsford LD, Bissonette DJ, Jannetta PJ, Sheptak PE, Zorub DS. Anterior surgery for cervical disease. *J Neurosurg.* 1980;53:1–11.
7. Thorell W, Cooper J, Hellbusch L, Leibrock L. The long-term clinical outcome of patients undergoing anterior cervical diskectomy with and without intervertebral bone graft placement. *Neurosurgery.* 1998;43:268–274.
8. Tajima T, Sakamoto H, Yamakawa H. Diskectomy cervicale percutanee. *Revue Med Orthoped.* 1989;17:7–10.
9. Richard J, Lazorthes Y, Verdie JC. Chemonucleolyse discale cervicale. Paper presented at: Gieda Rachis; December 15, 1994; Paris.
10. Theron J, Huet H. Nucleotomie cervicale. Paper presented at: Gieda Rachis; December 15, 1994; Paris.
11. Zucherman J; Implicito D, Vessa P. Percutaneous cervical discectomy. Paper presented at Eleventh annual meeting of the North American Spine Society; October 25, 1996, Vancouver.
12. Herman S, Nizard RS, Witvoet J. La discectomie percutanée au rachis cervical: rachis cervical degeneratif et traumatique. *Exp Sci [Fr].* 1994:160–166.
13. Hoogland T, Scheckenbach C. Low-dose chemonucleolysis combined with percutaneous nucleotomy in herniated cervical disks. *J Spinal Disord.* 1995;8:228–232.
14. Siebert W. Percutaneous laser discectomy of cervical disk: preliminary clinical results. JCI *Laser Med Surg.* 1995;13:205–207.
15. Hellinger J. Nonendoscopic percutaneous 1064 Nd:YAG laser decompression. Paper presented at: Third Symposium on Laser-assisted Endoscopic and Arthroscopic Intervention in Orthopaedics; October 11, 1994; Zurich.
16. Chiu JC, Clifford TJ, Greenspan M. Percutaneous microdecompressive endoscopic cervical diskectomy with laser thermodiskoplasty. *Mt Sinai J Med.* 2000;67:278–282.
17. Knight MTN, Goswami A, Patko JT. Cervical percutaneous laser disc decompression: preliminary results of an ongoing prospective outcome study. *J Clin Laser Med Surg.* 2001;19:3–8.
18. Macnab I. Negative disc exploration: an analysis of the causes of nerve–root involvement in sixty-eight patients. *J Bone Joint Surg Am.* 1971;53:891–903.

7

Posterior Cervical Microendoscopic Diskectomy and Laminoforaminotomy

ADNAN SIDDIQUI AND KENNETH S. YONEMURA

Posterior cervical disk surgery is a well-established and highly effective means of ameliorating disk- and bone-associated compression of cervical nerve roots. It was first proposed by Spurling and Scoville[1] in 1944 and remains a procedure of choice for posterolateral disk herniations and focal foraminal stenosis, as well as for patients for whom anterior approaches are contraindicated or associated with increased risk. Despite the effectiveness of the posterior approach, the popularity of the anterior diskectomy procedure has risen steadily. The anterior approach requires an acceptance of the potential risks to the anterior midline structures (e.g., the esophagus and trachea, recurrent laryngeal nerve, and such vascular structures as the carotid artery and its branches).[2] In addition, the anterior approach requires near complete disk removal, leading to premature disk space collapse and potential cervical kyphosis. To circumvent this problem, the routine performance of fusion with anterior diskectomy has become standard. The reduction in mobility seen with fusion is associated with an acceleration of degenerative changes at adjacent levels.[3]

The classic open posterior cervical approach necessitates a moderate-sized incision to develop the relatively deep dissection for visualization of the junction of the lamina with the lateral mass and the underlying neural foramen. Because of the sensitivity of the posterior cervical musculature, the dissection and retraction of ipsilateral and at times bilateral paraspinous musculature can result in significant postoperative pain and muscle spasm. Both anterior and posterior approaches can be performed in the outpatient setting, but posterior approaches can be associated with a longer inpatient postoperative course due to incisional pain.

It is therefore very appropriate that initial minimally invasive techniques in spine surgery have attempted to harness the posterior cervical approach, with its relative simplicity and lack of complicated adjacent anatomy, to see if there is a benefit to reducing the extent of the incision and muscle dissection. Reduction in approach-related incisional morbidity has been clearly documented in the laparoscopic experience over the past several decades, and natural progression dictates that this technology be extended to spinal surgical techniques. Minimally invasive surgery is in many ways synonymous with endoscopic techniques that allow visualization of deep structures through small portals in the external body wall. Emphasis is placed on pathology in the case of minimally invasive posterior cervical disk surgery, which results in unilateral radiculopathy, as compared with those that result in central canal stenosis presenting with myelopathy.

Classic open treatment of cervical spondylosis has employed both anterior and posterior procedures. Anterior procedures include diskectomy with or without fusion, corpectomy with reconstruction, and, more recently, foraminotomy.[4] Smith and Robinson[5] initially described the anterior diskectomy procedure in 1955. This approach allows for direct decompression of osteophytes and disk herniations regardless of the location relative to the dorsally located spinal cord and nerve root. The anterior approach relies on naturally occurring dissection planes in the anterior strap muscles, which minimizes potential approach-related morbidity, and thus negates many of the advantages of endoscopic treatment. Anterior percutaneous techniques have had some proponents, but they increase the potential risk to the carotid artery, jugular vein, and esophagus as compared with open surgery. A variation of the anterior approach (i.e., the anterior foraminotomy procedure) allows for preservation of a majority of the disk, thus obviating the need for fusion, but requires dissection immediately adjacent to the ipsilateral vertebral artery, raising some concerns about injury to vascular structures as well as the sympathetic chain.

Posterior procedures include laminectomy, laminoplasty, and foraminotomy. These posterior procedures generally allow for indirect decompression, with the exception of foraminal disk herniations amenable to direct removal. Approach morbidity from posterior procedures can be significant, and weakening of the posterior elements can lead to instability. Spurling and Scoville[1] initially proposed the posterior approach to cervical disk disease in 1944. Several studies indicated postoperative axial neck pain ranging from 18 to 40%,[6,7] and one study failed to include this factor in the outcome.[8] The frequently quoted prospective comparison of anterior versus posterior approaches by Herkowitz et al[9] had 90% and 75% good to excellent results for both approaches, respectively. It is interesting to note that if the patients were evaluated for resolution of radicular symptoms alone, the results for posterior approaches were good to excellent in 85 to 90% of the cases. This indicated that the major difference in the two approaches was incisional and dissectional morbidity from the open surgical technique.

A major innovation allowing for minimally invasive procedures is the development of small-diameter glass rod endoscopes with high resolution. These devices allow for improved visualization of the deep structures through small portals, thereby minimizing soft tissue trauma. The associated development of various endoscopic delivery systems and instrumentation has provided the means for accomplishing such minimally invasive surgery in the cervical spine as the microendoscopic diskectomy (MED) procedure. These innovative procedures are not expected to replace open procedures entirely, but rather to provide surgeons with additional options for treating certain specific problems in the cervical spine. The decisional algorithm to offer anterior versus posterior procedures, single versus multiple levels, and fusion versus decompression alone is often complicated and is beyond the scope of this chapter.

Indications

Due to the limited exposure of endoscopic techniques, the pathology should ideally be unilateral and restricted to a single level or to two contiguous nerve root levels. Cervical MED is effective for removal of foraminal soft disk herniations, as well as foraminal stenosis from osteophytic spurs or facet arthropathy, including synovial cysts. Endoscopic foraminotomy has been shown to produce an equivalent or slightly larger decompression as compared with standard open surgery.[10] Additional indications include multilevel foraminal stenosis without central stenosis, persistent foraminal stenosis after an anterior diskectomy with fusion, and root compression in situations in which anterior approaches may be relatively contraindicated. These anterior issues include the presence of a tracheostomy, history of prior cervical radiation therapy, and disk herniations at the cervicothoracic junction (C7–T1 or T1–T2), as shown in Figure 7–1.

Cervical radiculopathy may be associated with significant axial neck pain, but it should not be confused with patients suffering from axial neck pain without nerve root or spinal cord symptoms. Cervical discogenic pain resulting in axial neck pain with referred, nonradicular arm pain is controversial and may require diskography for evaluation; however it is ultimately not amenable to posterior endoscopic treatment.

The presence of a brachial plexopathy is frequently ignored in favor of cervical disk disease or distal peripheral nerve entrapment (e.g., the ulnar or median nerve). Shoulder pain with radiation into multiple dermatomal levels, weakness of the hand intrinsics, aggravation with arm elevation, and the absence of significant cervical disk disease should trigger the inclusion of thoracic outlet syndrome into the differential diagnosis.

Positioning

Surgery may be performed in the prone or sitting position. After general endotracheal anesthesia is induced, the patient is positioned, and narcotics are avoided to minimize postoperative nausea. The authors' series were initially performed prone with transverse rolls utilized rather than a frame to minimize kyphosis over the cervicothoracic junction. The sitting position (Fig. 7–2) is currently preferred based on a reduction in blood loss and improved visibility, resulting in reduction in operative time. The sitting position also improves the ability to assess the cervicothoracic junction with the fluoroscope (see Fig. 7–1C). Because of the limited size of the exposure and short duration of surgery, the risk of air embolus is negligible, and a central line or precordial Doppler is therefore not needed. A Foley catheter is placed for cases involving multiple levels or bilateral procedures. A prophylactic single dose of intravenous antibiotic (cefazolin or vancomycin) is given at the start of the procedure.

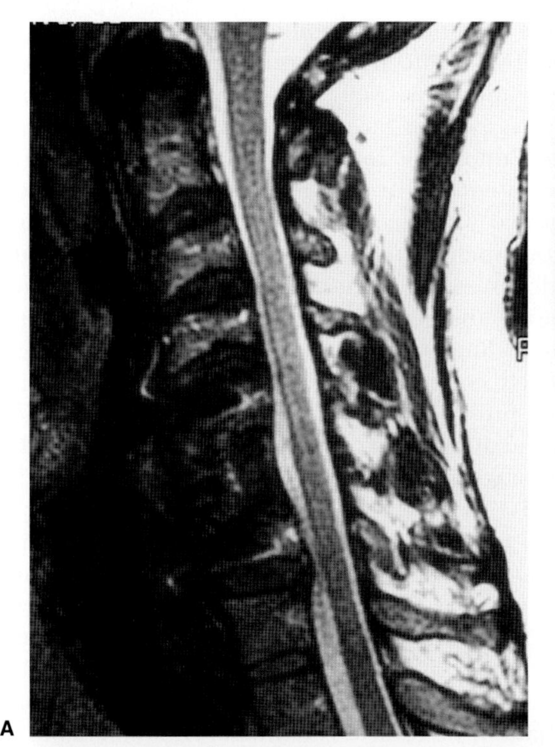

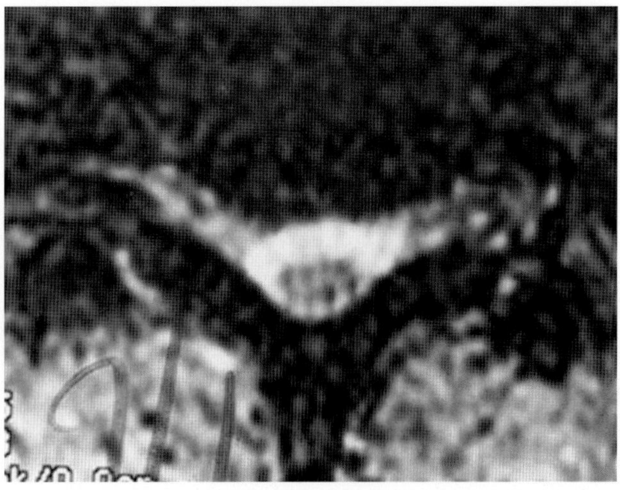

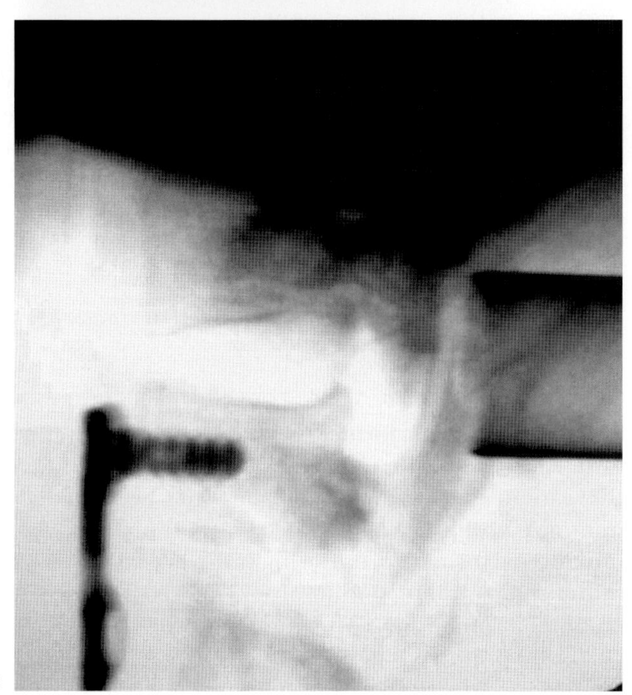

FIGURE 7–1 A 38-year-old patient with junctional spondylosis below a prior C5–C7 fusion. **(A)** Axial magnetic resonance imaging at C7–T1 showing a foraminal disk herniation involving the right C8 foramen. **(B)** Intraoperative fluoroscopic image showing the position of the tubular retractor over the C7–T1 facet joint at the time of surgery. **(C)** Fluoroscopic image showing the cervicothoracic junction.

Surgical Equipment and Setup

Lateral fluoroscopy is used after placement of an 18-gauge spinal needle to confirm the correct level. The fluoroscope can be placed under the drapes because rotation into the anteroposterior (AP) plane is not needed or feasible. The video monitors are placed contralateral to the side of the disk pathology, with the scrub technician on the ipsilateral side. Anesthesia personnel are positioned toward the patient's feet behind the fluoroscope.

Available endoscopic systems include the Flexposure system from Endius (Plainville, MA) and the METRx system by Sofamor Danek (Memphis, TN). The METRx system was chosen for cervical cases because of the

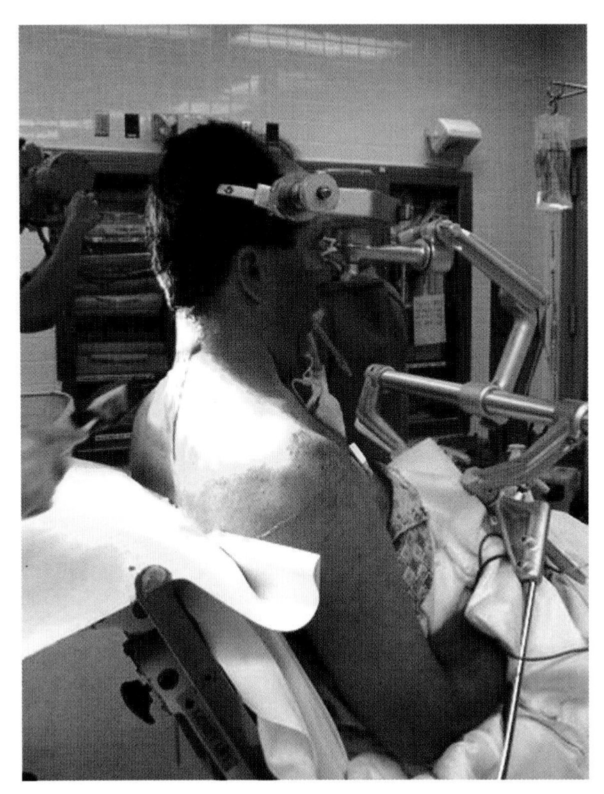

FIGURE 7–2 Use of the Mayfield head holder and table adaptor for placement in the sitting position.

availability of downsized instrumentation needed for cervical cases. Both systems use a tubular retractor to deliver an endoscope for visualization and provide a corridor to manipulate surgical instruments. The equipment includes a guidewire that is inserted under fluoroscopic guidance to the correct level onto the desired facet joint. A series of nested sequential dilators are used to create an access corridor. The METRx system is supplied with 16 and 18 mm tubular retractors, but a custom 14 mm tubular retractor has been used for cervical cases to reduce the muscle dissection and retraction. Both the tubular retractor and the endoscope are then fixed to the operating table through adjustable arms. Typical soft tissue and bone instruments have been lengthened for use through the tubular retractor and anodized to eliminate reflective glare. These include curettes, Kerrison rongeurs, pituitary rongeurs, Penfield retractors, nerve hooks, and bipolar cautery, among others. The METRx endoscope has a 25-degree viewing angle, and that of the Endius endoscope is 30 degrees; both provide an improved viewing angle and eliminate obscuration of the operative field, noted with use of the operating microscope. Both endoscopes use glass rod-lens technology, and the clarity of the images compensates for the lack of a three-dimensional image.

Surgical Technique

Following placement in the sitting position, an 18-gauge needle is placed over the correct foraminal level and confirmed with fluoroscopic images. A 1.5 cm incision is made ~2 cm lateral to the midline. If accessible, the fascia is incised with monopolar cautery to facilitate passage of the dilators to the interlaminar space. A K-wire is then passed to the appropriate facet joint, over which a series of dilators is used to create an operative corridor to the spine (Fig. 7–3). The initial dilator is used as a dissector to detach muscular and ligamentous attachments (Fig. 7–4). A 14 mm tubular retractor is then placed over the last dilator (Fig. 7–5) and secured to the operating table with a modified Greenberg articulated arm. Because of the reduced size of the cervical spine, the larger 16 mm tubular retractor has been avoided to prevent excessive resection of the facet joint.

The endoscope is then mounted within the tubular retractor (Fig. 7–6), with visualization of the appropriate interlaminar space and facet joint (Fig. 7–7). The 25-degree viewing angle of the endoscope provides a panoramic view of the epidural space and eliminates the

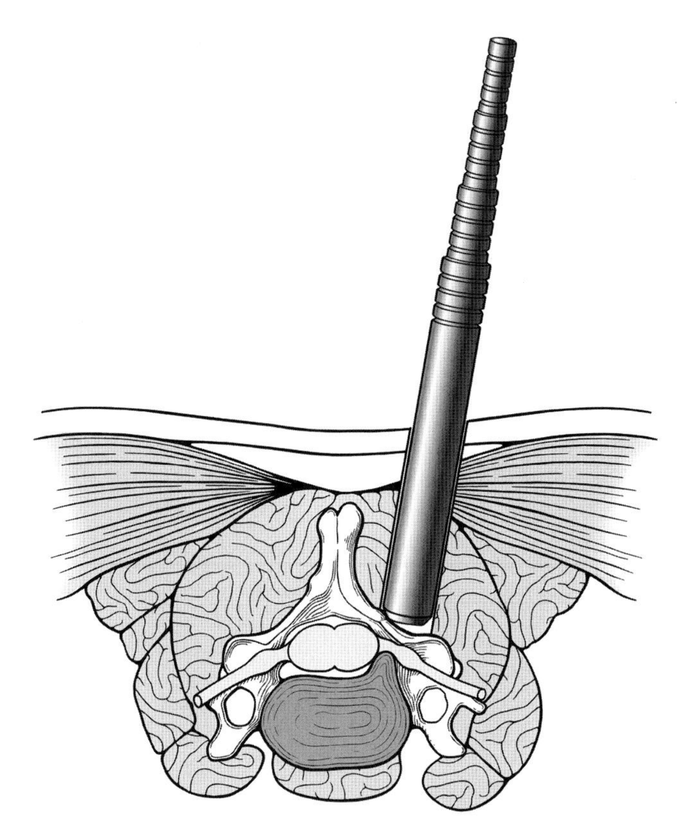

FIGURE 7–3 A K-wire is placed over the appropriate facet joint under fluoroscopic guidance. A series of dilators are then used to create the operative corridor to the interlaminar space.

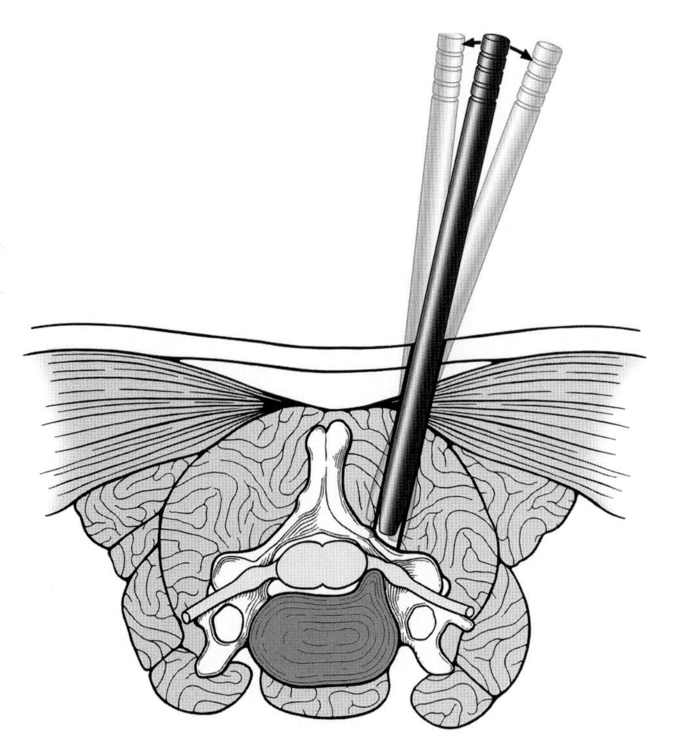

FIGURE 7–4 After removal of the K-wire, the tip of the smallest dilator is used to dissect soft tissue from the lamina and the interlaminar space.

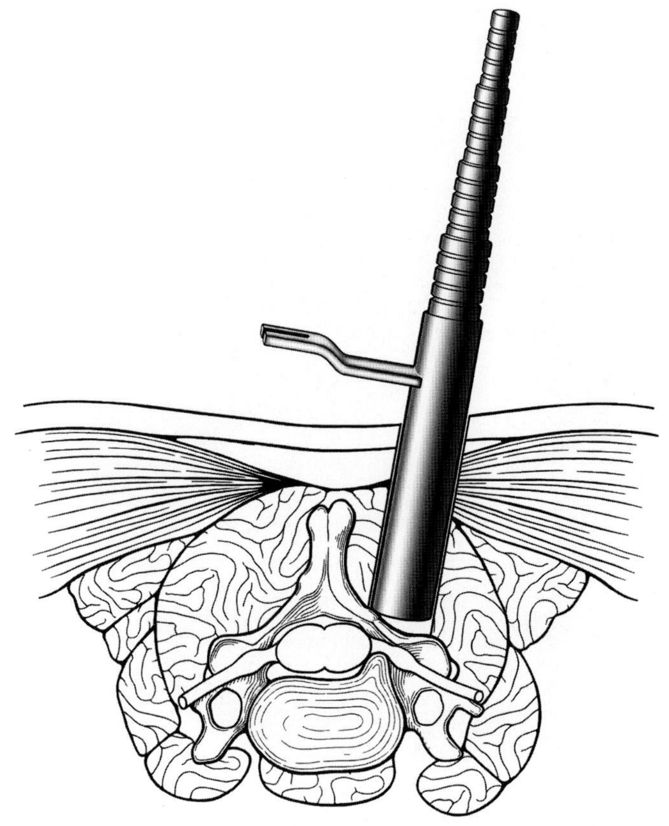

FIGURE 7–5 A tubular retractor is placed over the last dilator. Retractors are available in sizes ranging from 14 to 18 mm.

obscuration of the operative field that occurs if the operating microscope is used with bayoneted instruments.

The inferolateral margin of the superior lamina and medial facet joint of the superior vertebral segment are first cleared of soft tissue using bipolar long-tipped cautery, and the ligamentum flavum is separated from the laminar edge using an endoscopic curette. A hemilaminotomy is then performed with a high-speed drill and Kerrison rongeurs. The superior facet of the lower vertebral body is visualized laterally below the initial laminotomy and requires medial resection for access to the exiting nerve root.

The epidural space is entered laterally, with resection of the ligamentum flavum and coagulation of the epidural plexus overlying the exiting nerve root. A careful dissection of the ligamentum flavum and removal of an adequate amount of bone decrease the likelihood of dural injury and tears. Kerrison rongeurs are used to accomplish the foraminotomy, and a 90-degree version should be used medially to reduce the potential for a dural tear. After a foraminotomy is performed, a small nerve hook may be used to palpate the medial aspect of the superior and inferior pedicles to define the boundaries of the foramen and lateral margin of the canal. The nerve root is then mobilized using a small Penfield dissector to allow further removal of pathology. Dissection in the axilla of the nerve root usually uncovers the disk herniation or osteophyte, but a disk herniation can occasionally be found at the shoulder of the nerve due to the shape and angulation of the joint of Luschka. In the case of a soft disk herniation, the decompression is complete once the contained or free fragment of disk is removed, and exploration of the disk space is not necessary. Osteophytic spurs are generally not amenable to resection and are treated with a generous foraminotomy (Fig. 7–8). An arthritic, enlarged facet may also be the culprit, and it may be partially resected either through a high-speed drill or Kerrison rongeurs. Once the nerve root has been decompressed, this is confirmed through placement of the nerve hook or Woodson dissector through the foramen along the nerve root. The tubular retractor is removed after ensuring hemostasis, and the fascia is closed with a single absorbable suture. The skin is closed with subcuticular stitches, and a small volume of 0.25% bipuvicaine with epinephrine is injected into the paravertebral muscles.

The patient is then moved to the outpatient recovery area and discharged home, usually in 3 to 4 hours. Discharge mediations include antispasmodics for neck spasm and oral opioids for breakthrough pain.

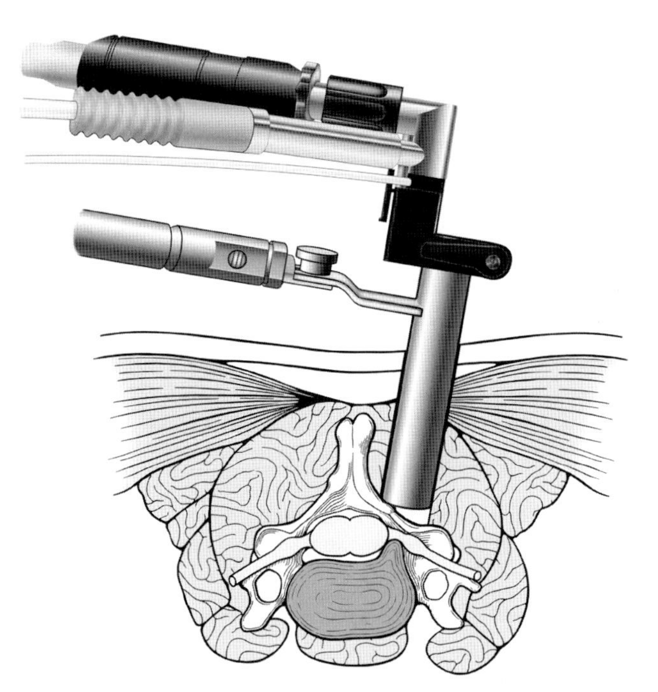

FIGURE 7–6 An articulated arm mounted to the operating table is used to stabilize the tubular retractor. The endoscope is then advanced into the tubular retractor. The depth of endoscope within the retractor determines the degree of magnification.

Results

In the authors' initial series, 14 patients (nine males and five females) underwent posterior cervical MED with minimum 1.5 years follow up. Two patients presented with symptomatic synovial cysts at C7–T1, and the remainder had spondylosis with or without an associated

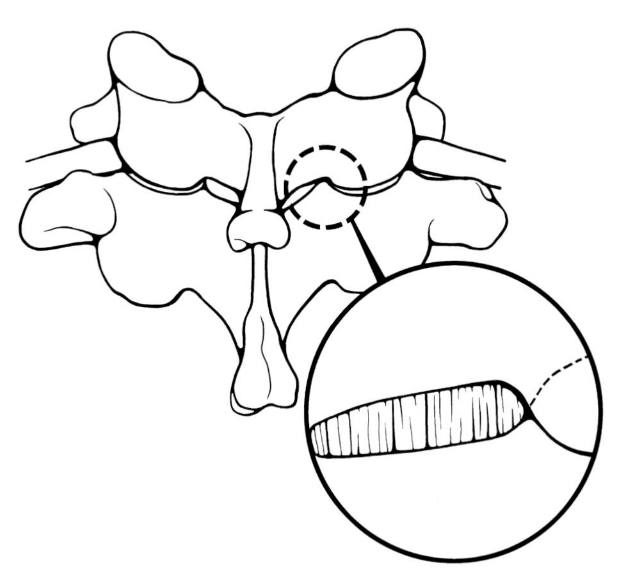

FIGURE 7–7 Scope view of the interlaminar space showing lamina/lateral mass junction over the nerve root, as well as medial facetectomy required for the laminoforaminotomy.

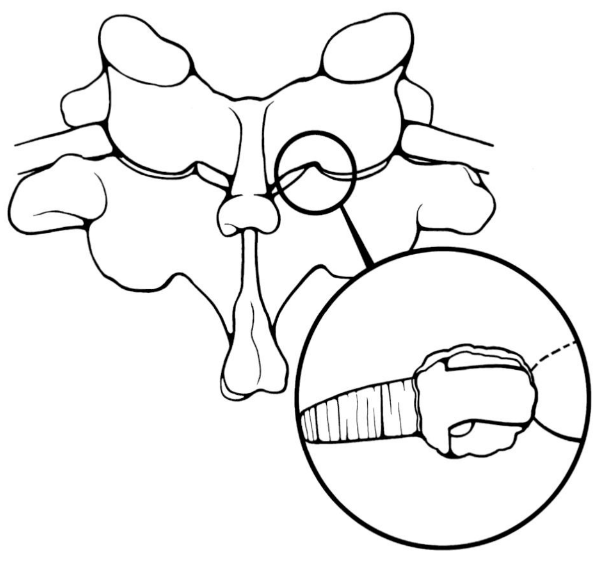

FIGURE 7–8 Following bone and ligament removal, instruments and dissectors can be placed through the tubular retractor for removal of the disk herniation, as demonstrated below the exiting nerve root.

soft disk herniation (see Fig. 7–8). Twelve had single-level surgery, and two required two-level procedures. All surgeries were performed on an outpatient basis. Thirteen noted complete resolution of radicular symptoms by the first week, and 12 denied the presence of any significant postoperative neck pain. By the sixth postoperative week, axial neck pain had resolved in the remaining two patients.

Complications included one recurrent disk herniation, blood loss greater than 800 cc on one occasion, and one patient with a contralateral neurogenic thoracic outlet syndrome from operative positioning. There was also one open conversion early in the series due to osteophytic foraminal stenosis, which at the time of open exploration had been adequately decompressed with the MED procedure alone. These complications were all noted in patients who were positioned prone.

The Neck Disability Index was used to assess outcomes, with a mean entry score of 41/65. The mean score was 12/65 at last follow-up, indicating a marked improvement in function and ability to perform daily activities. This 29-point difference is striking because a 10-point difference is felt to be significant in some studies.

The results of this technique reveal a definite improvement over historical controls. There has been virtual elimination of postoperative axial neck pain and uniform resolution of cervical radiculopathy. There has been one open conversion and one recurrent disk herniation requiring an anterior fusion. There have been no long-term neurologic deficits, and significant improvement was confirmed with the Neck Disability Index.

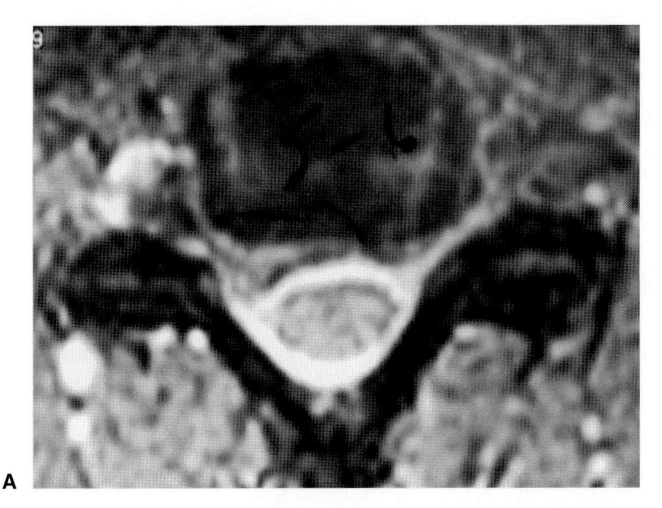

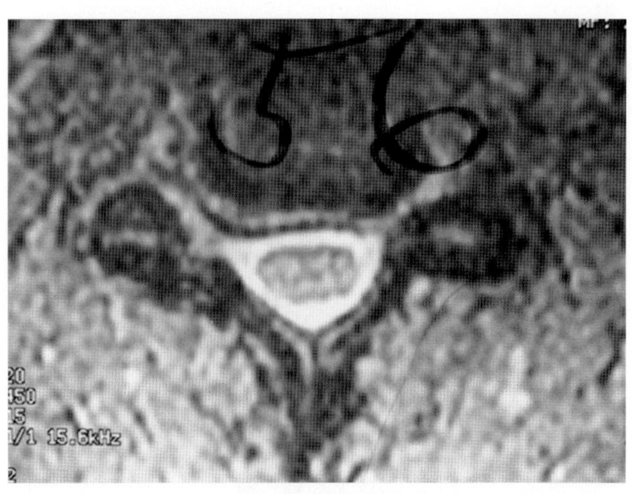

FIGURE 7–9 A 42-year-old patient with clinical symptoms of a right C6 radiculopathy. Magnetic resonance imaging (MRI) scan shows a paramedian disk herniation on the right at C5–C6 **(A)** Postoperative MRI showing decompression of the disk herniation. **(B)** Note the lack of paraspinal muscle trauma above the site of the foraminotomy.

Adamson[11] reported on 100 consecutive posterior cervical microendoscopic diskectomies for unilateral cervical radiculopathy from foraminal stenosis or lateral disk herniation. The author used the sitting position with good-to-excellent outcomes in 97% of patients. Adamson compared the results with open posterior or anterior cervical procedures and surmised that posterior cervical MED procedures were superior because of preservation of cervical motion segment, a much faster return to unrestricted activity, and a much lower incidence of complications.

Fessler and Khoo[12] reported on 25 patients who underwent posterior cervical MEDs, as compared with 26 patients who underwent open cervical laminoforaminotomy for foraminal stenosis from osteophytes or lateral disk herniation. They noted a marked reduction in blood loss, earlier recovery, shorter hospital stay, and fewer narcotics in patients who underwent MED. They noted similar outcomes when evaluating radiculopathy, neck pain, sensory, and motor status. The most remarkable feature was the relative absence of incisional neck pain, which was the most common cause of prolonged hospital stays for patients undergoing open procedures.

Complications and Avoidance

Our complications have included one recurrent disk herniation, blood loss greater than 800 ml on one occasion, and one patient with a contralateral neurogenic thoracic outlet syndrome from operative positioning. All these cases were performed with prone positioning. Our shift to the sitting position has resulted in a marked decline in blood loss, averaging 150 ml because of the reduction in epidural venous engorgement. Visualization is further facilitated through flow of blood out of the horizontal tubular retractor rather than pooling in the operative field in the prone position. Fessler and Khoo[12] have also documented a reduction in blood loss and operative times by employing the sitting position.

Although we have not experienced an intraoperative durotomy, Adamson[11] described two such cases from his series of 100 cervical MEDs, and Fessler and Khoo[12] reported three such cases in their series of 25 patients, as well as a single case of a superficial wound infection. Adamson did not place lumbar drains for his cases of cerebrospinal fluid (CSF) leak, whereas Fessler and Khoo performed 2 to 3 days of lumbar drainage in all cases. No long-term pseudomeningocele or CSF leak–related symptoms have thus far been reported. Given the small size of the incisional exposure, the potential for development of a symptomatic pseudomeningocele is small, and wound closure alone should be sufficient. Fessler and Khoo[12] also reported a single case of superficial wound infection.

Although no reports have been seen to date, the guidewire must be passed with fluoroscopic guidance to avoid the risk of inadvertent medial passage through the interlaminar space, with potential damage to the spinal cord or the exiting nerve root. A similar deviation laterally may result in injury to the vertebral artery or the venous plexus, with resultant bleeding and hematoma-related complications or arterial dissection and possible stroke. The lateral mass/facet joint complex is therefore the appropriate place for the guidewire and dilators placement, and the guidewire must be in contact with bone prior to passage of the dilators.

Posterior cervical microendoscopic diskectomy and laminoforaminotomy can be performed safely, with results comparable to the open posterior approach. MED avoids the approach-related morbidity encountered in open posterior approaches to the posterior paraspinal muscles. The advantages of the microendoscopic approach have been discussed, but the potential for recurrent disk herniations, the added time for surgery, and the requisite learning curve for endoscopic techniques must be taken into consideration.

Endoscopic equipment has evolved to hybrid systems that create a working corridor that facilitates recognition of key anatomic structures. For spinal procedures, the ability to identify normal structures is of paramount importance because an open working space (e.g., in laparoscopic techniques) does not exist in the cervical spine. The ability to affect a surgical cure with less destruction of normal structures is clearly a desirable goal. New technology has miniaturized the operative field and created a need for greater understanding of both normal and especially variant anatomy. Although the acceptance of various minimally invasive techniques may not be universal, the trend remains positive in limiting some of the destructive effects of operative exposure and has favorably affected many open surgical techniques.

REFERENCES

1. Spurling RG, Scoville WB. Lateral rupture of the cervical intervertebral disc: a common cause of shoulder and arm pain. *Surg Gynecol Obstet.* 1944;78:350–358.
2. Chesnut RM, Abitbol JJ, Garfin SR. Surgical management of cervical radiculopathy: indication, techniques, and results. *Orthop Clin North Am.* 1992;23:461–474.
3. Katsuura A, Hukuda S, Saruhashi Y, Asajimas S. Kyphotic malalignment after anterior cervical fusion is one of the factors promoting the degenerative process in adjacent intervertebral levels. *Eur Spine J.* 2001;10:320–324.
4. Johnson JP, Filler AG, Mcbride DQ, Batzdorf U. Anterior cervical foraminotomy for unilateral radicular disease. *Spine.* 2000;25: 905–909.
5. Smith GW, Robinson RA. Anterolateral cervical disc removal and interbody fusion for cervical disc syndrome. *Bull Johns Hopkins Hosp.* 1955;96:223–224.
6. Krupp W, Schattke H, Muke R. Clinical results of the foraminotomy as described by Frykholm for the treatment of lateral cervical disc herniation. *Acta Neurochir (Wien).* 1990;107:22–29.
7. Woertgen C, Holzschuh M, Rothoerl RD, Haeusler E, Brawanski A. Prognostic factors of posterior cervical disc surgery: a prospective, consecutive study of 54 patients. *Neurosurgery.* 1997;40:724–728.
8. Zeidman SM, Ducker TB. Posterior cervical laminoforaminotomy for radiculopathy: review of 172 cases. *Neurosurgery.* 1993;33: 356–362.
9. Herkowitz HN, Kurz LT, Overholt DP. Surgical management of cervical soft disc herniation: a comparison between the anterior and posterior approach. *Spine.* 1990;15:1026–1030.
10. Roh SW, Kim DH, Cardosci AC, Fessler RG. Endoscopic foraminotomy using MED system in cadaveric specimens. *Spine.* 2000;25: 260–264.
11. Adamson TE. Microendoscopic posterior cervical laminoforaminotomy for unilateral radiculopathy: results of a new technique in 100 cases. *J Neurosurg.* 2001;95(suppl 1):51–57.
12 Fessler RG, Khoo LT. Minimally invasive cervical microendoscopic foraminotomy: an initial clinical experience. *Neurosurgery.* 2002; 51(suppl 5):37–45.

8

Microendoscopic Cervical Laminectomy and Laminoplasty

MICK J. PEREZ-CRUET, MICHAEL Y. WANG, AND DINO SAMARTZIS

Compression of the spinal cord from cervical spondylosis was first described in 1911 by Bailey and Casamajor[1] and in 1928 by Stookey,[2] who described a patient made quadriplegic from cervical spinal stenosis compressing the spinal cord. It was 1952, however, when Brain and colleagues[5] described the role of vascular supply to the spinal cord and the manifestation of myelopathic symptoms, that cervical stenosis causing myelopathy was identified as a distinct entity. Lees and Turner[4] further noted the lengthy clinical course of the disease accompanied with a long duration of nonprogressive disability.

Cervical spondylosis is an insidious, progressive disease process that presents with several symptoms frequently refractory to conservative nonoperative treatment (Fig. 8–1). Nevertheless, controversy exists over the optimal choice of surgical treatment for this disorder. Despite nonoperative therapy, posterior decompression is an appropriate treatment option for patients with progressive symptoms; however, traditional methods of cervical decompressive laminectomy require stripping of the posterior cervical muscular, as well as ligamentous attachments to the spine. In so doing, patients experience considerable postoperative pain from muscle spasms and muscle injury. Some patients will go on to develop iatrogenic swan neck deformity, which is particularly prevalent in younger individuals undergoing multilevel posterior cervical decompression. Relatively recent improvements in posterior spinal instrumentation (i.e., lateral mass plates and screw-rod constructs) have made fusion more attractive (Fig. 8–2); however, this method adds considerable cost to the procedure, does nothing to reduce iatrogenic muscle and ligamentous injury, and can result in considerable complications from poor screw placement.

The laminoplasty technique attempts to widen the spinal canal diameter by preserving the posterior spinal elements (i.e., the spinous processes and laminae), while maintaining the dynamic motion of the cervical spine (Fig. 8–3). Open-door expansile laminoplasty was developed by Hirabayashi[5] in 1977 to treat compression of the cervical spinal cord; since then, it has become a treatment of choice for ossification of the posterior longitudinal ligament. Various modifications of this procedure were subsequently developed, all with the aim of increasing the cross-sectional area of the cervical spinal canal.[6,7] Laminoplasty is now most commonly used to address myelopathy due to multilevel degenerative cervical spondylosis. When compared with multilevel laminectomy without fusion, several human and animal studies have found laminoplasty to be superior.[8–10]

When comparing laminoplasty with anterior decompressive procedures, neurologic improvement rates from myelopathy are similar.[11–15] Anterior approaches are advantageous because extrinsic compression is more predominantly ventral and sagittal deformities can be corrected more effectively; however, laminoplasty also offers distinct advantages over anterior surgery when treating multilevel disease. Since there is no formal intersegmental fusion, the incidence of adjacent segment disk degeneration is reduced and there is no risk of a failed arthrodesis. Laminoplasty is also typically performed over four to six spinal segments, so even moderately stenosed segments of the cervical spine are treated without incurring additional morbidity. In addition, complications associated with extensive anterior neck exposures (e.g., laryngeal palsy and dysphagia) are avoided.

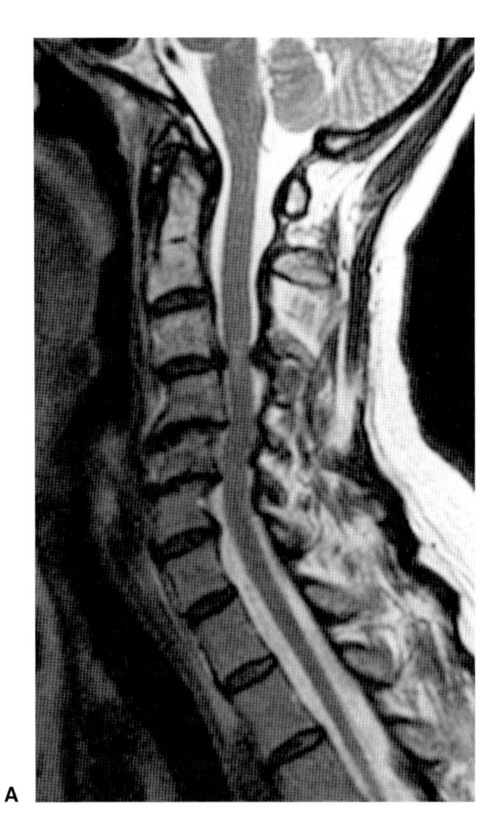
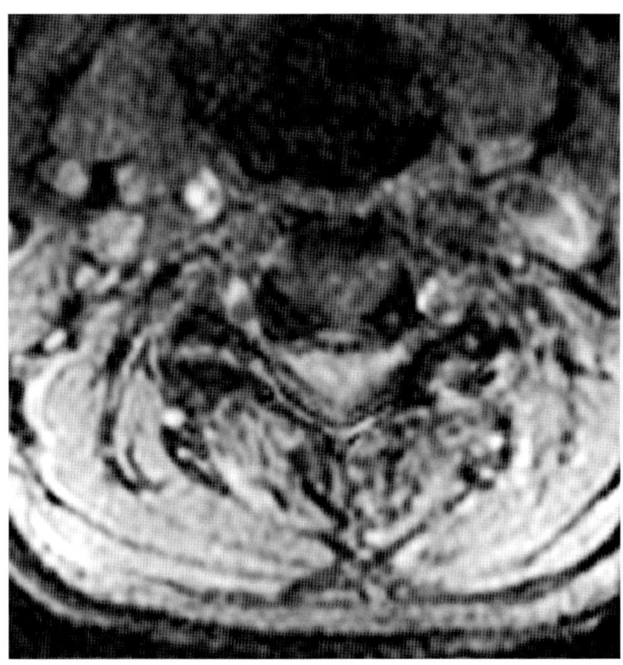

Figure 8–1 T2-weighted magnetic resonance imaging. **(A)** Sagittal, **(B)** axial at C3–C4 level showing cervical spinal cord compression in a patient suffering from cervical spondylotic myelopathy. Note signal changes in the spinal cord at the C3–C4 level.

Despite the advantages of laminoplasty, postoperative axial neck pain and loss of lordosis remain significant drawbacks of this procedure.[16] These complications may be related to the detachment of muscular and ligamentous insertions of the spine when using a posterior approach, and attempts have been made to minimize the soft tissue dissection for surgical exposure. Shiraishi and Yato[17] described a modification of French door laminoplasty that preserves the muscular attachments to the laminae and spinous processes in an attempt to surmount these problems. Tani et al[10] modified the open-door technique so that the midline ligaments remain attached to the spinous processes, which are osteotomized from the laminae in an osteoplastic fashion. Although these techniques preserve the ligamentous anatomy, they still require extensive muscular stripping off the periosteum.

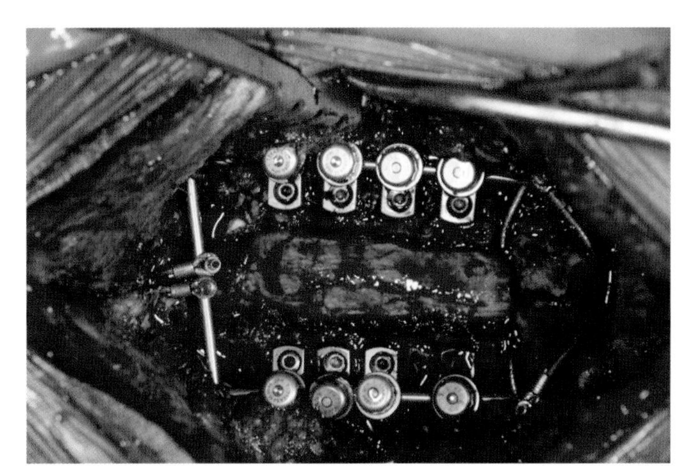

FIGURE 8–2 Intraoperative view showing decompressed spinal cord via laminectomy and lateral mass rod-screw construct overlying fusion bed.

A minimally invasive microendoscopic cervical laminectomy and laminoplasty techniques were developed to address many of the issues encountered with more traditional posterior cervical decompressive approaches (i.e., significant muscle, ligamentous, and bone removal; postoperative pain; and iatrogenic instability). The effectiveness of these techniques was first tested in cadaveric specimens before being applied in the clinical setting. This chapter will review both the cadaveric study and initial clinical experience with these techniques.

Anatomy and Pathophysiology

The cervical spine consists of seven vertebrae. The first two vertebrae (i.e., the atlas and axis) compose the high cervical region and are considered integral components of the craniovertebral junction. These vertebrae are unique in structure and are rarely involved in the degenerative process of cervical spondylosis. Cervical vertebrae C3

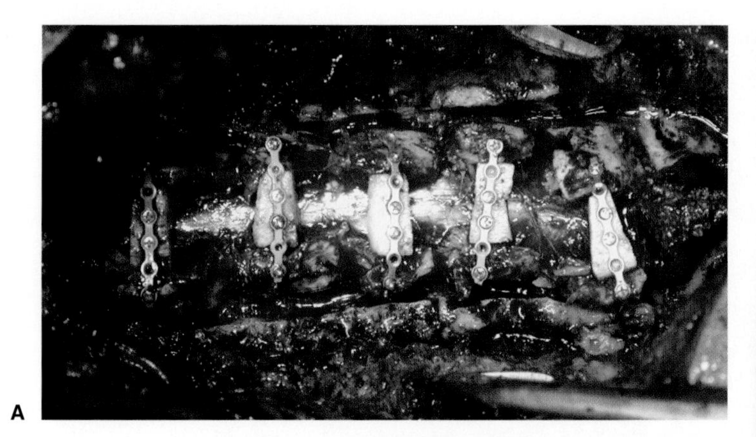

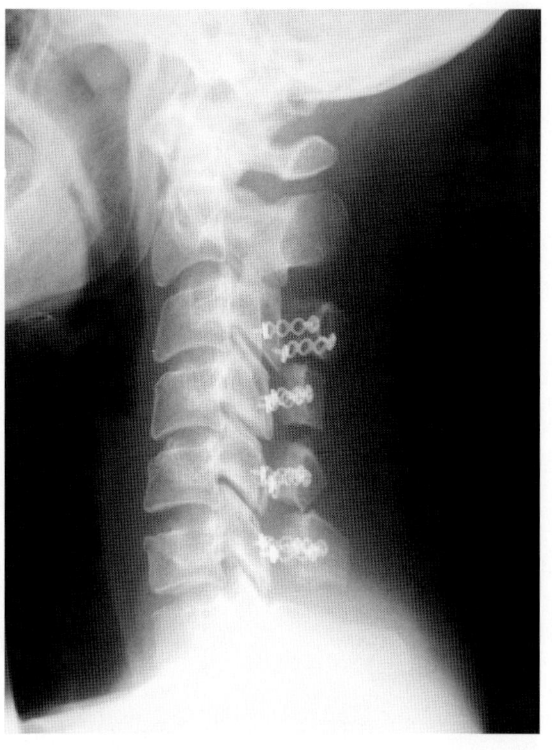

FIGURE 8–3 Laminoplasty technique from C3 to C7 levels. **(A)** Intraoperative decompression of the spinal cord by hinging posterior bone elements toward the left side, and plates to maintain open the hinged segments. **(B)** Postoperative lateral plain x-ray of construct.

through C7, which are otherwise known as the subaxial spine, are distinct from the high cervical vertebrae by the presence of uncovertebral joints and the morphology of the vertebral bodies. The lateral masses of the cervical spine are composed of superior and inferior articular processes, which are thinnest at the C6 and C7 level and have dimensions that increase from depth to height to width.[19] The spinal canal has a triangular configuration with a varied sagittal diameter of ~17 to 18 mm from C3 to C6 to 15 mm at C7.[20–23] In vitro biomechanical testing has determined that the anterior column of the cervical spine transmits 36% of the applied load, whereas each pair of facets transmits 32% of the total load, stressing the importance of the posterior structures in cervical stability.[24]

The diameter of the spinal cord is not uniform in the cervical spine region. The spinal cord occupies one half of the spinal canal at the level of C1. At the C5 to C7 level, the cord expands and occupies three fourths of the canal diameter, which increases the incidence of cord compression at the lower cervical spine. Cailliet[25] determined that cervical spinal canal stenosis is more uniform and restrictive in the diagonal anteroposterior diameter than the transverse. Spinal canal size is a predisposing factor to symptomatic cervical stenosis. Those patients with congenitally smaller canals are potentially at increased risk. A canal AP diameter less than 13 mm has been established as a diagnostic standard of medullary symptoms from spondylotic encroachment.[25,26]

The anterior spinal artery (ASA) provides 60 to 70% of the cervical spinal cord's vascular supply.[27] Although the ASA's midsagittal position is at risk from direct compression from disk protrusion or degenerative hypertrophies, its segmental medullary feeders provide collateral blood flow to enhance cord perfusion. Mannen[28] and Jellinger[29] reported that the lower cervical arteries are more predisposed to artherosclerotic changes.

The normal cervical spine has a sagittal lordotic curvature mainly attributed to the intervertebral disk height, which accounts for 22% of the overall length of the cervical spine. The disk space height is greatest at the anterior aspect of the interspace and accounts for the natural lordotic curvature of the cervical spine. Motion is greatest at the intervertebral disks, and compressive and tensile forces are distributed throughout the cervical spine. Loss of cervical lordosis is often attributed to dehydration of the intervertebral disks and may contribute to altered biomechanical forces throughout the cervical spine, resulting in reactive hyperostosis changes of the adjacent vertebral end plates and development of a spondylotic bar resulting from posterior disk protrusion. Posterior disk herniation may contribute to impingement of the exiting nerve root and produce radiculopathic symptoms. In combination, these physiologic alterations may contribute to overriding of the uncinate processes, leading to destruction of the uncovertebral joint space. Further progression of this degenerative process may lead to subsequent hypertrophy of the facet joints and ligamentum flavum and ossification of the posterior longitudinal ligament. Moreover, manifestation of pain is attributed to compression or stretching of the sinuvertebral nerve and altered integrity or distortion of the apophyseal facet joints, ligamentous elements, and cervical musculature. Furthermore, hypermobility at the adjacent levels may further induce hypertrophy at the respective motion segment and threaten encroachment on the spinal cord and nerve roots.

In addition, the pincher phenomenon entails dynamic contributions that are additive to cord encroachment. In flexion, the AP diameter decreases 2 to 3 mm, and the superior rim of the posterior vertebral body produces tension on the spinal cord. Although tension of the spinal cord is minimized in extension, the cord is susceptible to compression by buckling of the ligamentum flavum. Lateral motion of the neck on the side of compression may further reduce foraminal diameter and produce or exacerbate symptoms. In addition, compensatory subluxation may develop above the level of the rigid spondylotic segment.

Cadaveric Studies and Techniques of Minimally Invasive Laminectomy

Multiple studies of unilateral lumbar laminotomy have demonstrated successful bilateral decompression for spinal stenosis. These investigations involved extensions of the open surgical procedure, which uses a laterally placed incision to access a contralaterally directed trajectory.[30] In this manner, a high-speed drill, Kerrison rongeurs, and curettes can be used to undercut the inner surface of the laminae, affecting a central decompression while preserving all of the midline musculoligamentous structures. In initial clinical studies, effective spinal canal enlargement with concomitant symptom alleviation approximated the results with open surgery. Cadaveric studies using a similar approach have demonstrated that this technique is also feasible in the cervical spine and can result in canal expansion averaging 43%.[31]

Five cadaveric specimens were imaged pre- and postoperatively with CT/myelogram. Approximately 50 cc of Omnipaque contrast agent was injected into the subdural space of the cervical spine, followed by CT imaging. In the cadaver laboratory, the cadaver specimen was placed on a radiolucent table in the prone position with the lateral fluoroscopic C-arm in place. The C4–C5 level was first identified with a spinal needle and lateral fluoroscopic imaging, and a small incision was made ~2 cm lateral to the midline. A K-wire was then passed under fluoroscopic visualization and docked on the C4–C5 lamina-facet junction. The initial muscle dilator was passed over the K-wire and docked securely on bone, and the K-wire was removed. Subsequent dilators were then passed, and an 18 mm diameter tubular retractor was passed over the final dilator and locked in place. The muscle dilators were removed, and

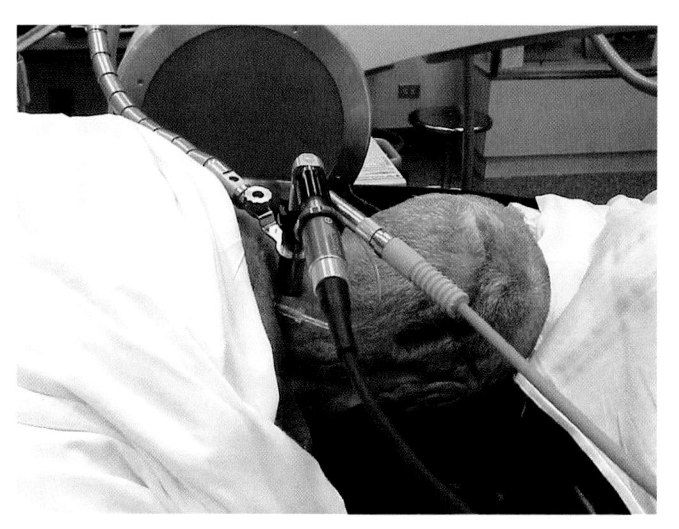

FIGURE 8–4 Endoscopic assembly in place with tubular retractor (Medtronic Sofamor Danek, Memphis, TN) in a cadaveric specimen.

the endoscopic assembly white balanced, focused, and passed down the tube for visualization during the case (Fig. 8–4, Medtronic Sofamor Danek, Memphis, TN). The soft tissue overlying the lamina and medial facet was removed using a Bovie cautery. Fluoroscopic imaging in both the AP and lateral projections was used to aid in proper surgical orientation and location. With the endoscopic assembly facing away from the surgeon, the ipsilateral lamina was removed using a high-speed drill and Kerrison punch. This allowed for good visualization using the 30-degree angulation of the endoscope, as well as for ipsilateral cervical foraminotomy. Wanding the tubular retractor-endoscopic assembly rostral and caudal, a multilevel (up to four levels) unilateral laminectomy was performed (Fig. 8–5) Once the ipsilateral laminectomy was performed, the endoscope was repositioned, facing the surgeon on the tubular retractor. This allowed for contralateral cervical decompression. The spinous process was identified, and drilling of the underside of the spinous process and contralateral lamina was performed. This maintained the bony integrity of the spinous process and contralateral lamina without any muscular or ligamentous removal; therefore, much of the bone, muscular, and ligamentous integrity was presented. This may reduce the incidence of postoperative muscle pain, spasms, and iatrogenic instability seen in more traditional approaches. Postoperative CT-myelogram confirmed adequate cervical-decompression (Fig. 8–6). Open cadaveric dissection revealed adequate spinal cord decompression, while preserving much of the posterior bony and muscular attachments of the cervical spine (Fig. 8–7).

Initial Clinical Experience

The initial clinical experience has been performed on patients with one- and two-level cervical stenosis.

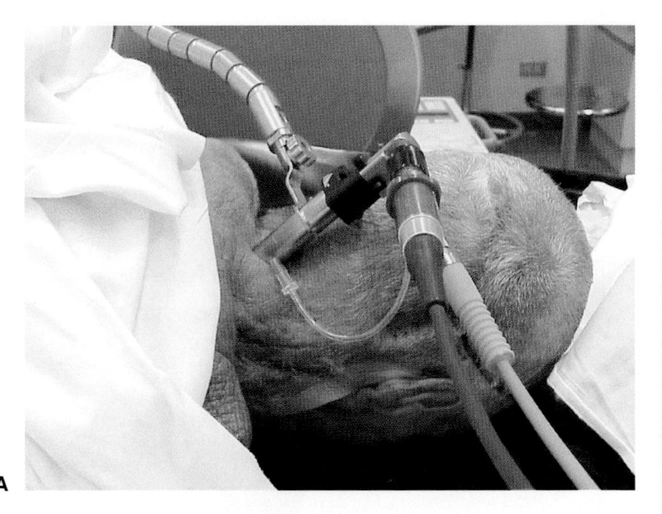

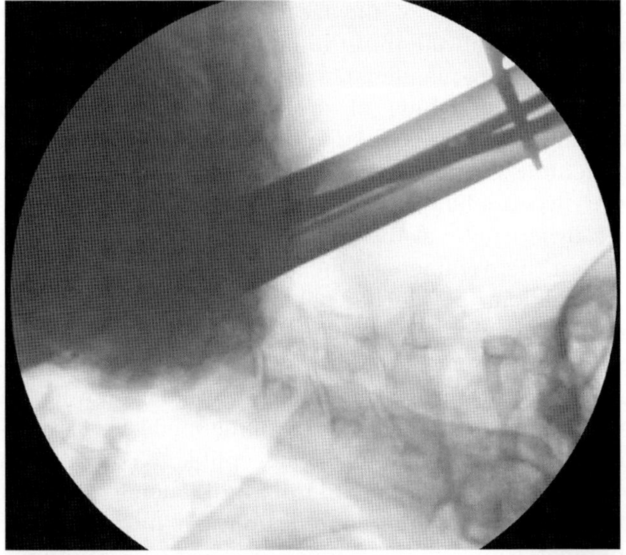

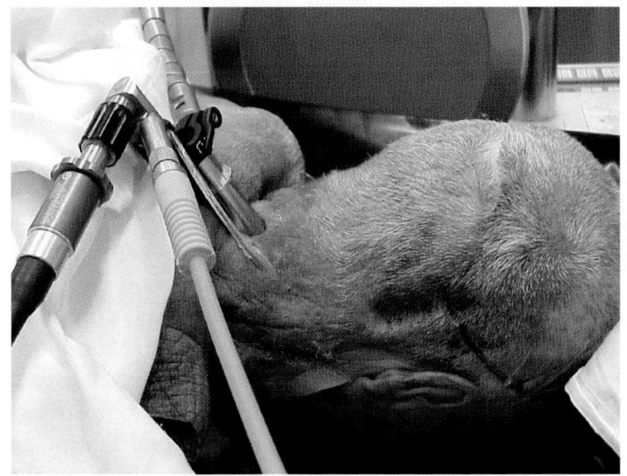

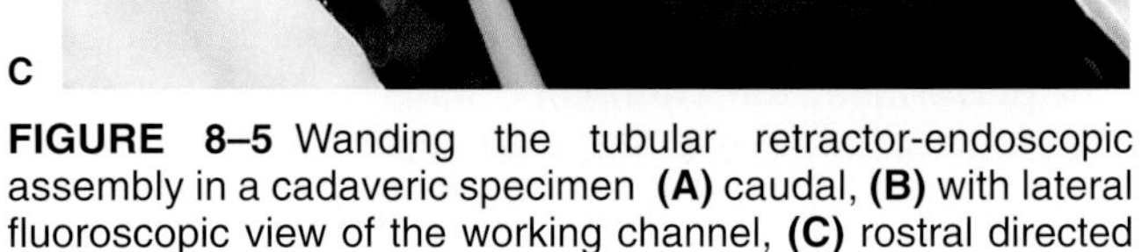

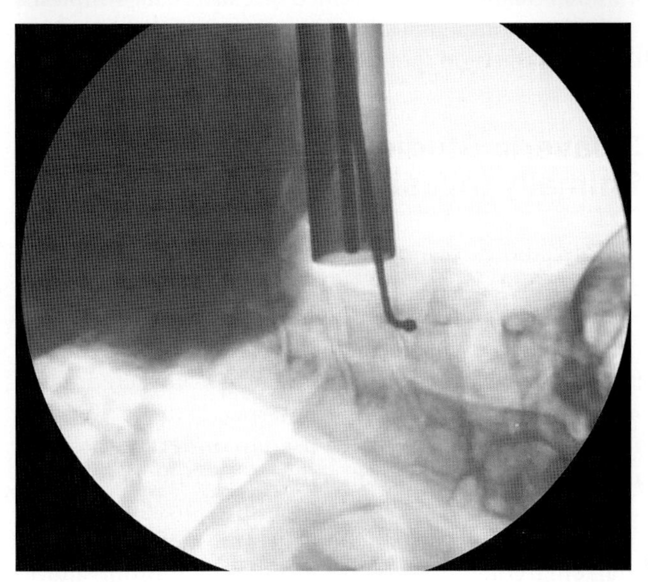

FIGURE 8–5 Wanding the tubular retractor-endoscopic assembly in a cadaveric specimen **(A)** caudal, **(B)** with lateral fluoroscopic view of the working channel, **(C)** rostral directed working channel, **(D)** with lateral fluoroscopic view of the working channel.

Case Illustration

A 52-year-old male presented with right C6 radiculopathy and neck pain. Preoperative MRI revealed stenosis at the C5–C6 level, with a posterior osteophyte causing spinal cord compression. We use an awake, fiberoptic intubation technique in all patients to minimize the risk of iatrogenic cord injury during intubation. The patient's clinical exam is briefly assessed after intubation, prior to sedation. After successful intubation, monitoring lines for intraoperative somatosensory evoked potentials (SSEPs) and motor evoked potentials (MEPs) are placed, and the patient is monitored during positioning. Although this is not infallible, we routinely use intraoperative SSEP and MEP monitoring in laminectomy patients. The patient's head is secured in a Mayfield three-pin head holder, and the patient is then turned in a controlled fashion onto the OR table. The patient in this case underwent a posterior decompressive cervical unilateral laminectomy and right C5–C6 foraminotomy. Intraoperative images revealed the spinal cord and foraminotomy. The patient had resolution of his arm and neck pain postoperatively and returned to work full time.

Cadaveric Studies and Technique of Minimally Invasive Laminoplasty

Our initial studies of minimal access surgery necessarily began in the cadaver laboratory. To investigate mini-

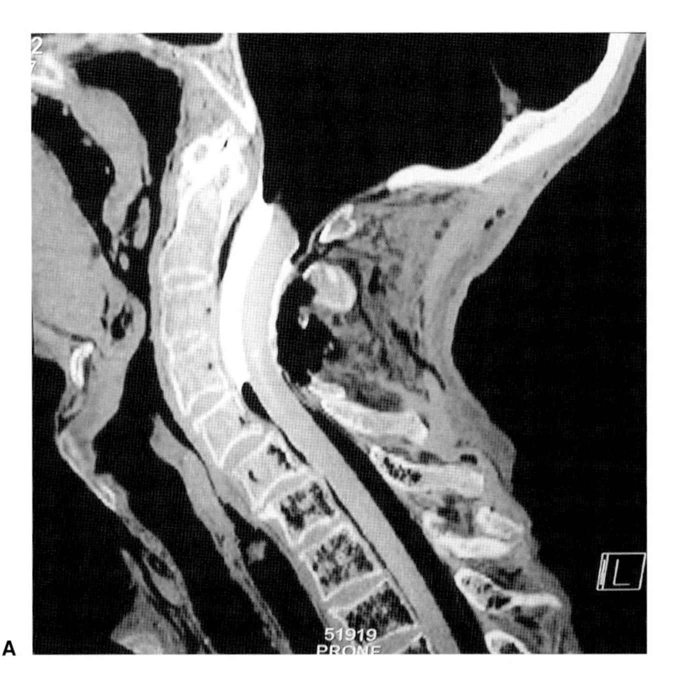

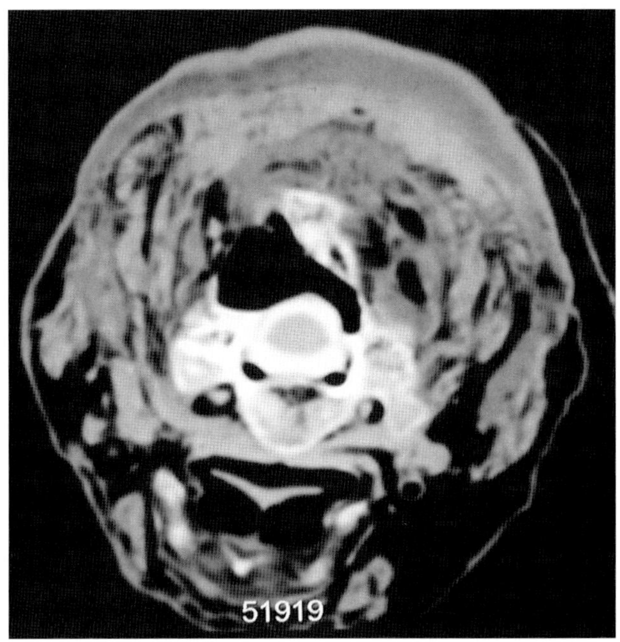

A B

FIGURE 8–6 Postoperative CT-myelogram confirmed adequate cervical decompression. **(A)** Sagittal CT myelogram reconstructed images and **(B)** axial image.

mally invasive laminoplasty, six formalinized human cadavers underwent preoperative spiral axial CT scans from C3 to C7 with 3 mm cuts. None of the cadavers showed evidence of ossification of the posterior longitudinal ligament or spinal stenosis. Stab incisions 2 cm long were made bilaterally at C4–C5 and C5–C6, 2 cm lateral to the midline. A Steinmann pin was then placed into each of these incisions to obtain a medially directed trajectory to the lamina-facet junction. The METRx MD-tubular dilator retractor (Medtronic Sofamor Danek, Memphis, TN) system was then inserted and dilated up to the 22 mm diameter port. The laminae and facets were then visualized, and any intervening soft tissue was removed with pituitary rongeurs. By manipulating the tubular retractor to favor either a rostral or a caudal trajectory in the sagittal plane, exposure of one or two segments above and below the level of the incision was possible. Visualization was aided by the use of an operating microscope. A 3 mm longitudinal trough at the lamina-facet junction was drilled with a G8–130 bit (Medtronic Midas Rex, Fort Worth, TX) through both the inner and outer cortices. This process was repeated through each of the four incisions to prepare for dorsal elevation of the five laminae from C3 to C7. On the open-door side of the laminoplasty, the ligamentum flavum was removed at the lamina-facet junction with a 1 mm Kerrison rongeur. The ligamentum flavum was left undisturbed on the hinge side to prevent collapse of the dorsal construct into the spinal canal. The laminae were then lifted en bloc from this side with a curved curette, and a 10 mm length spacer was fashioned at C4 and C6 from rib allograft inserted to maintain the dorsal elevation of the laminae (Fig. 8–8).

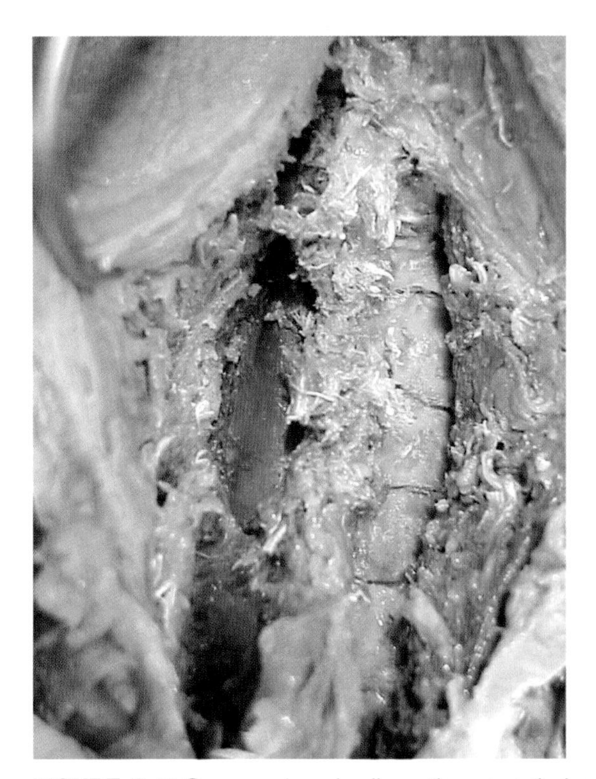

FIGURE 8–7 Open cadaveric dissection revealed adequate spinal cord decompression, while preserving much of the posterior bony and muscular attachments of the cervical spine.

Postprocedure spiral axial CT scans were obtained from C3 to C7 with 3 mm cuts (Fig. 8–9). CT images were

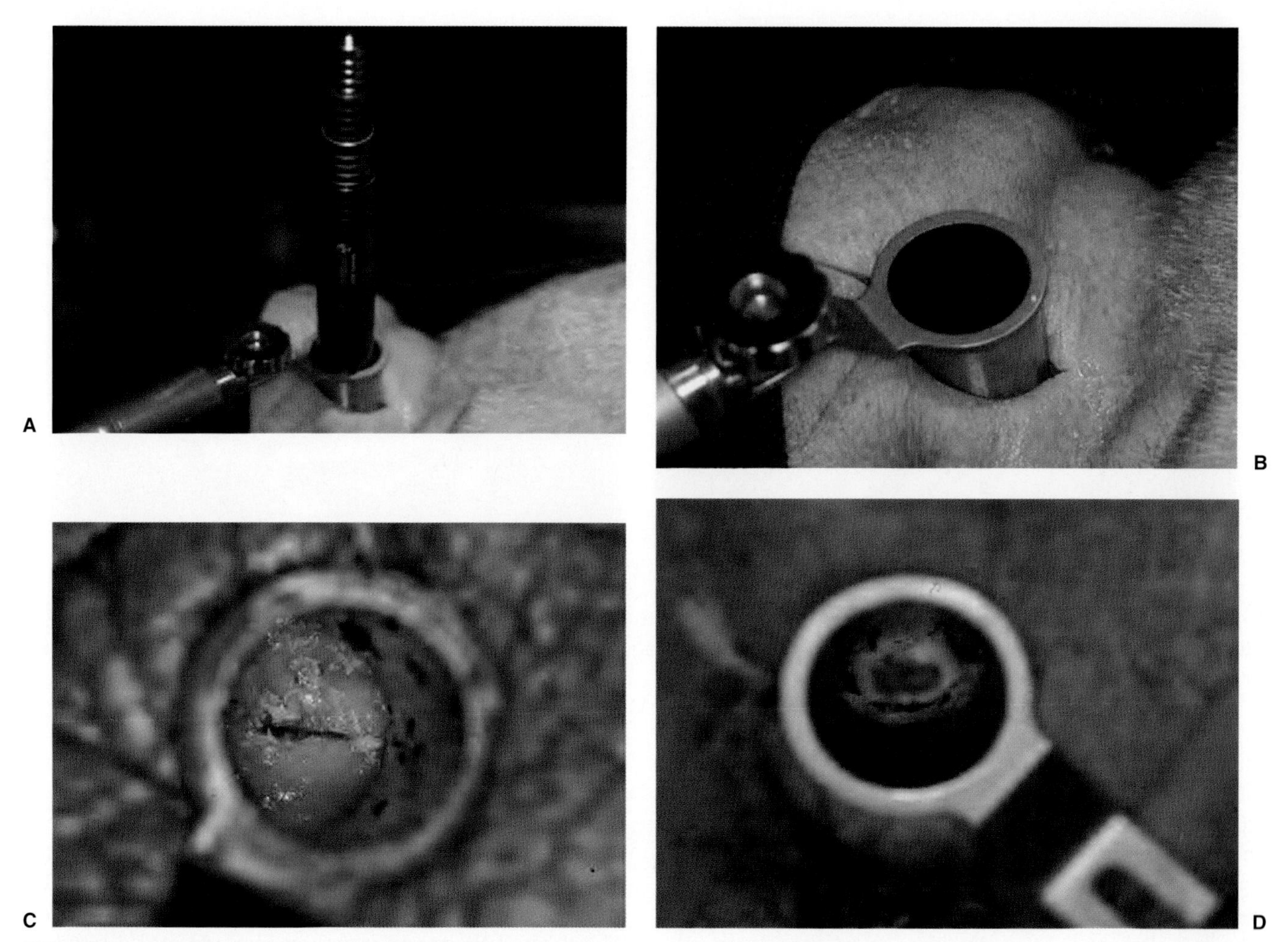

FIGURE 8–8 (A,B) Placement of METRx MD dilators in the cervical spine. **(C)** View of a facet joint through the tubular retractor. **(D)** A 10 mm rib allograft placed between the lamina and facet.

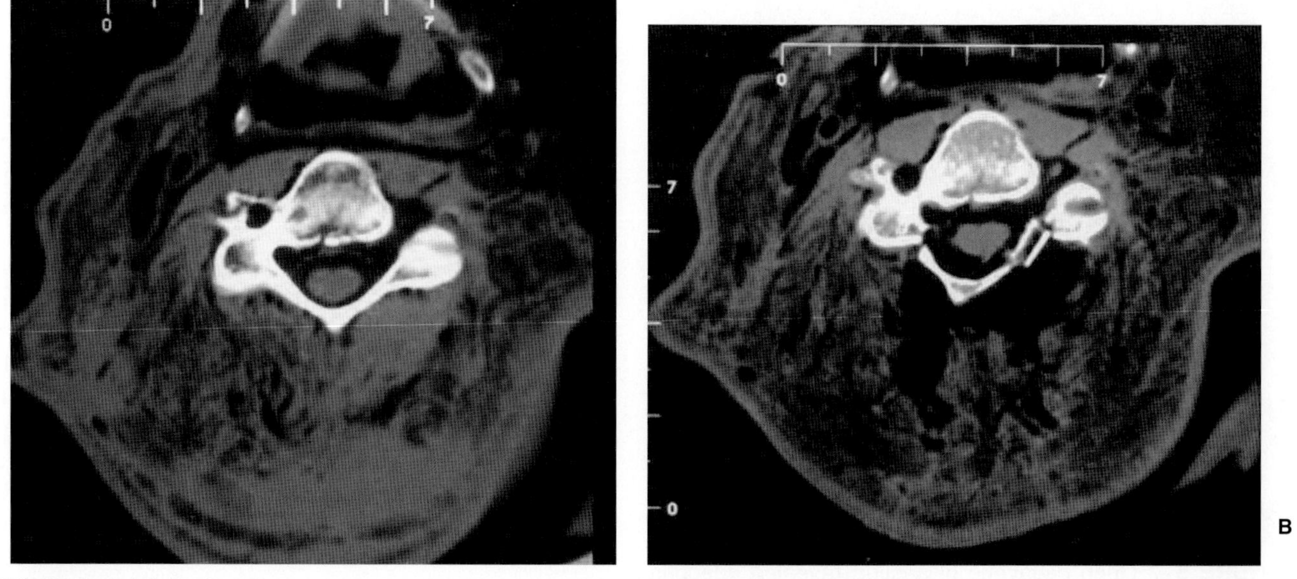

FIGURE 8–9 (A) Cadaveric preoperative axial CT scan at C5. **(B)** CT scan after placement of a 10 mm rib allograft to elevate the lamina.

TABLE 8–1 Morphologic Changes in the Spinal Canal following Minimally Invasive Laminoplasty

	Preoperative		Postoperative	
	Area (cm^2)	Sagittal Diameter (cm)	Area (cm^2)	Sagittal Diameter (cm)
Specimen # 1	2.19	1.15	3.01	1.80
Specimen # 2	2.32	1.21	2.89	1.66
Specimen # 3	2.53	1.35	3.13	1.60
Specimen # 4	1.99	1.38	3.27	1.89
Specimen # 5	1.94	1.20	3.10	1.70
Specimen # 6	1.95	1.16	3.14	1.63
Average	2.15	1.24	3.09	1.71
Increase in canal size			43%	38%

then digitally analyzed using ImageJ software (National Institutes of Health, Bethesda, MD). Image measurements were obtained directly from the CT scans and were calibrated to the reference scale on the CT images by determining pixels per millimeter. Midsagittal dimensions were measured at the C5 level, and the canal area was estimated from a computer-drawn perimeter of the inner bony margins. Statistical analysis was performed with a paired *t*-test.

All six cadaver spines were reconstructed successfully using this minimally invasive approach. Exposure, drilling, elevation of the laminae, and spacer placement could be accomplished through a total of four stab incisions (two bilaterally) in each case. Exposure of three or four adjacent laminae via a single incision was accomplished without difficulty, and a 10 mm high rib allograft was successfully placed to maintain elevation of the lamina in each case. The difficulty of the procedure was directly related to the depth of the retractor needed to span the skin surface to laminar distance. Those cadavers with thick, muscular necks required the longer 5 cm tubular retractor, and placement of the rib graft was considerably more difficult in these specimens. No dural violations were evident.

The preoperative spinal canal area averaged 2.15 cm^2, and sagittal diameter averaged 1.24 cm at the C5 level. Postoperative spinal canal area averaged 3.09 cm^2 and sagittal diameter averaged 1.71 cm at the C5 level (Table 8–1). This reflected a 43% increase in spinal canal area and a 38% increase in sagittal diameter. These changes reflected a significant increase in canal diameter ($p = .0001$) and area ($p = .0004$).

TABLE 8–2 Minimally Invasive Laminoplasty Patients

	Age	Pathology	Pre	Post	Complications
Patient # 1	43 M	Cervical spondylotic myelopathy	3	2	None
Patient # 2	58 F	Cervical spondylotic myelopathy	4	2	None
Patient # 3	63 M	Cervical spondylotic myelopathy	3	1	None
Patient # 4	60 F	Cervical spondylotic myelopathy	2	2	Dural tear

Minimally Invasive Laminoplasty Clinical Experience

Our initial experience with minimally invasive laminoplasty is limited to four patients (Table 8–2). All procedures were performed to treat cervical spondylotic myelopathy with associated gait abnormalities. The surgical procedure was identical to the cadaveric study, with laminar osteotomies performed from C3 to C7 (Fig. 8–10). Spacers were placed at C4 and C6.

There was a mean improvement of 1.25 points on the Nurick score. Complications were limited to a single case with a dural laceration. This was treated without primary repair and did not result in transcutaneous CSF leakage. Technical challenges encountered included difficulty with lifting of the laminae, limiting the spacer height to less than 11 mm (Fig. 8–11).

Discussion

Cervical spondylosis may be the most common underdiagnosed spine disorder whose true incidence is unknown. The majority of patients present in the fifth decade of life, but the condition is not limited therein and is indiscriminant of age and degree of disease manifestation.[32,33] Levels below C3–C4 are primarily affected, with predominance at C5–C6, followed by C6–C7 and C4–C5.[34] Spondylotic manifestations are evident radiologically in 25 to 50% of the population by age 50, and they are seen in as many as 85% of individuals by their mid-60s.[35,36] Several disorders may mimic the symptoms of cervical spondylosis and need to be differentiated for proper diagnosis. Such disorders include torticollis, athetosis, chronic dystonia, cerebral palsy, syringomyelia, low-pressure hydrocephalus, cerebral hemisphere lesion, amyotrophic lateral sclerosis, Down syndrome, multiple sclerosis, and neoplastic lesions.

Several variables have been reported to affect surgical outcome, including patient age, duration of symptoms, levels of myelographic block, extent of cord signal change, severity of myelopathy, transverse area of the spinal cord, and canal diameter.[37–42] Compression of the spinal cord can be due in part to pathology located anterior, posterior, or lateral to dynamic factors.

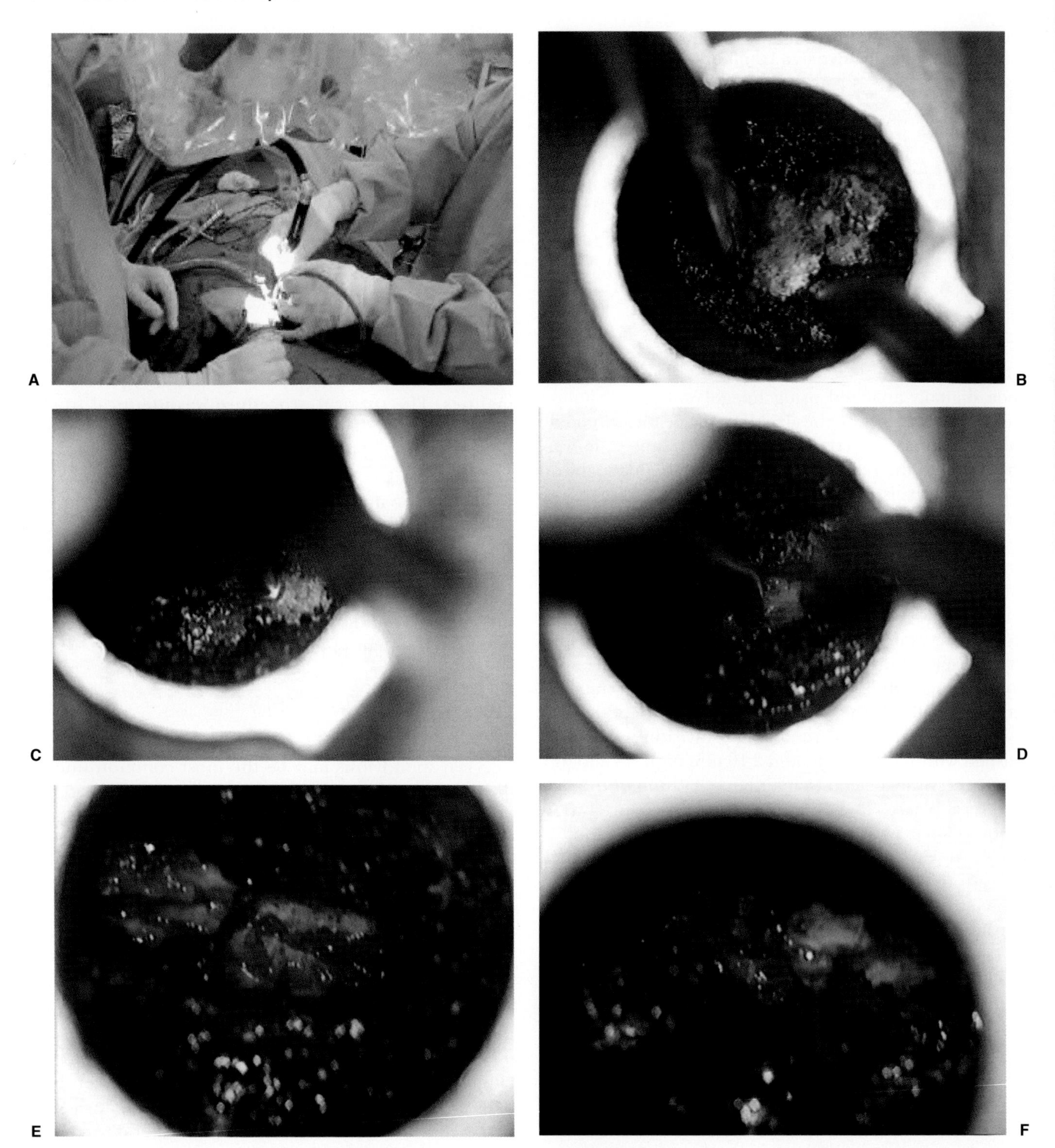

FIGURE 8–10 **(A)** View through the operating microscope showing **(B)** exposed lamina-facet junction, **(C)** drilling of lamina, **(D)** palpation of ligamentum flavum, **(E)** exposed dura with epidural vein, **(F)** lifting of lamina with curette,

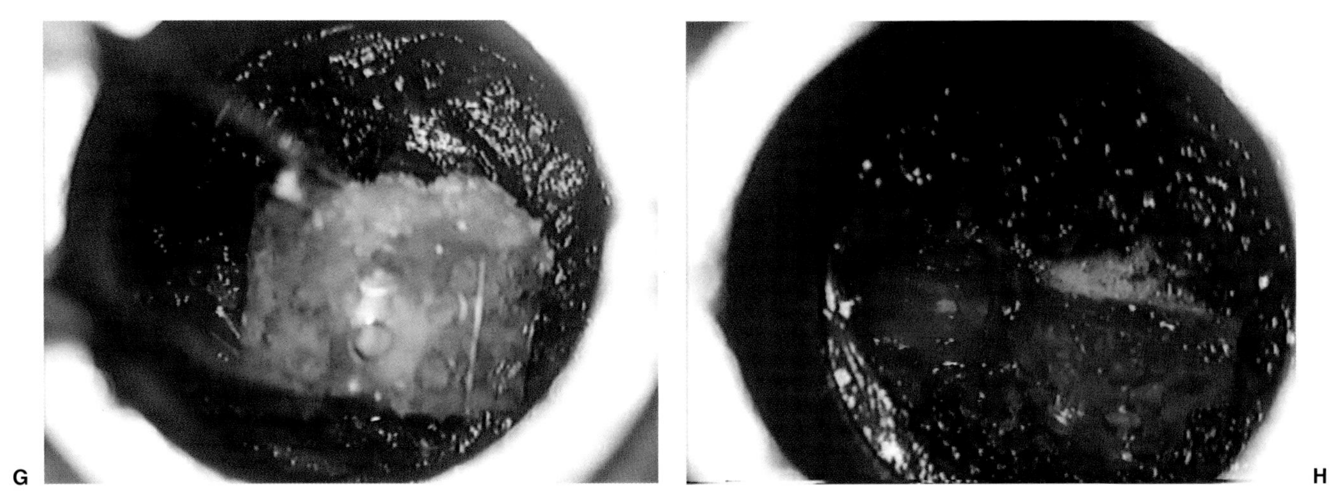

FIGURE 8–10 (*Continued*) **(G)** initial spacer placement, and **(H)** final spacer position.

Surgical treatment can be by either an anterior or a posterior approach. The anterior approach consists of decompression and interbody or strut grafting with or without instrumentation.[43–46] The posterior approach consists of laminoplasty or laminectomy with fusion with or without internal fixation. The selection of the approach is often dependent upon surgeon preference, the source of cord compressing (i.e., either anterior or posterior), the age of the patient, the number of vertebral levels involved, and maintenance of lordotic alignment. The anterior approach is recommended in cases of kyphotic curvature. The posterior approach is preferred in cases with preserved lordosis and more than three levels of involvement. The principle advantage to the posterior approach is its relative ease and familiarity by most spinal surgeons. This approach has been clearly established as a safe and effective means of decompressing the cervical spinal cord and nerve roots.[47–49] Nonetheless, the efficacy of any surgical approach is to maintain spinal stability and provide sufficient decompression without compromise to sagittal balance.

Cervical laminectomy may result in instability and progressive kyphotic deformity in some adults, particularly when extensive resection of facets has been performed.[50,51] In particular, progressive kyphotic deformity and cervical instability are common in children following laminectomy.[50,52,53] Bone grafting and internal

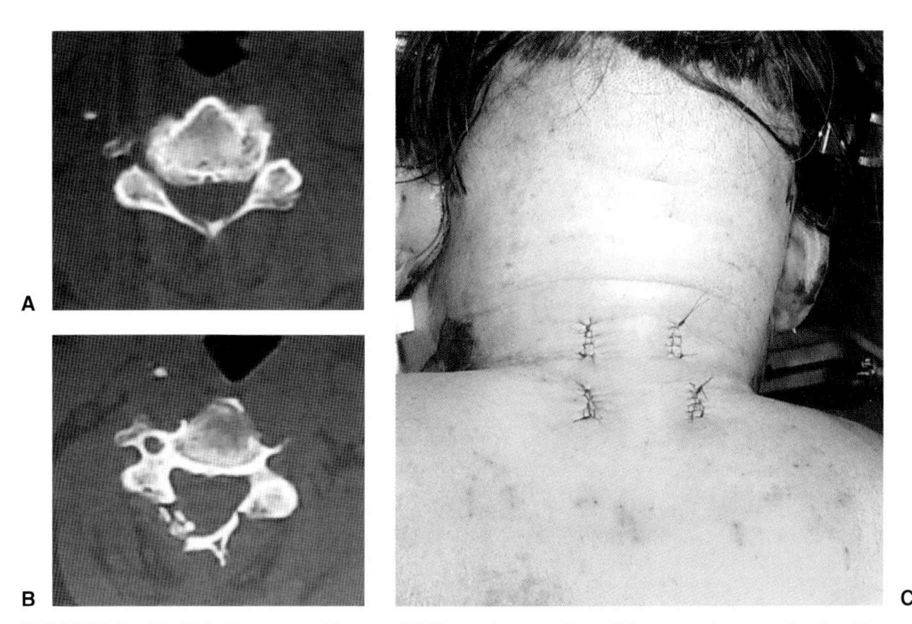

FIGURE 8–11 **(A)** Preoperative and **(B)** postoperative CT scans in a patient with cervical spondylotic myelopathy who underwent minimally invasive cervical laminoplasty. **(C)** Four skin incisions used for access in the posterior neck.

fixation using lateral mass plates have been reported to prevent the development of postlaminectomy instability and deformity.[54] Some authors believe development of a postlaminectomy membrane may yield late deterioration after laminectomy with or without fusion.[55]

Postoperative Kyphosis

Although cases of symptomatic postlaminectomy kyphosis are well described, their incidence and relevance are unclear in the literature.[56] The addition of fusion to the laminectomy procedure obviates these concerns.[54,57] Three groups of patients are at significant risk of developing postlaminectomy instability or spinal deformity: individuals under 25 years of age, trauma cases, and laminectomies combined with extensive facet dissection.[57]

The development of postlaminectomy kyphosis is a significant risk in younger patients.[50,58,59] According to Cattell and Clark,[50] children are predisposed to instability due to skeletal and ligamentous laxity, neuromuscular imbalance, and the formation of bone deformities as a consequence of osseous development. Adults may not be susceptible to similar patterns of spinal degeneration because of ligamentous changes with aging. Yasuoka et al[53] report 90% of patients less than 15 years of age undergoing cervical or cervicothoracic laminectomy developed kyphotic spinal deformity. All patients less than 15 years of age with cervical laminectomy alone developed kyphosis. Significantly fewer patients older than 15 years of age developed spinal deformity after laminectomy. Excluding trauma cases and cases with facetectomy, no adult patient developed spinal deformity significant enough to require fusion.[52]

In adult patients, development of postlaminectomy spinal deformity clearly correlates with facet disruption or resection. In cadaver studies, resection of greater than 50% of the facet joint and capsule is associated with acute instability.[60,61] Herkowitz[62] reported a 25% incidence of kyphotic deformity within 2 years following cervical laminectomy and partial bilateral facetectomies. Capsule resection alone also results in increased cervical motion in cadaver studies.[63] Less severe destabilization of the cervical spine, perhaps yielding slowly progressive deformity in spinal alignment, may be expected with less severe facet joint and capsule injury.

Many cases have been reported of symptomatic postlaminectomy cervical kyphosis. Development of instability and spinal deformity may produce late deterioration in postlaminectomy patients.[63–65] Adams and Logue[66] correlated late deterioration in laminectomy patients with increased postoperative cervical spine motion. Numerous series attest to a late deterioration in postlaminectomy patients, with some series reporting up to 50% of patients affected;[66–68] however, kyphotic deformities may remain asymptomatic. Kaptain et al[69] reported a postlaminectomy kyphosis rate of 21% and noted no correlation between postoperative alignment and clinical outcome. In their report of long-term follow-up of cervical laminectomy patients, Crandall and Gregorius[49] found significant rates of early and late deterioration. They did not emphasize development of instability in their patient population; instead, they offered only limited radiographic follow-up.

Laminectomy with Fusion and Instrumentation

Due to concerns over postoperative worsening of spinal alignment following laminectomy alone, the addition of fusion to the procedure was added to prevent delayed malalignment and loss of sagittal balance. A variety of fusion techniques have been offered in the literature, including facet wiring, lateral mass plate fixation, and polyaxial screw and rod fixation. All share the goal of immediate cervical fixation to promote bone fusion.

Goel et al[51] demonstrated in a cadaver model that posterior facet wiring limits the immediate instability generated by laminectomy. Kumar et al[54] found no instability, progression of spinal deformity, or late clinical deterioration after laminectomy with lateral mass plate fusion in a long-term follow-up of laminectomy with fusion patients.

Appropriate application of lateral mass plating screws has been scrutinized in an attempt to obtain proper placement, avoid neural and vascular injury, and ascertain optimal fixation. Two widely used techniques by Roy-Camille and Magerl have been established as relatively safe and effective;[70] however, in a comparison of these two techniques by Heller et al,[70] a 10.8 and 26.8% risk for nerve root injury was found to exist with the Roy-Camille and Magerl techniques, respectively. Moreover, the technique by Magerl was noted to have fewer facet joint violations, but proper screw trajectory was difficult to obtain at the cervicothoracic junction. To address such concerns, An et al[19] proposed an alternative to these established screw placement techniques and noted that anatomical variations do exist, accounting for inconsistent interfacet distances commonly implemented as markers in screw trajectory methods. Nonetheless, instrumentation-related complications are always a concern, as well as the potential for loss of cervical alignment, nerve injury, facet penetration, pseudarthrosis, and iatrogenic foraminal stenois.[71–73] Lateral mass plating, however, has the capability for restoring lordosis.[74–76] Coupled with fusion, lateral mass plating further minimizes the risk of kyphotic deformity and instability. Kumar et al[54] presented 25 patients with lateral mass plate fusion, with follow-up on average at 47.5 months after laminectomy. Most patients presented with gait difficulty, upper extremity and hand weakness, and sensory disturbances. Eighty percent of patients had good outcomes, and 76%

of patients had improved myelopathy scores. Moreover, no patient developed spinal deformity and patients with preoperative kyphosis or S-shaped deformities remained stable. There were no late deteriorations.

Laminoplasty

Cervical laminectomy has been an established procedure providing sufficient decompression; however, extensive cervical laminectomy pitfalls entail sagittal curvature alterations that may contribute to progressive kyphotic deformity, instability resulting in compromise or destruction of bony or ligamentous structures, and scar tissue or perineural adhesions. Cervical laminoplasty has been developed in an attempt to diminish the complications and poor outcomes associated with laminectomies. Hattori[77] first described laminoplasty in 1973 by his illustration of a Z-shaped method. The procedure generated interest in this technique and led to numerous laminoplasty variations, primarily from Japan, which are best classified as Z-shaped, midline or bilateral, and unilateral. The laminoplasty technique preserves posterior bony elements and spinoligamentous structures and minimizes muscle detachment, thus reducing the event of postoperative kyphotic deformity and instability often associated with laminectomy. Multilevel radiculopathy, myeloradiculopathy, and multilevel cerebrospinal meningitis (CSM) are indications for laminoplasty; however, an anterior approach is preferred for bilateral radiculopathy. Laminoplasty is thought to be a viable option if cervical lordosis is maintained with minimal to no preexisting neck pain. Additional indications for using the laminoplasty technique include involvement of more than three vertebral levels, CSM in younger patients, ossification of the posterior longitudinal ligament, and thickening of the ligamentum flavum.

Although various laminoplasty techniques have been developed and vary based on the location of the "hinge" to maintain the opening, an "open door" or unilateral laminoplasty is a common procedure whose initial exposure and intraoperative patient positioning are the same as the aforementioned laminectomy technique. The unilateral laminoplasty involves removal of the tips of the spinous processes of the involved levels and bilateral thinning at the lamina-facet junction to the inner cortex with a high-speed burr.[78] An opening is selected based on the patient's dominant symptomatic side, and a hinge is maintained by preserving the inner cortical laminar layer. A vertebral spreader is then used to open the canal by reflecting the ipsilateral cut lamina, spinous process, and contralateral "green sticked" lamina to the contralateral side in an open-hinged fashion. As the canal is opened, the ligamentum flavum and soft tissue adhesions are carefully resected. It is often necessary to cut the most caudal and rostral ligamentous attachments to hinge the posterior spinous structures freely. Once opened, bone grafts, struts, sutures, plating, or a combination of such can be used to maintain the opening.

Although the risks of instability still remain, complications associated with laminectomy are reduced with laminoplasty. Matsunaga et al[79] noted that laminectomy had a 33% incidence of a buckling-type alignment, compared with 6% following laminoplasty. Unlike laminectomy following fusion and instrumentation, range of motion is preserved following laminoplasty.[10,80] This may be an advantage, particularly in younger patients with CSM. Nevertheless, complications may exist with laminoplasty and may arise in open-door settling, epidural hematoma formation, and nerve root injury.[81]

Several techniques exist for the treatment of cervical stenosis. Posterior approaches do afford the advantage of being familiar to spine surgeons. The techniques of laminectomy, laminectomy with fusion and instrumentation, and laminoplasty have advantages and disadvantages, as reviewed in this chapter; however, these traditional techniques require extensive muscle dissection, resulting in muscle denervation, atrophy, and postoperative pain. The microendoscopic cervical laminectomy and laminoplasty procedures described in this chapter are encouraging further development of less-invasive spinal techniques that result in less postoperative pain, quicker recoveries, maintainance of dynamic spinal motion, and reduced iatrogenic instability by maintaining the normal musculature, bone, and ligamentous anatomy of the cervical spine. Further clinical studies are required in accessing the clinical efficacy of these techniques for the treatment of cervical stenosis.

REFERENCES

1. Bailey P, Casamajor L. Osteoarthritis of the spine as a cause of compression of the spinal cord and its roots. *J Nerve Ment Dis* 1911;38:588.
2. Stookey B. Compression of the spinal cord due to ventral extradural cervical chordomas. *Arch Neurol Psychiatry* 1928;20:275–291.
3. Brain WR, Northfield D, Wilkinson M. The neurological manifestations of cervical spondylosis. *Brain* 1952;75:187–225.
4. Lees F, Turner JWA. Natural history and prognosis of cervical spondylosis. *Br Med J* 1963;2:1607–1610.
5. Hirabayashi K. Expansive open-door laminoplasty for cervical spondylotic myelopathy (Japanese). *Jpn J Surg* 1978;32:1159–1163.
6. White AA, Panjabi M. Biomechanical considerations in the surgical management of cervical spondylotic myelopathy. *Spine* 1988;13:856–860.
7. Baisden J, Voo LM, Cusick JF, et al. Evaluation of cervical laminectomy and laminoplasty. A longitudinal study in the goat model. *Spine* 1999;24:1283–1288; discussion 1288–1289.
8. Fields M, Hoshijima K, Feng A, et al. A biomechanical, radiologic, and clinical comparison of outcome after multilevel laminectomy or laminoplasty in the rabbit. *Spine* 2000;22:2925–2931.
9. Heller J, Edwards W, Murakami H, et al. Laminoplasty versus laminectomy and fusion for multilevel cervical myelopathy. *Spine* 2001;26:1330–1336.

10. Herkowitz HN. A comparison of anterior cervical fusion, cervical laminectomy, and cervical laminoplasty for the surgical management of multiple level spondylotic radiculopathy. *Spine* 1988; 13:774–780.
11. Kawakami M, Tamaki T, Iwasaki H, et al. A comparative study of surgical approaches for cervical compressive myelopathy. *Clin Orthop* 2000:129–136.
12. Lee TT, Manzano GR, Green BA. Modified open-door cervical expansive laminoplasty for spondylotic myelopathy: Operative technique, outcome and predictors for gait improvement. *J Neurosurg* 1997;86:64–68.
13. Yonenobu K, Hosono N, Iwasaki M, et al. Laminoplasty versus subtotal corpectomy. A comparative study of results in multisegmental cervical spondylotic myelopathy. *Spine* 1992;17:1281–1284.
14. Yoshida M, Tamaki T, Kawakami M, et al. Indication and clinical results of laminoplasty for cervical myelopathy caused by disc herniation with developmental canal stenosis. *Spine* 1998;23:2391– 2397.
15. Hosono N, Yonenobu K, Ono K. Neck and shoulder pain after laminoplasty: A noticeable complication. *Spine* 1996;21:1969– 1973.
16. Shiraishi T. Skip laminectomy—a new treatment for cervical spondylotic myelopathy, preserving bilateral muscular attachments to the spinous processes: a preliminary report. *Spine J* 2002;2: 108–115.
17. Shiraishi T, Fukuda K, Yato Y, et al. Results of skip laminectomy-minimum 2-year follow-up study compared with open-door laminoplasty. *Spine* 2003;28:2667–2672.
18. Tani S, Isoshima A, Nagashima Y, et al. Laminoplasty with preservation of posterior cervical elements: surgical technique. *Neurosurgery* 2002;50:97–101; discussion 101–102.
19. An HS, Gordin R, Renner K. Anatomic considerations for plate-screw fixation of the cervical spine. *Spine* 1991;16 (Suppl):S548– S551.
20. Boijsen E. The cervical spinal canal in intraspinal expansive processes. *Acta Radiol* 1954;42:101–115.
21. Burrows EH. The sagittal diameter of the spinal canal in cervical spondylosis. *Clin Radiol* 1963;14:1963.
22. Chrispin A, Lees F. The spinal canal in cervical spondylosis. *J Neurol Neurosurg Psychiatry* 1963;26:166–170.
23. Panjabi MM, Duranceau J, Goel V, et al. Cervical human vertebrae: Quantitative three-dimensional anatomy of the middle and lower regions. *Spine* 1991;16:861–869.
24. Pal GP, Sherk HH. The vertical stability of the cervical spine. *Spine* 1988;13:447–449.
25. Cailliet R. Neck and Arm Pain. 2nd ed. Philadelphia: F.A. Davis Co.; 1981.
26. Ferguson RJL, Caplan LR. Cervical spondylotic myelopathy. *Neurol Clin* 1985;3:373–382.
27. Parke WW. Correlative anatomy of cervical spondylotic myelopathy. *Spine* 1988;13:831–837.
28. Mannen T. Vascular lesions in the spinal cord of the aged. *Geriatrics* 1966;21:151–160.
29. Jellinger K. Spinal cord arterioscleroses and progressive vascular myelopathy. *J Neurol Neurosurg Psychiatry* 1967;30:195–206.
30. Khoo LT, Fessler RG. Microendoscopic decompressive laminotomy for the treatment of lumbar stenosis. *Neurosurg* 2002;51:146–154.
31. Perez-Cruet M, Sandhu F, Kelly K, et al. Minimally invasive multilevel decompressive cervical laminectomy. Paper presented at: Annual Meeting of the AANS/CS Joint Spine Section; March 3–5, 2003; Tampa, FL.
32. Clarke E, Robinson PK. Cervical myelopathy: a complication of cervical spondylosis. *Brain* 1956;79:483–510.
33. Crandall PH, Batzdorf U. Cervical spondylotic myelopathy. *J Neurosurg* 1966;25:57–66.
34. DePalma AF, Rothman R. The Intervertebral Disk. Philadelphia: WB Saunders; 1970.
35. Friedenberg ZB, Miller WT. Degenerative disease of the cervical spine. *J Bone Joint Surg* 1963;45A:1171–1178.
36. Payne EE, Spillane JD. The cervical spine: An anatomicopathological study of 70 specimens (using special techniques) with particular reference to the problems of cervical spondylosis. *Brain* 1957;80:571–596.
37. Fujiwara K, Yonenobu K, Ebara S, et al. The prognosis of surgery for cervical compression myelopathy. *J Bone Joint Surg [Br]* 1989;71: 393–398.
38. Koyanagi T, Hirabayashi K, Satomi K, et al. Predictability of operative results of cervical compression myelopathy based on preoperative computed tomographic myelography. *Spine* 1993;18:1958–1963.
39. Matsuda Y, Miyazaki K, Tada K, et al. Increased MR signal intensity due to cervical myelopathy: analysis of 29 surgical cases. *J Neurosurg* 1991;74:887–892.
40. Mehalic TF, Pezzuti RT, Applebaum BI. Magnetic resonance imaging and cervical spondylotic myelopathy. *Neurosurgery* 1990;26: 217–227.
41. Morio Y, Teshima R, Nagashima H, et al. Correlation between operative outcomes of cervical myelopathy and MRI of the spinal cord. *Spine* 2001;26:1238–1245.
42. Wada E, Yonenobu K, Suzuki S, et al. Can intramedullary signal changes on MRI predict surgical outcomes in cervical spondylotic myelopathy? *Spine* 1999;24:455–461.
43. Bohler J. Sofort und Frubehandlung traumatischer Querschmnitt lahmungen. *Z Orthopad Grengebiete* 1967;103:512–528.
44. Bohler J, Gaudernak T. Anterior plate stabilization for fracture-dislocations of the lower cervical spine. *J Trauma* 1980;20:203–205.
45. Cloward RB. The anterior approach for ruptured cervical discs. *J Neurosurg* 1958;15:602–617.
46. Robinson R, Smith G. Anterolateral cervical disc removal and interbody fusion for cervical disc syndrome. *Bull Johns Hopkins Hosp* 1955;96:223–224.
47. Benzel EC, Lancon J, Kesterson L, et al. Cervical laminectomy and dentate ligament section for cervical spondylotic myelopathy. *J Spinal Disord* 1991;4:286–295.
48. Carol MP, Ducker TB. Cervical spondylitic myelopathies: surgical treatment. *J Spinal Disord* 1988;1:59–65.
49. Crandall PH, Gregorious FK. Long-term follow-up of surgical treatment of cervical spondylotic myelopathy. *Spine* 1977;2:139–146.
50. Cattell H, Clark GL. Cervical kyphosis and instability following multiple laminectomies in children. *J Bone Joint Surg* 1967;49:713–720.
51. Katsumi Y, Honma T, Nakamura T. Analysis of cervical instability resulting from laminectomies for removal of spinal cord tumor. *Spine* 1989;14:1171–1176.
52. Yasuoka S, Peterson HA, Laws ER, et al. Pathogenesis and prophylaxis of postlaminectomy deformity of the spine after multiple level laminectomy: Difference between children and adults. *Neurosurgery* 1981;9:145–152.
53. Yasuoka S, Peterson HA, MacCarty CS. Incidence of spinal column deformity after multilevel laminectomy in children and adults. *J Neurosurg* 1982;57:441–445.
54. Kumar V, Rea GL, Mervis LJ, et al. Cervical spondylotic myelopathy: Functional and radiographic long-term outcome after laminectomy and posterior fusion. *Neurosurgery* 1999;44:771–778.
55. LaRocca H, MacNab I. The laminectomy membrane. *J Bone Joint Surg* 1974;56:545–550.
56. Herman J, Sonntag VKH. Cervical corpectomy and plate fixation for postlaminectomy kyphosis. *J Neurosurg* 1994;80:963–970.
57. Goel V, Clark CR, Harris KG, et al. Kinematics of the cervical spine: Effects of multiple total laminectomy and facet wiring. *J Ortho Res* 1988;6:611–619.
58. Fager CA. Results of adequate posterior decompression in the relief of spondylotic cervical myelopathy. *J Neurosurg* 1973;38:684– 692.
59. Haft H, Ransohoff J, Carter S. Spinal cord tumors in children. *Pediatrics* 1959;23:1152–1159.
60. Raynor RB, Pugh J, Shapiro I. Cervical facetectomy and its effects on spine strength. *J Neurosurg* 1985;63:278–282.

61. Zdeblick T, Zou D, Warden KE, et al. Cervical stability after foraminotomy. *J Bone Joint Surg* 1992;74:22–27.
62. Zdeblick T, Abitbol JJ, Kunz DN, et al. Cervical stability after sequential capsule resection. *Spine* 1993;18:2005–2008.
63. Albert T, Vacarro A. Postlaminectomy kyphosis. *Spine* 1998;23: 2738–2745.
64. Yonenobu K, Fuji T, Ono K, et al. Choice of surgical treatment for multisegmental cervical spondylotic myelopathy. *Spine* 1985;10: 710–716.
65. Yonenobu K, Okada K, Fuji T, et al. Causes of neurologic deterioration following surgical treatment of cervical myelopathy. *Spine* 1986;11:818–823.
66. Adams C, Logue V. Studies in cervical spondylotic myelopathy: II the movement and contour of the spine in relation to the neural complications of cervical spondylosis. *Brain* 1971;94:569–586.
67. Ebersold M, Pare MC, Quast LM. Surgical treatment for cervical spondylotic myelopathy. *J Neurosurg* 1995;82:745–751.
68. Mikawa Y, Shikata J, Yamamuro T. Spinal deformity and instability after multilevel cervical laminectomy. *Spine* 1987;12:6–11.
69. Kaptain G, Simmons NE, Replogle RE, et al. Incidence and outcome of kyphotic deformity following laminectomy for cervical spondylotic myelopathy. *J Neurosurg (Spine)* 2000;93:199–204.
70. Heller JG, Carlson GD, Abitbol JJ, et al. Anatomic comparison of the Roy-Camille and Magerl techniques for screw placement in the lower cervical spine. *Spine* 1991;16:S552–S557.
71. Fehlings MG, Cooper PR. Posterior plates in the management of cervical instability: Long-term results in 44 patients. *J Neurosurg* 1994;81:341–349.
72. Grob D, Dvorak J, Panjabi MM, et al. The role of plate and screw fixation in occipitocervical fusion in rheumatoid arthritis. *Spine* 1994;19:2545–2551.
73. Heller JG, Silcox HD, Sutterlin CE. Complications of posterior cervical plating. *Spine* 1995;22:2442–2448.
74. Anderson PA, Henley MB, Grady MS, et al. Posterior cervical arthrodesis with AO reconstruction plates and bone graft. *Spine* 1991;16 (Suppl):S72–79.
75. Cooper RP. Posterior stabilization of the cervical spine using Roy-Camille plates: A North American experience. *Orthop Trans* 1988;12:43–44.
76. Ebraheim NA, An HS, Jackson WT, et al. Internal fixation of the unstable cervical spine using posterior Roy-Camille plate: Preliminary report. *J Orthop Trauma* 1989;3:23–28.
77. Hattori S. A new method of cervical laminectomy. *Centr Jpn J OrthopTraumatic Surg* 1973;3:792–794.
78. Hirabayashi K, Watanabe T, Wakano K, et al. Extensive open-door laminoplasty for cervical stenotic myelopathy. *Spine* 1983;6:693– 699.
79. Matsunaga S, Sakou T, Nakanisi K. Analysis of the cervical spine alignment following laminoplasty and laminectomy. *Spinal Cord* 1997;37:20–24.
80. Morio Y, Yamamoto T, Teshima R, et al. Clinicoradiographic study of cervical laminoplasty with posterolateral fusion or bone graft. *Spine* 2000;25:190–196.
81. Ozunal RM, Delamarter RB. Cervical laminoplasty for cervical myeloradiculopathy. *Oper Tech Orthop* 1996;6:38–45.

9

Endoscopic Posterior Fixation of the Cervical Spine

LARRY T. KHOO, MICHAEL Y. WANG, AND TOORAJ GRAVORI

Several internal fixation techniques have been developed for the posterior fixation of the subaxial cervical spine.[1] These techniques include the use of interspinous wiring with bone graft, the use of metallic plates affixed to the lateral masses with screws, interlaminar (i.e., Halifax) clamps, Daab plates, hook plates, and hook and rod constructs (i.e., Harrington) for long facet fusions.[2] McAfee and Bohlman's interspinous wiring techniques in multilevel fusions was more commonly used. In this technique, three wires are used and passed through holes made at the spinolaminar junction and around the rostral border of the rostral spinous process (Fig. 9–1A).[3–5] Biomechanical studies have verified the strength of this construct, and case reviews have described excellent union with this technique.[6–9] In cases of severe posterior column injury, the dorsal spinolaminar sites are also often unavailable for use, and Luque rectangles with facet wiring were often used (Fig. 9–1B). Advantages of this triple-wire technique included the ability to bridge large dorsal column defects (e.g., after tumor resections), afford segmental fixation at every level, and provide greater torsional and rotational stability.[10,11] In 1979, Roy-Camille and co-workers described a technique of cervical posterior instrumentation in which plates were fixed with screws to the lateral processes of the cervical spine (Fig. 9–1C).[12,13] This technique proved to be significantly stronger on biomechanical testing.[14–16] Subsequent authors described a 95 to 100% fusion rate with this technique when combined with autogenous bone grafting.[17–19] Anderson et al[20] went on to modify Roy-Camille's screw trajectory of dead-on center in the facet aiming inward to one where the screws are started 1 mm medial to the facet center and angled 30 degrees upward and 10 degrees outward. In the cervical spine, the screws are placed into the lateral masses, but the lateral masses evolve into the transverse processes in the thoracic spine, which may be insufficiently strong for screw placement.[21–25] Dissatisfaction with the quality of lateral mass screw fixation at C7 and T1 subsequently led several groups to use lower cervical spine and thoracic pedicle fixation for several spinal disorders.[1,2,26–32] In a calf model, Kotani et al[33] compared several midcervical reconstruction systems and found that transpedicular screws increased the stability of fixation more than any of the other constructs.

Newer instrumentation systems use two rods and variable screw islets at each level. These include Cervi-Fix (Synthes; Paoli, PA), StarLock (Fig. 9–1D) (Synthes), Summit (Depuy Acromed; Raynham, MA), and Vertex (Medtronic Sofamor Danek; Minneapolis, MN) (Fig. 9–1E). These systems vary by the angulation of their screws and in the degree of the constraint placed at the screw-rod interface. The polyaxial tulip or islet connectors of the screws are able to angle medially, laterally, and straight, with varying degrees of rotational freedom in each direction. As such, segmental fixation is more easily achieved via a top-loading approach, thereby making the possibility of minimally invasive posterior cervical fixation possible.

Minimally Invasive Rationale and Evolution

The past decade has witnessed an explosion of minimally invasive surgical techniques. In particular, there has been great excitement in the field of spinal surgery

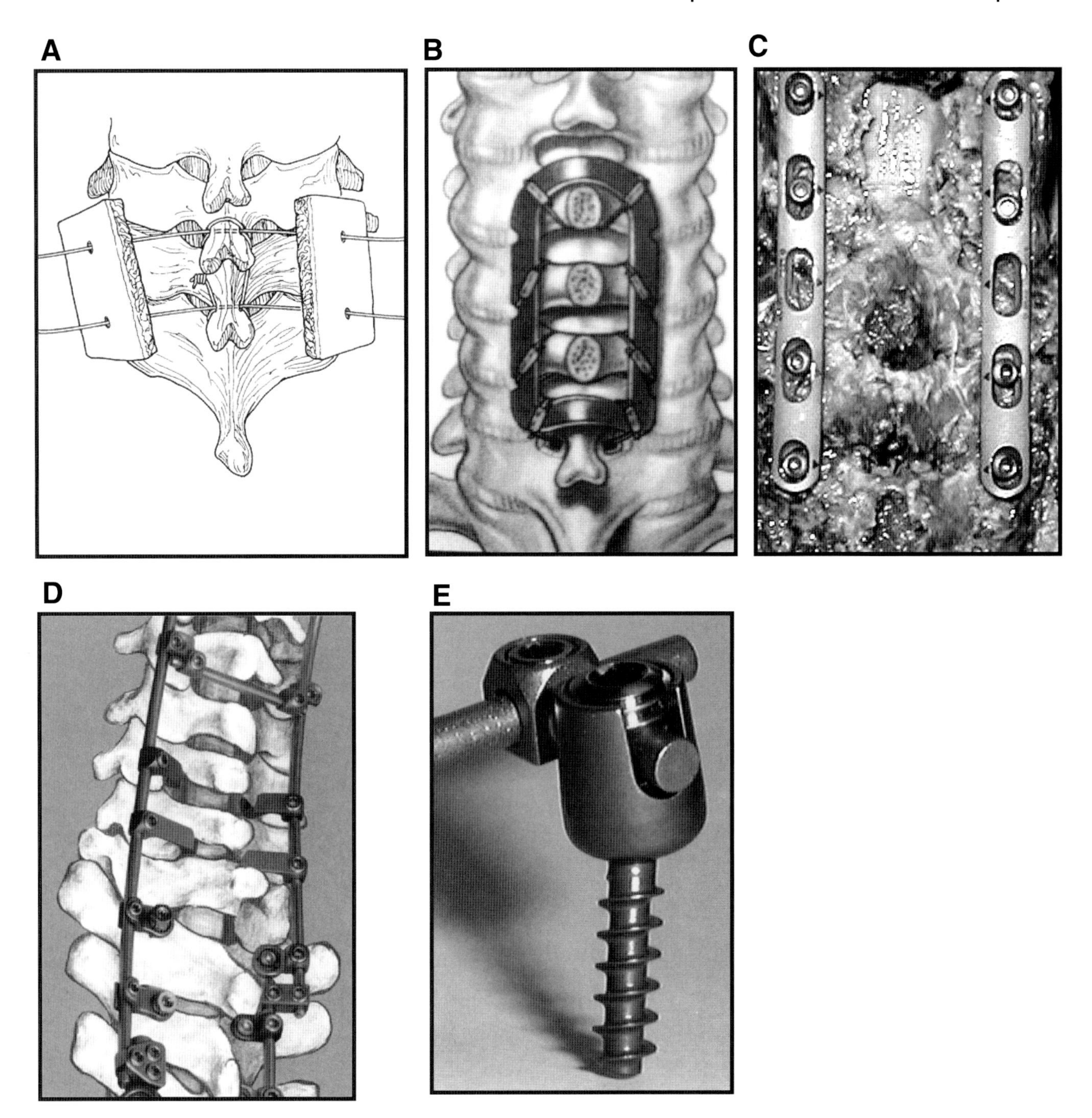

FIGURE 9–1 Numerous posterior cervical fixation techniques have been used with varying degrees of success over the years. One of the earliest was the interspinous triple-wire technique **(A)** popularized by Bohlman and colleagues. Sublaminar wiring was similarly commonly used and could be combined with a Luque-type construct for additional rigidity **(B)**. Popularity of these semi-rigid constructs was eventually supplanted by the use of posterior lateral mass screw-plate fixation **(C)**. The original unconstrained lateral mass screw-plate systems have since been supplanted by more rigid screw-rod and polyaxial screw-rod constructs **(D,E)**.

over minimal access technology due to the significant approach-related morbidities encountered by spine surgeons. Open surgery of the posterior spine requires stripping of muscles and ligaments simply for bony exposure. In the cervical and lumbar spine, this subperiosteal dissection devitalizes muscles and detaches key muscular and ligamentous insertions, disrupting the posterior musculoligamentous dynamic tension band. These drawbacks serve as the impetus driving minimally invasive surgery of the posterior spine.

Ideal minimal access surgery should be (1) safe and effective, (2) accessible to surgeons newly acquiring the technique, and (3) economically comparable to conventional surgeries. For these reasons, tubular dilator retractors have been developed for posterior spinal procedures. Multiple systems are now commercially available, and all have similar characteristics. These instruments essentially involve fluoroscopic placement of a guidewire through fascial and muscular structures followed by sequential dilation up to a final diameter of 14 to 24 mm. The putative advantage of using tubular dilator retractors is that the soft tissues are spread sequentially and not incised or stripped. Visualization can then be accomplished directly, with surgical loupes and a headlight, through the operating microscope, or via endoscopy. These systems are thus quite versatile, inexpensive, and easily accessible to most surgeons. They are particularly appealing because the surgeon can use standard surgical instruments and choose from a variety of methods for visualization and illumination.

As already summarized, decompressive and fixation techniques of the posterior cervical spine have been well established for a variety of indications, including trauma, tumor, infection, degenerative disease, arthritides, and deformity.[34–36] Often, however, the extensive dissection and stripping of the posterior musculature and ligaments are far greater than the actual size of the pathology. Indeed, the superficial and musculoligamentous exposure is often three to four times the size of the actual working target area. As a consequence of such iatrogenic injury, the popularity of some procedures has been limited because the postoperative disability from the approach often exceeds the intensity of the patient's preoperative symptoms.

As one such example, the effectiveness of posterior cervical laminoforaminotomy for decompression of the lateral recess and neural foramen has been well documented in numerous publications over the last four decades.[37–40] For cases of isolated radiculopathy from either a lateral disk or an osteophyte, 93 to 97% of patients experienced symptomatic improvement by simply freeing the nerve root via decompressive laminoforaminotomy and removal of the disk and/or osteophyte.[38,41,42] Enthusiasm for the operation was tempered by the significant cervical muscular pain and spasm that often followed. The use of wider incisions for adequate visualization and the need for significant paraspinous muscle dissection were blamed for this postoperative pain syndrome that resulted in a slower recovery course. Microendoscopic foraminotomy (MEF) represents the modern evolution of the classic operation with a minimally invasive approach and high-magnification direct endoscopic visualization.[43] Developments in percutaneous surgical access, optical technology, neuroanesthetic techniques, and noninvasive imaging modalities have brought posterior foraminotomy into a new millennium of spinal surgery. By minimizing the amount of tissue trauma and muscle injury, the MEF procedure overcomes the limited visualization, postoperative pain, muscle spasm, and prolonged disability that served to limit the open foraminotomy operation. It is most important that several authors have consistently demonstrated the ability of the MEF operation to achieve the same clinical results as that of the classical open procedure[44] with far less postoperative pain and shorter functional recovery times.

Through the same corridor of tubular access, the lateral masses of the posterior cervical spine are readily visualized. Two adjacent lateral masses can typically be accessed through a 20 or 22 mm working portal. With the advent of some of the newer types of expandable access portals, including FlexPosure (Endius; Plainville, MA) and Xpand (Medtronic Sofamor Danek), up to three lateral masses can be instrumented through a single exposure. This led us to begin placement of top-loading polyaxial screws through the tubular portals for the purposes of posterior cervical lateral mass fixation. In our experience, the first such case was that of a 35-year-old male who suffered from a unilateral jumped facet with persistent radicular numbness and pain. A single 18 mm working portal was docked over the perched facet complex that was then drilled out and realigned intraoperatively. Local bone from the lamina, spinous process base, and facet was then packed into the denuded joint space. A short AO fragment plate was then placed into position and fixated with two 14 mm unicortical screws. At 1 year, no motion was demonstrated at this C5–C6 segment on flexion-extension films as measured at the spinous process tips.[45] To our knowledge, this was one of the first such reported cases of minimally invasive lateral mass fixation. Since this initial experience in 2001, this technique of minimally invasive posterior cervical fixation (MI-PCF) has been applied in several other cases requiring lateral mass fixation with excellent clinical and radiographic results.[46,47] The widespread popularity of simple top-loading polyaxial screw systems has also greatly facilitated the MI-PCF procedure.

Anatomic Considerations

There are various methods for placement of screws into the lateral masses. Roy-Camille initially described screw placement directed forward and outward 10 degrees.[12,17] A second technique popularized by Magerl starts at a point medial to the center of the facet and directs the screw 25 degrees laterally and 40 to 60 degrees cephalad (Fig. 9–2A).[48] Haid and colleagues[49] described a technique in which the entrance point is 1 mm medial to the center of the lateral mass, with the screws angled 15 to 20 degrees cephalad and laterally 30 degrees (Fig. 9–2B,C). An et al[50] studied these drilling techniques in cadaveric

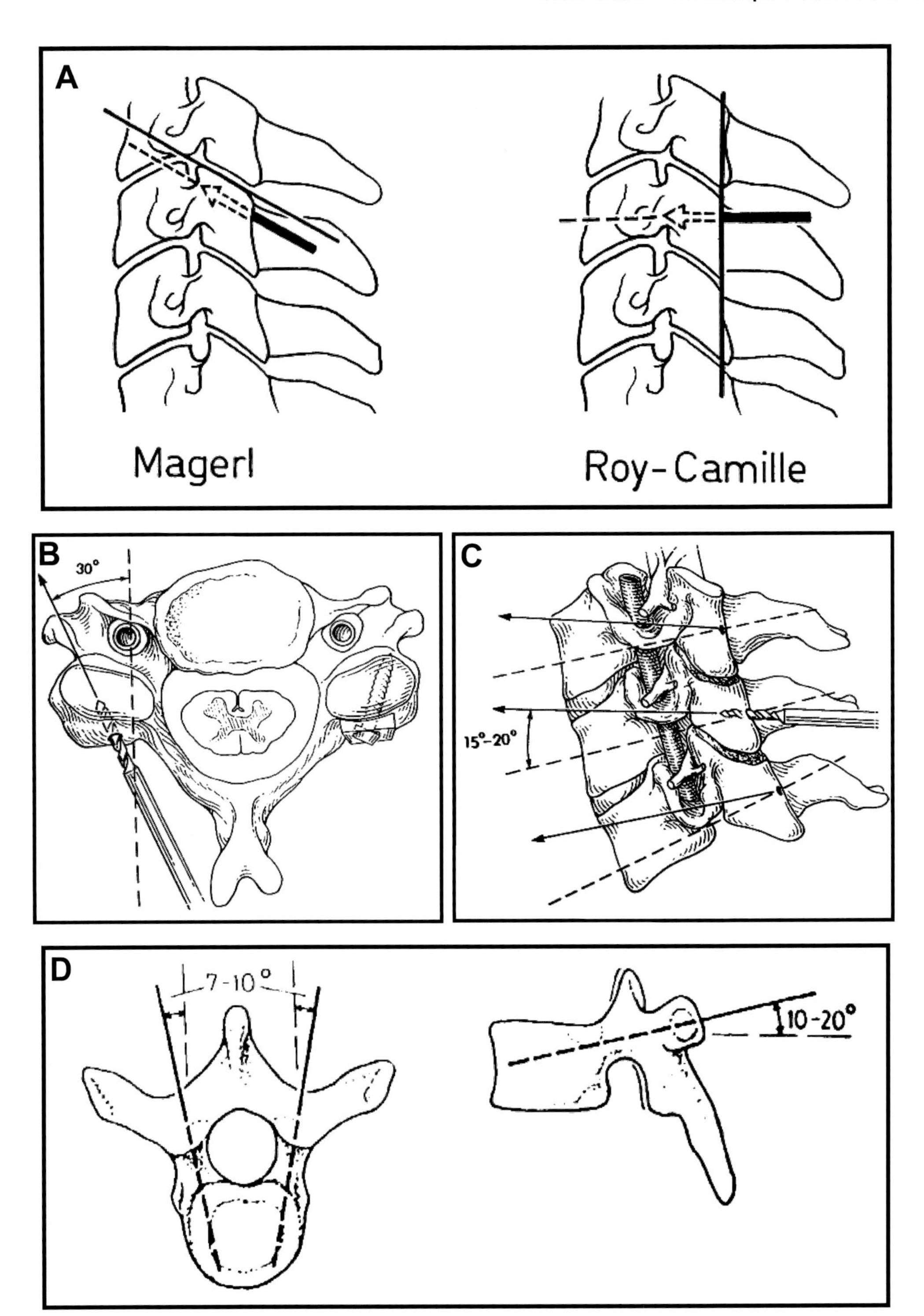

FIGURE 9–2 Lateral mass screw fixation as originally described by Roy-Camille utilized an orthogonally directed screw placement that potentially carried a risk of vertebral artery injury **(A)**. This was subsequently modified by Magerl et al, who described a rostral and lateral trajectory to avoid this important structure **(B,C)**. Because the C7 lateral mass is often minimal in size, pedicle fixation is often needed in this transitional area. The C7 pedicle typically has a 7- to 10-degree medial inclination and a 10- to 20-degree rostrocaudal angle as well **(D)**.

specimens. They found that more cephalad and medial trajectories increased the risk of neurologic injury. They verified the findings of Haid et al and also recommended starting 1 mm medial to the center of the lateral mass, with the screws angled 15 to 20 degrees cephalad and laterally 30 degrees.

Lateral mass screw fixation offers particular advantages over other techniques from C3 to C6, where the lateral mass is typically generous and broad. It can be readily applied in cases of posterior element incompetence (e.g., lamina fracture, laminectomy, and spinous process removal or fracture). Furthermore, it is useful for a wide range of pathologies, including posttraumatic instability, neoplasms, and degenerative instability, and for multilevel cervicothoracic stenosis. It is also biomechanically more resistant to rotation than are wired constructs. Although there is a risk of potential neurovascular injury, proper use of the technique is associated with an extremely low incidence of complication (4 to 6%). Lateral mass plating, however, is primarily an in situ fixator system and cannot be used for reduction of a significant kyphosis. Significant anterior compression, kyphosis, or cases with very poor bone quality in the lateral masses may best be treated with an anterior approach instead.

The C7 and thoracic pedicle is oriented in a posterolateral to anteromedial direction by ~10 degrees along most of the thoracic spine (Fig. 9–2D).[51,52] There is a slight anterior and lateral angulation of the pedicle at T12. It is recommended that fluoroscopy be available to assist in the proper trajectory. If the dorsal elements are intact, then a small laminotomy may be performed to enable direct palpation of the medial aspect of the pedicle. It is also important to note that the thoracic pedicle height is greater than the width; therefore, smaller diameter pedicle screws should be used in the thoracic region as compared with the lumbar spine. The entry site for the pedicle screw is identified by the intersection of a horizontal line connecting the transverse processes with a vertical line connecting the middle of the facet joints. A high-speed drill with a cutting burr is used to remove the cortical surface overlying the entry point.

Open surgical stabilization and fusion of the posterior cervical spine, however, suffer from several drawbacks. A relatively long midline neck incision is needed to obtain the appropriate cephalad drill trajectory. This can lead to complaints of postoperative neck pain from the muscular dissection, which detaches the semispinalis cervicis and multifidus muscles. Standard exposures can also cause substantial blood loss, muscular atrophy, large cosmetic defects, and unintended “creeping fusions.”

The technique of minimally invasive lateral mass screw placement was developed because of these drawbacks. Minimally invasive techniques have already been described in the lumbar spine for diskectomy, laminectomy, anterior fusion, posterior fusion, and pedicle screw placement. In the cervical spine, foraminotomies have successfully been performed through tubular dilator retractor systems. In these reports, the exposure of multiple cervical laminae and facet joints was safely accomplished through a single small incision on each treated side.

Surgical Anatomy

The posterior neck musculature consists of three layers: superficial, intermediate, and deep. The superficial layer is composed of the trapezius, splenius capitis, and semispinalis capitis muscles; the intermediate layer is composed of the levator scapulae, spinalis cervicis, longissimus capitis, and inferior oblique capitis muscles; and the deep layer is composed of the rotator cervicis brevis, rotator cervicis longus, and interspinalis cervicis muscles. Because all of these muscles are primarily responsible for neck extension, lateral bending, and rotation, their fibers run in a longitudinal or oblique fashion. Thus, placement of sequentially dilating tubes can be accomplished primarily by muscle splitting and stretching without cutting, thus minimizing tissue trauma.

The minimally invasive technique for screw placement does not differ substantially from open methods after exposure of the lateral mass. The nerve roots exiting the neural foramina are more likely to be encountered by screw trajectories in the lower half of the lateral mass, and the vertebral arteries are more likely to be encountered by screw trajectories in the medial half of the lateral mass. Thus, the technique focuses on placing the screw into the upper lateral quadrant of each lateral mass.

Screw length should allow full penetration of the outer cortex and cancellous bone and, in cases of trauma, bicortical screw purchase. Lengths typically vary between 12 and 16 mm but depend on the patient’s specific morphology, the presence of dorsal osteophytes, and screw trajectory. Preoperative measurements from CT scans can be helpful if bicortical screw purchase is desired, but violations of soft tissues by overly lengthy screws are seldom problematic if the trajectory is correct.

Surgical Procedure

Anesthesia and Positioning

Following the induction of general endotracheal anesthesia, adequate intravenous access is secured. Local anesthesia, combined with intravenous sedation, is inadequate for most cases because there is a substantial risk of injury to the spinal cord and nerve roots should there be any accidental movement during the procedure. Patients can be postioned in either a sitting or a prone position for the

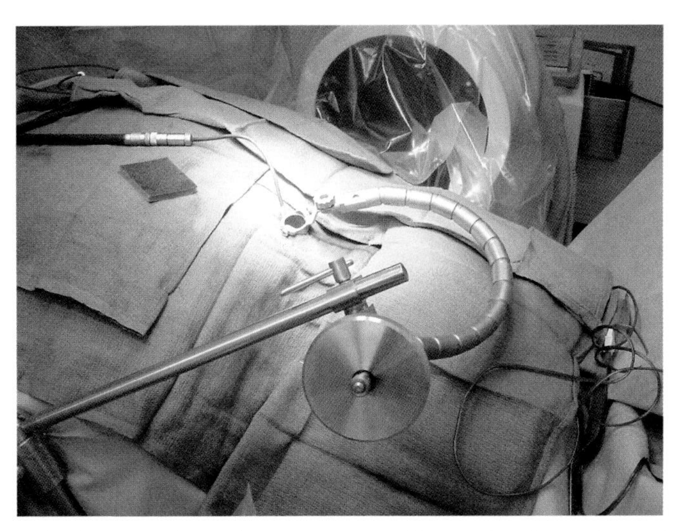

FIGURE 9–3 Operating room setup. The patient is positioned prone in a Mayfield skull clamp. Lateral fluoroscopic guidance is used for localization and screw placement, and the tubular retractor is held in position by a snake arm.

MI-PCF procedure. In our experience, an intermediate semi-sitting or heavily tilted head-up position is helpful to reduce epidural venous engorgement and intraoperative blood loss. Either way, it is recommended that the head be rigidly affixed in Mayfield pins (Fig. 9–3).

After positioning the patient, utmost care should be directed to ensuring that the cervical spine and neck musculature are not kinked or held in an unfavorable position. The neck, chin, and chest must be allowed to remain loose and free of compression. For cases with a high risk of venous air aspiration, a central venous pressure (CVP) catheter was placed into the right atrium in anticipation of blood loss and possible venous air embolus. Precordial Doppler monitoring can also be used to detect such air emboli within the atrium. As our facility and experience with this surgical technique have grown, we no longer routinely place a CVP catheter due to the brevity and minimal blood loss of the operation. We have to date had no cases of symptomatic air embolus during the MI-PCF procedure. We similarly do not typically place a Foley catheter for routine cases. We usually utilize intraoperative somatosensory evoked potential (SSEP) monitoring of the operated dermatome as well as of distal distributions to examine spinal cord integrity. Electromyographic recordings can also be used to assess motor integrity of the involved root. After the initial induction of anesthesia, we have refrained from the use of neuromuscular paralytics to allow for improved feedback from the nerve root during the operation.

For most cases, a single intraoperative dose of either Ancef or vancomycin is used. We do not routinely employ Solumedrol or other glucocorticoids for neural protection MI-PCF procedures. The fluoroscopic C-arm is brought into the surgical field so that real-time lateral fluoroscopic images can be easily obtained. AP fluoroscopic images can be obtained during initial Steinmann pin localization if additional confirmation in the coronal plane is desired.

Tubular Dilation and Exposure

Skin incision planning is important for the success of the procedure. Because typical lateral mass screws are normally angled 20 to 30 degrees medial to lateral and 20 to 30 degrees rostral to caudal, the ultimate trajectory of the working portal must also match this inclination. As such, lateral fluoroscopy is essential for safe and appropriate guidance. After positioning of the patient, a Steinmann pin is placed lateral to the neck to exactly parallel the facet in question (Fig. 9–4A). The appropriate skin incision entry point can then be marked in the sagittal plane. On average, this skin entry point lies two to three segments below the target level. In the axial plane, the entry point typically lies at the midline level, which closely approximates the typical trajectory used during open lateral mass fixation (Fig. 9–4B).

Under fluoroscopic guidance, a thin Steinmann pin is inserted through the posterior cervical musculature and fascia down to the target facet and two adjacent lateral masses. The skin entry point is chosen so that the pin trajectory will be parallel to the facet joint in the sagittal plane, placing the entry point two to three spinal segments below the level of interest. In the axial plane, the entry point is in the midline of the neck. The pin trajectory is thus directed in a superior and lateral direction, approximating the desired screw orientation (Fig. 9–5). Particular caution should be taken at this point to ensure that the guidewire is docked on bone to avoid inadvertent dural penetration. It is better to err laterally during this docking maneuver to prevent entering the wide interlaminar space. The pin ideally should rest in the medial aspect of the facet complex (Fig. 9–6A). Although we have not routinely done so, AP radiographic images can be obtained to guarantee proper pin positioning. Once the guidewire is docked on the facet in question, the skin incision should be extended above and below the Steinmann pin for a total length of ~2.0 cm. The skin edges are retracted, and the cervical fascia is incised using Metzenbaum scissors. Care should be taken not to cut muscle fibers during this procedure because this can cause unnecessary blood loss. This sharp opening of the fascia allows for easier passage of the sequential dilating cannulas with a minimum of force. If a barrier such as Ioband has been placed on the skin, it should be dissected away from the skin edges to prevent plastic sequestra that can occur during placement of the percutaneous dilators.

The series of dilators are then sequentially inserted through the neck soft tissues, over which a tubular working channel is inserted (Fig. 9–6B,C). A variety of

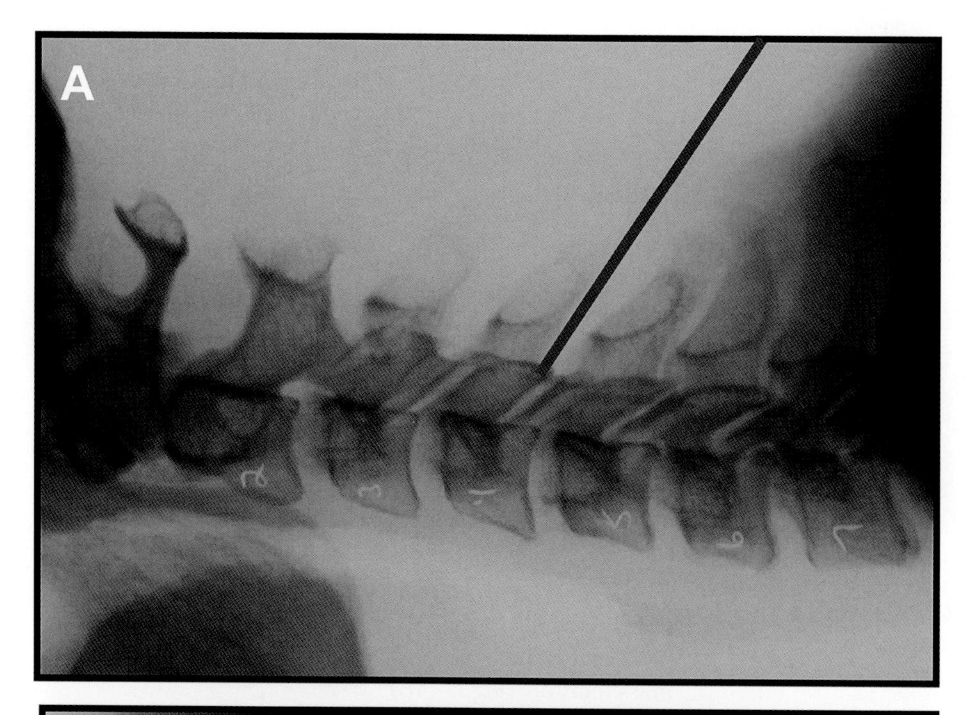

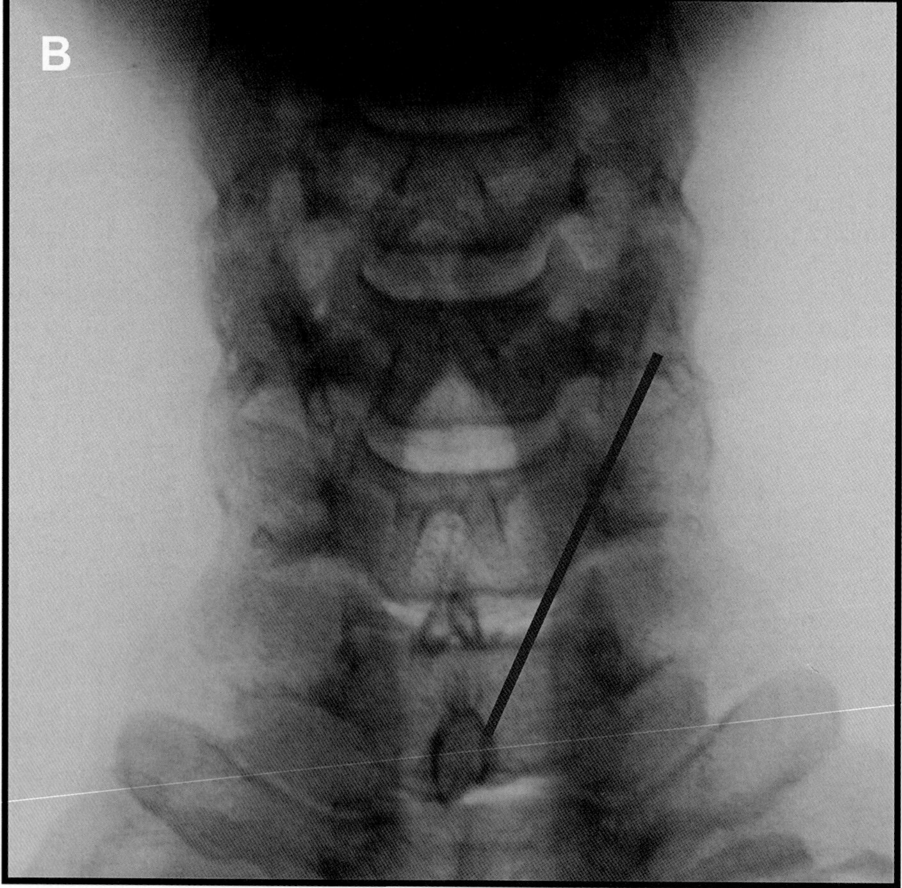

FIGURE 9–4 Utilizing lateral fluoroscopic guidance, the Steinmann pin is gradually advanced in a trajectory parallel to the target facet joint **(A)**. As such, the typical skin incision is located one or two spinal segments below the level to be instrumented. Under anteroposterior fluoroscopy, the trajectory begins at the midline and aims superiorly and laterally **(B)**.

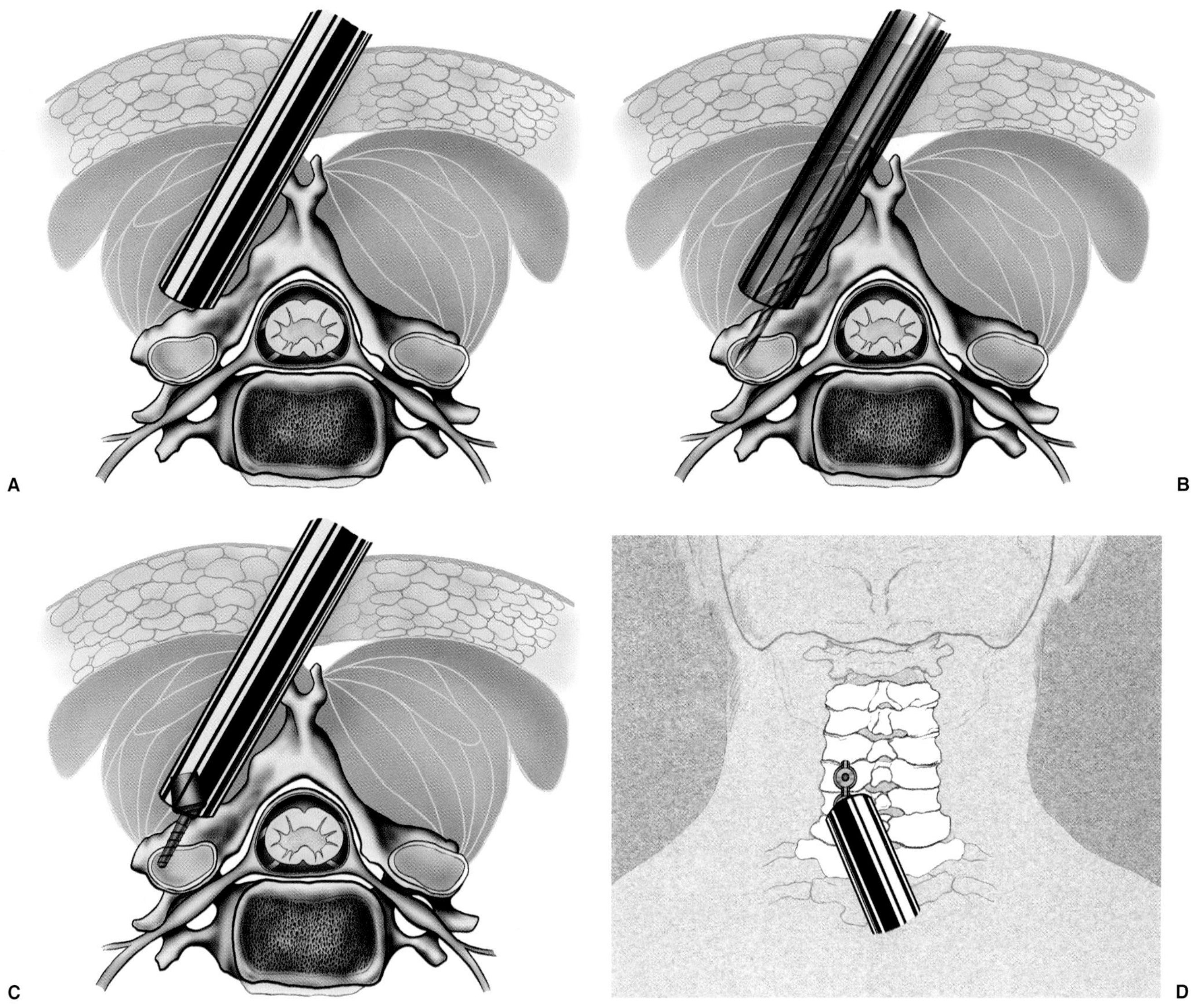

FIGURE 9–5 Surgical technique. **(A–C)** Axial projection showing positioning of the tubular dilator retractor through a single midline incision to ensure a trajectory aimed laterally, followed by drilling of a pilot hole and screw placement. **(D)** Posterior view.

working cannulas can be employed for this purpose. These include such fixed 20 or 22 mm tubular portals as the METRx MD tubular access system (Medtronic Sofamor Danek; Fig. 9–6D)) and Access system (Spinal Concepts; Austin, TX). As an alternative, such expandable cannulas as the Xpand system (Medtronic Sofamor Danek; Fig. 9–7A,B) and the FlexPosure cannulas (Endius; Plainville, MA) can provide a greater working space and more forgiving approach angles for instrumentation placement. Real-time lateral radiographic images should be obtained as often as needed to ensure a proper working trajectory throughout this process (Fig. 9–7C,D). The working channel (tubular retractor) is then attached to a flexible retractor affixed to the operating table-side rail and locked in position at the junction of the lamina and lateral mass. For the majority of the tubular access systems already mentioned, either direct visualization with loupes/microscope or an endoscope can be used for visualization (Fig. 9–8A). For cases of simple facet dislocation, it is our preference to employ simple loupe magnification combined with an intratubular light source (Radiance; Medtronic Sofamor Danek) because multiple viewing angles are needed for drilling of the facet, reduction of the dislocation, and placement of the lateral mass screws. For cases where extensive laminotomy, partial facetectomy, and foraminotomy are necessary; however, a high-quality operating microscope should be used to provide improved visualization and safety. If employed, the endoscope should be white-balanced and an antifog agent should be applied

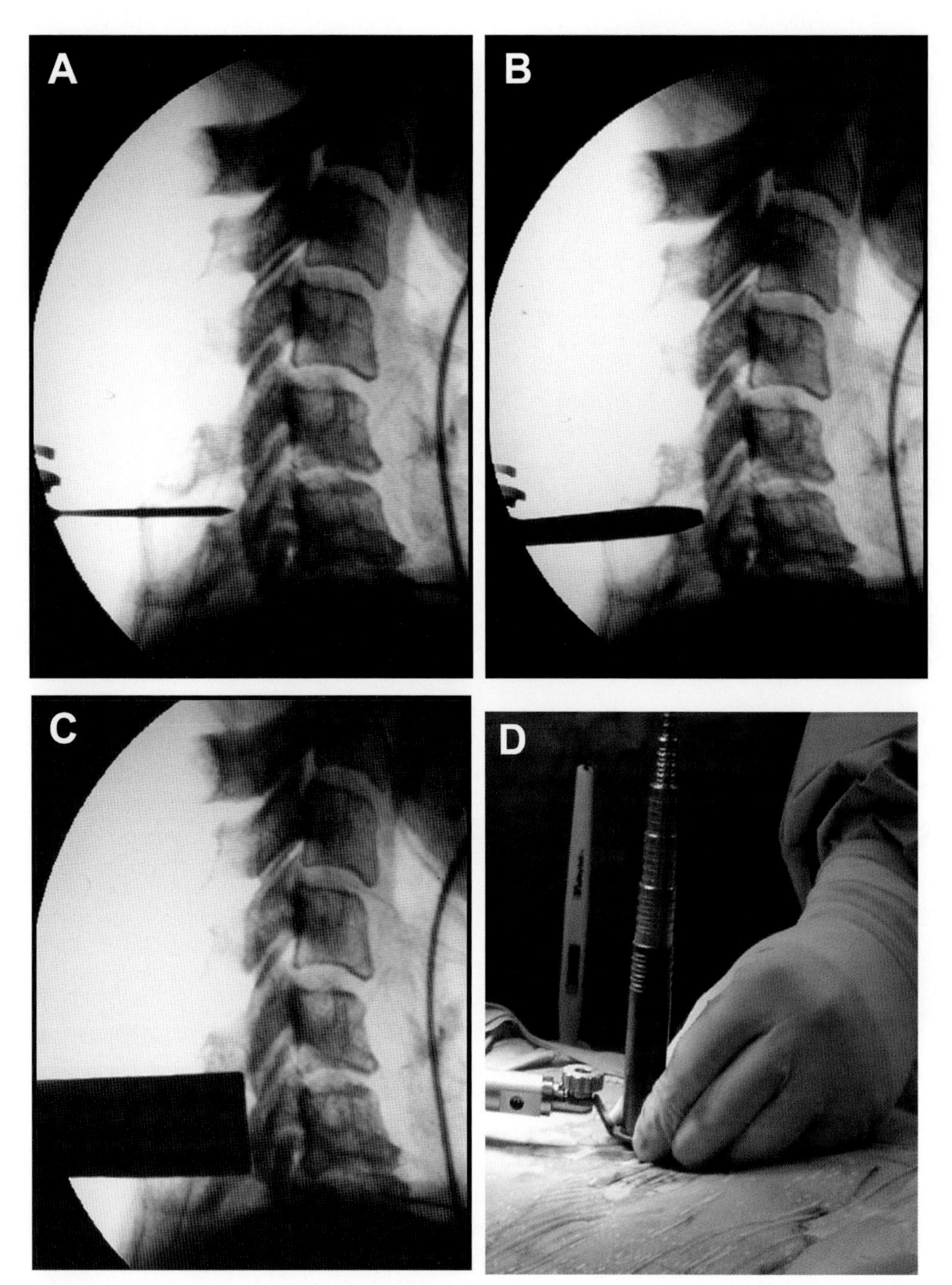

FIGURE 9–6 After placement of the Steinmann pin **(A)**, sequential tubular dilation is completed to achieve a final working portal of 20 to 22 mm in diameter **(B–D)**.

to the lens. The endoscope is then attached to the tubular retractor via a circular plastic friction couple or mounting stage.

For the placement of lateral mass plates, the soft tissue dissection must fully expose the facet joints and lateral borders of the lateral masses. This is readily accomplished with a shielded monopolar cautery combined with pituitary rongeurs. All capsular ligaments and soft tissue around the facets are removed. The facet joints above and below the involved ligaments should be left intact to prevent late instability or fusion at those levels. There is frequently bleeding from the venous plexus lateral to the lateral masses, which can be stopped using bipolar electrocautery. Caution should be exercised to avoid overly aggressive cautery in this region to avoid inadvertent injury to the vertebral artery. Gentle tamponade with Gelfoam and a cottonoid will often effectively stop bleeding from this troublesome venous plexus. We have found

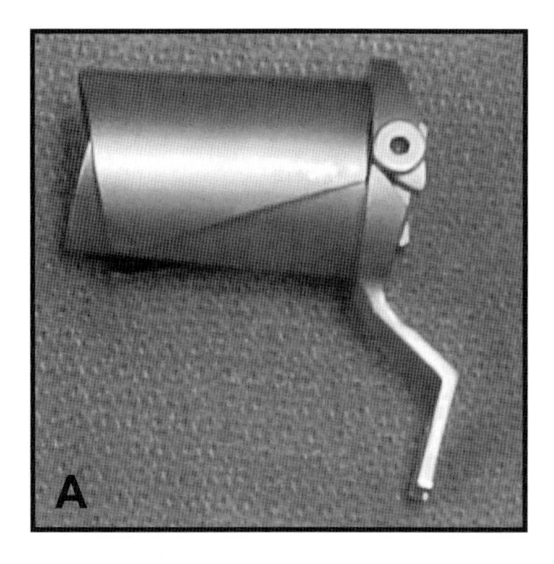

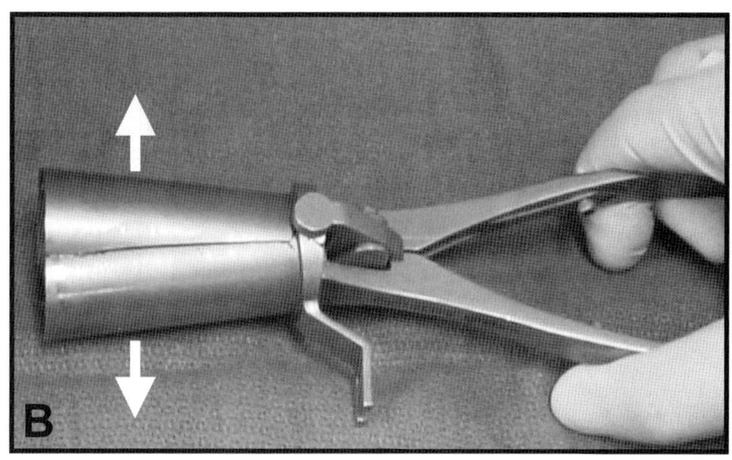

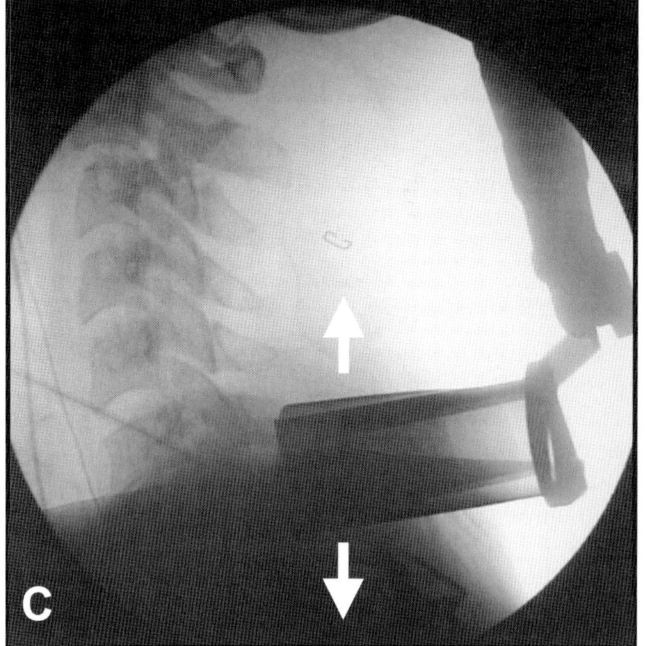

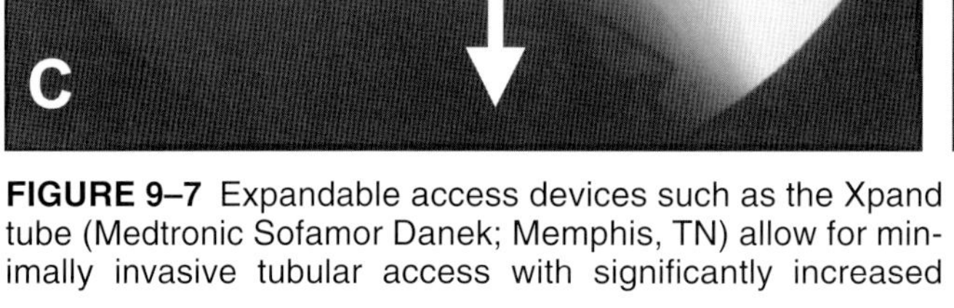

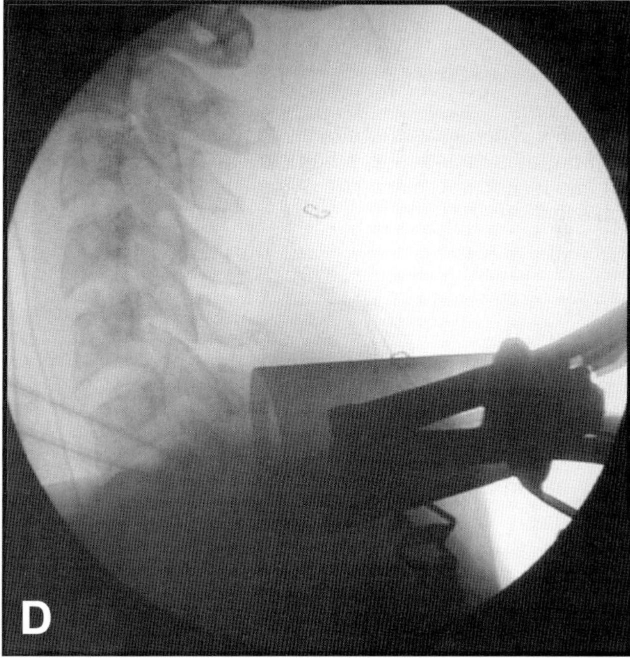

FIGURE 9–7 Expandable access devices such as the Xpand tube (Medtronic Sofamor Danek; Memphis, TN) allow for minimally invasive tubular access with significantly increased working space at depth **(A,B)**. Under lateral fluoroscopy, tubular expansion allows for visualization of two adjacent lateral masses **(C,D)**.

the use of powdered Gelfoam granules combined with thrombin delivered through a narrow plastic catheter to be extremely effective during the MI-PCF procedures.

For cases where facet realignment has been achieved either from closed reduction or an anterior surgical procedure, the lateral mass screws can simply be placed in an in situ fashion. Open reduction can be performed if closed reduction of a facet dislocation is not successful (Fig. 9–8B). A high-speed drill is used to remove part of the superior articular process of the inferior vertebrae. A Penfield-type instrument can then be inserted within the facet and rotated to bring the subluxed lateral mass up and back. This usually allows the facets to realign in their anatomical state. An alternative method that we have used on several occasions is simply to disengage the Mayfield head holder after drilling of the facet lip edges. Gentle in-line traction, appropriate anterior translation, and counterrotation opposite to the mechanism of injury are typically effective at restoring the normal anatomic alignment of the facet complex. It is highly recommended that SSEP monitoring combined with root surveillance at the pathologic level be used

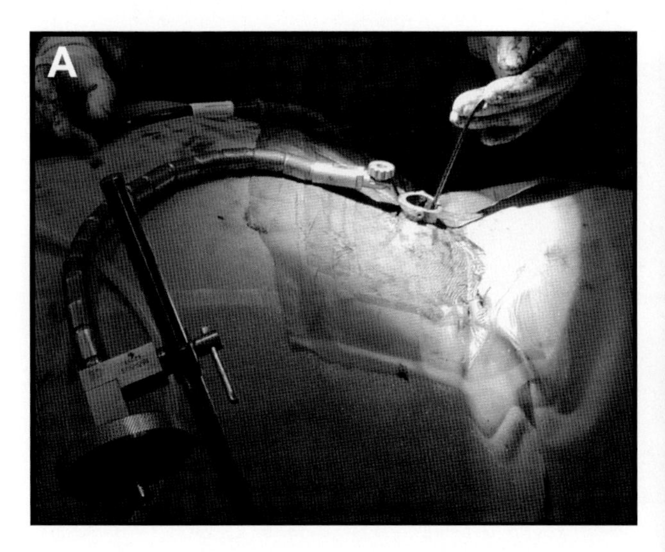

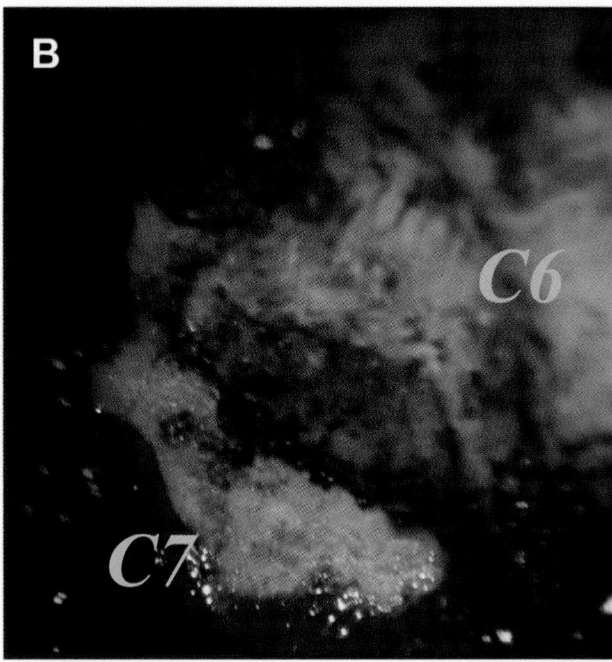

FIGURE 9–8 After access and radiographic confirmation, the working portal is mounted to a bed-mounted flexible arm retractor and locked into place **(A)**. Operative visualization can be achieved via loupe magnification, operating microscope, or high-resolution surgical endoscope. For cases of cervical jumped facet, the reversed relationship of the facets can be seen after soft tissue exposure **(B)**.

during such maneuvers. The Mayfield holder is then relocked and the facet complex fused in situ after packing of the joint space.

Should neural decompression be necessary, the screw sites are marked, drilled, and tapped prior to removing the laminae. Bleeding from these holes can be controlled by sealing them with bone wax at this point. This method protects the dura and spinal cord during drilling. The entry point is approximately 1 mm medial to the center of the lateral mass. The outer cortex is pierced with either an awl or a high-speed drill. This reduces the chance that the drill will slip over the lateral mass instead of entering the bone during screw placement. Fourteen or 16 mm length 3.5 mm diameter screws are typically used, depending on the size of the lateral masses, which can be measured on the CT scan or estimated from lateral fluoroscopy intraoperatively. As described earlier, for C3 to C6 (and sometimes C7), we prefer to drill the holes with a 15- to 20-degree cephalad angle and a 30-degree lateral trajectory. This rostral angle targets the transverse process and decreases the chance of violation of uninvolved joints. Given the angle of the tubular access, this is typically directly in-line with the trajectory of the working channel. The vertebral artery usually lies anterior to the valley created by the junction of the lamina and the lateral mass. By starting 1 mm medial to the center of the lateral mass and directing the drill laterally, there is less risk to the vertebral artery and nerve roots. After drilling, the dorsal cortex can be tapped using the 3.5 mm cancellous tap if desired. Because the majority of the new polyaxial screws are self-tapping, this step is not essential, in our experience. For a detailed account of the decompression technique, we would refer readers to the relevant literature.[46]

The joint cartilage from the facets is removed prior to instrumentation, and the joint is decorticated using a high-speed drill with a small matchstick-type bit. Although there is a wide body of literature demonstrating successful arthrodesis without the use of bone graft, we generally advocate the use of bone graft within the facets as well as over the decorticated laminofacet junctions. Cancellous autologous bone from the iliac crest is then packed into the facet joints. As an alternative, we now typically avoid iliac crest grafting by harvesting bone and bone dust obtained during facet drilling, laminotomy, and foraminal decompression. This graft is then combined in a one-to-one ratio with an appropriate bone extender, as is supported by the scientific literature (e.g., demineralized bone matrix or calcium triphosphate substitutes). Bone graft should also be packed in and around the construct.

After denuding the facet and placement of bone graft, the appropriate length lateral mass screw is then

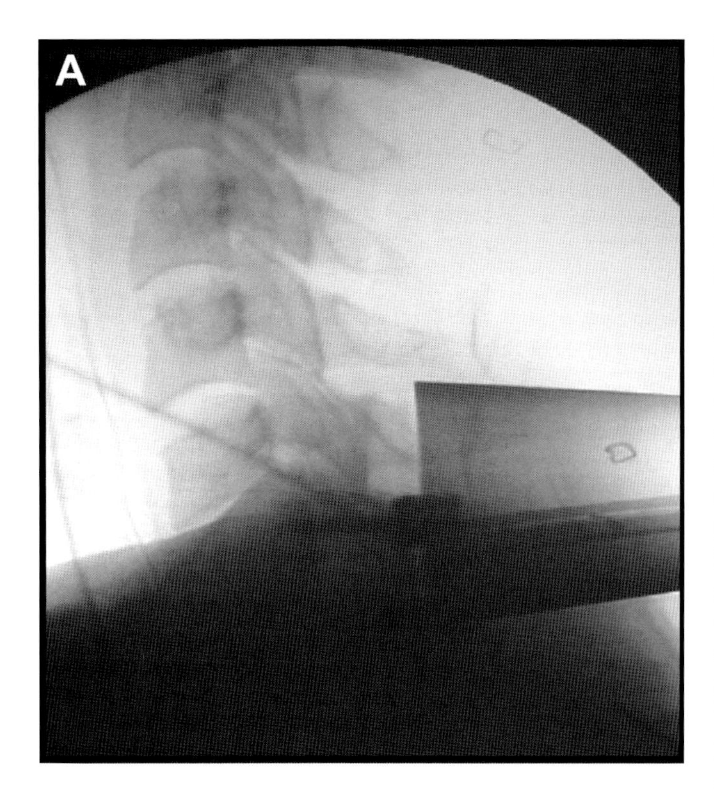

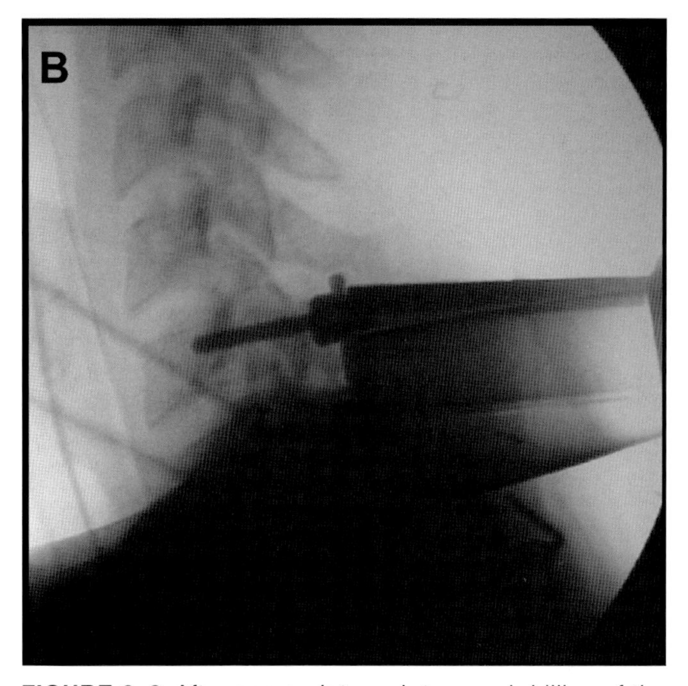

FIGURE 9–9 After appropriate awl, tap, and drilling of the screw trajectory, sequential confirmation under direct visualization and lateral fluoroscopy is accomplished prior to screw placement. The first screw is placed **(A)**, and the tubular retractor is then loosened to allow for migration of the portal over the second screw entry trajectory. The second screw is then placed **(B)**. Here the screws have been placed utilizing a trajectory between that of Roy-Camille and Magerl.

inserted under both direct visualization and fluoroscopic guidance (Fig. 9–9A). The tubular retractor arm usually must be relaxed at this point to allow easy acquisition of the second screw trajectory. Careful attention must be paid to avoid raising the tubular portal too much and letting soft tissue excursion obscure the exposure. The second screw is then placed in the manner already detailed (Fig. 9–9B).

A pedicle or lateral mass screw may need to be used at C7. The C7 lateral mass is much thinner than the rostral lateral masses, which can make screw placement difficult. There is usually no vertebral artery in the transverse foramen at this level. This often permits safe pedicle screw placement here and at T1. For C7 pedicle screw placement, the drill is angled 25 to 30 degrees medially, and perpendicular to the rostral-caudal plane. It is important to look at the preoperative CT scan to assess the pedicle size and gauge the appropriate angle. A 4.0 mm cortical screw of 20 to 22 mm length is typically used. A small laminotomy can be made to palpate the pedicle directly for safe placement of the screw. For T1 pedicle screw placement, the angle is usually 10 to 15 degrees medially and 5 degrees caudally. Cervical pedicle screws may attain greater pullout strength than lateral mass screws due to the greater length and circumferential cortical purchase. They may also be used in levels where the lateral mass is fractured or unusable. Gradual maneuvering of the working tubular portal will be needed in such cases to obtain this opposite-type trajectory.

At this point, an appropriate-sized rod is then inserted into the top of the polyaxial screws and locked into place (Fig. 9–10). The rod diameter varies from 3.2 to 3.5 mm, depending on the specific system used. At this point, the rod is inserted in a vertical fashion and then gradually rotated into one screw head at a time. Rod placement is more technically challenging when fusing three adjacent segments, but careful dorsal elevation of the tubular retractor system off of the facet joint creates adequate space for rod manipulation and placement (Fig. 9–11). The tubular retractor often needs to be released at this point to allow for slight elevation of the portal off the lateral masses above the level of the screw heads. This maneuver will help to facilitate placement of the rod in a rostral-caudal orientation. For this reason, the expandable cannulas are particularly useful at providing a larger working space. For such third-generation posterior cervical instrumentation systems as CerviFix (Synthes), StarLock (Synthes), Summit (Depuy Acromed), and Vertex (Medtronic Sofamor-Danek), there are subtle variations regarding the exact types of connectors, offsets, and locking devices used. We would refer readers to the individual instrumentation guides from each manufacturer regarding these differences in technique. Nevertheless, the

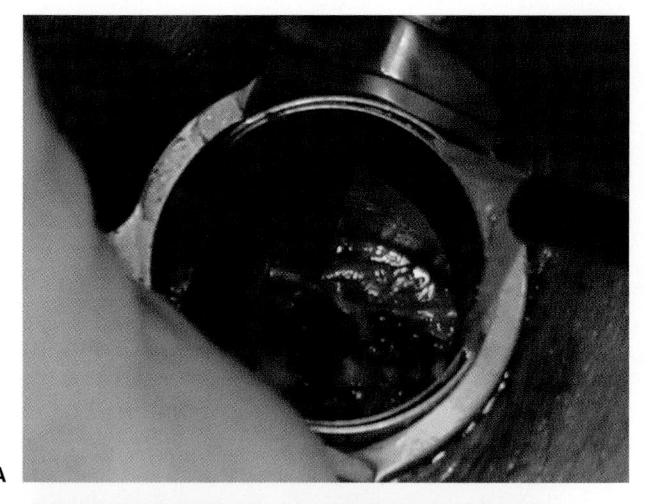
A

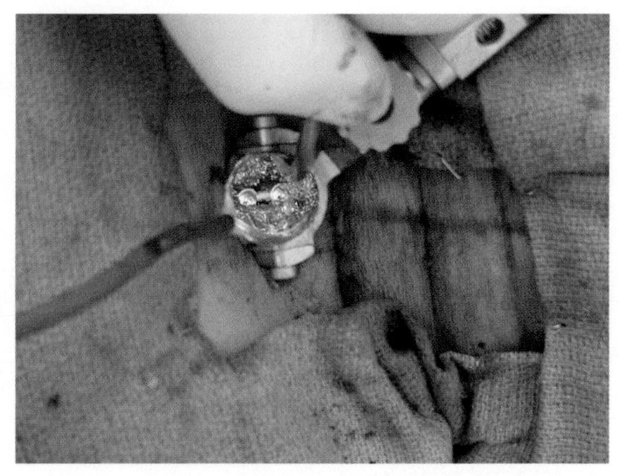

B

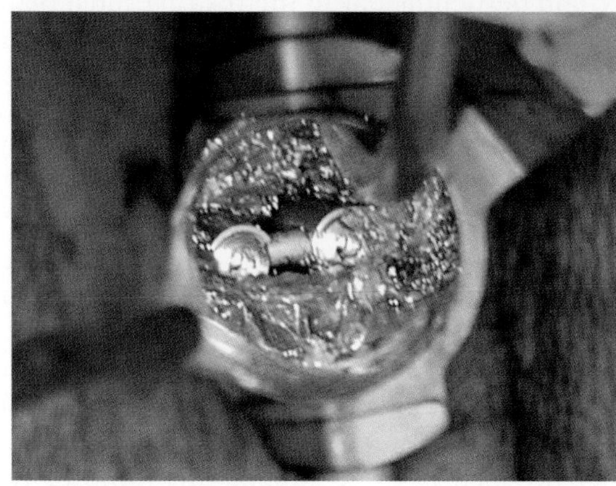
C

FIGURE 9–10 **(A)** Intraoperative view down tubular retractor showing two lateral masses with intervening facet joint. **(B)** View of polyaxial 16 mm lateral mass screws and rod in place. **(C)** Magnified.

appropriate locking or set screws are placed at this point, and the construct is completed (Fig. 9–12A). Appropriate lateral and AP fluoroscopy should be used to confirm proper bony alignment and construct placement. The tubular retractor is then removed. For cases where bilateral fixation is needed, the exact same steps of Steinmann pin placement, tubular dilation, decompression, and instrumentation can be accomplished through the same midline incision and a contralateral trajectory.

Closure

Meticulous hemostasis should be obtained by a combination of bipolar cautery and gentle tamponade with thrombin-soaked Gelfoam pledgets for cases with epidural bleeding. The area is then copiously irrigated with lactated ringers impregnated with bacitracin antibiotics. Although optional, we have usually placed a small pledget of Gelfoam soaked with Solumedrol gently over decompression defects, if present. Use of epidural morphine paste or similar cocktails is reasonable if there is no evidence of dural erosion or tear. Such agents may help to reduce postoperative pain and allow for more rapid recovery and ambulation.

The tubular retractor and endoscope are then cautiously removed, and a routine closure of the fascia and skin is performed. Antibiotic irrigation should be used to wash this soft tissue corridor copiously prior to placing sutures. Because the defect is typically quite small, only a limited amount of closure need be performed, and a drain is not needed. A Vicryl-type reabsorbable stitch is used to closure the lumbodorsal fascia in a figure 8. Marcaine (0.25%) is used to inject the skin edges and superficial musculature prior to closure. Inverted 2–0 Vicryl stitches are used to close the subcutaneous layer. A 4–0 clear Vicryl subcuticular closure is then used to reapproximate the skin carefully, with care paid to avoid inversion of the edges. Either Steri-Strips or Dermabond can then be used to cover the skin (Fig. 9–12B). Dermabond is attractive because it keeps the skin edges closely approximated for a 7- to 10-day period, and it provides a waterproof barrier. The patient can thus shower almost immediately after surgery.

Direct repair is difficult for cases where a CSF leak has occurred because the durotomy is small and the access is

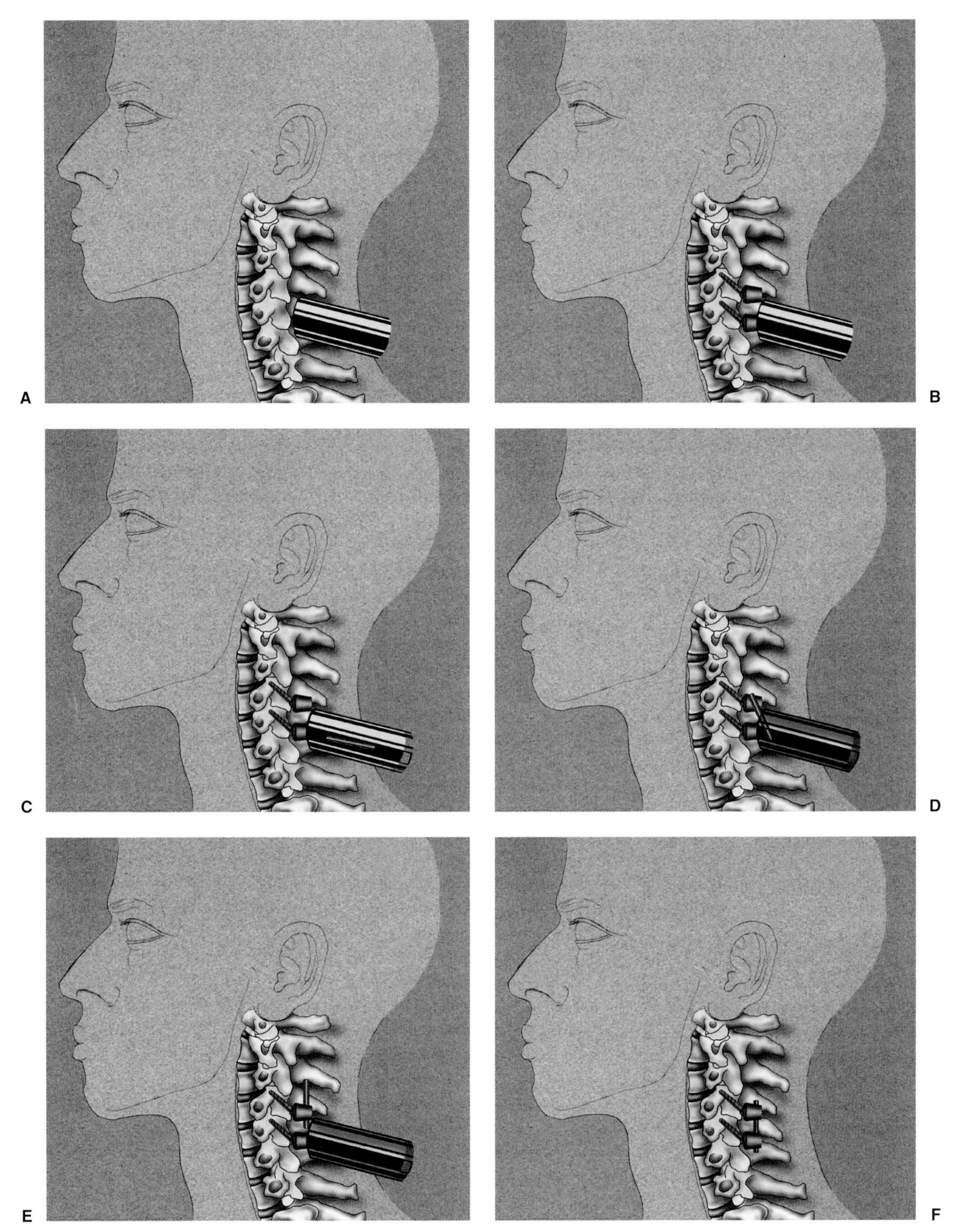

FIGURE 9–11 Rod advancement through tubular dilator if rod length exceeds the tube diameter. **(A)** Tube positioning. **(B)** Screw placement. **(C–F)** Rod advancement.

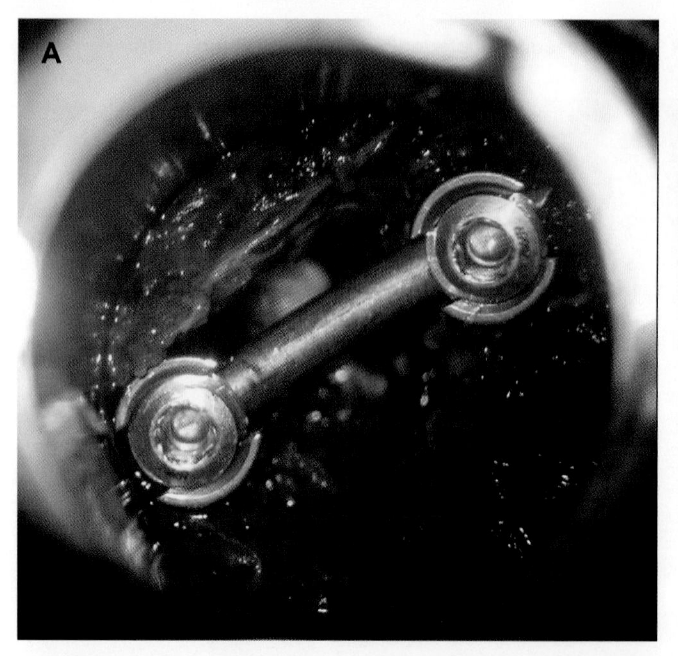

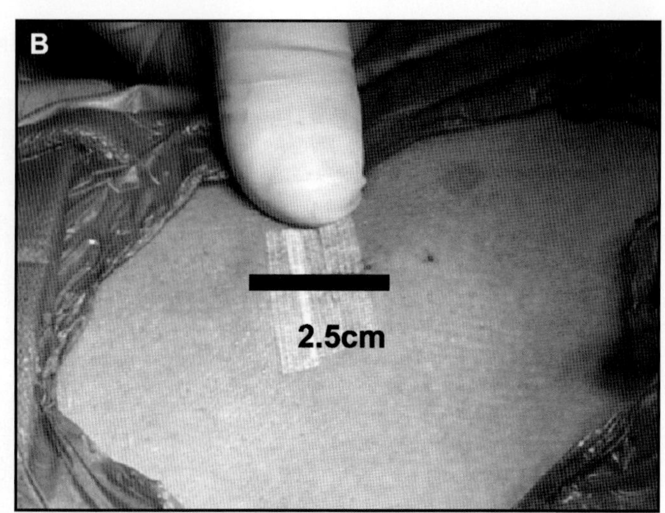

FIGURE 9–12 An appropriately sized rod is cut and secured into the polyaxial screw heads. After completion of the construct **(A)**, the tubular working channel is collapsed and removed. Skin closure is accomplished with a few resorbable stitches in multiple layers for a typical final incision length of 2 to 3 cm **(B)**.

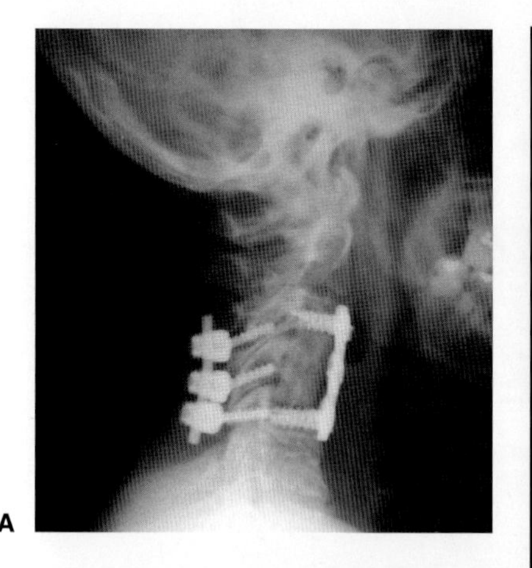

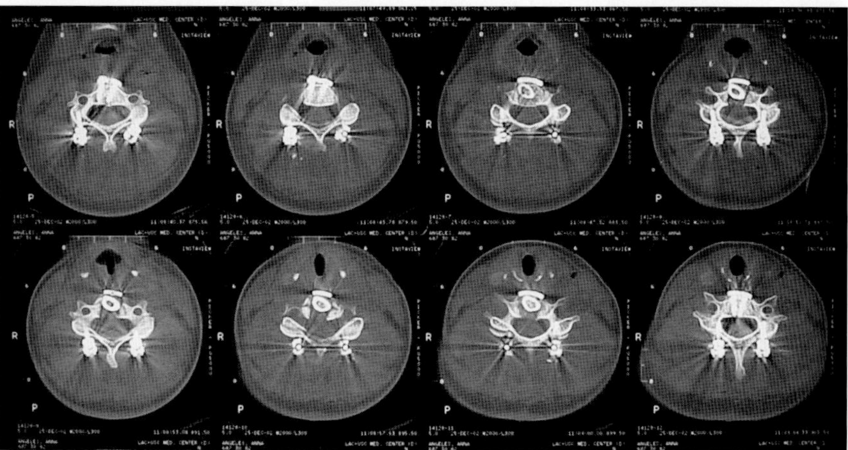

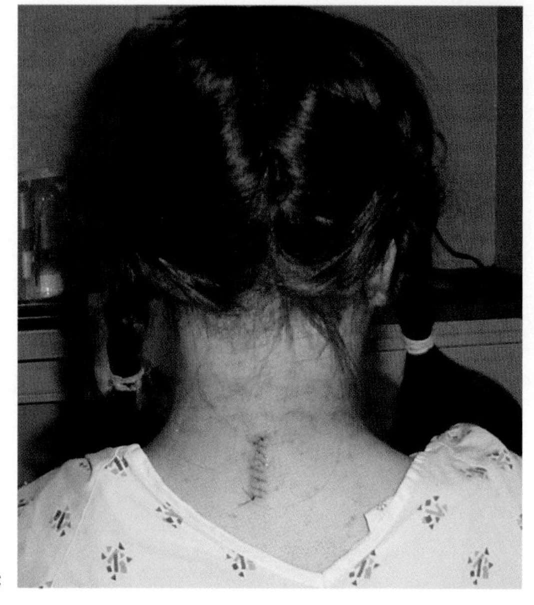

FIGURE 9–13 An 18-year-old female sustained a C4 burst fracture after a motor vehicle accident, but remained neurologically intact. CT scan and MRI demonstrated a comminuted vertebral body fracture with three-column injury. The posterior cervical spine was instrumented and fused from C3 to C5 in a minimally invasive fashion following anterior cervical corpectomy and plating. **(A)** Postoperative lateral x-ray images. **(B)** Immediate postoperative CT scan showing bilateral screw placement without violation of neural or vascular structures and no disruption of the posterior soft tissues. **(C)** Single midline 2 cm surgical incision in the posterior neck at the C7 level.

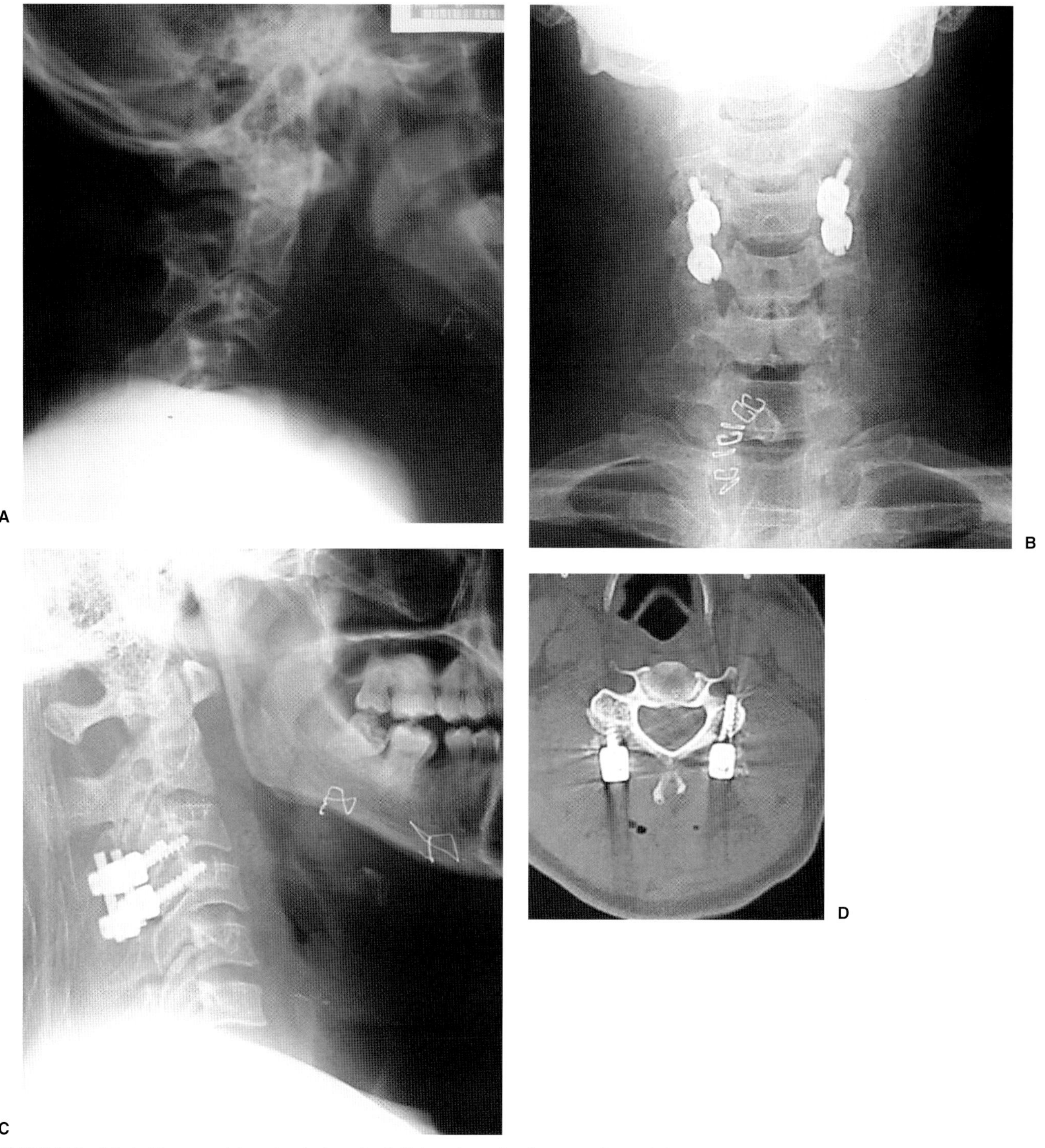

FIGURE 9–14 A 43-year-old male victim of a fall developed bilaterally jumped facets but remained neurologically intact. **(A)** Preoperative lateral x-ray demonstrated C3–C4 subluxation. The patient was taken to the operating room following partial reduction in traction, where drilling of the C4 superior facets allowed intraoperative reduction with placement of C3–C4 lateral mass screws. **(B)** Postoperative lateral x-ray. **(C)** AP x-ray showing staples with skin incision three levels below the fusion. **(D)** Postoperative CT scan.

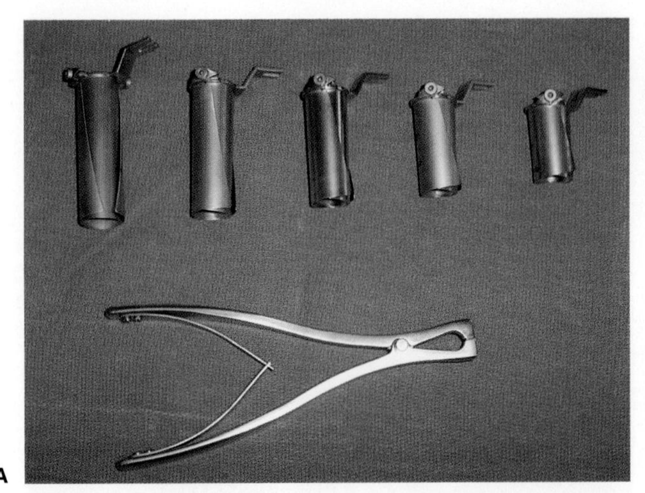

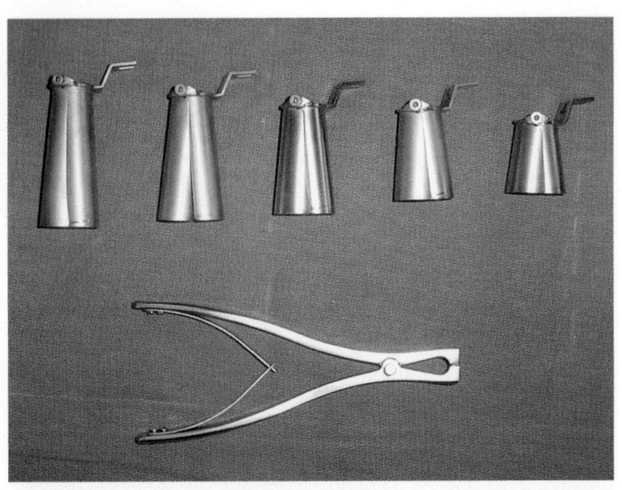

FIGURE 9–15 Expandable tubular dilator retractors allowing greater distal exposure through a smaller skin incision for minimally invasive posterior exposure of lordotic regions of the spine. Tubes **(A)** unexpanded and **(B)** expanded.

limited. Thus, we have routinely employed a lumbar drain for 2 to 3 days postoperatively to help closure of the small dural tear. Such adjuncts as fibrin glue, fat, or muscle grafts can also be used. Spinal headaches and nausea associated with the lumbar drainage can be treated symptomatically with nonsteroidal anti-inflammatory medications and bed rest. For large dural tears, direct repair can be attempted if specialized instruments are available for use through the endoscopic tube. Castro-Viejo-type needle holders and long forceps are particularly useful in this regard. In rare instances, conversion to an open procedure may be necessary to close large dural violations. To date, we have not had problems with delayed pseudomeningoceles or CSF leaks after simple lumbar drainage.

Clinical Experience

Our initial experience with minimally invasive cervical fixation consists of 10 patients followed to radiographic fusion. Six underwent single-level fusions, and four underwent two-level fusions (Fig. 9–13). Instrumentation was performed at the C3 to C7 segments. In three cases screw placement was unilateral due to lateral mass fractures; in the remainder the instrumentation was bilateral. Seven cases were posterior supplementations of anterior fusions, and three were stand-alone posterior constructs.

Seven of the cases were due to traumatic pathology. Cervical burst fractures and fracture dislocations were treated with combined anterior and posterior fusion. In three cases with bilaterally jumped facets treatment consisted of drilling and removal of the superior facet through the tubular dilator retractor (Fig. 9–14). This was followed by intraoperative reduction and hardware placement with fusion. Three cases were posterior supplements to an anterior corpectomy for neoplasia.

All procedures were accomplished successfully with the use of 18 to 22 mm tubular dilator retractors. There were no complications or new neurologic deficits, and proper hardware placement was confirmed with CT scanning. In one case, the C6 screw was positioned somewhat laterally with penetration of the lateral cortex of the lateral mass. Fusion was confirmed in all cases with dynamic x-rays and CT scans.

Current tubular dilator dimensions limit this minimally invasive approach to one- or two-level fusions. Longer segment constructs are currently not feasible due to difficulties with rod placement; however, the development of elliptical expandable tubular dilators (Fig. 9–15) may allow longer constructs to be placed safely because the final diameter of tubular access ports is limited by the short length of the cervical muscles. As the technology proliferates to overcome this problem in the lumbar spine, similar systems will be developed for cervical instrumentation. Strategies such as arc rod systems and polymerizing connecting rods are allowing true percutaneous transpedicular instrumentation in the lumbar spine. This promising technology ultimately may allow placement of longer segment cervical constructs in a minimally invasive fashion.

Radiographic guidance is essential for safe screw placement, and fluoroscopic images may be inadequate for the lower cervical spine in patients with a short neck, large body habitus, or muscular shoulders. Image-guided systems surmount this problem and allow for virtual representation of the spine without the need for

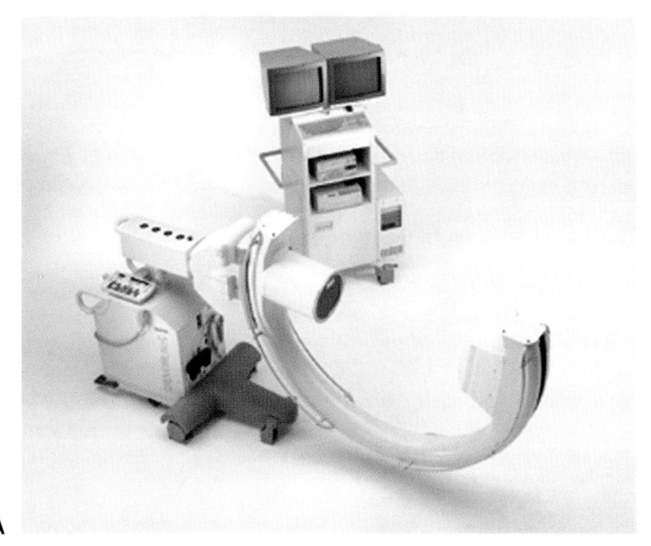
A

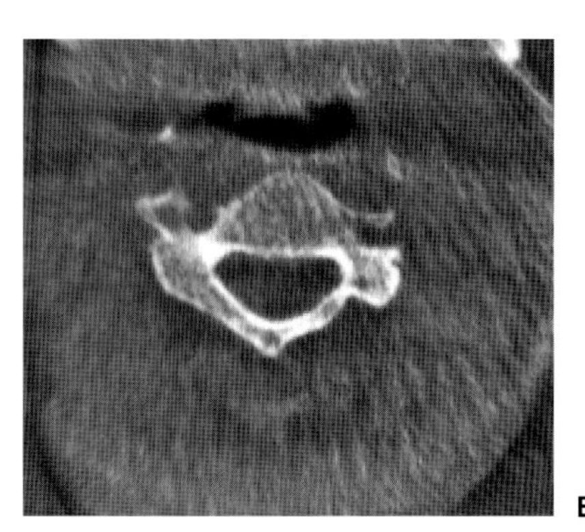
B

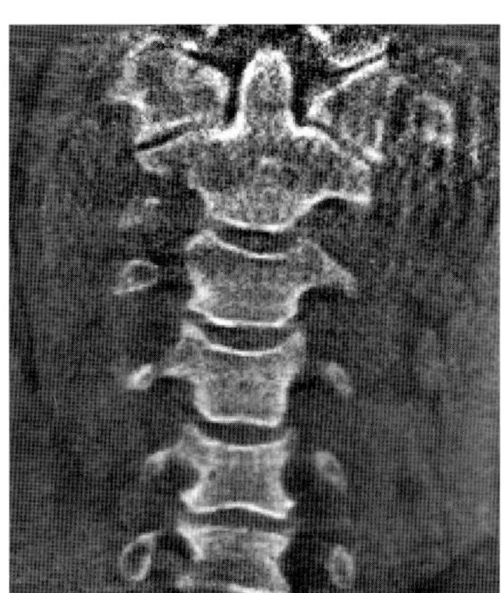
C

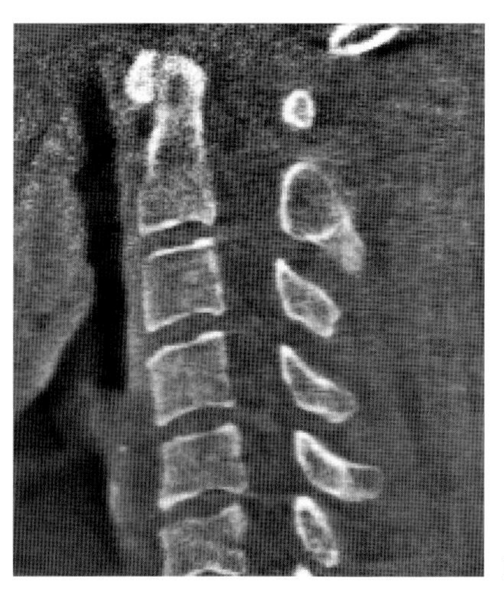
D

FIGURE 9–16 Concentric fluoroscopic unit (SIREMOBIL Iso-C) for acquiring intraoperative axial CT resolution images. **(A)** Motorized C-arm unit capable of automated movement through a 190 degree arc to acquire 100 x-ray images. **(B–D)** Actual intraoperatively acquired image of the cervical spine in axial, coronal, and sagittal orientations.

real-time x-rays. However, differences in the intersegmental relationships between vertebrae in preoperative image acquisition and final operative positioning affect the accuracy of current commercially available systems. These inaccuracies are exaggerated in cases with abnormal intersegmental motion or in patients requiring fracture reduction.

The emergence of three-dimensional fluoroscopic imaging allows for intraoperative acquisition of axial CT renderings of the spinal column (Fig. 9–16). These images are less hampered by superimposed soft tissues, making minimally invasive screw placement in the lower cervical spine accessible. Furthermore, because the images are acquired intraoperatively, screw trajectories can be confirmed by guidewire placement prior to final instrumentation. Amalgams of 3D intraoperative imaging modalities with frameless navigation systems will ultimately make percutaneous placement of cervical instrumentation safe and accessible.

REFERENCES

1. Chapman JR, Anderson PA, Peipin C, et al. Posterior instrumentation of the unstable cervicothoracic spine. *J Neurosurg.* 1996;84: 552–558.
2. Aebi M, Thalgott JS, Webb JK. *AO ASIF Principles in Spine Surgery.* New York: Springer; 1998.
3. Bohlman HH. Acute fractures and dislocations of the cervical spine: an analysis of three hundred hospitalized patients and review of the literature. *J Bone Joint Surg.* 1979;61A:1119–1142.
4. Cahill DW, Bellegarrigue R, Ducker TB. Bilateral facet to spinous process fusion: a new technique for posterior spinal fusion after trauma. *Neurosurgery.* 1983;13:1–4.
5. Callahan RA, et al. Cervical facet fusion for control of instability following laminectomy. *J Bone Joint Surg Am.* 1977;59:991–1002.

6. McAfee PC, Bohlman HH, Wilson WL. Triple wire technique for stablization of acute cervical fracture dislocation. *Orthop Trans.* 1986;10:455–456.
7. Perin NL, Cusick JF. Interspinous, lamina, and facet fusion. In: Benzel EC, ed. *Spine Surgery: Techniques, Complication Avoidance, and Management.* New York: Churchill-Livingstone; 1999:257–263.
8. Stauffer ES. Wiring techniques of the posterior cervical spine for the treatment of trauma. *Orthopedics.* 1988;11:1543–1548.
9. Sutterlin CE, McAfee PC, Warden KE, Rey RM, Farey ID. A biomechanical evaluation of cervical spinal stabilization methods in a bovine model: static and cyclical loading. *Spine.* 1988;13: 795–802.
10. Coe JD, Warden KE, Sutterlin CE III, et al. Biomechanical evaluation of cervical spinal stabilization methods in a human cadaveric model. *Spine.* 1989;14:1122–1131.
11. Maurer PK, Ellenbogen RG, Ecklund J, et al. Cervical spondylotic myelopathy: treatment with posterior decompression and Luque rectangle bone fusion. *Neurosurgery.* 1991;28:680–684.
12. Roy-Camille R, Saillant G, Berteaux D, et al. Early management of spinal injuries. In: McKibbin B, ed. *Recent Advances in Orthopedics.* Edinburgh: Churchill-Livingstone; 1979:57–87.
13. Roy-Camille R, Saillant G, Mazel C. Internal fixation of the unstable cervical spine by posterior osteosynthesis with plates and screws. In: The Cervical Spine Research Society Editorial Committee, eds. *The Cervical Spine.* 2nd ed. Philadelphia: Lippincott-Raven; 1989:390–404.
14. Benzel EC. Construct design. In: Benzel EC, ed. *Biomechanics of Spine Stabilization: Principles and Clinical Practice.* New York: McGraw-Hill; 1995:163–172.
15. Gill K, Paschal S, Corin J, et al. Posterior plating of the cervical spine: a biomechanical comparison of different posterior fusion techniques. *Spine.* 1988;13:813–816.
16. White AA, Panjabi MM. Biomechanical considerations in the surgical management of the spine. In: White AA, Panjabi MM, eds. *Clinical Biomechanics of the Spine.* 2nd ed. Philadelphia: Lippincott-Raven; 1990:511–639.
17. Cooper PR, Cohen A, Rosiello A, et al. Posterior stabilization of cervical spine fractures and subluxations using plates and screws. *Neurosurgery.* 1988;23:300–306.
18. Ebraheim N, An HS, Jackson WT, et al. Internal fixation of the unstable cervical spine using posterior Roy-Camille plates: preliminary report. *J Orthop Trauma.* 1989;3:23–28.
19. Khoo L, Chu F, Hedman T, Samudrala S. Biomechanical comparison of fixation techniques across the cervicothoracic junction. Paper presented at: Annual Meeting of the North American Spinal Society; October 2000; New Orleans.
20. Anderson PA, Henley MB, Grady MS, et al. Posterior cervical arthrodesis with AO reconstruction plates and bone graft. *Spine.* 1991;16(suppl 3):72–79.
21. Chapman J, Anderson PA. Posterior plate fixation of the cervicothoracic junction. *Techn Orthop.* 1994;9:80–85.
22. Halliday AL, Zileili M, Stillerman CB, Benzel E. Dorsal thoracic and lumbar screw fixation and pedicle fixation techniques. In: Benzel EC, ed. *Spine Surgery: Techniques, Complication Avoidance, and Management.* New York: Churchill-Livingstone; 1999; 1053–1064.
23. Papadopolous SM, Fessler RG. The thoracic spine. In: Benzel EC, ed. *Spine Surgery: Techniques, Complication Avoidance, and Management.* New York: Churchill-Livingstone; 1999:157–168.
24. Sawin PD, Traynelis VC, Goel VK. Cervical spine construct design. In: Benzel EC, ed. *Spine Surgery: Techniques, Complication Avoidance, and Management.* New York: Churchill-Livingstone; 1999:1129–1140.
25. Simpson JM, An H. Posterior exposures of the thoracic spine. In: An HS, Riley L III, eds. *An Atlas of Surgery of the Spine.* New York: Lippincott-Raven; 1998:31–43.
26. An HS, Vaccaro A, Cotler JM, et al. Spinal disorders at the cervicothoracic junction. *Spine.* 1994;19:2557–2564.
27. Dekutoski MB, Schendel MJ, Ogilvie JW, Olsewski JM, Wallace LJ, Lewis JL. Comparison of in vivo and in vitro adjacent segment motion after lumbar fusion *Spine.* 1994;15:1745–1751.
28. Delamarter RB, Batzdorf U, Bohlman HH. The C7–T1 junction: problems with diagnosis, visualization, instability and decompression. *Orthop Trans.* 1989;13:218.
29. Evans DK. Dislocations at the cervicothoracic junction. *J Bone Joint Surg [Br].* 1983;65:124–127.
30. Kramer DL, Ludwig SC, Balderston RA, Vaccaro AR, Foley KF, Albert TJ. Placement of pedicle screws in the cervical spine: comparative accuracy of cervical pedicle screw placement using three techniques. *Orthop Trans.* 1997;21:496.
31. Panjabi MM, Duranceau J, Goel V, et al. Cervical human vertebrae: quantitative three-dimensional anatomy of the middle and lower regions. *Spine.* 1991;16:861–869.
32. Stanescu S, Ebraheim NA, Yeasting R, et al. Morphometric evaluation of the cervico-thoracic junction: practical considerations for posterior fixation of the spine. *Spine.* 1994;19:2082–2088.
33. Kotani Y, Cunningham BW, Abumi K, McAfee PC. Biomechanical analysis of cervical stablization systems. *Spine.* 1994;19:2529–2539.
34. An HS, Coppes MA. Posterior cervical fixation for fracture and degenerative disc disease. *Clin Orthop.* 1997;335:101–111.
35. Johnson RM, Southwick WO. Surgical approaches to the spine. In: Rothman RH, Simeone FA, eds. *The Spine.* 2nd ed. Philadelphia: WB Saunders; 1982:67–187.
36. Robinson RA, Southwick WO. Indications and techniques for early stabilization of the neck in some fracture dislocations of the cervical spine. *South Med J.* 1960;53:565–579.
37. Aldrich F. Posterolateral microdiscectomy for cervical monoradiculopathy caused by posterolateral soft cervical disc sequestration. *J Neurosurg.* 1990;72:370–377.
38. Henderson CM, Hennessy RG, Shuey HJ, et al. Posterior-lateral foraminotomy as an exclusive operative technique for cervical radiculopathy: a review of 846 consecutively operated cases. *Neurosurgery.* 1983;13:504–521.
39. Murphey F, Simmons JCH, Brunson B. Cervical treatment of laterally ruptured cervical discs: review of 648 cases, 1939–1972. *J Neurosurg.* 1973;38:679–683.
40. Odom GL, Finney W, Woodhall B. Cervical disc lesions. *JAMA.* 1958;161:23–28.
41. Krupp W, Schattke H, Muke R. Clinical results of the foraminotomy as described by Frykholm for the treatment of lateral cervical disc herniation. *Acta Neurochi [Wien].* 1990;107:22–29.
42. Raaf JE. Surgical treatment of patients with cervical disc lesions. *J Trauma.* 1969;9:327–338.
43. Roh SW, Kim DH, Cardoso AC, Fessler RG. Endoscopic foraminotomy using MED system in cadaveric specimens. *Spine.* 2000;25(2): 260–264.
44. Fessler RG, Khoo L. Minimally invasive cervical microendoscopic foraminotomy (MEF): an initial clinical experience. *Neurosurgery.* 2002;51(5 suppl):37–45.
45. Khoo L. Cervical minimally-invasive spinal surgical techniques. Paper presented at Annual meeting of the AAISMS, 4th Global Congress on Minimally Invasive Spinal Surgery and Medicine; Nov. 20, 2003; Thousand Oaks, CA.
46. Khoo LT. Minimally-invasive posterior decompression and fixation of cervical jumped facets: an initial clinical experience in 11 patients. Paper presented at: Annual Meeting of the AANS/CNS Section on Disorders of the Spine and Peripheral Nerves; March 6, 2003; Tampa, FL.
47. Wang MY, Prusmack CJ, Green BA, Gruen PJ, Levi ADO. Minimally invasive lateral mass screws in the treatment of cervical facet dislocations: technical note. *Neurosurgery.* 2003;52:444–448.
48. Grob D, Magerl F. Dorsal spondylodesis of the cervical spine using a hooked plate. *Orthopade.* 1987;16:55–61.

49. Haid RW, Papadopoulos S, Sonntag V. Lateral mass plating for cervical instability. Paper presented at: Congress of Neurological Surgeons; October 22,1990; Los Angeles.
50. An HS, Gordin R, Renner K. Anatomic considerations for plate-screw fixation of the cervical spine. *Spine*. 1991;16:S548–S551.
51. Albert TJ, Klein GR, Joffe D, Vaccaro AR. Use of cervicothoracic junction pedicle screws for reconstruction of complex cervical spine pathology. *Spine*. 1998;23:1596–1599.
52. Bailey AS, Stanescus S, Yeasting R, et al. Anatomic relationships of the cervicothoracic junction. *Spine*. 1995;20:1431–1439.

SECTION THREE

Thoracic Spine

10

Thoracoscopic Diskectomy

J. PATRICK JOHNSON AND CRYSTAL D. ROGERS

Thoracoscopic diskectomy procedures emerged with technical advances in endoscopy and digital video imaging in the early 1990s, described as video-assisted thoracoscopic surgery (VATS) by researchers independently in Germany and the United States.[1] The advantages of thoracoscopy over thoracotomy have been described in the literature,[2–5] and thoracoscopy is generally accepted as the procedure of choice for treating thoracic disk lesions. The expanding use of thoracoscopic spinal procedures, however, now includes a variety of such applications as sympathectomy (Fig. 10–1), diskectomy, vertebral biopsy, anterior release, vertebral corpectomy, internal fixation, and tumor resection. This chapter will describe the indications and procedures for thoracoscopic diskectomy procedures.

These techniques largely simulate an open thoracotomy procedure in the sense that the trajectory through the chest cavity and the decompression of the spinal canal proceed in a similar manner as the open procedure. The minimal tissue retraction of the endoscopic procedure has reduced postoperative pain and hospitalization in our experience and is supported by results from previous studies.[6,7]

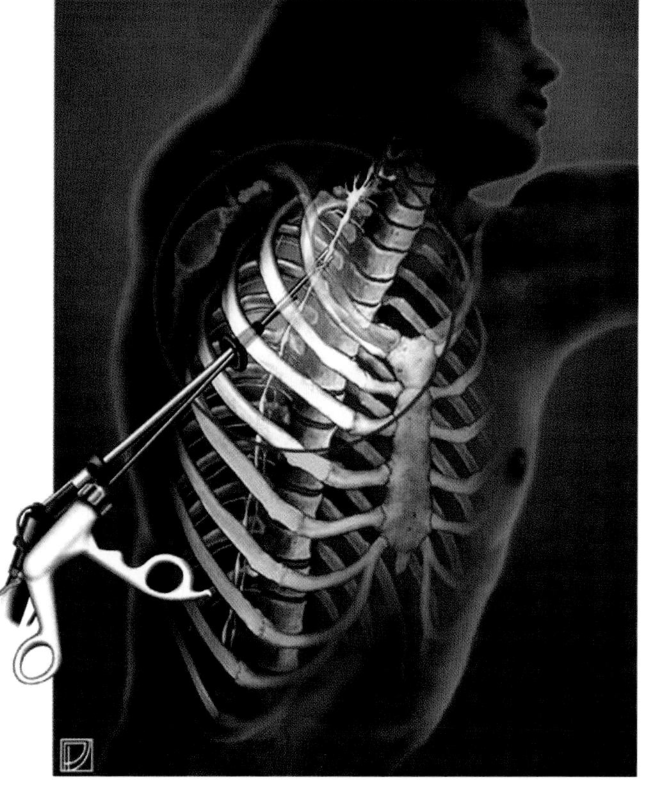

FIGURE 10–1 Illustrated thoracoscopic procedure for sympathectomy.

Indications for Thoracoscopic Diskectomy

The thoracoscopic diskectomy procedure is used to treat symptomatic thoracic disk herniation causing spinal cord and nerve root compression.[8,9] The indications for thoracoscopic diskectomy are essentially the same as are those for thoracotomy to treat primarily ventral lesions causing spinal cord compression and myelopathy.[10]

Radiculopathy due to thoracic disk herniation typically causes both axial back pain and radicular pain that manifests as paraspinal muscular spasms and bandlike

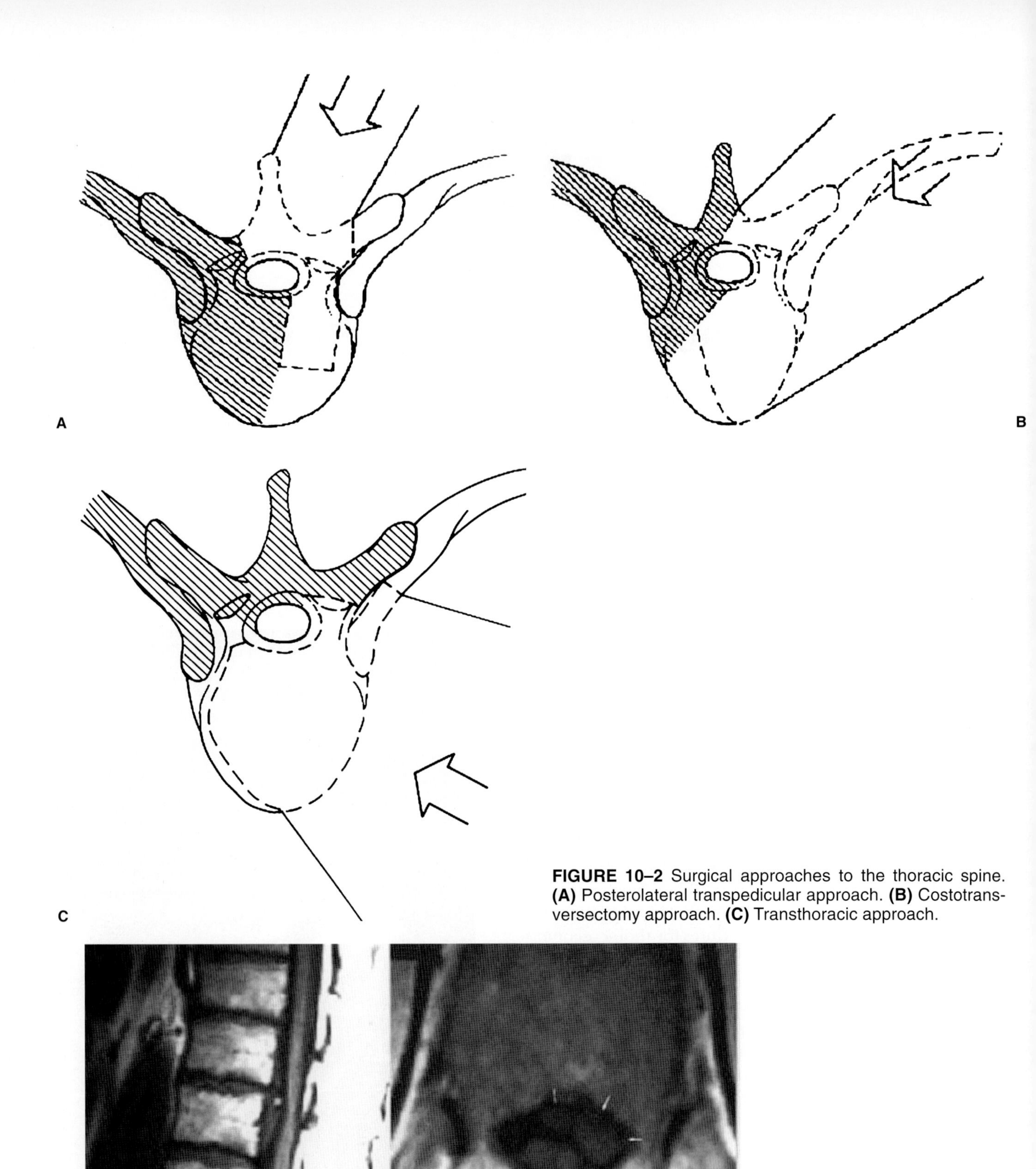

FIGURE 10–2 Surgical approaches to the thoracic spine. **(A)** Posterolateral transpedicular approach. **(B)** Costotransversectomy approach. **(C)** Transthoracic approach.

FIGURE 10–3 T-1 weighted MRI demonstrating a herniated thoracic disk located ventral and lateral to the spinal cord. **(A)** Sagittal and **(B)** axial images.

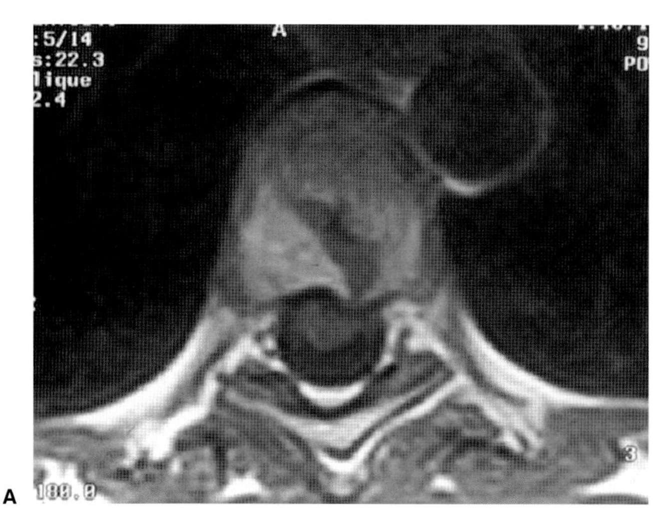

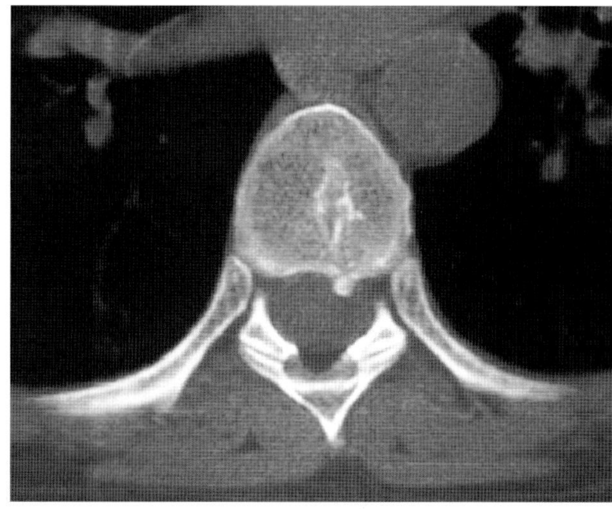

FIGURE 10–4 Calcified herniated disk causing radiculopathy demonstrated with MRI **(A)** and CT scan **(B)**.

radiating chest wall pain. Nonsurgical management of these lesions with nonsteriodal anti-inflammatories, epidural steroid injections, and physical therapy has been successful in treating many patients with solely radicular symptoms. Nonsurgical treatment of tolerable thoracic radiculopathy for 3 to 6 months is reasonable because a large proportion of cases will improve without surgical intervention. Failed nonsurgical treatment of patients with primarily radiculopathy symptoms can be treated with a thoracoscopic diskectomy procedure, but other posterior and posterolateral exposure techniques (i.e., transpedicular and costotransversectomy; Fig. 10–2A,B) are possible alternatives to a transthoracic exposure (Fig. 10–2C), depending on the exact location of the disk herniation. A thoracic disk compressing only the exiting nerve root can usually be treated with posterolateral approaches (Fig. 10–3), whereas a thoracic disk herniation that requires any retraction of the spinal cord should be considered for treatment primarily with an anterior (i.e., transthoracic) approach. An unusual case with a longstanding thoracic radiculopathy from a small calcified disk lesion ventral to the spinal cord is shown in Figure 10–4.

Myelopathy due to thoracic disk herniation is a clearer indication for surgical treatment, although there are some exceptions. There are several presentations of thoracic myelopathy with acute disk herniation and progressive neurologic deficit that require urgent surgical intervention, with timing dependent on each clinical situation (Fig. 10–5). Some patients have a more chronic progression of symptoms that may represent a calcified disk herniation (Fig. 10–6) or ossification of the posterior longitudinal ligament, as shown in Figure 10–7. Most patients with myelopathy due to thoracic disk herniation will require surgical intervention to prevent permanent neurologic impairment; however, cases of disk resorption and resolution of early and mild myelopathy symptoms have been described.

Back pain due to thoracic disk herniation and degenerative disk disease are the least clear indications for surgical intervention (Fig. 10–8). Establishing the diagnosis convincingly may be difficult, and the appearance of a degenerative disk on MRI is useful, but it is not clearly diagnostic. Additional studies to determine if a degenerative

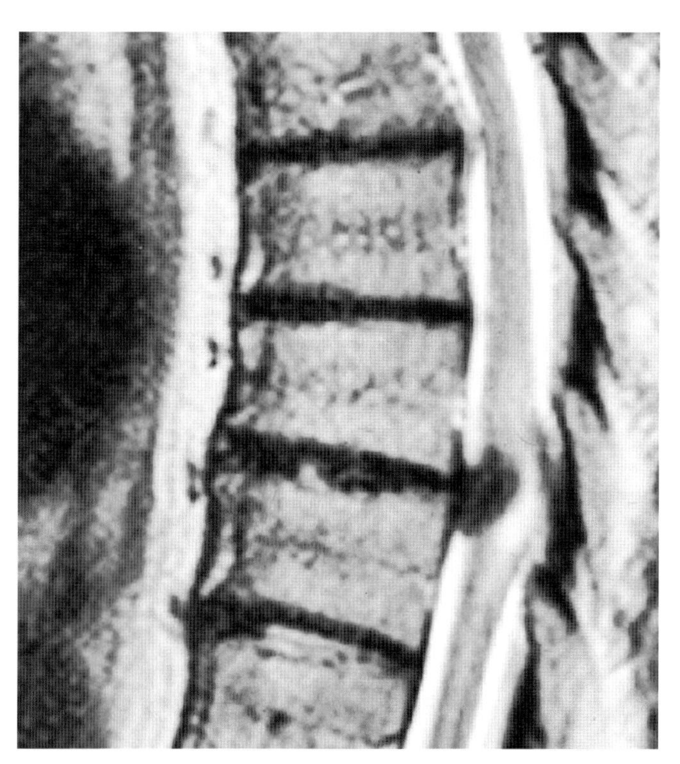

FIGURE 10–5 T-2 weighted MRI sagittal image of the thoracic spine demonstrated a large acute thoracic disk herniation causing severe spinal cord compression and neurologic deficit.

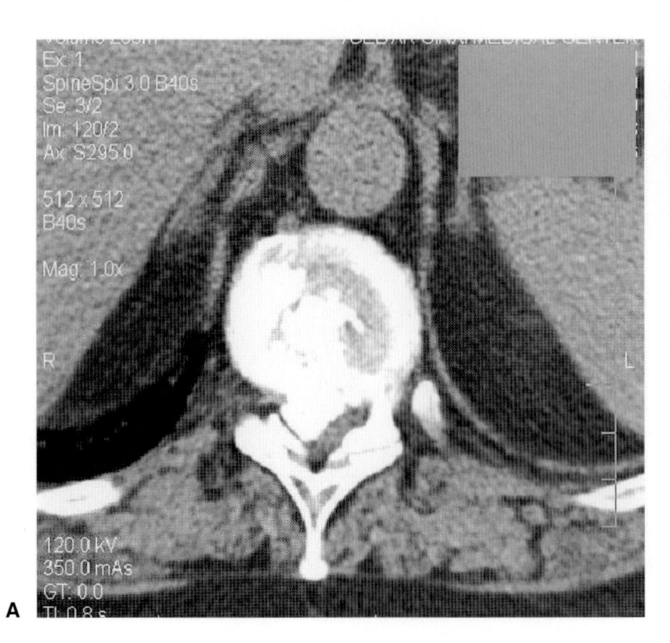

A

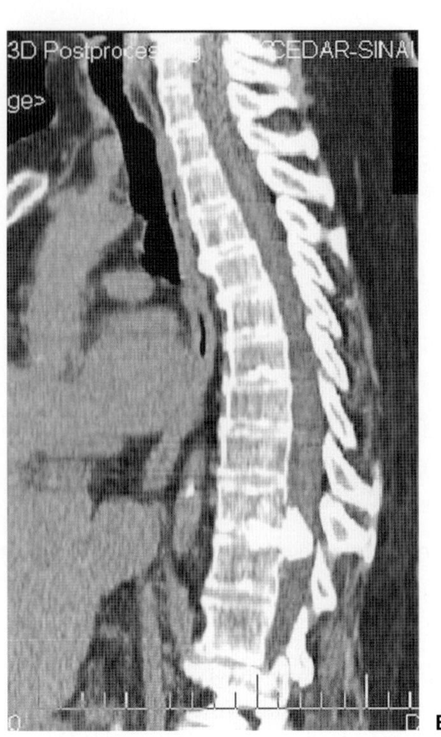

B

FIGURE 10–6 CT of thoracic spine **(A)** axial and **(B)** sagittal reconstructed images demonstrate a large calcified thoracic disk herniation causing slowly progressive symptoms of myelopathy.

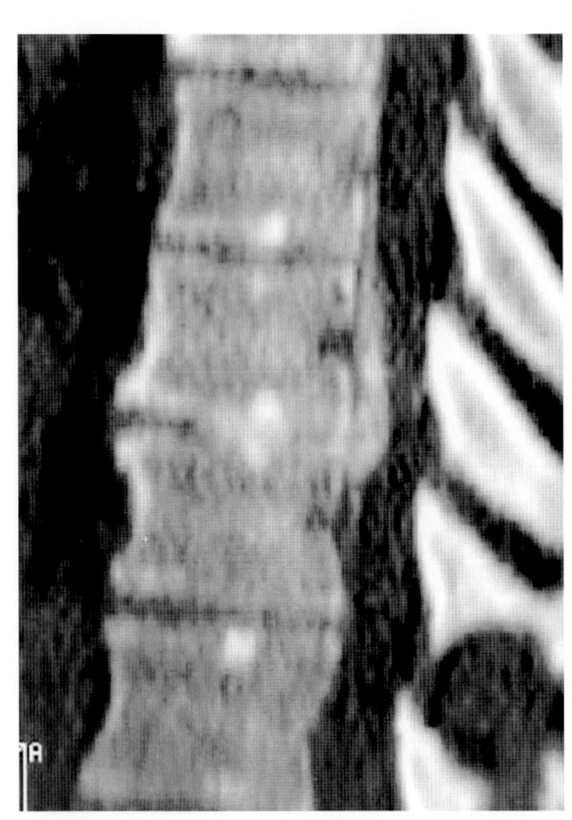

FIGURE 10–7 Sagittal reconstructed CT images of the thoracic spine demonstrates ossification of the posterior longitudinal ligament with severe myelopathy.

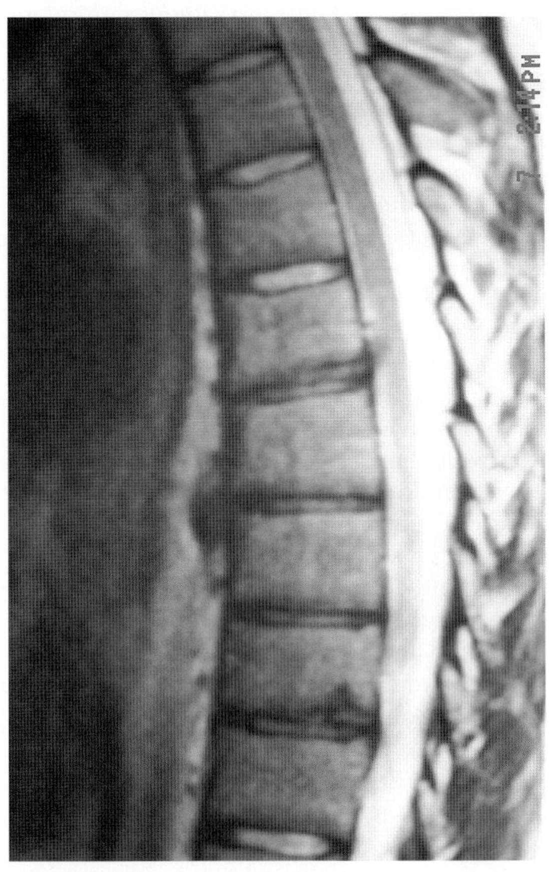

FIGURE 10–8 T-2 weighted image of the thoracic spine demonstrates degenerative thoracic disk disease causing axial back pain.

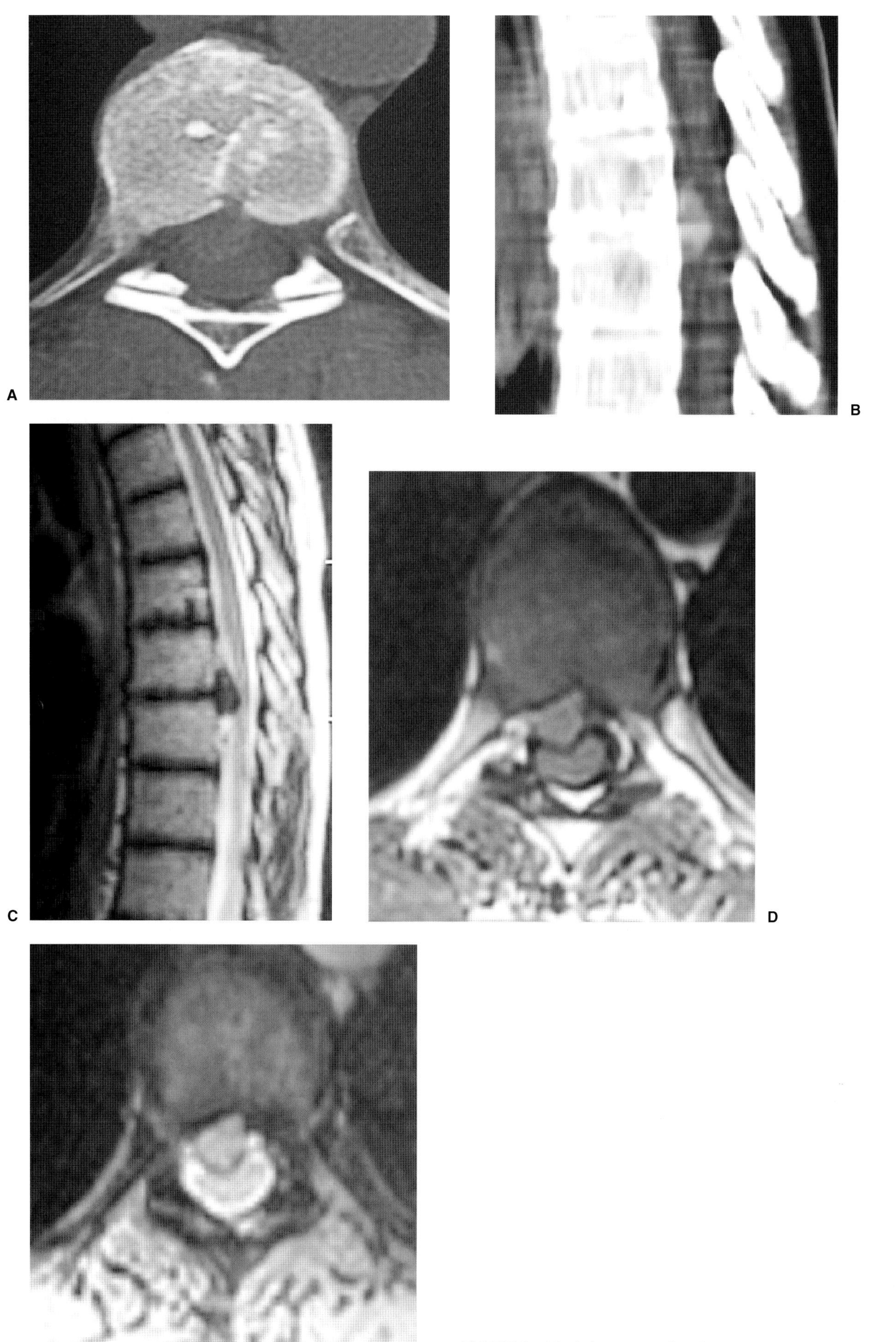

FIGURE 10–9 Large soft thoracic disk herniation poorly demonstrated with CT scan **(A,B)** and well demonstrated with MRI **(C–E).**

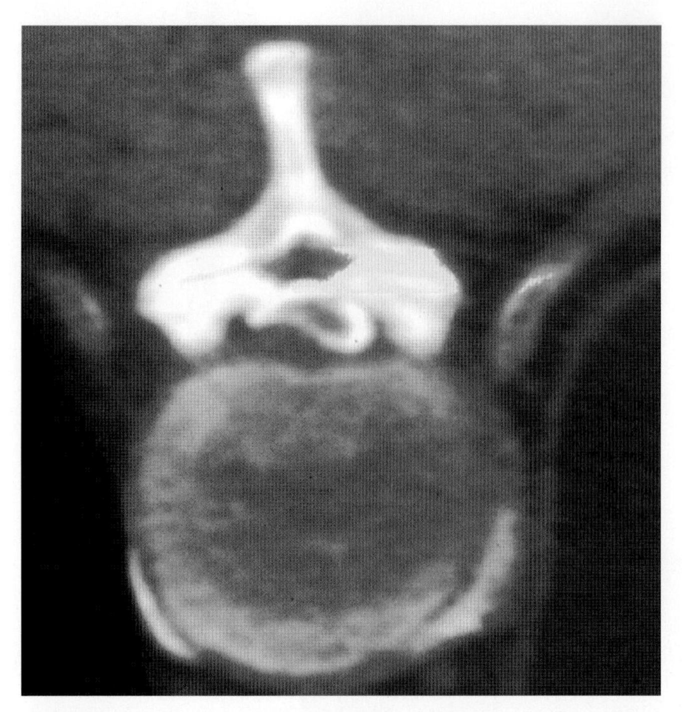

FIGURE 10–10 Postmyelopathy CT scan demonstrating herniated disk and severe spinal cord compression.

disk is the source of pain may require anesthetic blocks and/or diskography to generate as much diagnostic evidence as possible.

Imaging for Thoracic Disk Disease

Modern diagnostic imaging technologies available for the clinician to evaluate thoracic disk disorders are truly remarkable as compared with the past, when only myelography was available. Magnetic resonance imaging has been the primary method to survey the thoracic spine since the late 1980s because it is noninvasive and now easily obtained. It has superior soft tissue definition in multiple orthogonal views to visualize clearly the spinal cord and soft intervertebral disk herniation, as well as other adjacent soft tissue structures that may affect surgical decision making. Bony anatomy is not as well defined with MRI as it is with CT scanning (Fig. 10–9). Calcified disk lesions similarly are not appreciated as well with MRI, so CT is clearly the imaging study of choice in such cases (see Fig. 10–4). The sequence of imaging for a patient with a thoracic disk lesion is usually referral with an MRI completed and indicating the presumed lesion. Plain radiographs of the thoracic and lumbar spine should also be obtained prior to surgery to confirm the level(s) and 12 thoracic vertebrae that are present. CT scanning with or

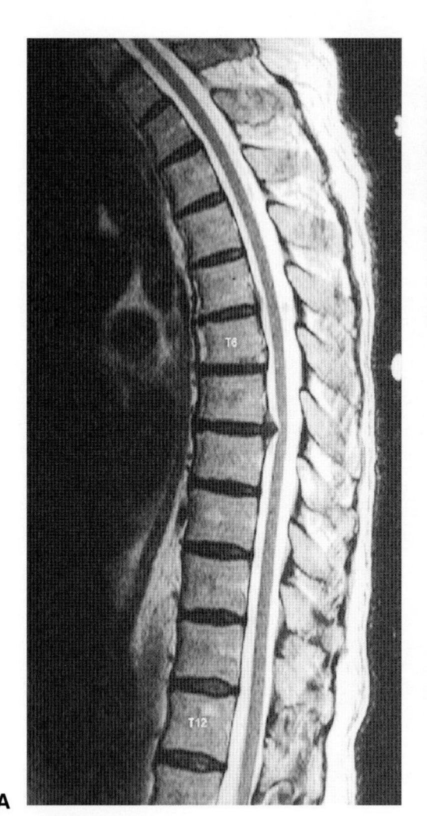

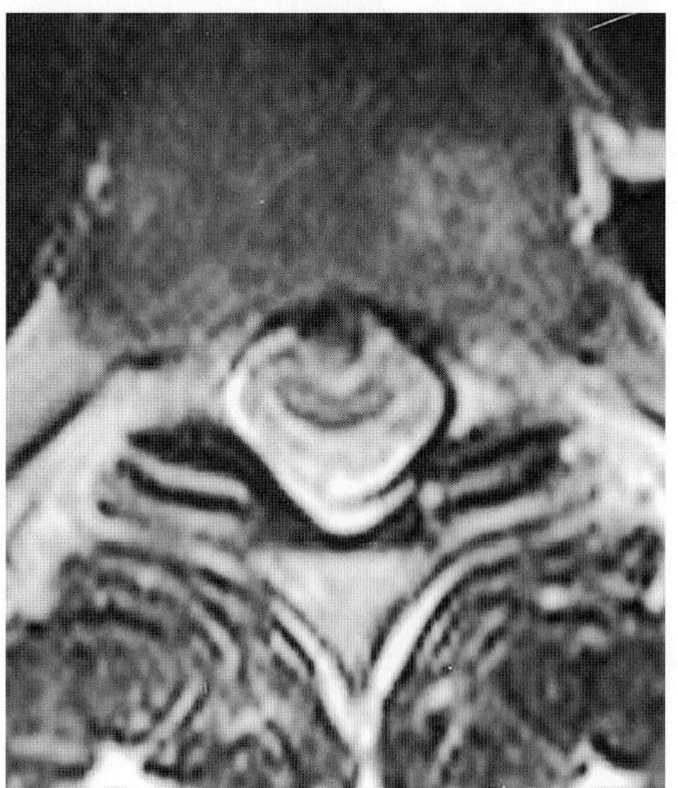

FIGURE 10–11 T-2 weighted MRI. **(A)** Sagittal and **(B)** axial images of the thoracic spine midline herniated disk requiring transthoracic approach for excision.

without myelography can be obtained to define the disk and vertebral lesion further (Fig. 10–10). CT scanning is ideal for imaging primarily bony architecture and further defining specific details of a lesion (e.g., a calcified thoracic disk). Myelography combined with CT scanning provides clear definition of the spinal cord and spinal nerves in relation to the bony and disk anatomy, and it remains superior to MRI in many respects. Nevertheless, the combination of both MRI and CT-myelography for patients with complex thoracic disk lesions provides the maximum preoperative diagnostic information available.

Surgical Decision Making for Thoracic Disk Lesions

Midline ventral lesions causing myelopathy are a clear indication for a transthoracic procedure (Fig. 10–11). Thoracotomy remains the index procedure for these lesions, and none of the posterior laminectomy, posterior transpedicular, or posterolateral costotransversectomy procedures is considered acceptable. Lesions that are ventral-lateral to the spinal cord may be considered for treatment with one of the posterolateral approaches, but they need to be considered carefully. Any retraction of the spinal cord from a posterolateral approach is an indication for an anterior approach. The number of levels treated (i.e., one vs. three) may be a relative indicator for the type of anterior procedures (i.e., thoracoscopy vs. thoracotomy), because the length of a multilevel thoracoscopic procedure may be significantly greater than that for an open thoracotomy.

Endoscopic Instrumentation Required for Thoracoscopic Diskectomy

The endoscopic equipment needed for a thoracoscopic diskectomy procedure is available in hospital operating rooms where general surgical and gynecological laparoscopy and/or general thoracic endoscopy is being performed.[11] The additional spinal instruments are readily obtainable. The endoscopes used are typically endoscope rod lenses (5 to 10 mm diameter) that have 0-, 30-, and 45-degree angles (Fig. 10–12). The lens attaches to the camera that is connected to the light source and video monitor, which are all usually located on the endoscopic cart.

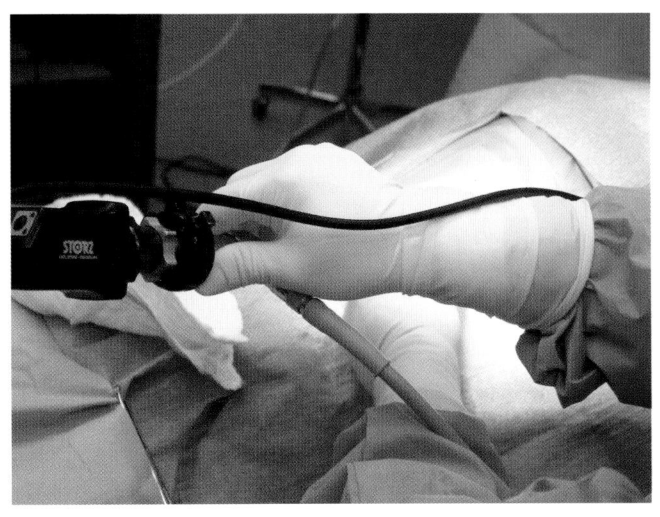

FIGURE 10–12 Surgical endoscope used for thoracoscopy.

The surgical drill is a longer version (8- to 10-in. shaft) of the standard spinal drill used for open procedures. A pistol grip provides some rotational and angular stabilization of the longer shaft instrument that we prefer (Fig. 10–13A). The burr we use is a larger round dissector (5 mm), or a coarse diamond burr can be used (Fig. 10–13B). Other surgical instruments needed are longer-version spinal instruments that are available as custom instrument trays with long, thin shafts (8 to 10 in.), Kerrison rongeurs, straight and

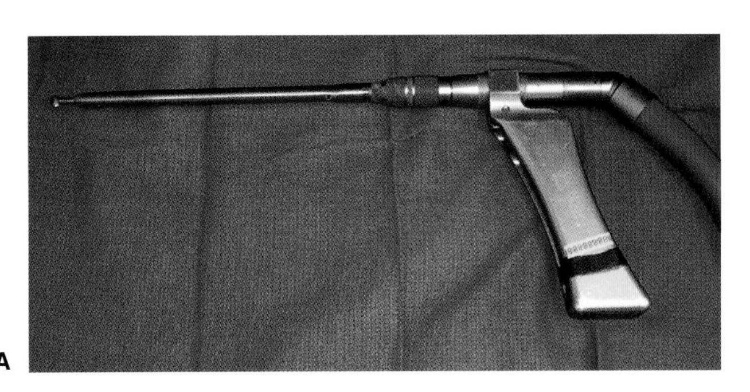

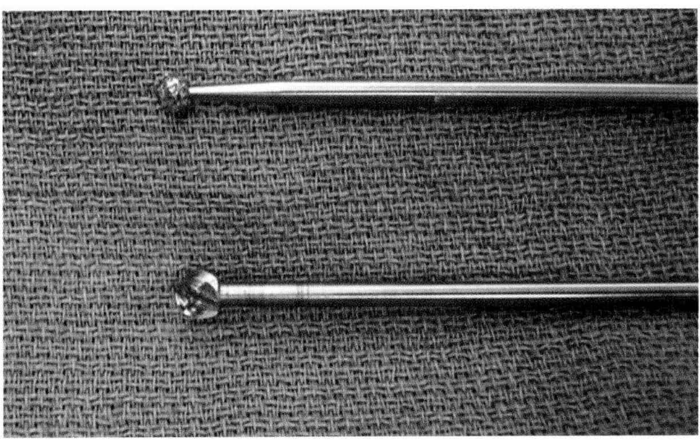

FIGURE 10–13 **(A)** Pneumatic drill with long (8 to 10 inches) shaft. **(B)** Coarse diamond cutting burrs (5 mm diameter) used for bone removal.

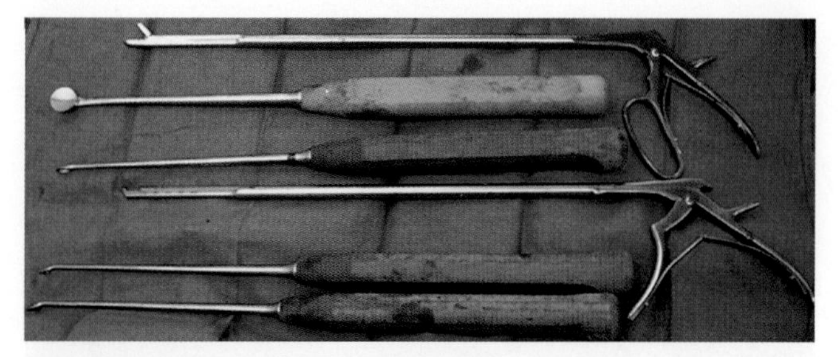

FIGURE 10–14 Long shaft thoracoscopic instruments (pituitary grasper, Kerrison rongeurs, and curettes).

angled curettes, pituitary grasper, nerve hook, Penfield number 4 dissector, and dental dissector (Fig. 10–14). A suction-irrigator is available from the standard endoscopic equipment, but a longer version of a Fraser-type suction is often used to maintain a clear operating field. Various cotton-tip applicators can be used as soft tissue dissectors and to apply bone wax.

Techniques for Thoracic Diskectomy

The procedure requires the induction of general anesthesia and the insertion of a double-lumen endotracheal tube for selective ventilation of the contralateral lung from the side of the procedure. The patient is then secured in a lateral position with the operative side up, and the arm is held in an "airplane"-type holder to expose the chest wall for a thoracotomy (Fig. 10–15). The operating room setup we use is shown in Figure 10–16, although several variations of this setup can be arranged. Standard anesthetic and spinal cord evoked potential monitoring techniques for thoracic endoscopic procedures are used. The spinal level and the portal sites are initially localized from a postpositioning AP chest radiograph. The patient is prepped for a thoracotomy in the event that conversion to thoracotomy is needed.

Three portals are placed in the chest wall in a triangular pattern, with the middle port perpendicular to the operated disk in the posterior axillary line. This port is

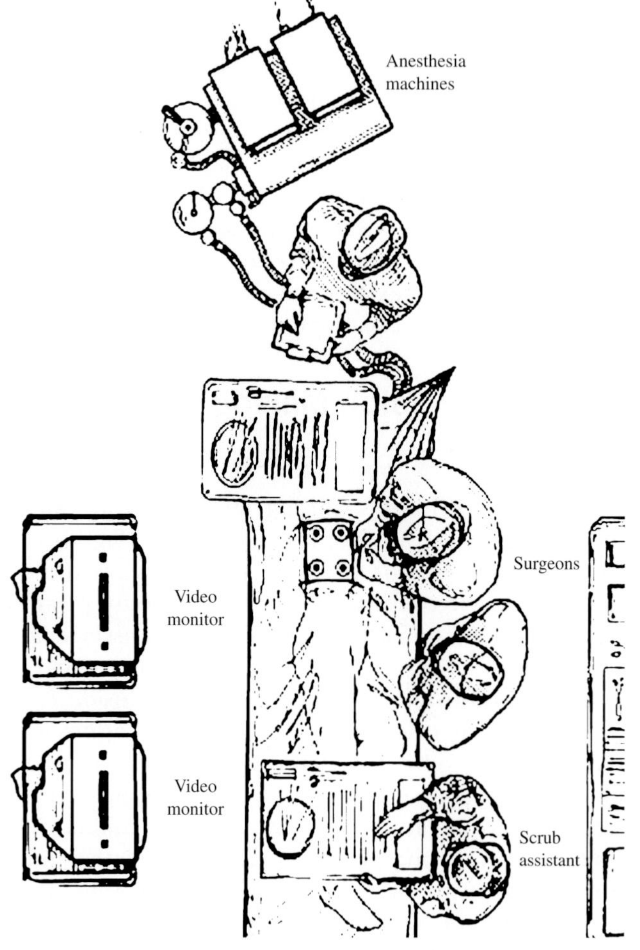

FIGURE 10–16 Operating room setup for thoracoscopic diskectomy.

usually used for the endoscope that overlies the operated disk (Fig. 10–17). The other two ports are placed in the anterior axillary line to complete the triangular pattern and serve as the working portals. The ports are soft, flexible 15 mm cannulas that reduce the incidence of intercostal nerve injury (Fig. 10–18).

Once the portals are placed, the lung is retracted anteriorly, whereas the table is tilted to allow the lung to

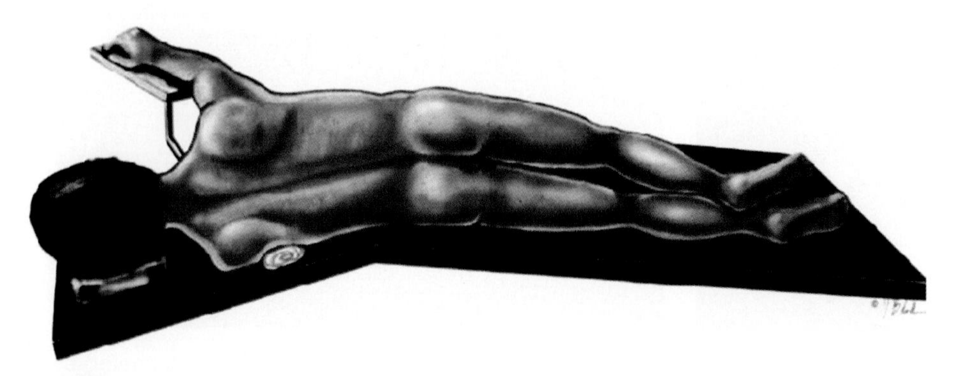

FIGURE 10–15 Lateral surgical position for thoracoscopic procedure.

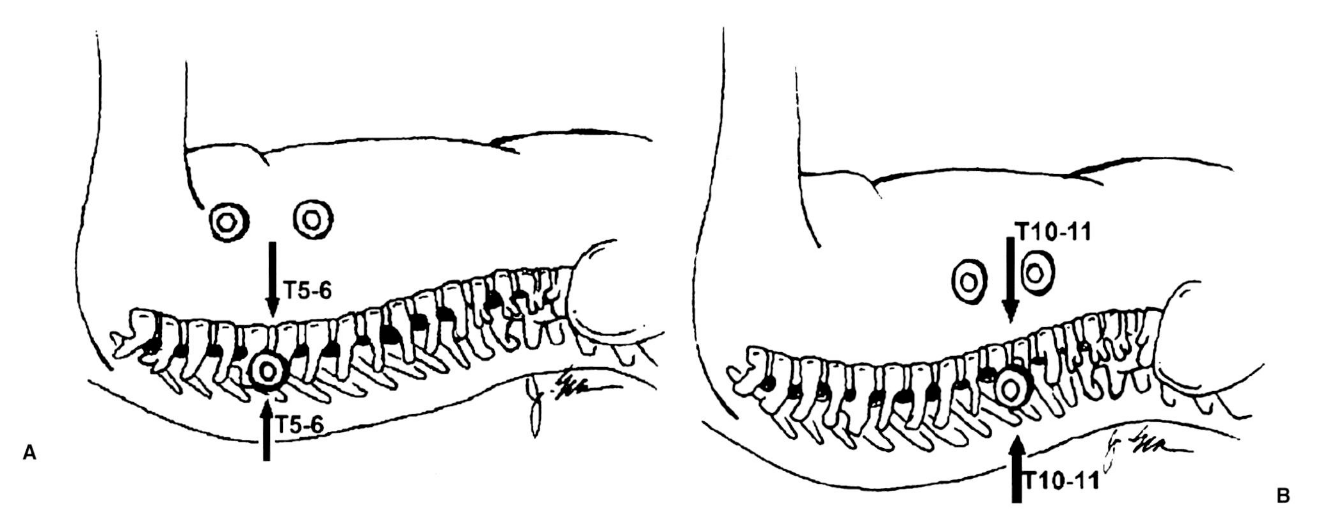

FIGURE 10–17 Portal position for thoracoscopic diskectomy at different levels.

fall away anteriorly. Further retraction of the lung can be accomplished manually by rotation of the operating table to allow the lung to fall forward, away from the vertebral column. Localization of the spinal level is confirmed with an anteroposterior radiograph using a Steinmann pin inserted into the presumptive disk space adjacent to the rib head overlying the disk space.

The adjacent segmental vessels are usually not divided because they are located in the midportion of the vertebral body (Fig. 10–19A). Nevertheless, they can be mobilized, coagulated, and divided if necessary with a monopolar or bipolar cautery device. The parietal pleura is opened widely over the rib head and over the disk space (Fig. 10–19B. The proximal end of the rib and the disk space are colinear and help to orient the surgeon during the procedure. The proximal 2 cm of the rib is removed using a high-speed drill to expose the lateral surface of the pedicle and neural foramen (Fig. 10–19C). The neural foramen contains epidural fat and is relatively small, with the segmental nerve and vessels traversing. The spinal cord dura is then exposed by drilling through the pedicle with a high-speed drill that also orients the surgeon during the remainder of the procedure. A round cutting bit (5 mm diameter) is typically used for the bone drilling. The drilling of the vertebral body is the most critical stage of the procedure; the potential for injury to the patient while achieving adequate bony removal to decompress the spinal canal is significant. The decompression requires drilling across the posterior aspect of the disk space and adjacent end plates that essentially undermine the floor of the spinal canal, creating a tunnel (Fig. 10–19D). The cortical bone on the ventral aspect of the spinal canal should remain intact until the drilling is completed because it protects the spinal cord. Bleeding from the cancellous bone from beneath the end plates can obscure visualization, and hemostasis during every stage of the procedure is essential. Bone wax applied with an endoscopic cotton tip applicator will effectively control bone bleeding. The drilling can be extended to the opposite pedicle and verified with an intraoperative radiograph. A disk fragment that has migrated either cephalad or caudally requires further drilling to undermine the spinal canal adequately for complete decompression. Once the drilling is completed, the floor of the spinal canal is removed with either small Kerrison rongeurs or sharp curettage, beginning where the pedicle was initially removed. After the bony cavity is created, the posterior longitudinal ligament is identified and opened with a blunt tip probe and subsequently resected with sharp endocurettes and Kerrison rongeurs (Fig. 10–19E). This often requires pulling soft disk material or cracking calcified disk into the defect created by the bony decompression. This procedure achieves complete decompression of the dura and spinal cord and spinal canal from a ventral-lateral endoscopic exposure (Fig. 10–19F).

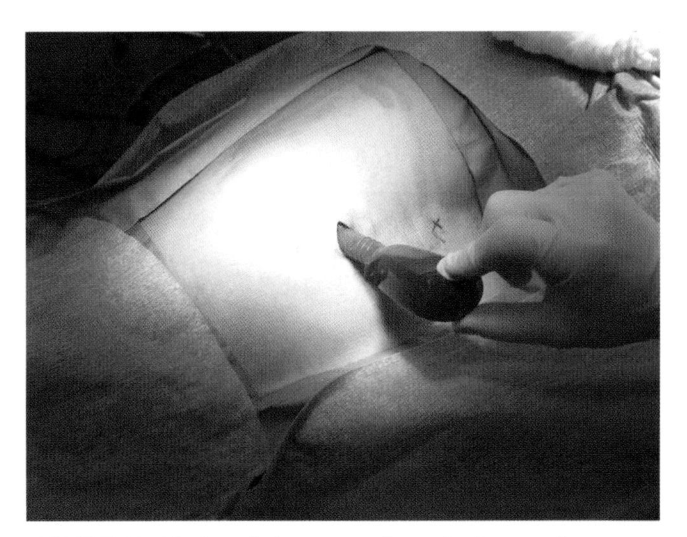

FIGURE 10–18 Portal placement through chest wall.

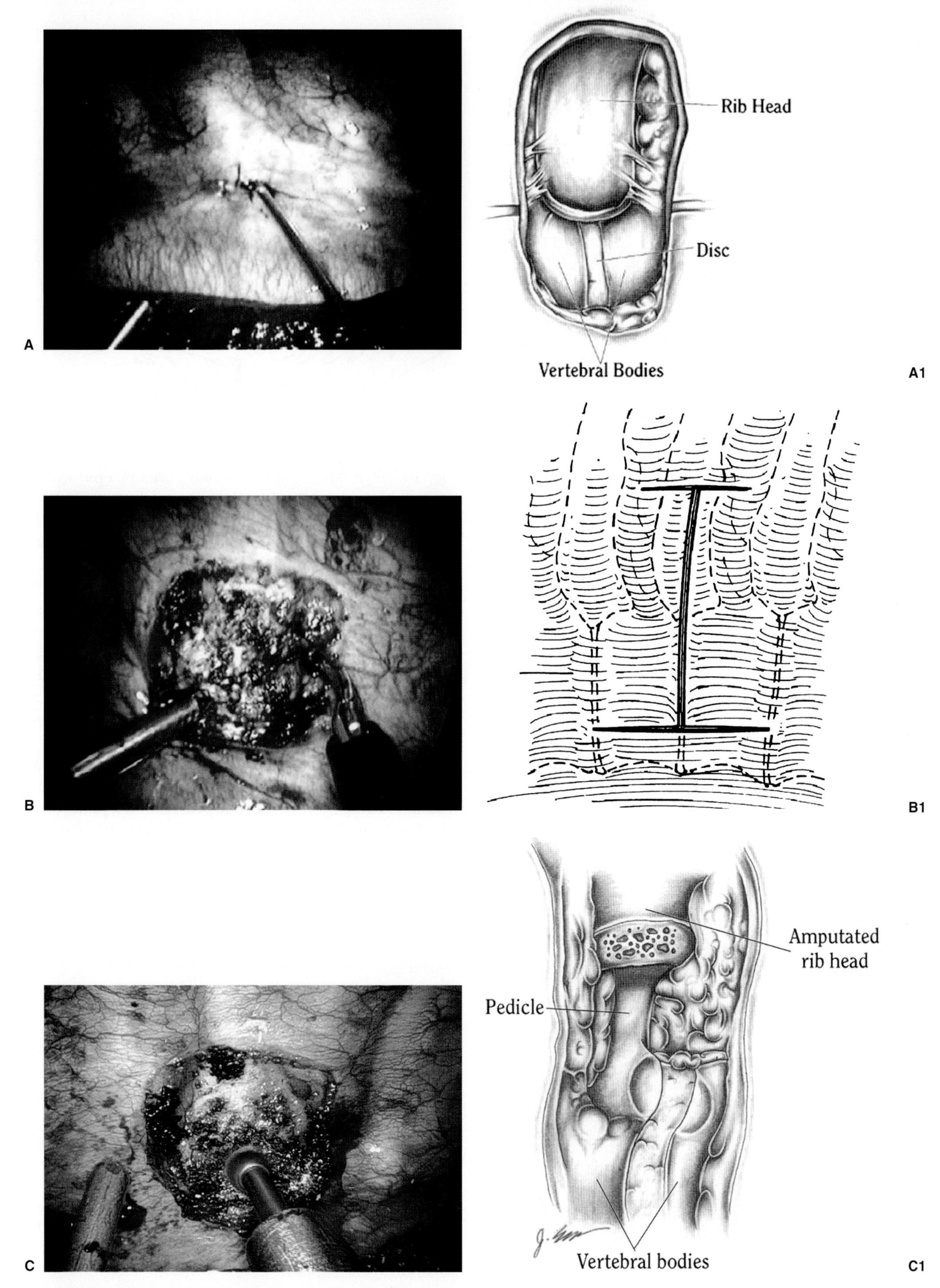

FIGURE 10–19 **(A)** Steinmann pin marker in disk space for radiographic localization. **(B)** Pleural incision over rib head and disk space. **(C)** Drilling of rib head and pedicle.

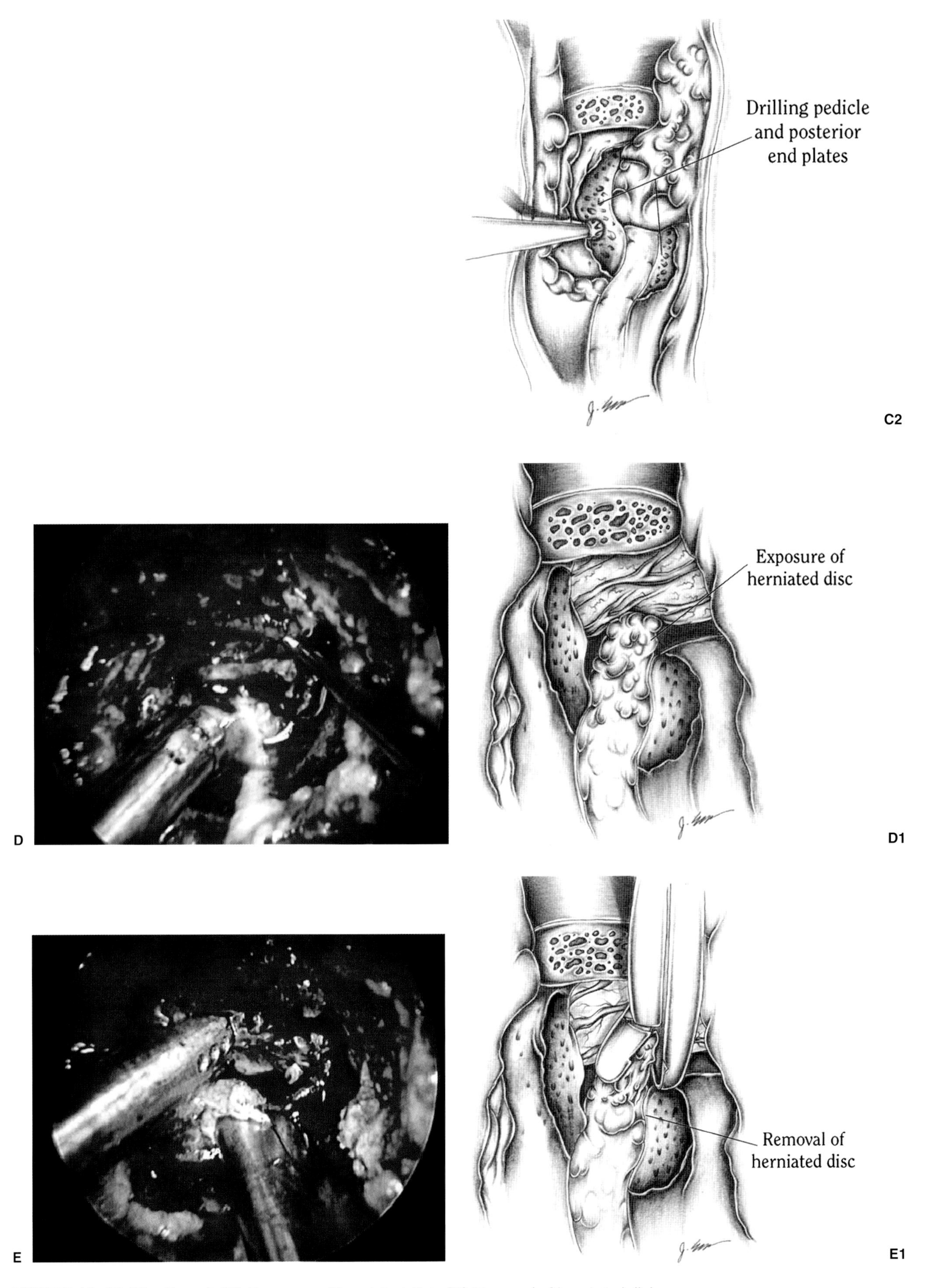

FIGURE 10–19 (*Continued*) **(D)** Exposure of herniated disk. **(E)** Removal of herniated disk.

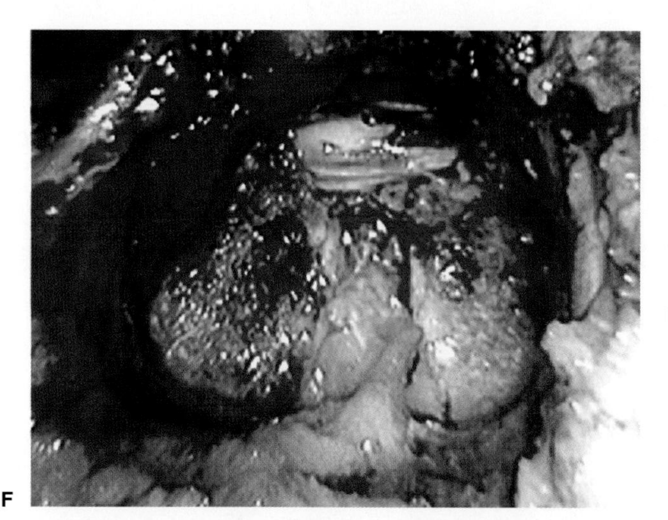

F

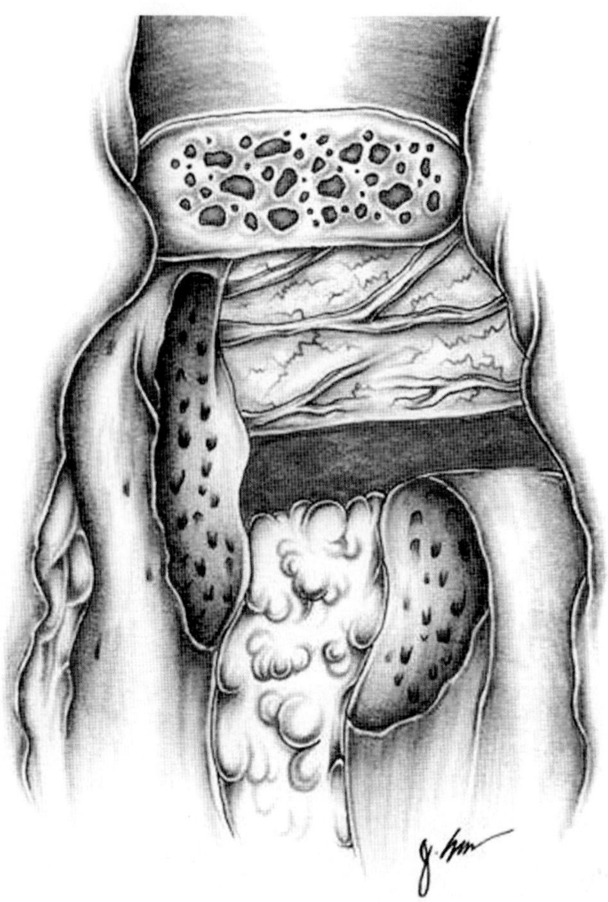

F1

FIGURE 10–19 (*Continued*) **(F)** Diskectomy completed and spinal cord decompressed.

Wound Closure and Postoperative Management

A chest tube is placed through the posterior portal with endoscopic guidance, and 20 cm H_20 suction is applied while the anesthesiologist reinflates the lung. The endoscopic ports are then removed, and the incisions are closed in anatomic layers with absorbable sutures. The patient is extubated at the end of the procedure, and a chest radiograph is obtained in the recovery room to ensure lung inflation. The patient is treated postoperatively with aggressive pulmonary toilet. The chest tube is removed when drainage diminishes to less than 100 ml per day, typically within 24 to 48 hours. Postoperative analgesia with oral narcotics is usually sufficient.

Complications

Complications from the thoracoscopic diskectomy procedure have been uncommon, and most were transient and not life-threatening.[12] Intercostal neuralgia was the most frequent transient complication, and it resolved in nearly all patients by 3 months. Hard plastic ports were used early in the series, and no permanent cases have occurred since changing to soft flexible ports. Other complications that occurred in our experience included pneumonia, recurrent disk herniation, and chylothorax. Pneumonia resolved with antibiotics and pulmonary toilet. Recurrent disk herniation is quite unusual and occurred in a patient who underwent thoracoscopic diskectomy for primarily radicular pain and a mild myelopathy. This patient was initially improved for 6 months, then had recurrent chest wall pain. A new disk fragment was found that was not present on the postoperative MRI. Thoracoscopic reexploration was converted to an open procedure because of dense adhesions, and the disk was removed uneventfully. Chylothorax with a persistent high output of whitish fluid from the chest tube occurred in one patient, despite the fact that no leak was noted at surgery. Treatment with no oral feedings, which provided elemental total intravenous parenteral nutrition for 2 weeks, and leaving the chest tube in place resolved the leak.

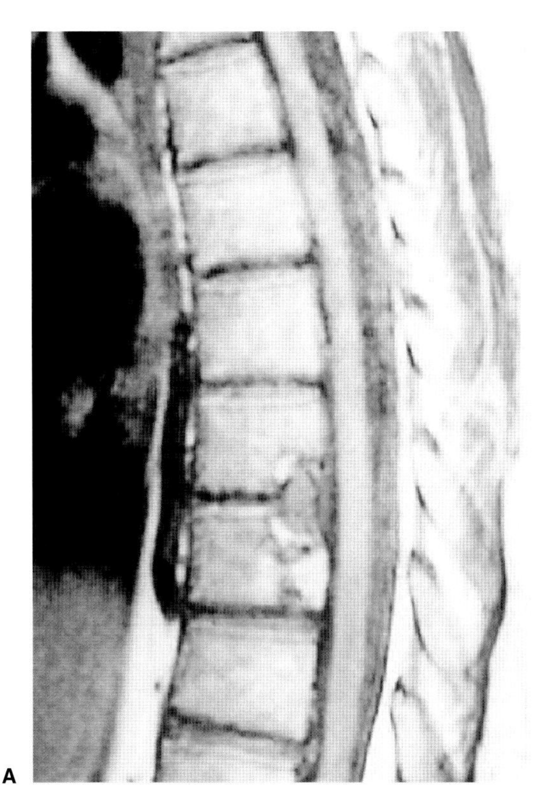

A

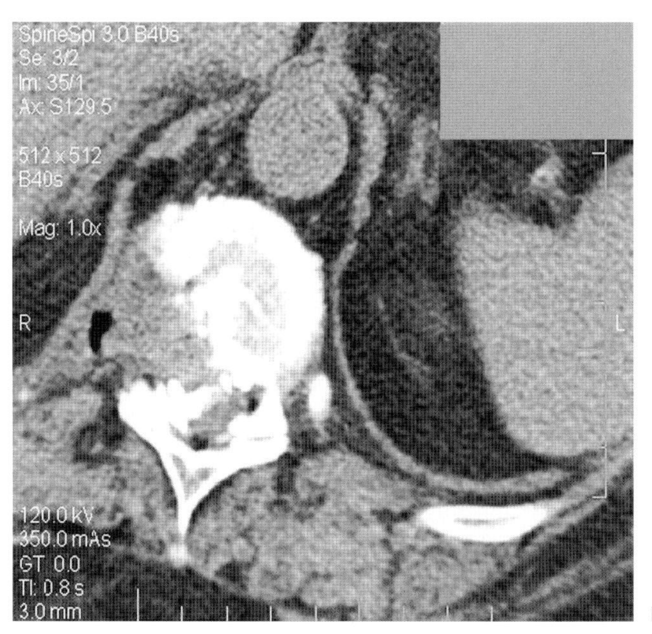

B

FIGURE 10–20 (A,B) Postoperative MRI after thoracoscopic diskectomy.

Advantages of Thoracoscopic Diskectomy

Thoracoscopic procedures for thoracic and pulmonary pathologies have been well established as the procedures of choice compared with thoracotomy and are considered to reduce morbidity, hospitalization, and complications. The advantages are mostly intuitive and obvious: to achieve a minimally invasive thoracic diskectomy (Fig. 10–20) and reduced pain due to small incisions (Fig. 10–21) that avoid rib retraction, and to reduce the risk of long-term post-thoracotomy pain syndromes that are difficult to treat. It is unlikely that a true randomized prospective study comparing thoracotomy with thoracoscopic diskectomy will occur because patients seeking minimally invasive procedures from surgeons skilled in these techniques would have a thoracotomy as a primary procedure.

Disadvantages of Thoracoscopic Diskectomy

The difficulty of thoracoscopic spinal surgery is the steep learning curve: The procedure requires the surgeon to convert a two-dimensional video image into a working three-dimensional field with appropriate spatial orientation. Endoscopically visualized anatomical landmarks were previously used exclusively to determine spatial ori-

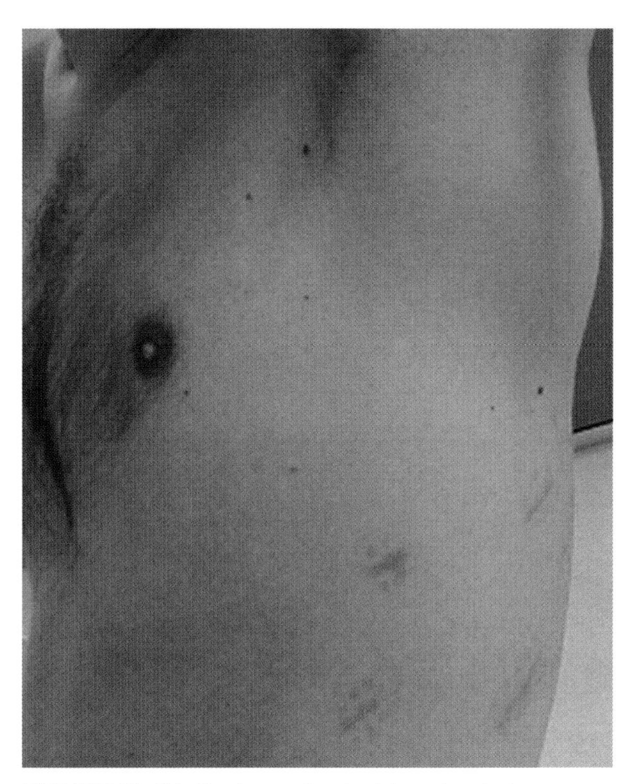

FIGURE 10–21 Postoperative incisions healed.

entation and proximity to critical structures. Additional depth perception was gained by using calibrated instruments. The length of the surgical instruments and the fulcrum effect that occurs through the portals in the chest wall create a whole new set of visual-motor skill challenges that must be acquired. It is also difficult for the surgeon to use instruments in each hand simultaneously to perform complex tasks; an experienced assistant is required.

Thoracoscopic diskectomy procedures have several distinct advantages over thoracotomy, including reduced surgical pain and morbidity and shorter hospitalization. We should emphasize the need for adequate training in the treatment of thoracic disk herniations, which requires that a surgeon have an adequate surgical volume to maintain an effective skill set for these procedures. Such alternatives as transthoracic, transpedicular, and costotransversectomy procedures clearly remain viable and effective techniques for appropriately selected cases by surgeons who are experienced in them but who have limited experience with thoracoscopic diskectomy procedures.

Acknowledgments

The authors wish to thank Josh Emerson for his artistic contributions and Samantha Phu for her assistance in preparing this chapter.

REFERENCES

1. Horowitz MD, Moossy JJ, Julian T, et al. Thoracoscopic discectomy using video assisted thoracoscopy. *Spine.* 1994;19:1082–1086.
2. Dajczman E, Gordon A, Kreisman H, et al. Long-term post-thoracotomy pain. *Chest.* 1991;99:270–274.
3. Dickman CA, Rosenthal D, Perin NI. *Thoracoscopic Spine Surgery.* New York: Thieme Medical Publishers; 1999.
4. Ferson PF, Landreneau RJ, Dowling RD, et al. Comparison of open versus thoracoscopic lung biopsy for diffuse infiltrative pulmonary disease. *J Thorac Cardiovasc Surg.* 1993;106:194–199.
5. Regan JJ, Mack MJ, Picetti GD III, et al. A comparison of video-assisted thoracoscopic surgery (VATS) with open thoracotomy in thoracic spinal surgery. *Today's Ther Trends.* 1994;2:203–218.
6. Johnson JP, Filler AG, McBride DQ. Endoscopic thoracic discectomy. *Neurosurg Focus.* 2000;9:11.
7. Oskouian. Johnson JP, Regan JJ. Thoracoscopic microdiscectomy. *Neurosurgery.* 2002;50:103–109.
8. Rosenthal D, Rosenthal R, de Simone A. Removal of a protruded thoracic disc using microsurgical endoscopy: a new technique. *Spine.* 1994;19:1087–1091.
9. Rosenthal D, Dickman CA. Thoracoscopic microsurgical excision of herniated thoracic discs. *J Neurosurg.* 1998;89:224–235.
10. Mack MJ, Regan JJ, Bobechko WP, et al. Application of thoracoscopy for disease of the spine. *Ann Thorac Surg.* 1993;56:736–738.
11. Regan JJ, McAfee PC, Mack MJ. *Atlas of Endoscopic Spine Surgery.* St. Louis, MO: Quality Medical Publishing; 1995.
12. McAfee PC, Regan JJ, Zdeblick T, et al. The incidence of complications in endoscopic anterior thoracolumbar spinal reconstructive surgery: a prospective multicenter study comprising the first 100 cases. *Spine.* 1995;20:1624–1632.

11

Posterolateral Endoscopic Thoracic Diskectomy

JOHN C. CHIU

Posterolateral endoscopic thoracic diskectomy (PETD) is an alternative procedure for treating symptomatic herniated thoracic disks through an endoscope to achieve less tissue trauma than is caused by current conventional thoracic disk surgery and thoracoscopic procedures. The purpose of this chapter is to demonstrate the indications, instrumentation, surgical technique, safety, and efficacy of this less-traumatic outpatient endoscopic procedure. In addition, lower-energy nonablative laser is applied for shrinkage and tightening of the disk (laser thermodiskoplasty). This minimally invasive spinal surgery has numerous advantages, but it requires thorough knowledge of the PETD procedure, the surgical anatomy, specific surgical training, and hands-on experience in a laboratory and working closely with an experienced endoscopic surgeon through its steep surgical learning curve. The rationale and technique of this minimally invasive percutaneous endoscopic operation to relieve symptoms of protruded thoracic disks are presented.

Spinal surgeons have long sought to find a procedure of choice by which to treat thoracic disk herniations.[1–12] The threat of spinal cord, neural, vascular, and pulmonary injury has stimulated many attempted approaches, including posterior laminectomy (seldom performed because it is too likely to result in neurologic injury), costotransversectomy, and transthoracic, transpleural, posterolateral, transfacet pedicle-sparing, transpedicular, and, more recently, transthoracic endoscopic and posterolateral endoscopic procedures.[1–6,11–13]

Many clever, minimally invasive surgical endoscopic thoracic procedures have been developed, including video-assisted thoracic surgery (VATS),[1] thoracic sympathectomy, and others attempting to reduce operative trauma.

In the past, surgery was not contemplated unless considerable cord compression and neurologic deficit were present.[5,6,11,12] A significant number of patients complain of thoracic spinal and paraspinal pain, intercostal or chest wall pain, upper abdominal pain, and occasionally low back pain due to thoracic disk protrusions without severe neurologic deficit or dramatic radiological abnormalities. With such improved diagnostic methods as MRI scans[8] (the method of choice), CT myelograms, and CT scans, the diagnosis of these thoracic disk protrusions is now far more common. Such patients usually receive some period of physical therapy, injection therapy, and analgesics, and, if not cured, are expected to live with their discomfort because potential severe postoperative complications are feared if usual surgical treatment is attempted.

PETD with laser thermodiskoplasty[11–13] evolved from minimally invasive techniques used in the lumbar and cervical areas,[10–16] and from the basic approach for performing thoracic diskography.[9] We also have utilized pre- or intraoperative diskograms and pain provocation tests on almost all cases to confirm the diagnosis and the appropriate levels to treat. This chapter will describe the technique, safety, and efficacy of a method for treating thoracic disk protrusions by outpatient PETD.

Indications

The PETD approach is indicated[12] in the following clinical situations:

- Pain in the thoracic spine, often radiating to the chest wall, with possible numbness and paresthesia in an intercostal distribution due to thoracic disk herniation

- No improvement of symptoms after a minimum of 12 weeks of conservative management
- MRI or CT scan positive for disk herniation, consistent with the level of clinical symptoms
- Confirmatory pre- or intraoperative diskogram and pain provocation test
- Multiple thoracic disks may be treated at one sitting[17–21]

Contraindications

The PETD approach is contraindicated in the following clinical situations:

- Severe cord compression or total block on radiographic studies
- Advanced spondylosis with severe disk space narrowing or osteophytes blocking entry into the disk space

Instruments and Preparation

This surgical equipment and these instruments[11–13] are necessary to perform PETD (similar to anterior endoscopic cervical microdiskectomy):

- Digital fluoroscopy equipment (C-arm) and monitor
- Full radiolucent C-arm/fluoroscopic carbon-fiber surgical table
- Endoscopic tower equipped with digital video monitor, DVT/VHS recorder, light source, photo printer, with trichip digital camera system (Fig. 11–1)

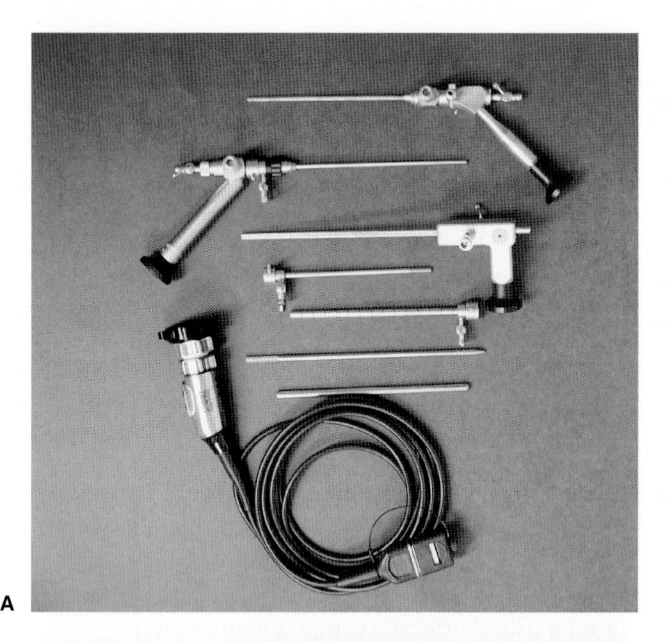
A

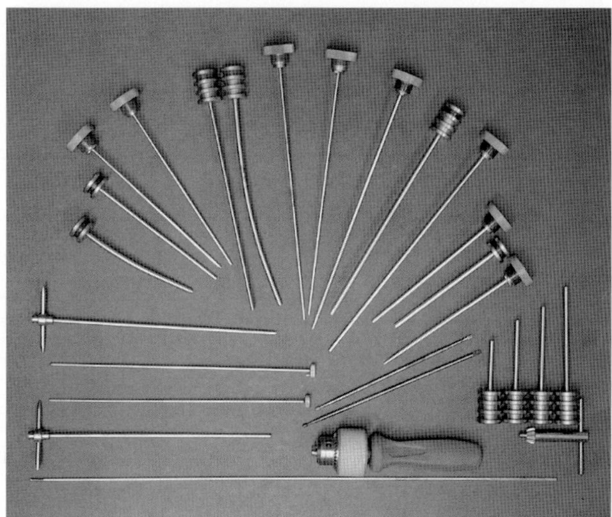
B

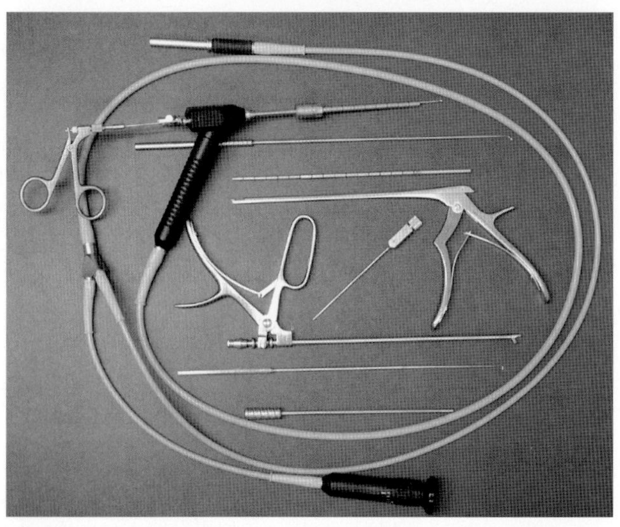
C

FIGURE 11–1 Posterolateral endoscopic thoracic diskectomy instruments. **(A)** Thoracic endoscopes (0-, 6-, and 30-degree) and trichip digital camera. **(B)** Endoscopic working cannula systems, trephines, rasp, and burrs. **(C)** Various types of forceps and rongeurs.

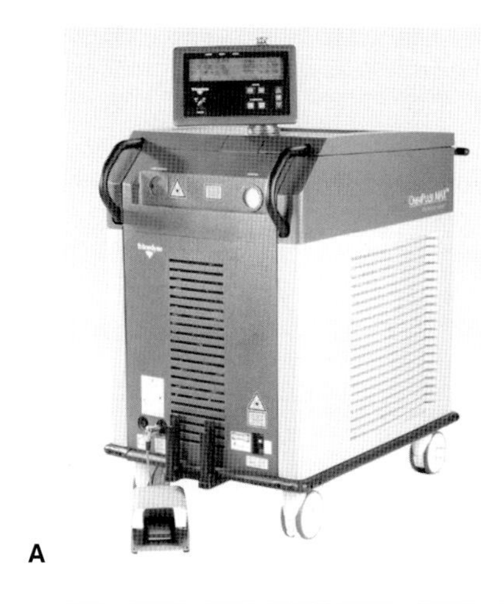
A

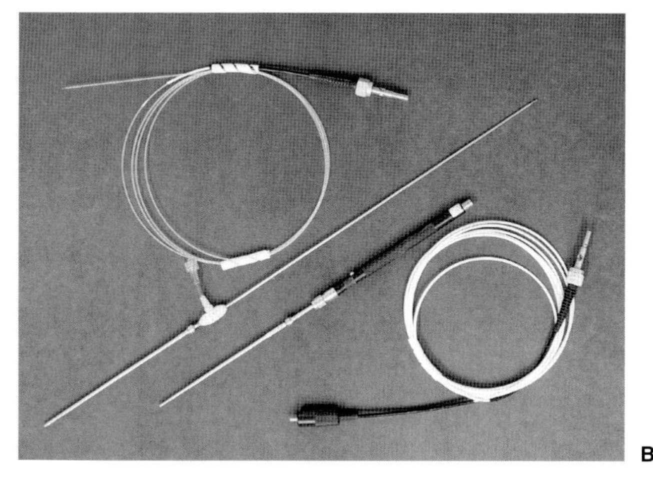
B

C

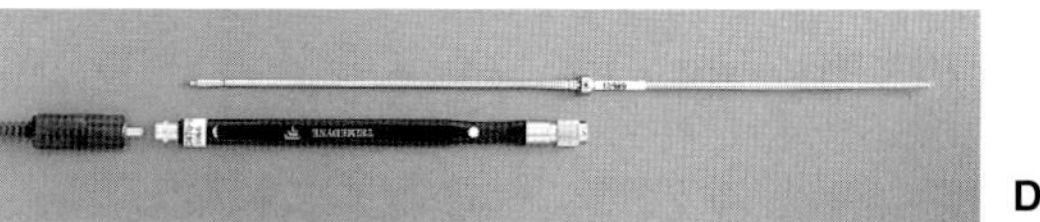
D

FIGURE 11–2 Holmium:YAG laser equipment for laser thermodiskoplasty. **(A)** An 85 W double-pulse holmium:YAG laser generator. **(B)** A 550 μm holmium bare fiber with flat tip, and right-angle (side-firing) probe. **(C)** Single-use side-firing probes. **(D)** Reusable short side-firing probes.

- Thoracic endoscopic diskectomy set (Karl Storz, Tuttlingen, Germany), including 4 mm 0-degree endoscope (Fig. 11–1)
- Thoracic operating endoscope, 3.5 mm 6-degree, and diagnostic endoscopes, 2.5 mm 0-degree and 30-degree (Fig. 11–1)
- Thoracic diskectomy sets (2.5 and 3.5 mm) (Blackstone Medical, Inc., Springfield, MA) with short and long diskectomes (Fig. 11–1)
- Endoscopic grasping and cutting forceps and scissors (Fig. 11–1)
- Endoscopic probe, knife, rasp, and burr (Fig. 11–1)
- More aggressively toothed trephines used for spurs and spondylitic ridges at the anterior and posterior disk space (Fig. 11–1)
- Holmium:YAG laser generator (Trimedyne; Irvine, CA) with and 550 μm holmium bare fiber with flat-tip right-angle (side-firing) probe (Fig. 11–2)

Anesthesia

The patient is treated in an operating room under local anesthesia and monitored for conscious sedation. The anesthesiologist maintains mild sedation, but the patient is able to respond. Two grams of Ancef and 8.0 mg of dexamethasone are given intravenously at the start of anesthesia. Surface EEG (SNAP; Nicolet Biomedical, Madison, WI, USA) provides added precision of anesthesia.

Patient Positioning

The patient is prone on the table with a radiolucent 20-degree angled sponge under the symptomatic side of the chest, angling it into an obliquely up position (Fig. 11–3A). The arms are supported on arm boards over the head. Because only local anesthesia and mild sedation are used, the extremities, buttocks, and shoulders are restrained from sudden motion with adhesive tape.

Localization

Levels are identified by counting under C-arm fluoroscopy from the twelfth rib up, and from C7 of the cervical spine down for upper level thoracic diskectomies. Radiopaque markers are placed on the skin at appropriate sites.[11–13] The midline, the levels, and the point of entry (operating portal) for surgery are marked on the skin with a marking pen (Fig. 11–3B). Using sterile technique, the level of the disk can be accurately identified by inserting an 18-gauge needle into a disk under fluoroscopic guidance (Figs. 11–3C, 11–4, 11–5). The portal of entry is to be marked at 4 to 5 cm away from the midline at the midthoracic area (T5–T8 inclusive) at the respective thoracic disk level, 6 to 7 cm from the midline at the lower thoracic area (T9–T12 inclusive), and at the upper thoracic area (T1–T4 inclusive). Positioning of the instruments is checked throughout the procedure

A

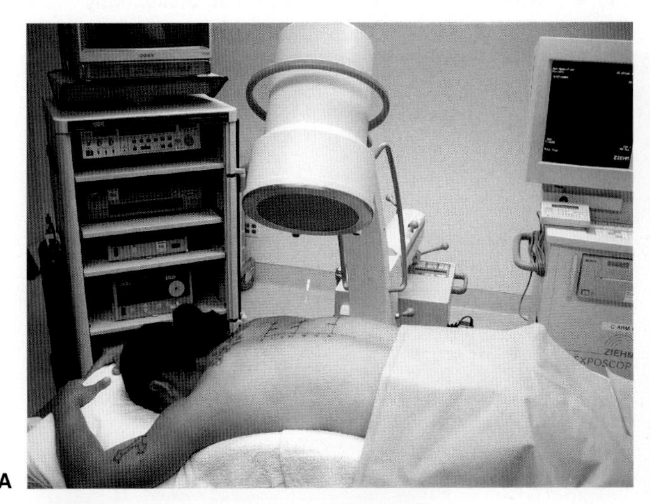

B

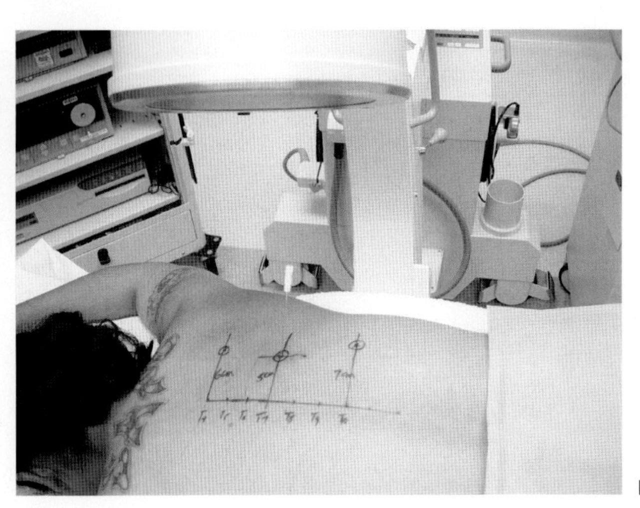

C

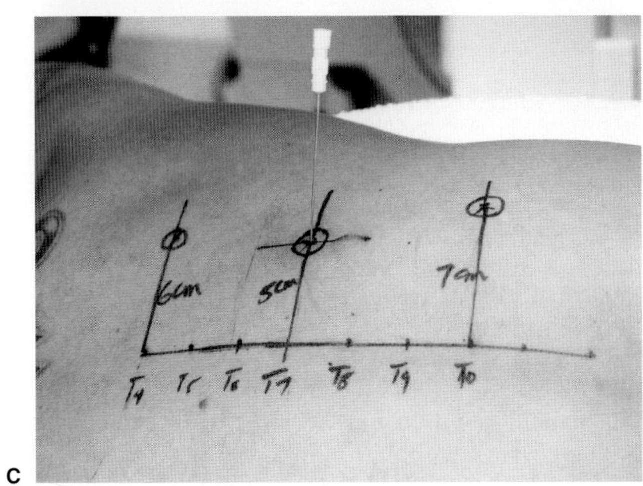

FIGURE 11–3 Patient positioning and localization. **(A)** Patient positioning. **(B)** Localization—skin marking. **(C)** Placement of needle (portal).

A

B

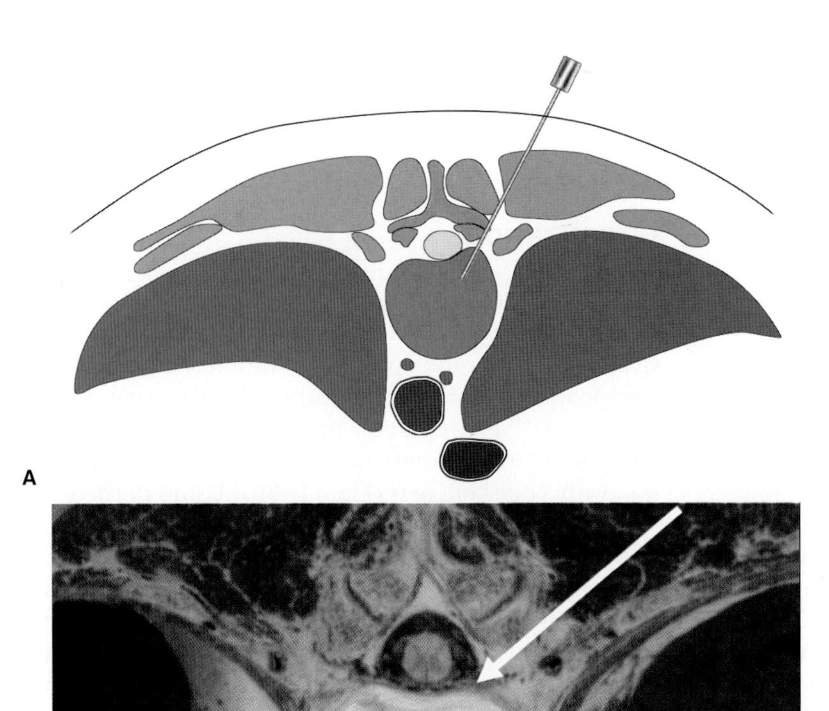

FIGURE 11–4 Surgical approach for posterolateral endoscopic thoracic diskectomy for needle and stylette placement into the disk. **(A)** Axial view illustration for needle placement. **(B)** Cross-section cadaveric cryomicrotome: posterolateral surgical approach.

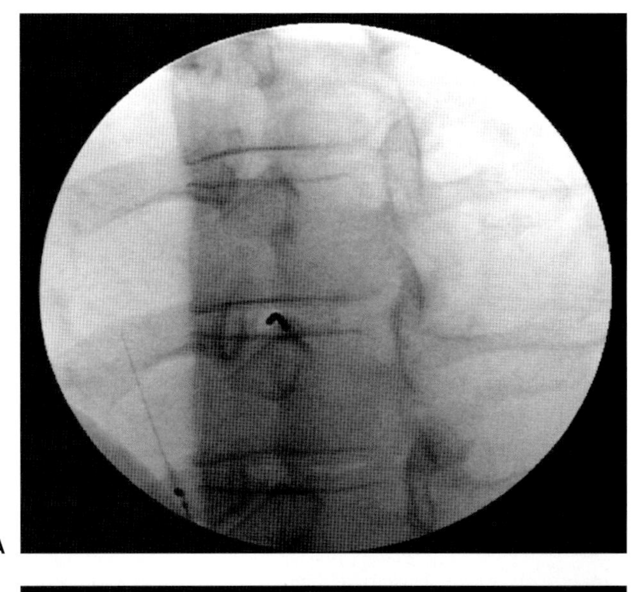
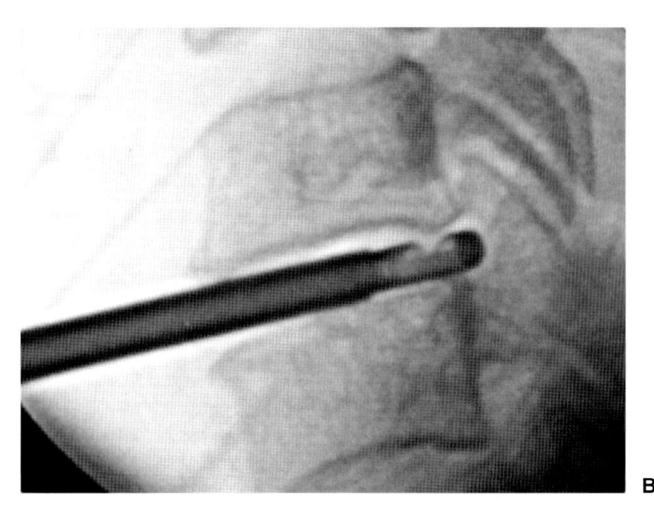
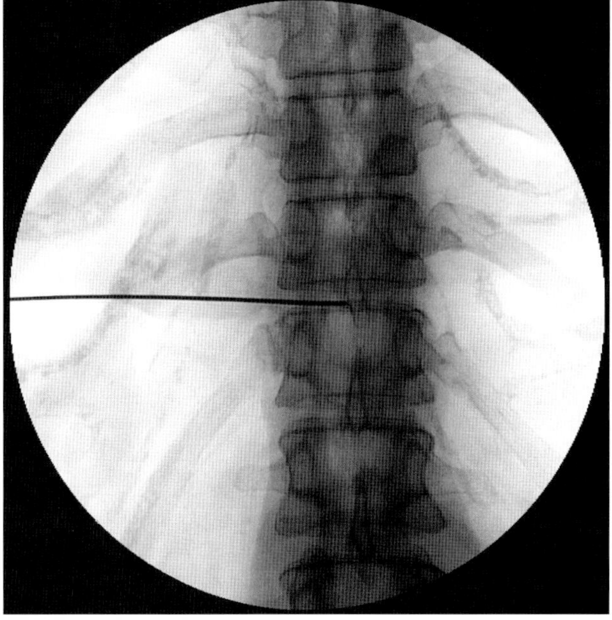
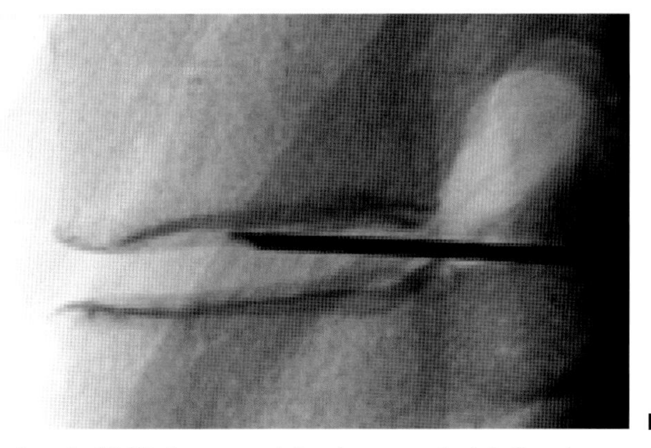
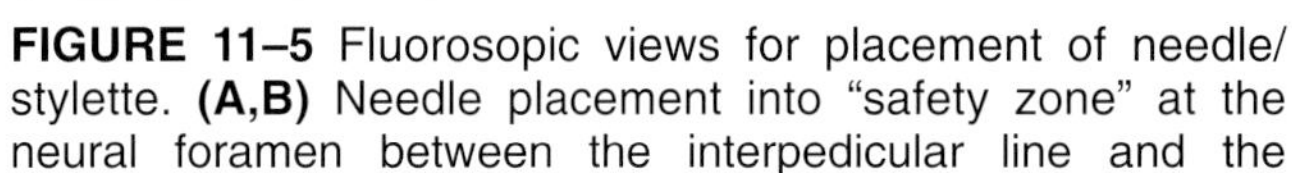

FIGURE 11–5 Fluorosopic views for placement of needle/stylette. **(A,B)** Needle placement into "safety zone" at the neural foramen between the interpedicular line and the rib head. **(C,D)** Incremental advance of stylette placement into center of the disk.

by C-arm fluoroscopy in two planes as needed. After the involved levels are identified, sterile needle electrodes are placed in the intercostal muscles innervated from those levels for continuous neurophysiological EMG monitoring,[22] with a ground electrode having been previously placed.

Surgical Technique

Under local anesthesia a beveled 20-gauge, 3.5-inch spinal needle is inserted into the portal of entry, as described under localization and fluoroscopic guidance (Fig. 11–5). The needle is incrementally advanced under C-arm fluoroscopic guidance at a 35- to 45-degree angle from the sagittal plane, targeting toward the center of the disk, into the "safety zone," between the interpedicular line medially and the rib head at the costovertebral articulation laterally,[11,12] and medial to the costotransverse junction (Fig. 11–5). During the needle insertion, one must keep the needle tip immediately along the medial aspect of the rib head to avoid entering the spinal canal medially, and medial to the costovertebral junction to avoid pleural puncture. After the anulus

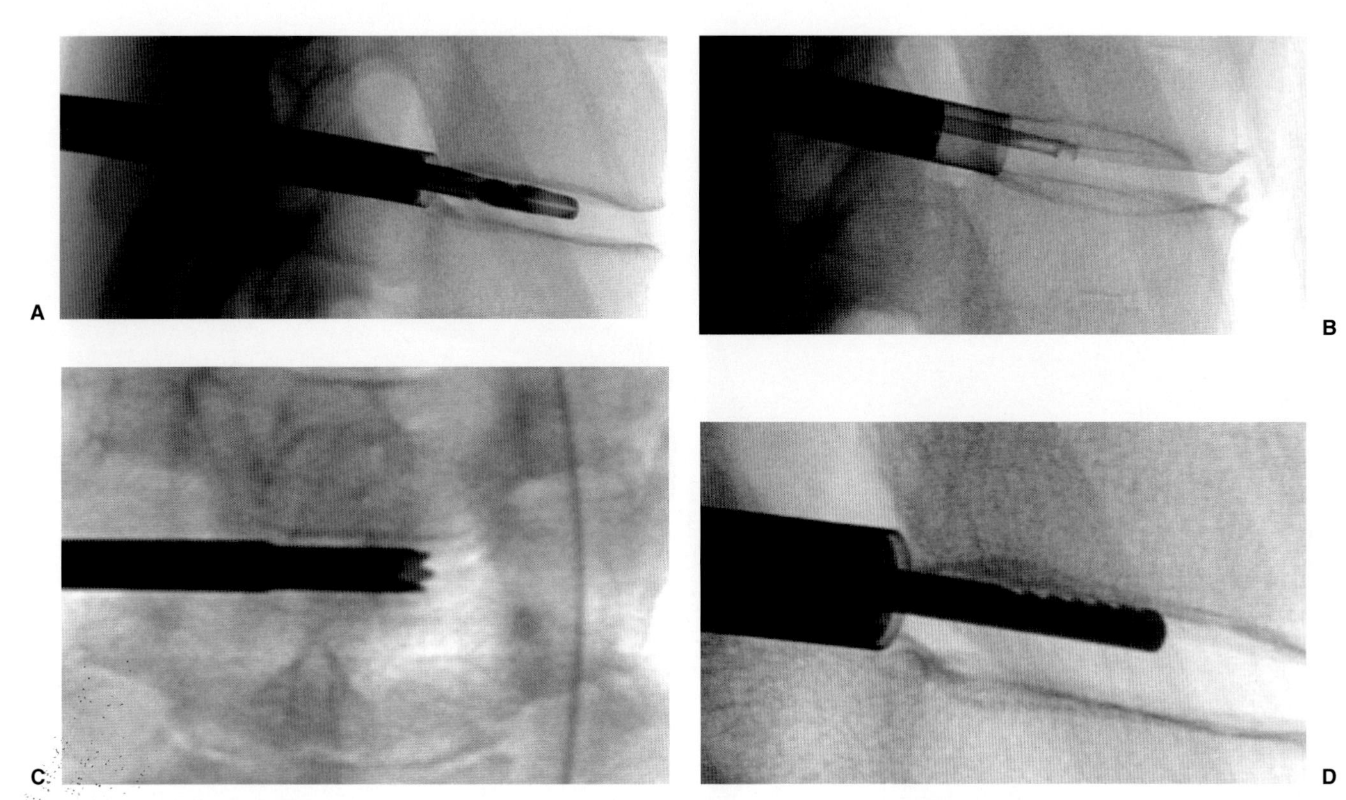

FIGURE 11–6 Fluoroscopic view of posterolateral endoscopic thoracic diskectomy (PETD) instruments. **(A)** Micrograsper forceps. **(B)** Trephine. **(C)** Side fire laser probe. **(D)** Endoscopic rasp.

is punctured, the needle is incrementally advanced to the center of the disk. The stylette of the spinal needle is removed. Isovue contrast (Bracco Diagnostics, Inc., Princeton, NJ) is injected, observing the ease and volume of injection, the fluoroscopic appearance in AP and lateral projections, and the patient's description of the location, concordance, and intensity of any pain produced. Surgery is performed if the diskogram and pain provocation tests are confirmatory.

A narrow 12-inch plain wire guide is passed into the center of the disk through the spinal needle placed for the diskogram. The needle is then removed. A 3 to 4 mm skin incision is made at the site. The diskectomy cannula containing its dilator is passed over the guidewire and is advanced to the anulus. A trephine replaces the dilator and incises the anulus. The cannula then advances a short distance into the disk space. The disk is decompressed using curettes, trephine, microforceps, diskectome, and the laser (Figs. 11–6, 11–7, 11–8, 11–9). Disk removal is aided by a rocking excursion of the cannula in a 25-degree arc, a "fan sweep" motion from side to side, that creates an oval cone-shaped area of removed disk totaling up to 50 degrees (Fig. 11–7).

During the procedure the endoscope is utilized for visualization, and under magnification additional disk material and osteophytes are removed with microcurettes, rasps, forceps, and diskectomes (Figs. 11–8, 11–9). Large spurs or a rib head obstructing entry to the disk space can be removed or can be perforated by a set of more aggressive-toothed trephines (Fig. 11–6). A holmium:YAG laser (Fig. 11–2) is used to ablate additional disk (500 J at 10 W, 10 Hz, 5 sec on and 5 sec off), then at a lower power setting (300 J at 5 W) (Table 11–1) to shrink and contract the disk, further reducing the profile of the protrusion and hardening the disk tissue, laser thermodiskoplasty[9] (Fig. 11–7). This may also cause sinovertebral neurolysis or denervation. The diskectome is again used briefly to remove charred debris. The disk space can be directly visualized by endoscopy for confirmation of disk decompression (Fig. 11–9). The probe and cannula are removed. Marcaine (0.25%) is infiltrated subcutaneously about the wound. A Band-aid is applied over the tiny wound.

Postoperative Care

The patient is checked neurologically prior to leaving the operating room. An upright portable chest x-ray done in the recovery room rules out a pneumothorax. Ambulation begins immediately after recovery, and the patient is usually discharged 1 hour after surgery. The patient may shower the following day. An ice pack is helpful. Mild analgesics and muscle relaxants

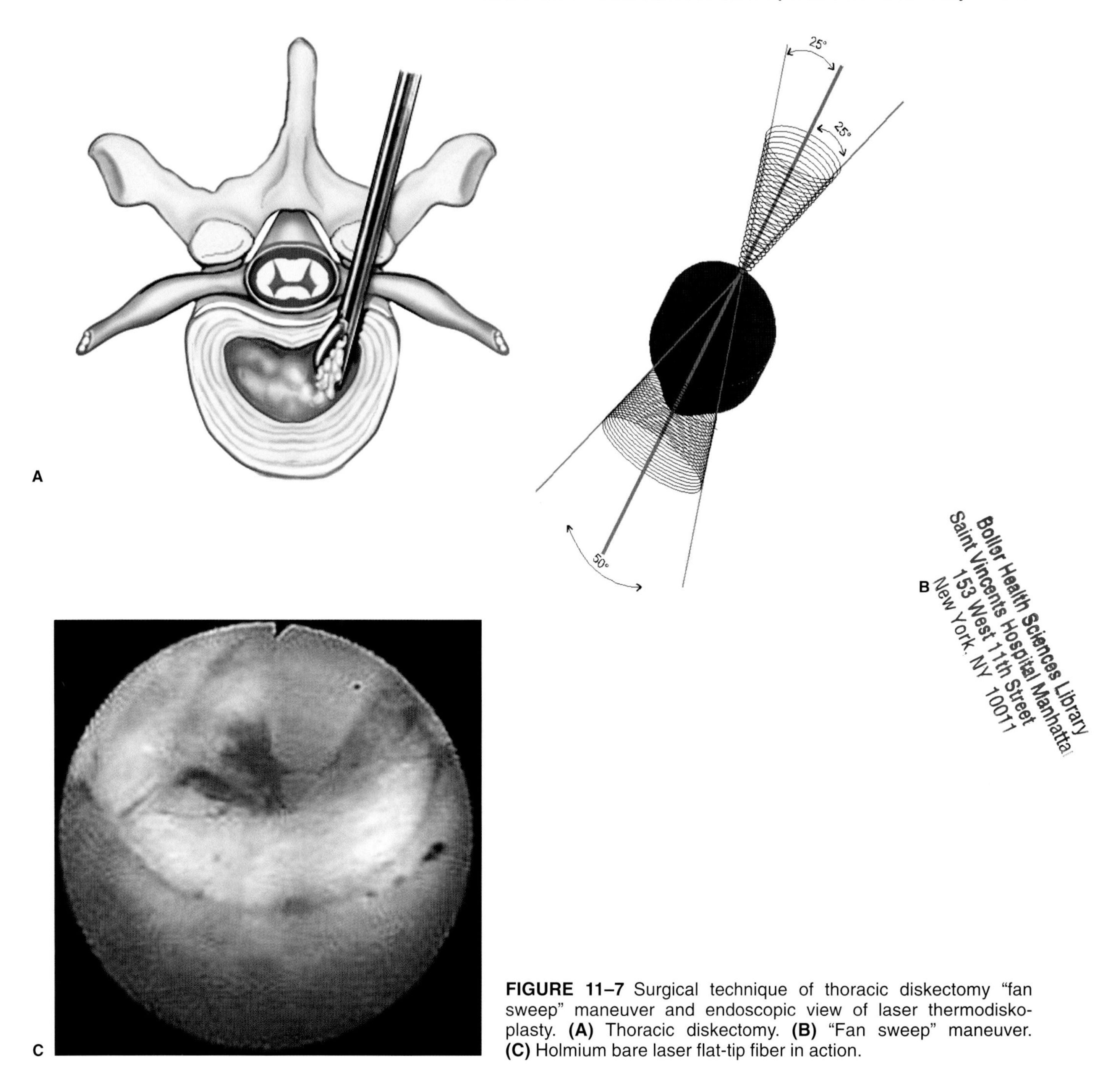

FIGURE 11–7 Surgical technique of thoracic diskectomy "fan sweep" maneuver and endoscopic view of laser thermodiskoplasty. **(A)** Thoracic diskectomy. **(B)** "Fan sweep" maneuver. **(C)** Holmium bare laser flat-tip fiber in action.

are required at times. A progressive exercise program begins the second postoperative day. Patients are usually allowed to return to work in 1 to 2 weeks, as long as heavy labor and prolonged sitting are not involved. Most patients found this procedure extremely gratifying.

Outcome

Ninety-six percent of 150 consecutive patients with a total of 197 herniated thoracic disks demonstrated good to excellent relief of symptoms. Six patients (4%) had persistent thoracic pain, although overall their pain improved. The patients postoperatively resumed usual activity in a few days, and full active lives in 3 to 7 weeks.[13]

Discussion

PETD is a minimally invasive surgical procedure for treating symptomatic herniated thoracic disks through an operating endoscope with much less tissue trauma

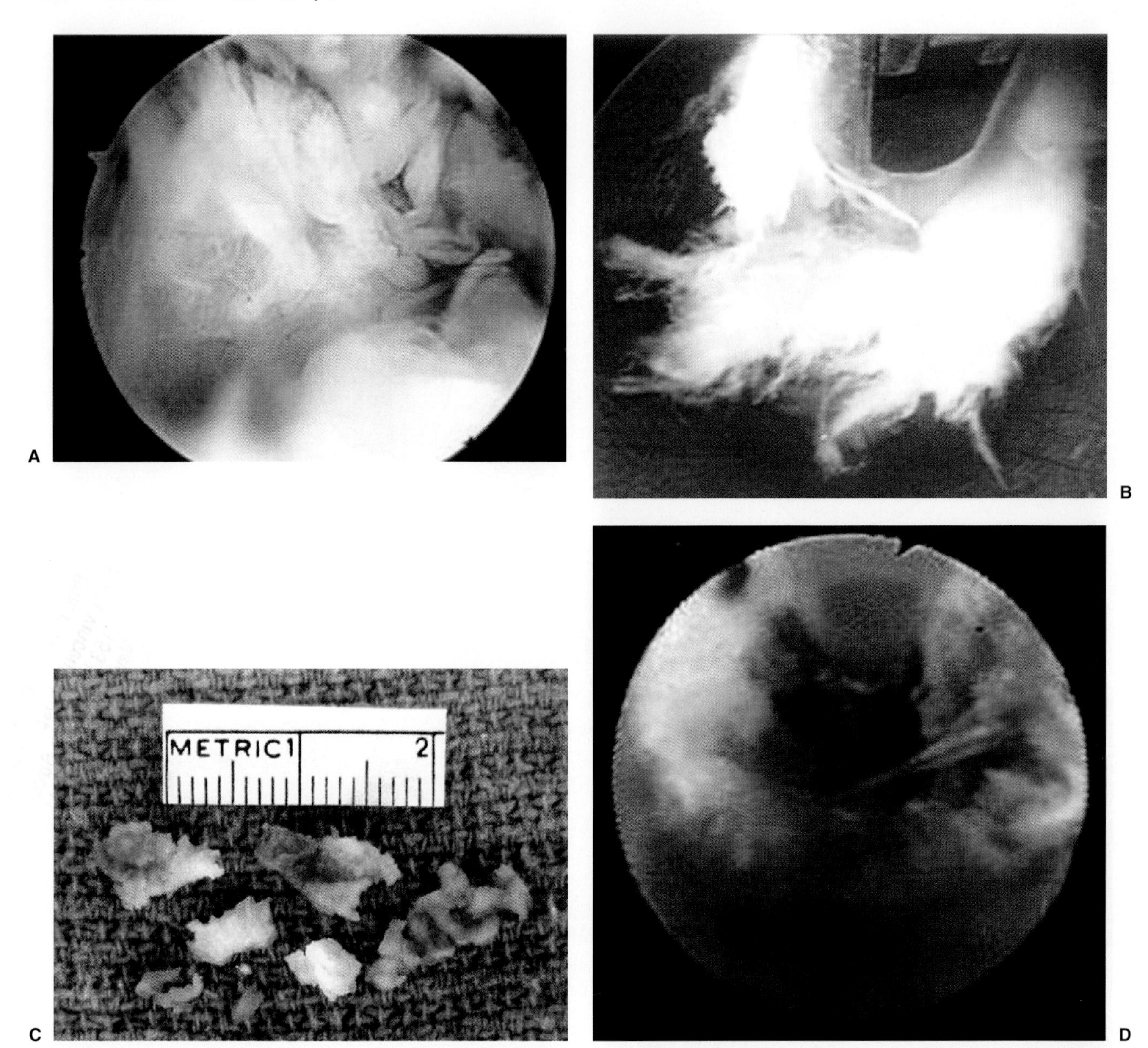

FIGURE 11–8 Endoscopic view of thoracic diskectomy. **(A)** Intradiscal endoscopic view. **(B)** Endoscopic disk removal with cutter forceps. **(C)** Disk fragments removed. **(D)** Laser application for disk decompression.

and zero mortality. It has numerous advantages, but it requires thorough knowledge of the surgical anatomy, the PETD procedure, specific surgical training, and hands-on experience in a laboratory and working closely with an experienced endoscopic surgeon through its steep surgical learning curve in order for a surgeon to become competent and avoid possible complications.

Complications and Avoidance

A thorough knowledge of the procedure and surgical anatomy of the thorax and thoracic spine, careful selection of patients, and preoperative surgical planning with appropriate diagnostic evaluations facilitate the PETD and prevent potential complications.[2,3,11,13] All potential complications of open approaches for thoracic disk surgery are possible but are rare or much less frequent[3,7,10,11,21,23] in PETD, with no rib resection or deliberate collapse of the lung required.

- **Pneumothorax, pulmonary injury, and postoperative atelectasis:** Pneumothorax is a potential complication in all approaches to thoracic disks, including PETD. The spinal needle should be introduced into the "safety zone" of the disk, with the interpedicular line medially and rib head laterally

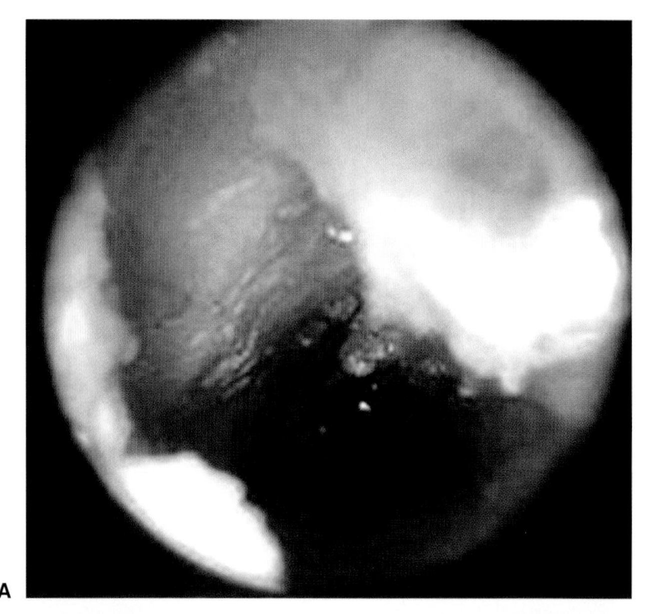

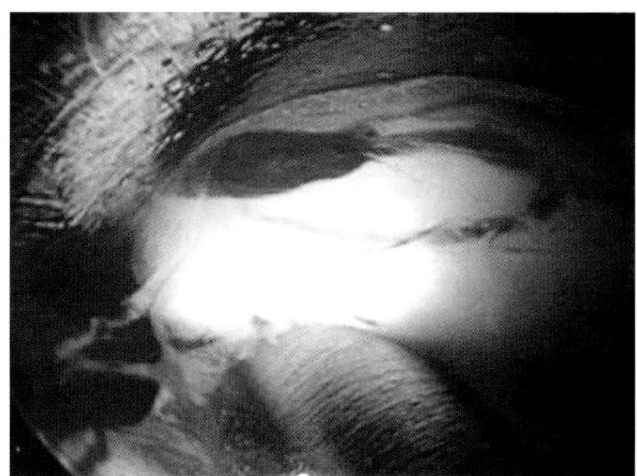

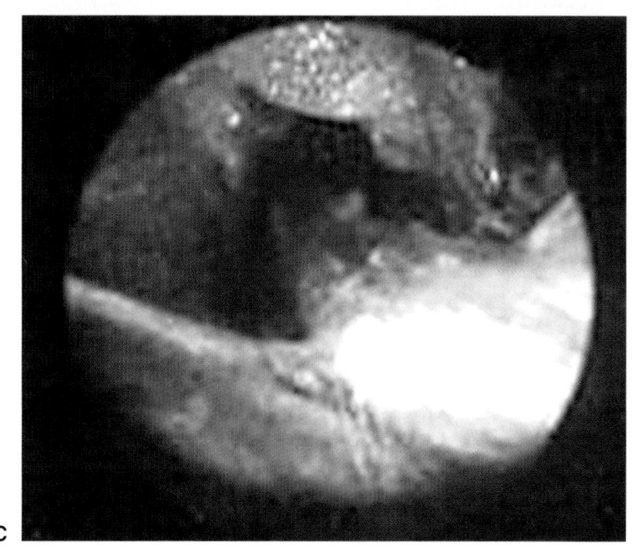

FIGURE 11–9 Endoscopic view after PETD. **(A)** After PETD, hollow disk defect and end plates are seen. **(B)** Grasper forcep for disk removal below the intercostal nerve. **(C)** Intercostal nerve after microdiskectomy.

at the neuroforamen, to protect it from penetrating the pleura. Direct endoscopic visualization helps to avoid pulmonary injury. Atelectasis is not a problem. Chest x-ray is obtained immediately after completing the operation to rule out pneumothorax and to initiate treatment if present.

TABLE 11–1 Laser Setting for Thoracic Laser Thermodiskoplasty*

	Stage	*Watts*	*Joules*
Thoracic	First	10	500
Thoracic	Second	5	300

*Nonablative levels of laser energy, at 10 Hz, 5 seconds on and 5 seconds off.

- **Infection:** Avoided by careful sterile technique, using prophylactic antibiotics IV intraoperatively, and the much smaller incisional area compared with open posterolateral and transthoracic approaches, as well as the multiport thoracoscopic approaches.
- **Aseptic discitis:** May be prevented by aiming the laser beam in a "bowtie" fashion to avoid damaging the end plates (at 6 and 12 o'clock).
- **Hematoma (subcutaneous and deep):** May occur with PETD but is minimized by careful technique, the small incision (3 mm), not prescribing aspirin or NSAIDs within 1 week prior to surgery, and application of digital pressure or an IV bag over the operative site for the first 5 minutes after surgery, and application of an ice pack thereafter.

- **Vascular injuries:** The thoracic aorta and its segmental branches, the intercostal artery and vein, the azygos, hemiazygos, and accessory hemiazygous veins are at risk in open procedures and lateral, anterior, and posterolateral approaches to thoracic disks. Strict adherence to the technique and knowledge of the applicable surgical anatomy should avoid such injuries. No vascular injury has been reported with PETD.
- **Neural injury:** Extremely rare with PETD; no spinal cord injuries have been reported. Nerve root injury (intercostal nerve) causing intercostal neuralgia, or chest pain, although possible, can be avoided with intraoperative neurophysiologic monitoring (EMG/NCV)[22] of intercostal muscles at and immediately below the operated levels. By using direct endoscopic visualization (Fig. 11–9), intercostal injury related to open chest surgery and thorascopic surgery can be avoided. No nerve injuries were noted in 300-plus cases at our center. The initial spinal needle placement can be onto the posterior, superior surface of the rib into the "safety zone" at the neuroforamen, avoiding the intercostal nerve lying in the inferior surface of the rib, in the costal groove. This maneuver and observing the strict boundaries of the interpedicular lines protect the spinal cord.
- **Sympathetic chain and rami communicantes:** Prone position for surgery avoids pressure on the brachial plexus, which can cause compression plexopathy. Complications are only a remote possibility; observing the surgical anatomy of the parathoracic area and keeping needle placement within the "safety zone" should sufficiently guard against this.
- **Excessive sedation:** Avoided by surface EEG monitoring, providing more precise estimation of the depth of sedation and reducing the amount of anesthetics, as well as preventing excessive or insufficient sedation. Patients are able to respond throughout the procedure, and this provides a further means of evaluating their level.
- **Improper localization:** A major complication of all disk surgeries is operating at the wrong level. Proper utilization of C-arm fluoroscopy for anatomical localization avoids complications caused by poor placement of instruments or operating at the wrong disk level. Routine pain provocation test and diskogram give additional verification of the proper level.
- **Dural tears:** These are common in all other approaches to the thoracic disk, but they have not been reported in PETD.
- **Soft tissue injuries** due to prolonged forceful retraction, as occurs in many disk operations, are not an issue with PETD.
- **Inadequate decompression of disk material:** Minimized by using multiple modalities and such instruments as forceps, trephines, diskectome, burr, and rasp, and by application of laser both to vaporize tissue and to perform thermodiskoplasty.

Advantages

The advantages[7,10–12,14,21] of PETD are numerous. They include:

- No general anesthesia required
- Commonly done under local anesthesia
- Small incision and less scarring without multiple or large incision
- Minimal blood loss
- Zero mortality
- No need of lung collapse or opening of the pleural cavity
- No postoperative pleural effusion, intercostal neuralgia, and pneumothorax
- No significant infection
- Avoiding injury to blood vessels
- No resection of rib
- No spinal fusion or fixation needed
- No dissection of muscle, bone, ligaments, or manipulation of the dural sac, spinal cord, or nerve roots
- Little or no epidural bleeding
- Minimal use of analgesics postoperatively
- Same-day outpatient procedure
- Less traumatic, both physically and psychologically
- Does not promote further instability of spinal segments
- Early return to usual activities, including work
- Costs less than conventional diskectomy
- Multiple-level diskectomy feasible and well tolerated[17–21]
- Least challenging to such medically high-risk patients as those with cardiopulmonary problems, the aged, and the morbidly obese
- Exercise programs can begin the same day as surgery
- Direct endoscopic visualization and confirmation of the efficacy of surgery, which contribute to a safe and effective outcome

Disadvantages

This technique is useful in select patients and is not appropriate for patients with severe thoracic disk extrusions causing cord compression with severe neurologic deficit (parparesis) and patients with severe congenital or acquired stenosis of the spinal canal. In patients with severe spondylosis and foraminal stenosis, this

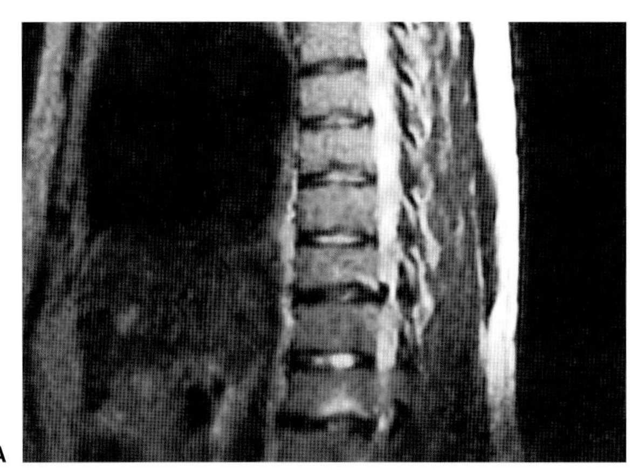
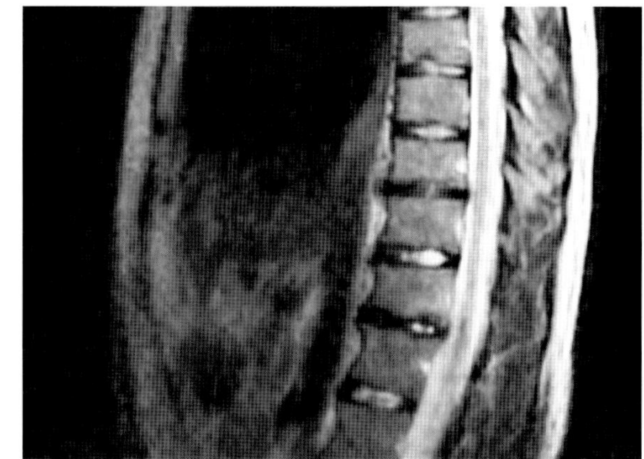

A B

FIGURE 11–10 Large herniated T10 and T12 disks, pre- and postoperative MRI scans.

technique may not be suitable because insertion of the endoscope may not be feasible.

Case Illustration

A 24-year-old man had complained for 2 months of intractable midback pain and muscle spasm. Past history was noncontributory. Parathoracic muscle spasm was palpable adjacent to the painful level. Neurologic examination showed hypalgesia in T10 and T12 dermatomes. MRI demonstrated two protruded thoracic disks (at T10 and T12 levels). Physical therapy, analgesics, and epidural steroid injections did not alleviate his discomfort. Chest x-ray demonstrated 13 thoracic vertebrae with 13 ribs, with seven cervical and five lumbar vertebrae. The patient was treated by PETD at T10–T11 and T12–L1. He had total relief of his symptoms postoperatively. Comparative preoperative and postoperative MRI scans showed the disappearance of the protruded disks (Fig. 11–10).

Posterior endoscopic thoracic diskectomy performed for symptomatic herniated thoracic disk with added laser "tightening" of the disk (thermodiskoplasty) is an easier, safe, and efficacious procedure. This minimally invasive, less-traumatic outpatient procedure results in less morbidity, more rapid recovery, and significant economic savings. The mortality rate was zero in a multicenter study[23] of percutaneous endoscopic spinal diskectomy (26,860 cases), and the morbidity rate was less than 1%, with patient satisfaction of more than 92% for thoracic disks. There are no reported spinal cord injuries, intercostal neuralgia, or dural tears, and no significant infection, vascular injury, or pulmonary complications.

PETD requires a knowledgeable and competent surgeon with a thorough appreciation of the surgical anatomy of the thorax and thoracic spine intercostal nerves and vessels, the relationship of the rib heads, pedicles, disk spaces, and spinal cord. To perform the procedure, the spine surgeon must have specific surgical training with hands-on experience in the laboratory, and, most importantly, must spend time working through the steep surgical learning curve with an endoscopic spinal surgeon expert at this procedure.

REFERENCES

1. Jaikumar S, Kim D, Kam A. History of minimally invasive spine surgery. *Neurosurgery*. 2002;51(2 suppl):1–14.
2. Jaikumar S, Kim D, Kam A. Minimally invasive spine instrumentation. *Neurosurgery*. 2002;51(2 suppl):15–22.
3. Perez-Cruet M, Fessler R, Perin N. Review: complications of minimally invasive spinal surgery. *Neurosurgery*. 2002;51(2 suppl): 26–36.
4. Fessler R, Khoo L. Minimally invasive cervical microendoscopic foraminotomy: an initial clinical experience. *Neurosurgery*. 2002;51(2 suppl):37–45.
5. Dickman C, Mican C. Thoracoscopic approaches for the treatment of anterior thoracic spinal pathology. *Barrow Neur Inst Quart*. 1996;12:4–19
6. Nicholas T, Curtis AD. Current management of thoracic disc herniation. *Cont Neurosurg*. 1996;18:1–7.
7. Chiu J, Clifford T, Princenthal R. The new frontier of minimally invasive spine surgery through computer assisted technology. In: Lemke HU, Vannier MN, Invamura RD, eds. *Computer Assisted Radiology and Surgery*. New York: Spring-Verlag; 2002: 233–237.
8. Simpson J. Thoracic disc herniation. *Spine*. 1993;18:872–877.
9. Schellhas KP, Pollei SR, Dorwart RH. Thoracic discography: a safe and reliable technique. *Spine*. 1994;18:2103–2109.
10. Chiu J, Clifford T, Greenspan M. Percutaneous microdecompressive endoscopic cervical discectomy with laser thermodiskoplasty. *Mt Sinai J Med*. 2000;67:278–282.
11. Chiu J, Clifford T, Sison R. Percutaneous microdecompressive endoscopic thoracic discectomy for herniated thoracic discs. *Surg Technol Int*. 2002;10:266–269.
12. Chiu J, Clifford T. Percutaneous endoscopic thoracic discectomy. In: Savitz MH, Chiu JC, Yeung AD, eds. *The Practice of Minimally Invasive Spinal Technique*. Richmond, VA: AAMISMS Education; 2000:211–216.
13. Chiu J, Clifford T. Posterolateral approach for percutaneous thoracic endoscopic discectomy. *J Min Inv Spinal Tech*. 2001:1:26–30.

14. Chiu J, Clifford T. Microdecompressive percutaneous discectomy: spinal discectomy with new laser thermodiskoplasty for non-extruded herniated nucleus pulposus. *Surg Technol Int.* 1999; 8:343–351.
15. Savitz MH. Same day microsurgical arthroscopic lateral approach laser assisted (small) fluoroscopic discectomy. *J Neurosurg.* 1994; 80:1039–1045.
16. Yeung AT, Chow PM. Posterior lateral endoscopic excision for lumbar disc herniation: surgical technique, outcome, and complications. *Spine.* 2002;27:722–731.
17. Boriani S, Biagini R, Delure F. Two level thoracic disc herniations. *Spine.* 1994;21:2461–2466.
18. Coleman R, Hamlyn P, Butler P. Anterior spinal surgery for multiple thoracic disk herniations. *Br J Neurosurg.* 1990;4:541–543.
19. Dickman C, Mican C. Multilevel anterior thoracic discectomies and anterior interbody fusion using a microsurgical thoracoscopic approach: case report. *J Neurosurg.* 1996;84:104–109.
20. Shikata J, Yamamuro T, Kashiwagi N. Multiple thoracic disc herniations: case report. *Neurosurgery.* 1988;22:1068–1070.
21. Chiu J, Clifford T. Multiple herniated discs at single and multiple spinal segments treated with endoscopic microdecompressive surgery. *J Min Inv Spinal Tech.* 2001;l:15–19.
22. Clifford T, Chiu J, Rogers G. Neurophysiological monitoring of peripheral nerve function during endoscopic laser discectomy. *J Min Inv Spinal Tech.* 2001;1:54–57.
23. Chiu J, Clifford T, Savitz MA, et al. Multicenter study of percutaneous endoscopic discectomy (lumbar, cervical and thoracic). *J Min Inv Spinal Tech.* 2001;1:33–37.

12

Endoscopic Transpedicular Thoracic Diskectomy

DAVID H. JHO AND HAE-DONG JHO

Minimalism for the surgical treatment of thoracic disk herniation has several surgical goals: cure or resolution of symptoms, minimal disruption of biointegrity, minimal risk from the surgical procedure itself, minimal chance of postoperative complications, rapid surgical recovery, and cost effectiveness. Regardless of the anatomical approach, surgical treatment must provide high rates of symptomatic resolution with low risks of intraoperative complications. Surgical results among the various posterolateral approaches have been comparable. As for surgical risks, spinal cord damage has been the most serious potential risk in thoracic disk surgery. Postoperative paraplegia was not uncommon when thoracic disk herniation was treated with the midline posterior laminectomy technique.[1] Surgical treatment for thoracic disk herniation via the posterior approach has gradually shifted from the traditional midline laminectomy to such posterolateral approaches as costotransversectomy, lateral extracavitary, and a transpedicular approach in an attempt to avoid catastrophic spinal cord injury.[2–9] The posterior surgical approaches have extended further laterally to provide a maximum ventral view of the spinal cord, which has significantly reduced the risk of intraoperative spinal cord damage; however, posterolateral surgical approaches often necessitate extensive surgical incision and tissue dissection. The least invasive among the various posterior approaches is the transpedicular approach, but because this approach is usually paramedian rather than posterolateral, the ventral aspect of the spinal cord is not directly visualized during surgical decompression. The transthoracic approach was also developed to avoid intraoperative spinal cord damage. Although the main advantage of this thoracotomy approach is direct access to the anterior aspect of the spinal cord, the thoracotomy procedure itself involves an extensive surgical incision and entrance into the pleural cavity. An endoscopic transthoracic approach has been developed to minimize invasiveness of the conventional thoracotomy technique[10]; however, this endoscopic transthoracic technique still necessitates three to four separate skin incisions in the chest wall and often requires postoperative chest tube drainage. The depth of the surgical tract is also very long, thus maneuvering such delicate surgical tools as a power drill can be challenging.

In an attempt to achieve the ideal surgical goals of minimalism for thoracic disk herniation, an endoscopic transpedicular approach was adopted. The transpedicular approach involves a relatively small skin incision and minimal tissue dissection. The required skin incision is 1.5 to 2 cm in length when an endoscope is adopted. The medial portion of the facet joint and rostral-medial one-third portion of the pedicle are removed to access the protruded disk under a 0-degree-lens endoscope. A 4 mm diameter rigid endoscope with a 70-degree lens is then mounted to a custom-made endoscope holder. The use of a 70-degree lens enables the surgeon to visualize the ventral aspect of the spinal cord directly.[3] Under this steady image provided by the mounted endoscope, decompression of the ventral spinal cord is executed utilizing 90-degree-curved surgical instruments. The invasiveness of this transpedicular thoracic diskectomy becomes quite comparable to that of cervical or lumbar microdiskectomy.[4] In this chapter, the details of endoscopic transpedicular thoracic diskectomy will be described.

Surgical Indications and Preoperative Tests

Surgical indications for endoscopic transpedicular thoracic diskectomy are as follows:

- Intractable thoracic pain that does not respond to conservative treatment (relative indication)
- Radiculopathy that does not respond to conservative treatment
- Myelopathy caused by spinal cord compression

Clinical symptoms of thoracic disk herniation can be divided into these three groups. The first group of symptoms can be considered thoracic spine symptoms due to local disruption of the anatomy. Thoracic spine symptoms may include midline thoracic pain, paramedian thoracic pain, and retrosternal pain. Because cervical spine pathology can also produce scapular or interscapular pain, upper thoracic disk herniation may mimic symptoms related to cervical disk disease. The second group of symptoms is radiculopathy related to compression of the nerve root or ganglion. The resulting focal muscle weakness can produce protrusion of the abdomen. The third group of symptoms is myelopathy caused by spinal cord compression. Surgical treatment is indicated in patients with myelopathy or radiculopathy unresponsive to trials of medical treatment; however, the sole presence of midline paramedian thoracic pain related to local disruption of the anatomy does not respond well to surgical treatment. Patients without radiculopathy or myelopathy must be fully aware that surgery may fail to relieve their thoracic pain. In addition to the clinical evaluation of symptoms, high-resolution MRI scans should be the diagnostic choice, although CT with myelography is still occasionally used (Fig. 12–1). As surgery on the correct level is absolutely essential in thoracic disk surgery, the sagittal scout film should include all levels of the spine. The levels of the thoracic spine in MRI are counted from the cervical spine; however, intraoperative corroboration of the correct level of pathology often involves fluoroscopic vertebral counting from the lumbar spine. Because anatomical variations are relatively common, a complete spine roentgenogram or MRI scout films are necessary.

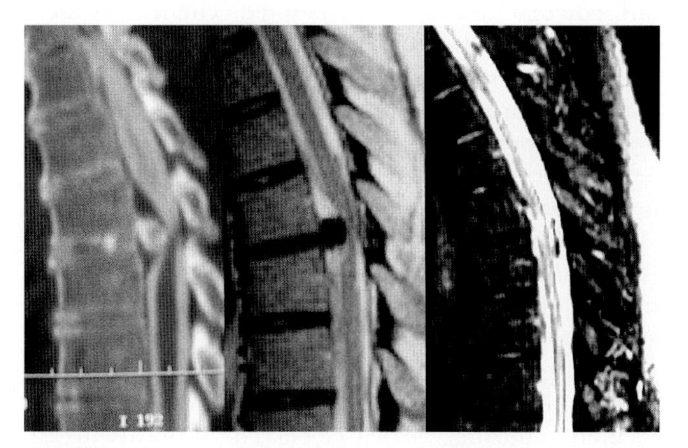

FIGURE 12–1 (A) Preoperative sagittal CT-myelogram and **(B)** sagittal T-2 weighted MRI of the thoracic spine (middle) disclose calcified disk herniation with severe spinal cord compression in a patient with radiculomyelopathy. **(C)** The postoperative sagittal MRI demonstrates excellent decompression of the spinal cord.

Surgical Instrumentation and Preparation

The following instruments are necessary to perform endoscopic transpedicular thoracic diskectomy:

- Fluoroscopic C-arm for localization of the correct operating level
- Zero-degree and 70-degree rod-lens endoscopes that are 4 mm in diameter
- Endoscope-light system and video-camera-monitor system
- Endoscope holder
- Endoscope lens cleansing device
- Slender high-speed drill
- Special curette system
- Diskectomy tools (e.g., various pituitary and Kerrison rongeurs)
- Disposable trocar, 1.1 or 1.5 cm in diameter
- Somatosensory monitoring system (SEP)

As previously mentioned, the use of a fluoroscopic C-arm is necessary for localizing and operating at the correct level of pathology. The endoscope used for this procedure is a 4 mm diameter, 18 cm length rod-lens rigid endoscope. A 3 mm endoscope can be used, but it does not produce a full-screen image. The image quality is much better with a 4 mm than a 3 mm endoscope. For the start of the endoscopic transpedicular approach, a 0-degree-lens endoscope is used. Disk removal in front of the spinal cord is then performed under a 70-degree-lens endoscope. An endoscope holder is an important tool for tightly securing the endoscope during disk removal because it allows the surgeon to use two hands simultaneously. Two different types of endoscope holders are currently available. The first is a manual holder, which has joints that need to be tightened manually. The other is a nitrogen gas-powered holder, which is controlled with one-touch buttons. An endoscope lens-cleansing device is an essential tool for intermittent cleaning of the lens and is controlled by a foot pedal. A slender power drill is another important tool; the shaft of the drill is ~5 mm, and the drill tip is a round 2 mm cutting bit. A special down-cutting curette system is used. A disposable

1.1 or 1.5 cm diameter trocar is threaded at the outer surface and has a stylet for introduction. Other instruments used are pituitary rongeurs (i.e., straight, curved-up, and curved-down), Kerrison rongeurs (i.e., 1 and 2 mm tips), French number 7 suction cannulas (i.e., straight and curved-down), and suction-coagulators. Somatosensory monitoring is also useful for monitoring intraoperative spinal cord function.

Anesthesia

General anesthesia with conventional orotracheal intubation is used. Because the operating time is usually 1 to 2 hours, Foley catheterization is not necessary.

Positioning

The patient is positioned 60 degrees ventrally inclined lateral, with the operating side facing up (Fig. 12–2). An axillary roll is placed, and a pillow is folded as a floating armrest with bear hugging. The legs are cushioned; the shoulders, pelvis, and legs are securely taped with 2-inch adhesive tapes. The operating level is corroborated using a fluoroscopic C-arm, and an 18-gauge spinal needle is placed obliquely under sterile conditions. The skin entry site of the spinal needle is 2 to 3 inches lateral from the midline, with the needle tip aiming at the upper edge of the pedicle. The surgeon and scrub nurse stand at the dorsal aspect of the patient. The video-system tower and the endoscope lens-cleansing motor are placed on the other side of the patient.

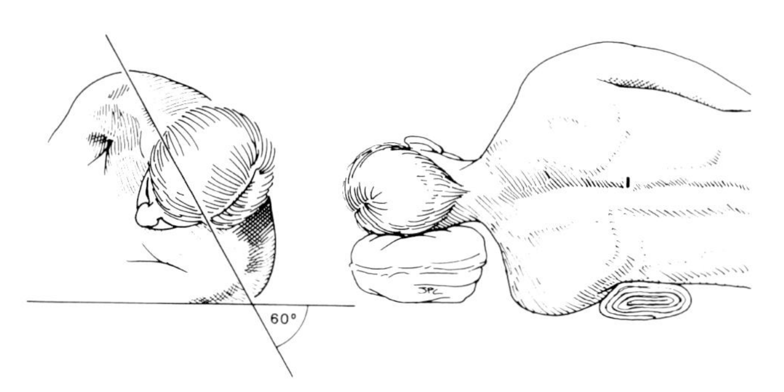

FIGURE 12–2 This schematic drawing demonstrates patient positioning. The patient is positioned lesion-side-up lateral decubitus. The patient is inclined forward at 60 degrees. An axillary roll is placed under the axilla to prevent neurovascular injury. The correct level of herniated disk is corroborated using fluoroscopic C-arm or roentgenogram.

Surgical Technique

The localizing spinal needle is left in position, while preparation and draping are done following aseptic technique. The endoscope system is assembled with a 0-degree lens, and the endoscope is mounted to the holder. A 1.5 cm (for the use of a 1.1 cm trocar) or 2 cm (for the use of 1.5 cm trocar) transverse skin incision is made laterally from the lateral margin of the corresponding spinous process. The paraspinal muscles are dissected from the spinous process, lamina, and transverse process using a small periosteal elevator. A localizing spinal needle is used again to confirm correct surgical trajectory and is then removed. A tubular threaded trocar measuring 1.1 or 1.5 cm in diameter is introduced, exposing the facet and lamina (Fig. 12–3). A smaller 1.1 cm diameter trocar is used in the approach to laterally herniated disks causing radiculopathy. The 0-degree-lens endoscope is mounted to the endoscope holder and introduced into the trocar. Endoscopic view will demonstrate surgical landmarks (e.g., the inferior edge of the lamina and inferior edge of the facet), and transverse process is confirmed. The medial portion of the facet, the very lateral portion of the lamina, and the rostral-medial one-third portion of the pedicle are removed with a high-speed drill. When the yellow

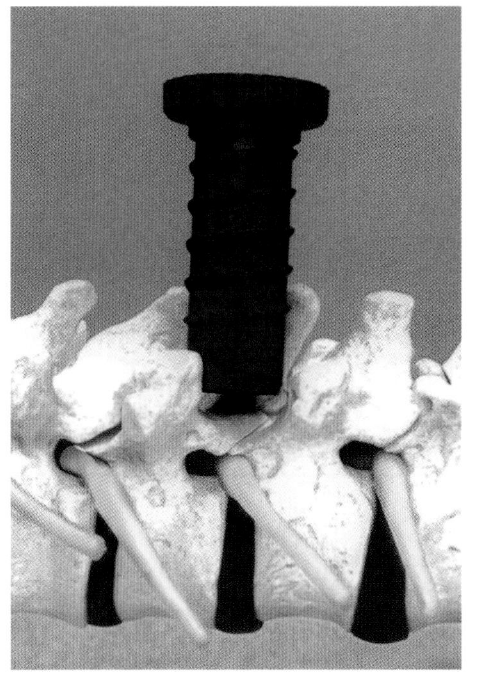

FIGURE 12–3 This photo shows placement of a 1.5 cm diameter threaded trocar (green) toward the thoracic disk in a thoracic spine model. The trajectory of a trocar is aimed toward the operating intervertebral disk. A 0-degree-lens endoscope will provide a view at the ipsilateral lamina and facet joint.

ligament is removed, a ~2 to 3 mm portion of the very lateral margin of the spinal cord dura mater is exposed. The nerve root can usually be identified rostral to the intervertebral disk, but it may occasionally be found just rostral to the resected portion of the pedicle. The nerve root compression can be identified at this point for radiculopathy. Using a high-speed drill with a 2 mm cutting bit, the lateral bony spurs rostral and caudal to the herniated disk are removed, creating a small cavity, ~5 mm in depth, in the posterior portion of the vertebral bodies. Limited exposure of the spinal cord dura mater will prevent the surgeon from injuring the spinal cord because the main portion of the spinal cord will still be covered by the remaining ipsilateral lamina. The exposed portion of the dura mater corresponds to the subarachnoid space. After a ~1 cm wide cavity is created at the lateral intervertebral disk space by resection of the bony spur and disk material, the 70-degree-lens endoscope is introduced.

The 70-degree-lens endoscope is mounted to the endoscope holder. It is used to visualize the ventral aspect of the spinal cord dura mater directly. Under this direct endoscopic visualization, the cavity created lateral to the spinal cord is extended further medially by removing disk material and bony spurs with down-biting curettes (Fig. 12–4). An extended tunnel is made underneath a thin layer of dorsally protruded disk and bony spur that is compressing the spinal cord. The shell of disk material and bony spur are pushed away from the spinal cord toward the created cavity and are removed using a long-

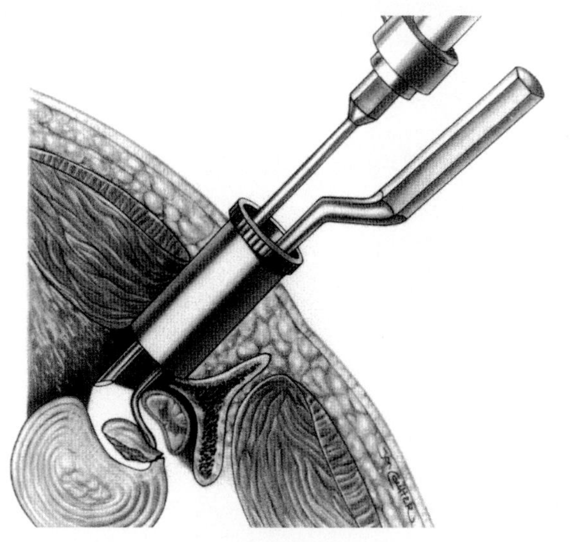

FIGURE 12–4 This schematic drawing depicts the placement of a 1.5 cm trocar retractor via a 2 cm paramedian transverse skin incision, the application of the 70-degree-lens endoscope, and the use of a right-angle down-biting curette for removal of the protruded disk ventral to the spinal cord. The patient is positioned right-side up and inclined 60 degrees ventral and lateral.

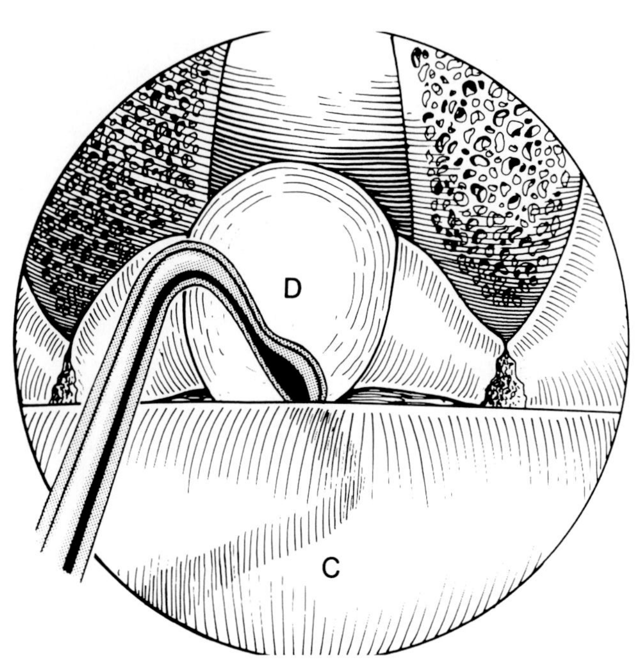

FIGURE 12–5 This schematic drawing demonstrates removal of a herniated disk in front of the spinal cord with use of a curved down-cutting curette under a 70-degree-lens endoscope. C, Spinal cord; D, herniated disk.

armed down-biting curette and a curved pituitary rongeur (Fig. 12–5). Because the common pathology in thoracic disk herniation is calcified disk or protruded bone spurs along the edges of the inter-vertebral disk rather than soft disk herniation, creating a small cavity anterior to the compressive pathology is an important step of surgical maneuvering to prevent spinal cord damage. Operating under the 70-degree-lens-endoscope image requires an advanced level of endoscopic technique. When adequate decompression has been performed, the ventrally concave curvature of the spinal cord dura mater bulges out ventrally to make a convex curvature toward the intervertebral space (Fig. 12–6). Bone bleeding is controlled with the application of bone wax, and the trocar retractor is removed. A couple of stitches are placed at the paraspinal fascia if possible, and local anesthetic is infiltrated to minimize postoperative incisional pain. Subcuticular skin closure is done, and a small bandage is applied. This transpedicular thoracic diskectomy can be performed on an outpatient basis or with overnight stay in the hospital.

Discussion

Patterson and Arbit first introduced the transpedicular approach to thoracic disk herniation in 1978.[7] Stillerman et al reported a similar surgical technique to thoracic disks and called their surgical maneuver a

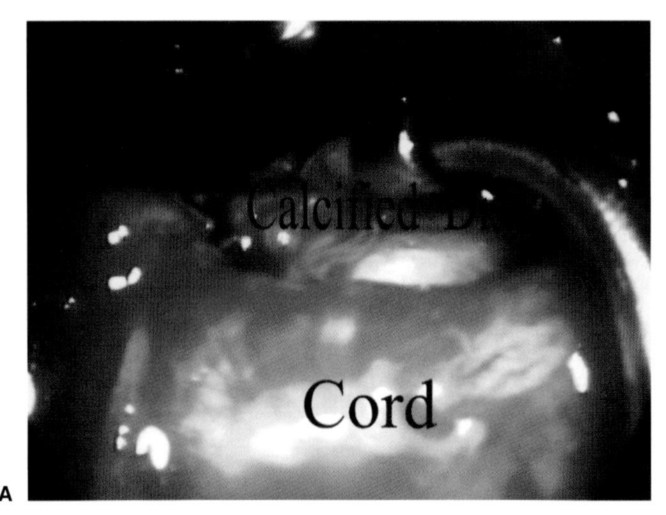

A

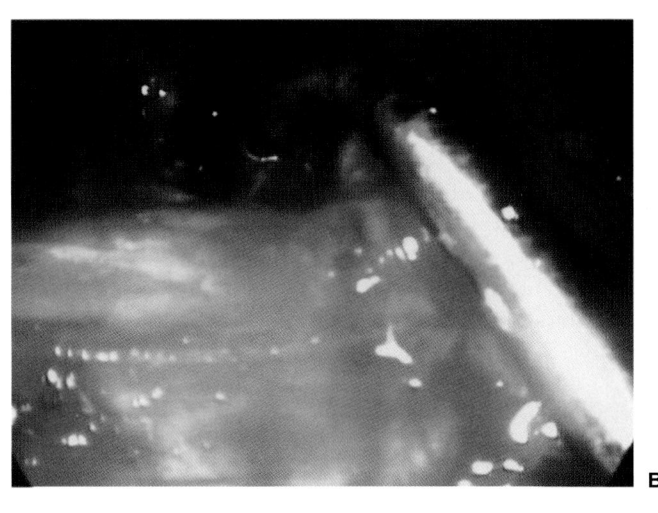

B

FIGURE 12–6 An intraoperative picture taken with a 70-degree-lens endoscope reveals a protruded calcified disk, which is indenting the ventral aspect of the spinal cord **(A)**. When the protruded disk is removed, the ventral aspect of the spinal cord dura mater bulges out toward the cavity created at the intervertebral disk space **(B)**. Surgical tools are curved to access the ventral aspect of the spinal cord.

transfacet pedicle-sparing approach.[9] The surgical procedure adopted in the authors' endoscopic transpedicular approach is very similar to that microscopic technique.[3] Minimally invasive surgical technique requires tremendous precision because the margin of error is so narrow that being a bit off the surgical target will lead to frustration and a possible surgical disaster. Accurate localization of the surgical target with the fluoroscopic C-arm is essential to achieve precision to the surgical target. The surgical landmark is the crossing point of a line drawn along the inferior margin of the facet process horizontally and a vertical line drawn along the midpoint of the facet joint. The crossing point of these two lines will lead to the rostral portion of the pedicle. Other landmarks are the transverse processes of adjacent vertebrae and the inferior margin of the lamina. The facet joint can be identified just medially between the transverse processes. The intervertebral disk in the thoracic spine is located at the level of the facet joint. To expose the intervertebral disk laterally to the spinal cord, the facet joint has to be partially removed. In addition, the rostral edge of the pedicle in the thoracic spine is so close to the intervertebral disk that the rostral-medial one-third portion of the pedicle at the lower vertebra has to be removed for adequate exposure of the superior bony edge of the lower vertebra adjacent to the intervertebral disk. The surgical procedure from the skin incision to trocar placement is fast and straightforward, lasting only a few minutes. The very lateral portion of the laminae and the medial portion of the facet joint are removed using a high-speed drill with a 2 mm cutting bit. Drilling of the bone under a 0-degree-lens endoscope requires practice because it is performed under a two-dimensional view, which eliminates visual depth perception. Surgical approach is made under a 0-degree-lens endoscope, and diskectomy ventral to the spinal cord is performed under a 70-degree-lens endoscope without normal depth perception. When a 3D endoscope is fully developed, endoscopic stereoscopic images will provide the surgeon with improved depth perception; however, a surgeon who is fully advanced in endoscopic surgery can have adequate perceptional surgical guidance even under a two-dimensional image using other visual and tactile cues. As Patterson and Arbit originally reported, it is important to create a small cavity lateral to the spinal cord first by removing the bony spur of the rostral and caudal vertebra in addition to the removal of the intervertebral disk before any attempt at removal of the disk is made medially.[7] A surgical exposure, however, should not produce postsurgical mechanical instability. The lateral portion of the facet joint has to be preserved for that purpose. In addition, the cavity created anterior to the herniated disk should not compromise the spinal integrity. The remaining disk in the intervertebral disk space is preserved, not disintegrated.

Operating under the 70-degree-lens endoscope is very difficult and confusing until the surgeon becomes skilled in endoscopic technique. The lateral 2 mm portion of the spinal cord dura mater is exposed, and this limited exposure of the spinal cord helps to avoid inadvertent spinal cord damage. In addition to the confusing view of the 70-degree-lens endoscope, the use of oddly curved surgical instruments may prove to be an initial technical challenge for the surgeon. An endoscope holder is essential to maintain a steady image on the monitor and to allow the surgeon to use both hands. An endoscope-cleansing device is another integral element in this technique. Although the endoscope cleaner that is commercially available at present is not yet ideal, it does significantly aid the surgeon in operating continuously without the frequent interruption of having to move the endoscope to clean a foggy or blood-stained lens.

Although we have not experienced any cases of intraoperative spinal cord damage, the main potential risk of this endoscopic transpedicular technique is still spinal cord damage. SEP monitoring has been used in all patients; however, its use does not preclude the development of spinal cord injury intraoperatively. The display of SEP changes occurs a few minutes after they actually happen. In addition, it provides only posterior column function of the spinal cord. Once a surgeon desires to use an endoscope through a posterior approach to the treatment of thoracic disks, a posterolateral extracavitary approach may be an easy operation to start with. With this wider and further lateral exposure, a surgeon can become accustomed to the use of a 70-degree-lens endoscope more easily. Once the surgeon's endoscopic skill has improved with practice, a more restricted surgical exposure such as a transpedicular approach can be applied. Endoscopic inspection of the ventral aspect of the spinal cord alone is not difficult. When decompression of the spinal cord is achieved, the spinal cord dura mater bulges out ventrally toward the diskectomy cavity, showing convexity on the endoscopic view. The lack of this dural ventral bulging means inadequate decompression of the spinal cord. Inadequate decompression of the spinal cord is obviously another potential undesired outcome, and nerve root damage is another possible complication. The lack of depth perception in two-dimensional endoscopic images may lead to injury of the nerve root while the facet joint is removed. When the surgeon becomes familiar with the surgical technique, the patient's postoperative recovery, the amount of surgical invasiveness, and the complexity of the surgical procedure may become comparable to that of cervical or lumbar diskectomy.

The endoscopic transpedicular approach provides a minimally invasive surgical option for treating thoracic disk herniation. Access to the ventral spinal cord is obtained through a 1.1 or 1.5 cm trocar with the use of a 0-degree-lens rigid 4 mm endoscope for visualization during drilling of the medial portion of the facet, lateral lamina, and rostral-medial pedicle of the lower vertebra. A mounted 70-degree-lens endoscope provides direct visualization of the ventral spinal cord during decompression of the spinal cord with 90-degree-curved surgical instruments. As adjuncts, fluoroscopic C-arm and somatosensory monitoring aid in the guidance of the surgical approach and in the detection of intraoperative complications, respectively. When skillfully performed, endoscopic transpedicular thoracic diskectomy provides high levels of symptomatic resolution and low complication risks.

REFERENCES

1. Arseni C, Nash F. Thoracic intervertebral disc protrusion: a clinical study. *J Neurosurg.* 1960;17:418–430.
2. Hulme A. The surgical approach to thoracic intervertebral disc protrusions. *J Neurol Neurosurg Psychiatry.* 1960;23:133–137.
3. Jho HD. Endoscopic microscopic transpedicular thoracic discectomy: technical note. *J Neurosurg.* 1997;87:125–129.
4. Jho HD. Endoscopic transpedicular thoracic discectomy. *J Neurosurg.* 1999;91:151–156.
5. Lardon SJ, Holst RA, Hemmy DC, et al. Lateral extracavitary approach to traumatic lesions of the thoracic and lumbar spine. *J Neurosurg.* 1976;45:628–637.
6. Le Roux PD, Haglund MM, Hemmy DC, et al. Thoracic disc disease: experience with the transpedicular approach in twenty consecutive patients. *Neurosurgery.* 1993;33:58–66.
7. Patterson RH, Jr, Arbit E. A surgical approach through the pedicle to protruded thoracic discs. *J Neurosurg.* 1978;48:768–772.
8. Perot PL, Jr, Munro DD. Transthoracic removal of midline thoracic disc protrusions causing spinal cord compression. *J Neurosurg.* 1969;31:452–458.
9. Stillerman CB, Chen TC, Diaz Day J, et al. The transfacet pedicle-sparing approach for thoracic disc removal: cadaveric morphometric analysis and preliminary clinical experience. *J Neurosurg.* 1995;83:971–976.
10. Rosenthal D, Rosenthal R, de Simone A. Removal of a protruded thoracic disc using microsurgical endoscopy: a new technique. *Spine.* 1994;19:1087–1091.

13

Thoracoscopic Management of Spinal Tumors

J. PATRICK JOHNSON

Thoracoscopic spinal surgeries for neurogenic and vertebral tumors are advanced procedures that are beyond the basic procedures of sympathectomy and the more complex procedures of diskectomy for spinal cord and spinal nerve decompression. The advances in endoscopic thoracic spinal procedures described in the previous chapter allow these techniques to be used for significantly more complex spinal disorders, including resection of neurogenic tumors and reconstruction of vertebral tumors.

The advantages of thoracoscopy over thoracotomy that have been described for the treatment of both spinal and nonspinal disorders are well known. Although thoracoscopic procedures have altered the treatment paradigm for many of these lesions, significant limitations to these procedures remain, particularly for the inexperienced endoscopic spinal surgeon. The procedures described here require the surgeon to have a working familiarity with more fundamental thoracoscopic procedures as a prerequisite to perform these more complex procedures with appropriate safety and efficacy. In this chapter, we will describe the indications and techniques for thoracoscopic resection of neurogenic tumors and vertebral tumors.

Indications

Neurogenic Tumors

The most common neurogenic tumors in the thoracic spine are schwannomas and neurofibromas; less frequently, there are other tumors of nerve origin arising from segmental intercostal nerves. They are typically benign tumors and are rarely malignant, presenting as the classic "dumbell" tumor, with a smaller component in the spinal canal causing spinal cord compression with a larger intrathoracic component (Fig. 13–1A,B). These tumors can also present with chest wall pain due to spinal nerve compression or may be discovered incidentally with a routine chest radiograph. Strategies for surgical resection of these tumors depend entirely on their anatomic location. Tumors that are found exclusively within the chest cavity arising from an intercostal nerve can be removed with thoracic endoscopic techniques (Fig. 13–1C). Tumors that extend into the neural foramen without an intraspinal component can still be removed with a thoracoscopic procedure; however, that portion of the tumor that extends into the spinal canal must be removed with a posterior laminectomy exposure and excision. The intraspinal tumor must also be evaluated as to whether the lesion is intradural or extradural. This can be determined with a postmyelography CT scan that will assist in defining the location in relation to the thecal sac. Tumors that do not extend into the spinal canal can be treated solely with an endoscopic procedure. If the tumor extends into the spinal canal, then a combined transthoracic and posterior tumor excision can be performed. We have performed these procedures simultaneously in a lateral position, which can expedite the procedure.

Vertebral Tumors

Vertebral tumors are primary or secondary neoplasms that affect the vertebral body and may result in either

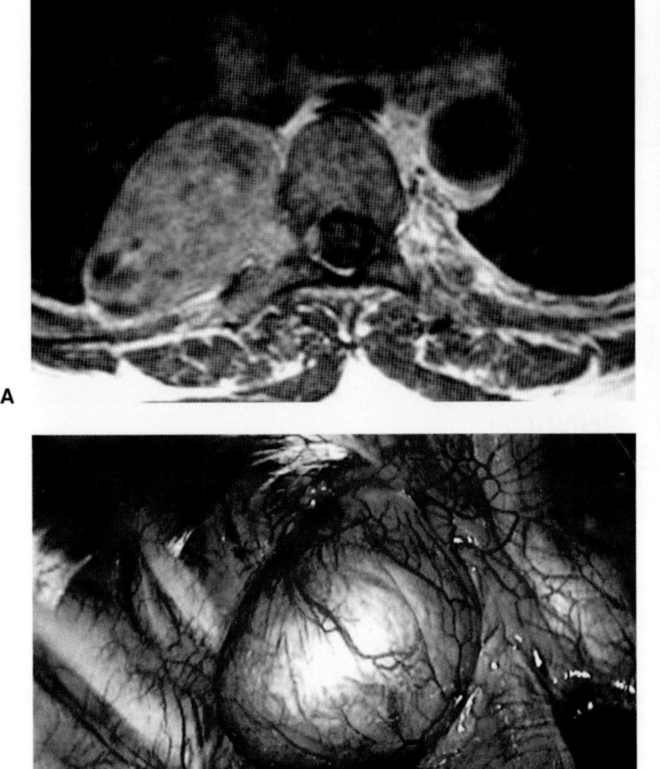

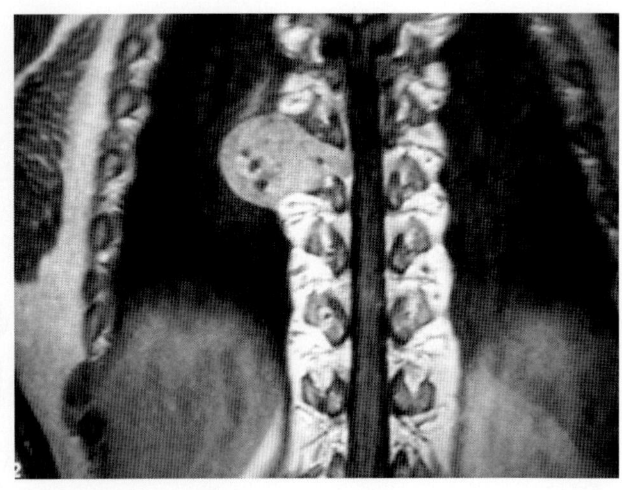

FIGURE 13–1 (A,B) Axial T2 MRI showing nerve sheath tumor with intrathoracic extension. **(C)** Thoracoscopic view of nerve sheath tumor.

vertebral collapse or tumor mass that compresses the spinal cord. The most common vertebral tumors are metastatic, and primary vertebral tumors are relatively rare (Fig. 13–2). These tumors, which previously required a thoracotomy, are potential candidates for thoracoscopic resection and reconstruction. They typically have a slowly progressive presentation pattern with onset of continuous unremitting pain. Neurologic deficits usually occur later in the clinical course and only rarely require urgent surgical intervention. These lesions have often been irradiated and have a wide range of variability in radiation responsiveness that generally depends on the tissue type and biologic behavior.

Imaging for Thoracic Spinal Tumors

Imaging for thoracic spinal neoplasms is essential for determining whether a lesion can be treated successfully with a thoracoscopic procedure. Magnetic resonance imaging (MRI) is the ideal method for surveying the thoracic spine due to superior soft tissue definition with orthogonal views to visualize the spinal cord, vertebral lesions, and adjacent anatomy that may include extension of the neoplasm that affects surgical decision making. Because bony anatomy is not as well defined with MRI techniques, CT (Fig. 13–2B) is useful to demonstrate the bony architecture of the vertebral column. Neurogenic tumors typically do not invade the vertebral column, but they can erode and enlarge the neural foramen where it exits the nerve in a classic dumbbell shape. Vertebral tumors from metastases or primary bony tumors cause destruction of the bony architecture that requires definition with CT imaging to determine the extent of tumor involvement and what tumor resection and reconstruction will be required. Most cases of thoracic spinal tumors require both MRI and CT scans to define the anatomic details fully for either an open or a thoracosopic procedure.

Plain radiographs of the thoracic and lumbar spine are always obtained preoperatively to determine deformity and for verification and comparison of intraoperative radiographs to confirm the level(s) operated.

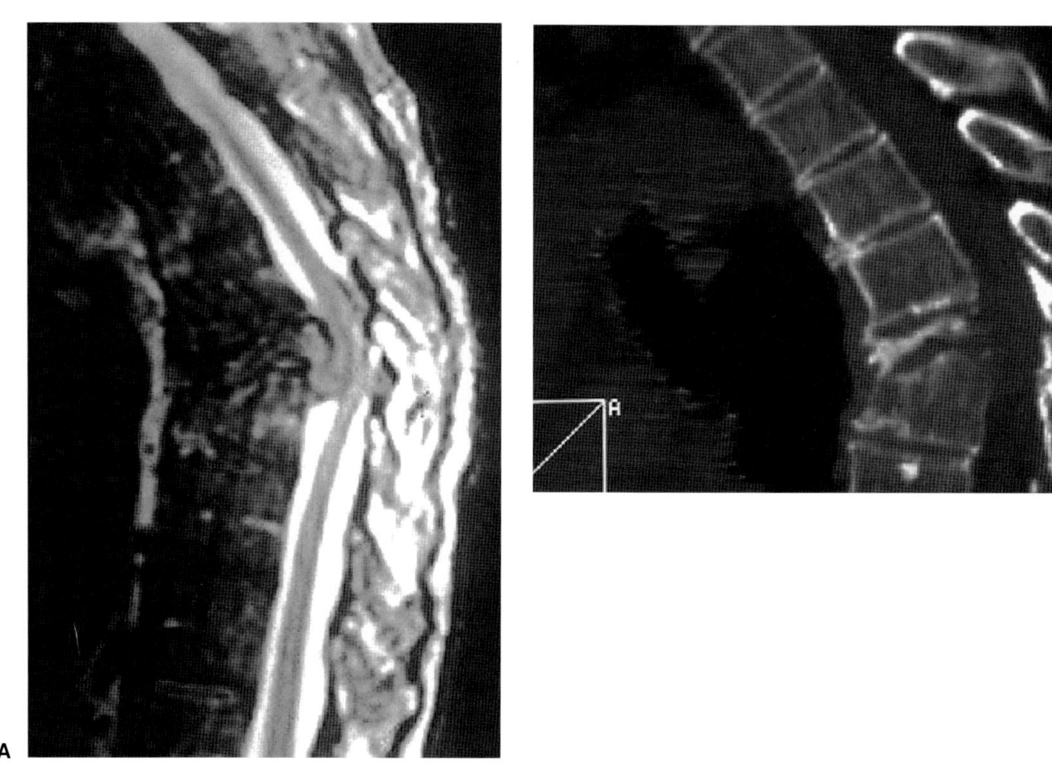

FIGURE 13–2 MRI **(A)** and CT **(B)** showing metastatic vertebral tumor causing compression fracture with kyphotic deformity.

Surgical Procedure

Description of Procedure

Thoracoscopic spinal procedures for diskectomy and sympathectomy have been well described previously and provide the basic thoracoscopic spinal surgical skills necessary to perform these more complicated procedures. The procedure begins with induction of general anesthesia and placement of a double lumen endotracheal tube for ventilation of the opposite lung during the operation. The patient is placed in a lateral position, with the operated side of the spinal column facing upward. The arm is held in an "airplane" holder to expose the chest wall. A preliminary anteroposterior chest radiograph is then obtained for localization of the spinal level and the portal sites. This assists in precise placement of the portal sites prior to prepping and draping, with the thoracoscope portal placed in the chest cavity perpendicular to the level of the pathology in the posterior midaxillary line. Two additional working ports are established in the anterior/midaxillary line rostral and caudal to the operated level. Soft portals are used to help reduce the incidence of intercostal nerve injury. Initial thoracoscopy includes retraction of the lung anteriorly that is facilitated by rotation of the operating table. The exact spinal level is then identified by placing a localizing needle into the disk spaces adjacent to the level of interest and obtaining another radiograph. This may be obviated in large neurogenic tumors that are clearly visible within the chest cavity.

Vertebral Tumor Removal and Reconstruction

A vertebral tumor resection usually requires a vertebrectomy procedure and exposure by reflecting the parietal pleura widely over the site of the pathology to expose the vertebra, rib heads, and disk spaces. The segmental vessels crossing in the midportion of the vertebral body can be coagulated and divided with clips and/or cautery. The rib head at the resection level is subsequently removed with the pneumatic drill to expose the pedicle, which is removed to expose the spinal canal (Fig. 13–3). A vertebrectomy to remove the tumor is then completed with curettage or a pneumatic drill (Fig. 13–4). The adjacent level disks can be removed with standard dissection techniques. The decompression is continued until the ventral aspect of the spinal cord is visualized. The anterior longitudinal ligament can be removed with a blunt tip probe and divided with Kerrison rongeurs to expose the dura. Bone bleeding is controlled with bone wax, and

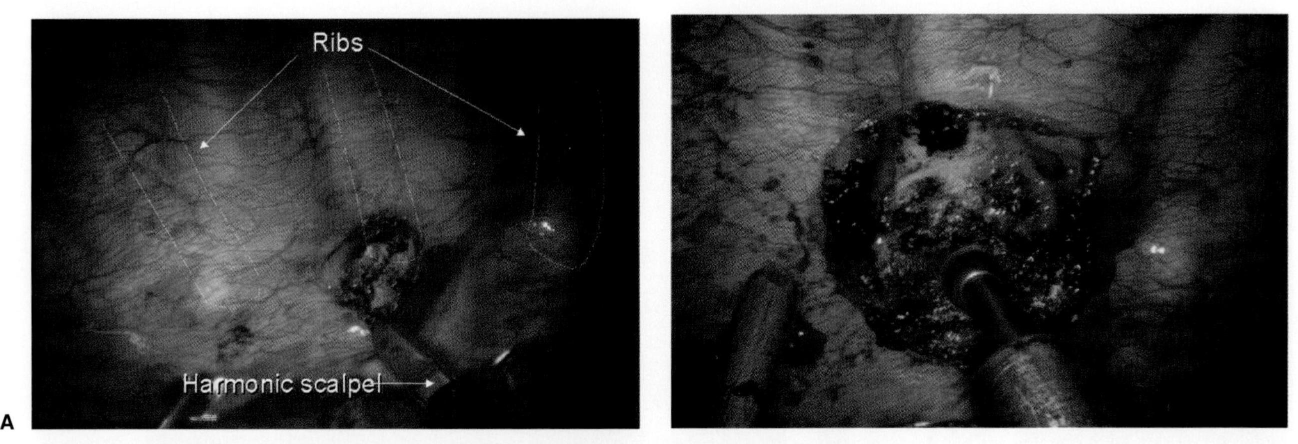

FIGURE 13–3 (A,B) Exposure and removal of the rib head for exposing the pedicle.

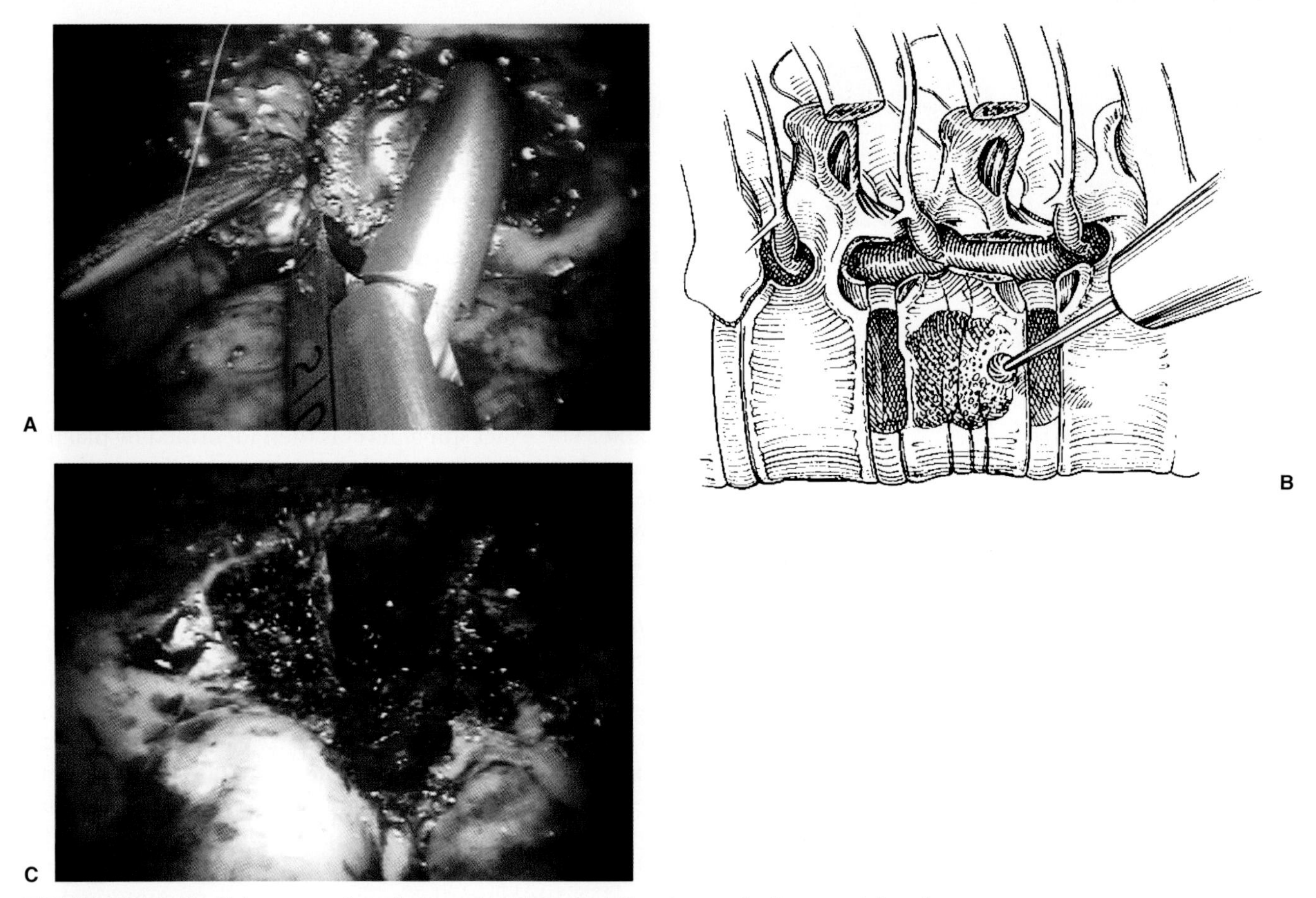

FIGURE 13–4 (A–C) Intraoperative photos and artist's depiction demonstrating a vertebrectomy.

epidural hemostasis is achieved with Gelfoam and/or bipolar cautery. Reconstruction of a vertebrectomy defect can be accomplished with either a bone graft or a titanium mesh cage, depending on the pathology (Fig. 13–5). We typically use a cage for metastatic tumors and either an autograft or an allograft for infectious cases that will progress to fusion. The vertebral implant is inserted into the chest through a slightly enlarged portal site. Instrumentation with a lateral plate or screw-rod construct can be used to secure the graft in place (Fig. 13–6). Additional portals may be required to place instrumentation with screw trajectories across the vertebral bodies and assemble a plate or screw-rod construct.

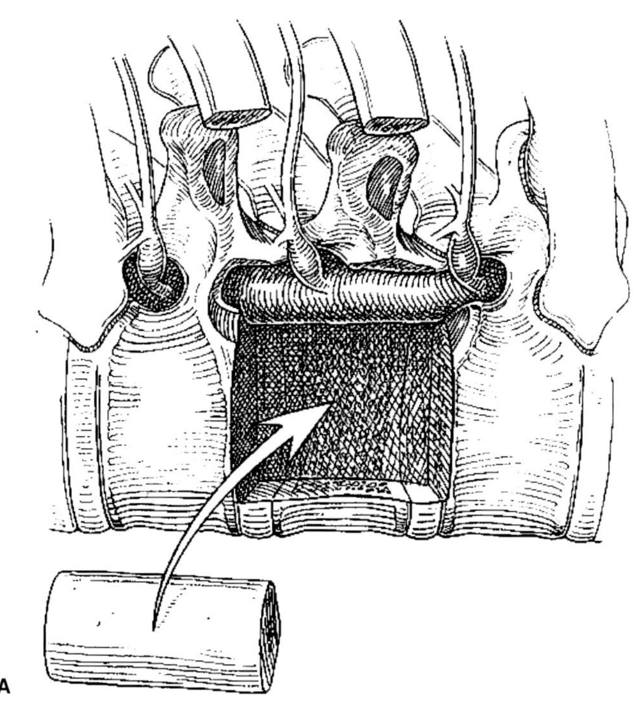

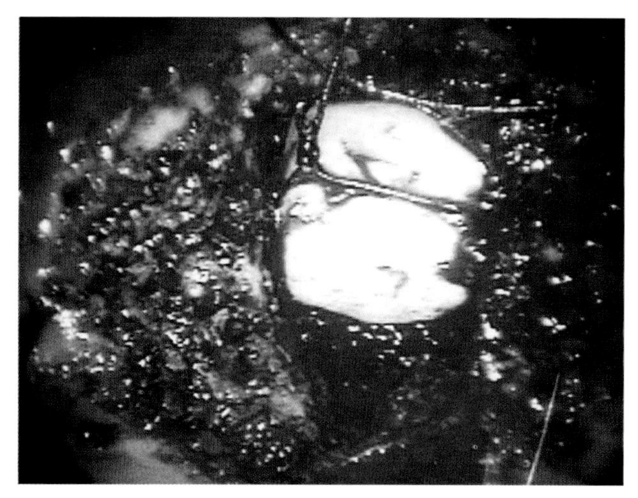

FIGURE 13–5 (A,B) Reconstruction with bone graft.

Nerve Sheath Tumor Resection

A spinal tumor resection of a neurofibroma usually does not require significant bone removal that involves vertebrectomy because these tumors are usually distinctly separate from the bony structure of the vertebra. The vertebra and rib may be eroded with an enlarged foramen that is seen in the classic dumbbell-shaped tumor. These tumors require exposure by opening the pleura widely to expose the full extent of the lesion. Small tumors can be removed en bloc, but larger tumors are removed by internal debulking with pituitary rongeurs, followed by dissection and mobilization of the capsule with surgical techniques similar to open procedures. Hemostasis in the tumor resection cavity can be achieved with bipolar cautery.

A number 20 French chest tube is inserted and externalized through one of the portals. The portals are removed,

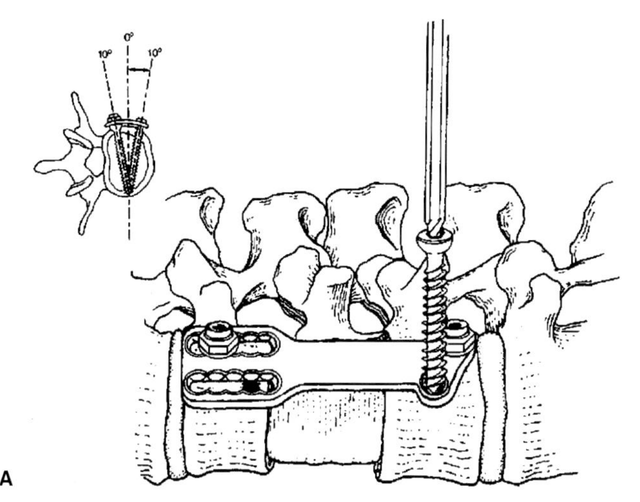

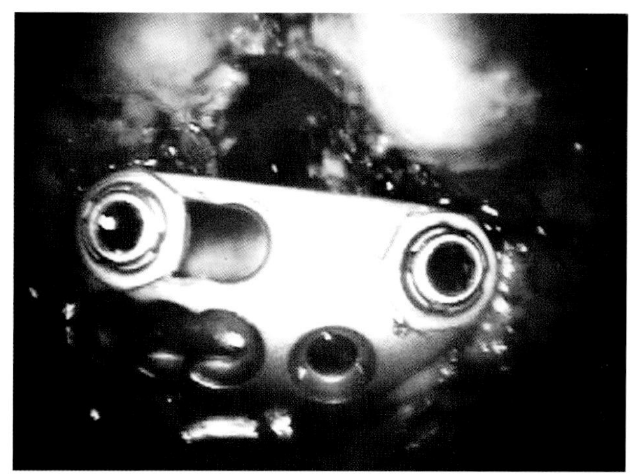

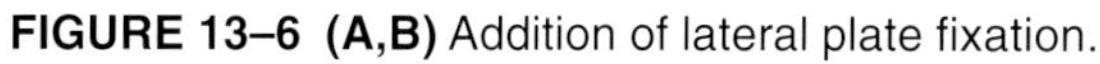
FIGURE 13–6 (A,B) Addition of lateral plate fixation.

and the incisions are closed in layers. Sterile dressings are subsequently applied. The chest tube is placed to suction in the operating room and to water seal in the recovery room; it is usually removed within 24 to 48 hours.

Thoracoscopy was initially introduced as a diagnostic tool for evaluation of pleural disease but has expanded greatly over the years now to include treatment of thoracic disk herniations, sympathectomies, vertebral biopsies, spinal deformities correction, and, lastly, corpectomies associated with trauma or tumor followed by reconstruction and stabilization. Over the past 2 decades, several clinical studies have found significant advantages of thoracoscopy over thoracotomy in terms of reduced postoperative pain, reduced intensive care unit and hospital stays, shortened recovery time, faster return to activity, and lower complication rates. Overall, the advantages of the thoracoscopic approach are numerous; however, when applied to cases of thoracoscopic tumor resection, reconstruction, and stabilization, a surgeon must have the added working familiarity with more fundamental thoracoscopic procedures as a prerequisite to perform these more complex cases.

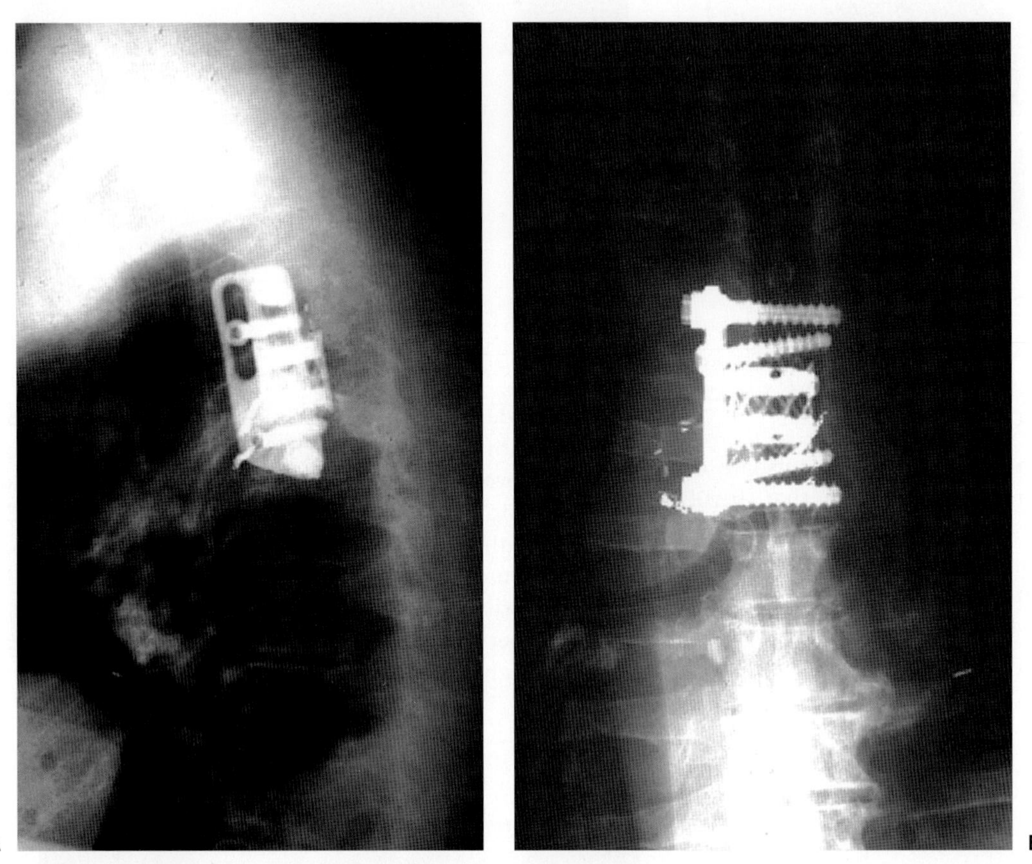

Figure 13–7 (A,B) Postoperative radiographs after thoracoscopic tumor vertebrectomy, cage reconstruction, and fixation.

14

Minimally Invasive Instrumentation, Correction, and Fusion of Primary Thoracic and Thoracolumbar Scoliosis

GEORGE D. PICETTI III AND MICHAEL YEE

Endoscopic spine surgery has made many advances and improvements, from its inception with biopsy and diskectomy in the early 1990s, to the present, with instrumentation, correction, and fusion of deformity.[1] Endoscopic or minimally invasive surgery has the advantage of improved visualization, decreased blood loss, decreased tissue trauma, decreased pain, and less time for rehabilitation; however, when performing endoscopic or minimally invasive surgery, one must adhere to the ultimate goals of the procedure to be performed and not do less because the incisions are smaller. One also must be well versed in the open technique before embarking on this endoscopic procedure.

After extensive experience at the Kaiser Sacramento (California) Spine Center with thoracoscopic anterior release and fusion for scoliosis, kyphosis, hemiepiphyseodesis, and hemivertebrectomy, we embarked on the development of a technique for endoscopic instrumentation, correction, and fusion of primary thoracic curves. From our previous work and that of others, we documented the benefits of thoracoscopic surgery, which included improved visualization, improved access to the extremes of the curve, decreased blood loss, decreased operating times, shorter hospital stay, faster return to school and activities, and decreased overall costs.[1,2]

Our goal in developing an endoscopic technique for the treatment of scoliosis is to perform a safe, reproducible, and effective procedure that is comparable to or better than a formal open technique. Goals for scoliosis surgery continue to be the restoration of spinal alignment and balance in all planes, as well as axial derotation.

At the Kaiser Sacramento Spine Center, we performed our first entirely endoscopic instrumentation, correction, and fusion for thoracic scoliosis in October 1996.[3] The first few cases were performed with rudimentary implants and instrumentation. As we have gained experience with the surgical technique, and as improvements have been made in the implants and instrumentation, advances in the procedure have continued.

Surgical Technique for Primary Thoracic Scoliosis

Intraoperative Preparation

Intraoperative somatosensory evoked potential (SSEP) and motor evoked potential (MEP) monitors are placed in standard fashion and checked. General anesthesia is administered with a double lumen intubation technique in adults and children weighing more than 45 kg. Children weighing less than 40 to 45 kg may require selective intubation of the ventilated lung. Once intubated, the patient is placed in the direct lateral decubitus position with the concave side of the curve positioned down. All bony prominences are checked and well padded. This body orientation provides a reference guide to estimate the direction of the anteroposterior and lateral guidewire and screw placement. The position is rechecked prior to beginning guidewire placement. The arms are both placed at 90 degrees to the body (Fig. 14–1).

The hips and shoulders are secured to the operating table with tape to ensure correct body position throughout the procedure. The C-arm is utilized in the posteroanterior and lateral plane to mark the sites for portal

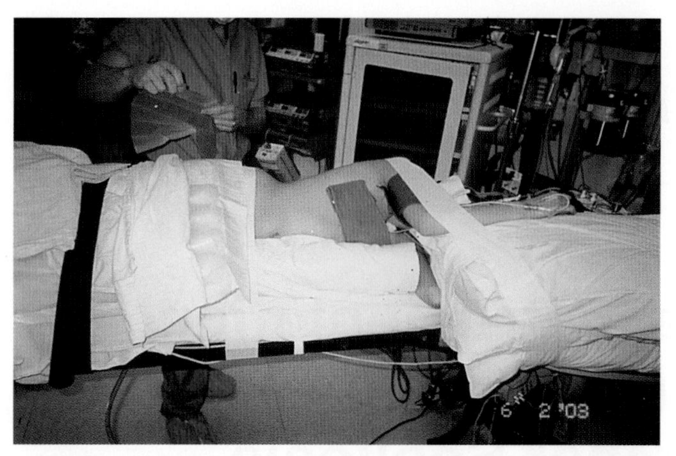

FIGURE 14–1 The patient is in the direct left lateral decubitus position. The arms and hips are taped onto the operating room table to maintain this position throughout the procedure.

placement (Fig. 14–2). The portal sites are cutaneously marked with a felt tip pen from the inferior to the superior ends of the Cobb angle. Two endoscopic monitors are necessary and are placed at the head of the operating table to allow visualization from both the anterior and posterior positions. The operating surgeon is positioned at the patient's back to allow anatomic orientation of the external landmarks visualized through the endoscope. In addition, this position allows all instruments to be directed away from the spinal cord and enables the surgeon to place the screws in line with the spinal rotation safely.

Incision and Portal Placement

Following deflation of the lung, an initial 1.5 cm incision is made at the level of the sixth or seventh intercostal space in line with the spine. The portal placement accounts for spinal rotation as determined preoperatively under C-arm control. Placement of the initial portal at this level will avoid injury to the diaphragm, which maintains a more caudal position. Digital inspection of the portal is performed to ensure lung deflation and the absence of pleural adhesions.

The endoscope is inserted into the initial portal and utilized for additional portal placement under direct visualization. The portals are positioned directly over the rib two interspaces apart, allowing access to two vertebral

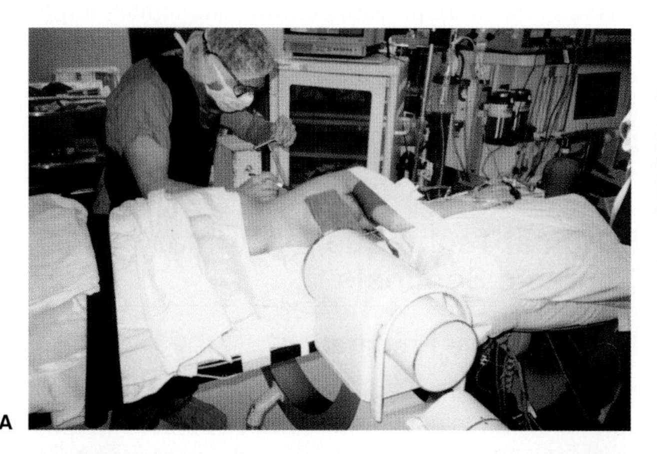

A

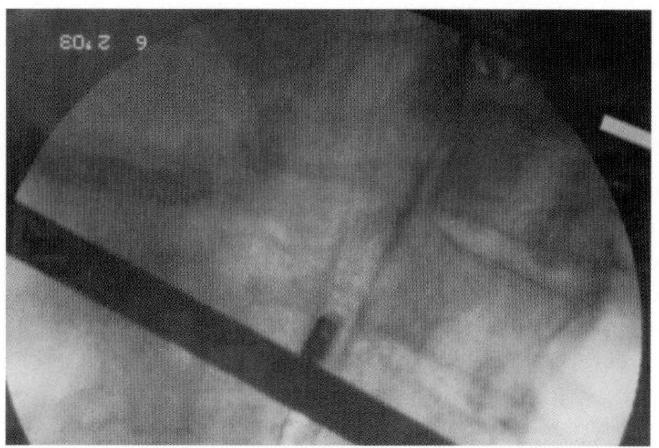

B

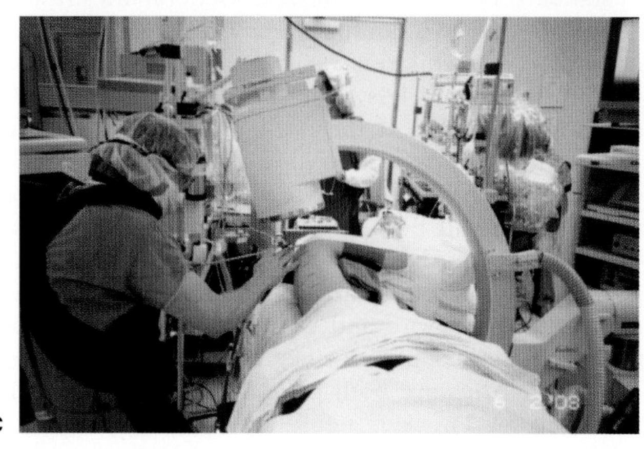

C

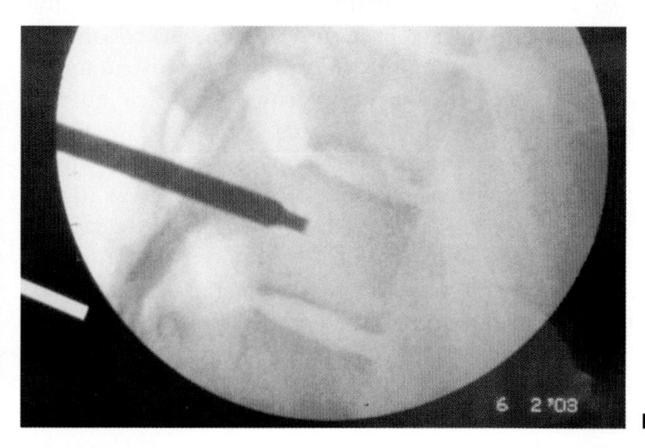

D

FIGURE 14–2 (A) The C-arm is placed in the posteroanterior plane at the distal level to be instrumented with a rod as a marker. A skin marker is used to notate the levels to be instrumented. **(B)** Posteroanterior C-arm image of the rod marker parallel to the end plates of the distal level. **(C)** Schematic drawing demonstrating the C-arm in position in the lateral plane using the rod marker to determine the portal location. **(D)** Lateral C-arm image demonstrating the rod marker at the level of the rib head; the portal will be made just anterior to this mark.

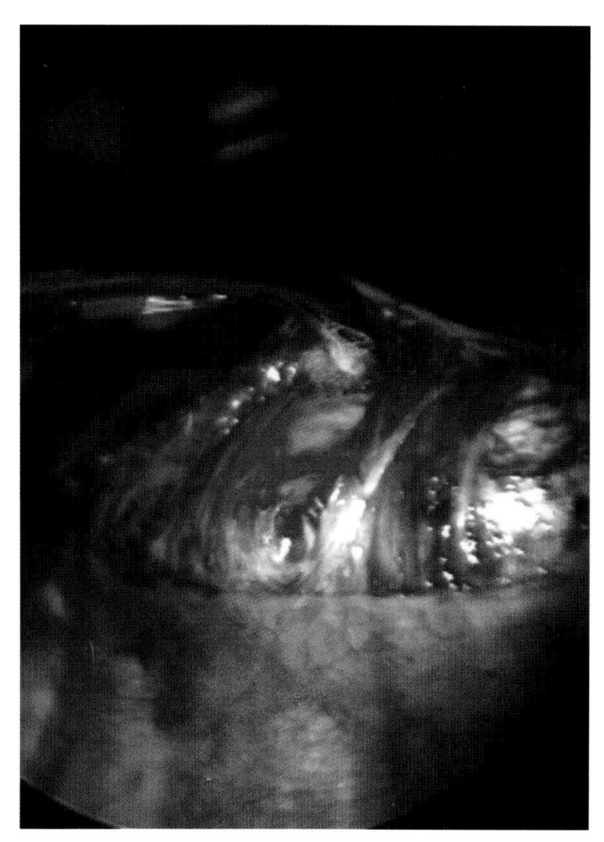

FIGURE 14–3 Intraoperative view through the endoscope. The pleura has been incised along the midline of the vertebral bodies and is reflected off the anterior longitudinal ligament.

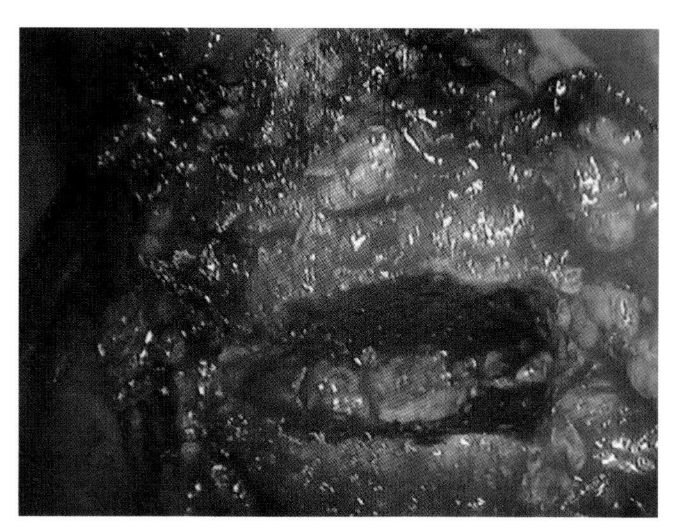

FIGURE 14–4 Intraoperative view through the endoscope of a diskectomy. The cartilage has been removed from the end plates, and the anterior longitudinal ligament has been thinned from inside the disk space.

levels from a single incision by moving the portal above and below the rib. Three to five incisions are needed, depending on the number of levels to be instrumented.

Spine Exposure

The pleura is incised longitudinally with electrocautery along the length of the spine to be instrumented. A hook electrocautery is placed on the pleura overlying an intervertebral disk, and a pleural opening is made. The pleura is elevated off the spine and incised. This maneuver allows for incision of the pleura along the spine segments to be instrumented and thus avoids injury to the segmental vessels. The pleura is further dissected anteriorly from the anterior longitudinal ligament and posteriorly from the rib heads (Fig. 14–3).

An x-ray is obtained as the first disk is removed, and a small shaver is placed into the disk space to the opposite side. This allows for determination of the level and will confirm complete diskectomy.

Diskectomy

The intervertebral disk anulus is incised with the cautery. A complete diskectomy is performed using standard or custom curettes and Kerrison and pituitary rongeurs to expose the chondral end plates. The removal of the disk and anulus extends anteriorly to the anterior longitudinal ligament and posteriorly to just behind the rib heads (Fig. 14–4). The anterior longitudinal ligament is thinned to a flexible remnant with a pituitary rongeur from within the disk space. By thinning the anterior longitudinal ligament, it can no longer limit spinal mobility; however, it is able to contain bone graft. The chondral end plates are removed, and the bony end plates are rasped to a homogeneous bleeding surface. The disk space is packed with Surgicel to provide hemostasis.

Bone Graft Harvest

On completion of the diskectomies, the portals are removed, and attention is directed toward rib bone graft harvest. At the level of each incision the rib is subperiosteally exposed with sequential retraction as far anteriorly and posteriorly as possible. A perpendicular cut using the endoscopic rib cutter is made in the superior aspect of the rib at the anterior and posterior extent of the rib dissection. The cuts are connected, with a straight osteotome removing the superior portion of the rib. Multiple rib sections are removed in a similar fashion and morcellized until sufficient graft is available. This technique maintains the integrity of the rib as well as protecting the intercostal nerve and decreasing postoperative pain.

Screw Placement

Body position and rotation are checked. The sterilely draped C-arm is brought into the operating field, and the base is placed parallel to the superior most vertebral body to provide an accurate image. The portals and

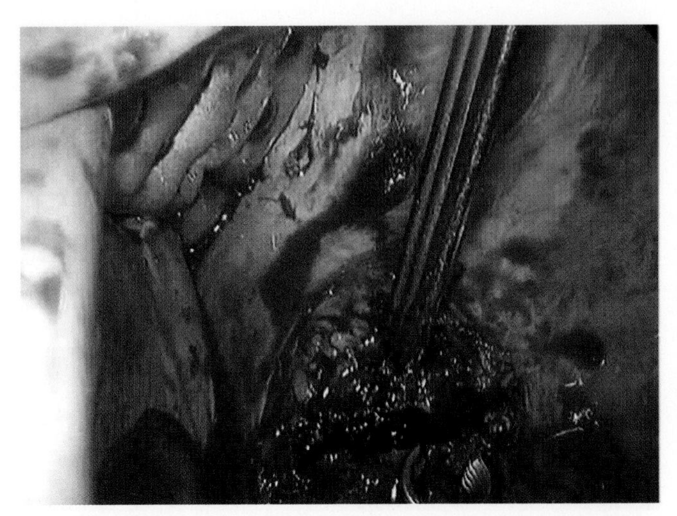

FIGURE 14–5 Intraoperative view through the endoscope showing the K-wire guide inserted onto the vertebral body.

endoscope are replaced. The segmental vessels are cauterized at the midvertebral level. Larger segmental vessels and the azygous system may be ligated with endoscopic vascular staples and transected.

The K-wire triple guide is placed centrally on the vertebral body and parallel to the end plates. The guide is placed anterior to the rib head, with a slight posterior to anterior inclination (Fig. 14–5). This position directs the wire away from the spinal canal, and the position can be monitored under biplanar fluoroscopic control.

Once the guide is correctly aligned, a K-wire is advanced into the vertebral body, engaging the opposite cortex. Fluoroscopic monitoring is used to avoid penetration of the opposite cortex and potential penetration of the K-wire into the contralateral segmental vessels and lung (Figs. 14–6, 14–7). The screw length is measured on the scale at the upper section of the K-wire

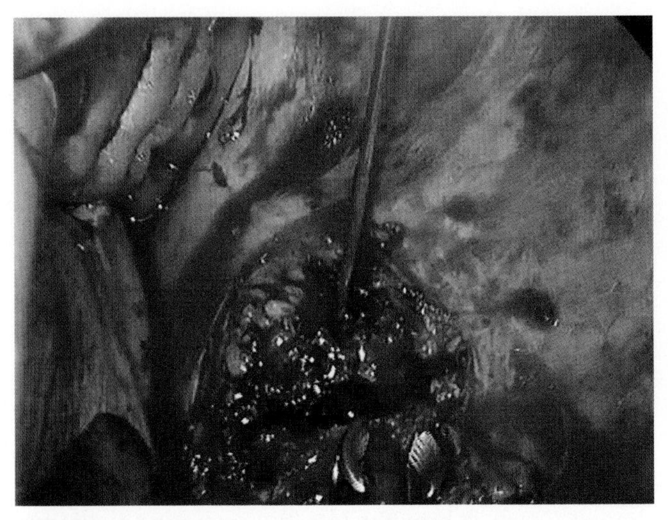

FIGURE 14–6 Intraoperative view through the endoscope showing the K-wire inserted into the vertebral body.

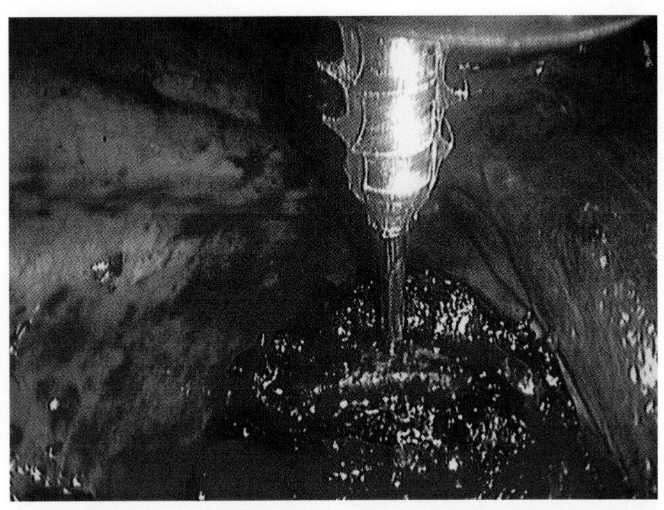

FIGURE 14–7 Intraoperative view through the endoscope showing the tap placed over the K-wire ready to be inserted into the vertebral body.

or determined by measuring the preoperative x-ray. The K-wire guide is removed, and the cannulated screw tap is advanced only into the near cortex of the vertebral body. If the use of a staple or a washer is desired, it can be inserted at this time. The K-wire is grasped to avoid cortical penetration during screw tap and screw advancement (Fig. 14–7). The appropriately sized screw is advanced over the guidewire, engaging the opposite cortex and seating the head against the valley of the vertebral body (Fig. 14–8). The guidewire is removed once

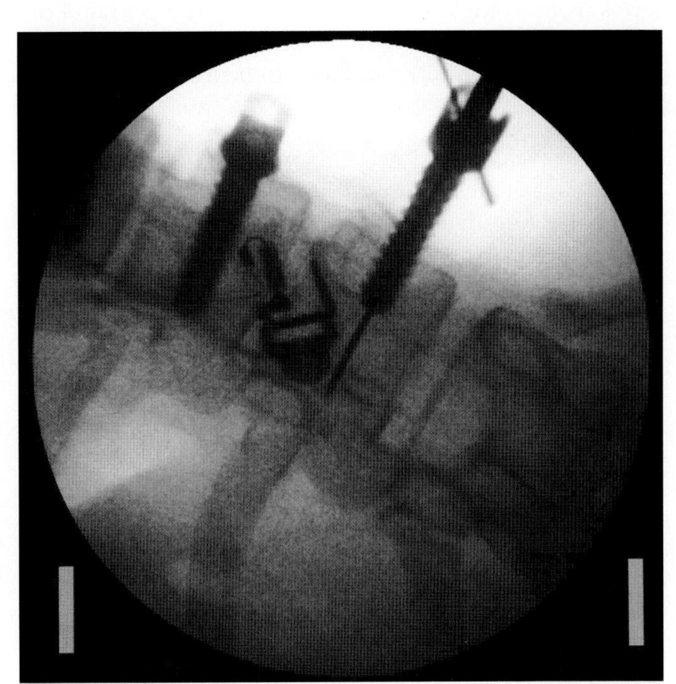

FIGURE 14–8 Intraoperative view through the endoscope showing a screw placed over the K-wire ready to be inserted into the vertebral body.

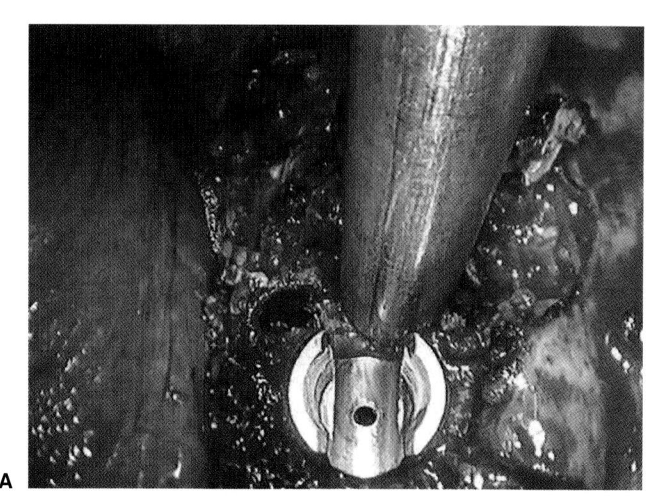

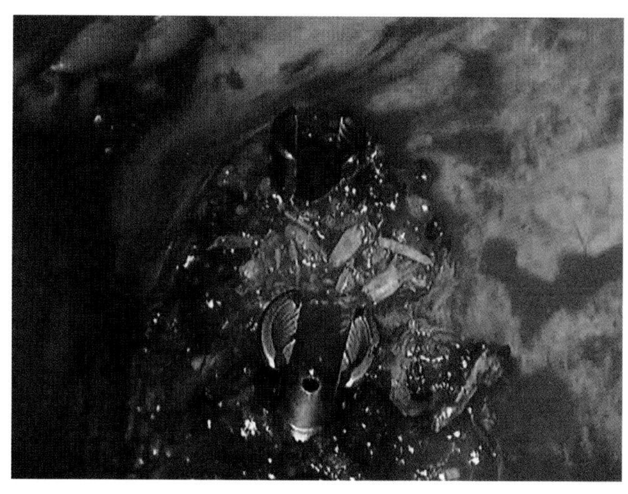

FIGURE 14–9 (A) Intraoperative view through the endoscope showing the bone graft funnel inserted into the disk space. **(B)** Intraoperative view demonstrating a disk space filled with bone graft and graft placed over the adjacent vertebral bodies.

the screw is advanced three fourths of the distance across the vertebral body. The screws can also be inserted without a K-wire or with image guidance. The rib heads are used as a reference for subsequent screw placement to ensure appropriate screw alignment, thus resulting in proper spinal rotational alignment. If each of the screws is placed in the same position of each vertebral body accounting for rotation, the screws will end in a V pattern and will aid in derotation of the spine during rod reduction. Screw depth placement must be accurate and at similar levels; otherwise, seating of the rod will be difficult. The screw depth can be checked with fluoroscopic guidance.

Bone Graft Placement

The Surgicel is sequentially removed from the intervertebral disk space prior to bone graft placement. The periosteum is incised anteriorly and posteriorly at each disk space. The periosteum is next elevated off the ends of the vertebral bodies. The end plates are rerasped, and the bone graft is delivered to the disk space using the graft funnel and plunger. The disk is partially filled, then a small tamp is used to push the graft to the opposite side to ensure complete filling of the space. Once the disk space has been filled, more graft is placed over the space and the adjoining area where the periosteum has been elevated (Fig. 14–9; this will allow for improved x-ray evaluation of the fusion postoperatively).

Rod Length and Placement

The rod length is measured with the endoscopic rod gauge, consisting of a fixed ball on the end of a flexible cable. The fixed ball is placed within the saddle of the inferior screw, and the end of the cable is then guided with a pituitary rongeur through the other screw heads to the superior screw. The cable is tightened, and the rod length is measured from the scale (Fig. 14–10).

A 4.5 mm titanium rod is cut to the premeasured length and placed freely within the chest cavity through the inferior incision. The rod is placed flush into the inferior screw saddle. This is performed to avoid protrusion into or puncturing of the diaphragm. The plug introduction tube is placed over the screw head, temporarily securing the rod (Fig. 14–11). The plug inserter is advanced through the plug guide and the plug is inserted into the vertebral screw, thus securing the rod to the vertebral screw. The inferior screw is the only plug that is initially completely tightened. The rod is next sequentially reduced into the saddles of the remaining screws with the rod pusher, and plugs are placed but not tightened.

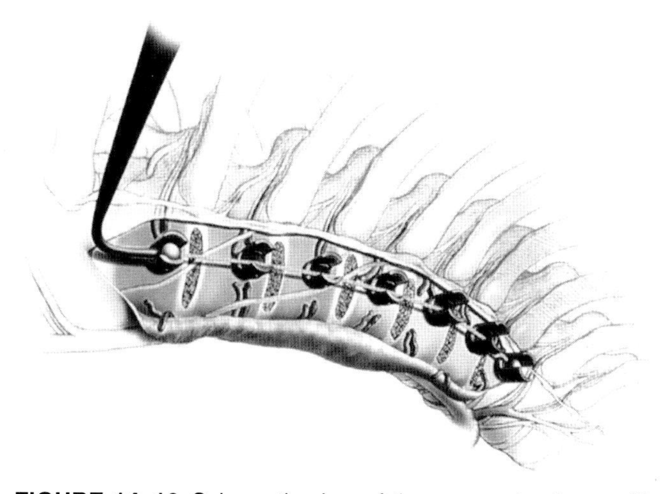

FIGURE 14–10 Schematic view of the screws in place, with the endoscopic rod measurer inserted through all of them. The rod length is determined by reading the scale at the top of the measurer.

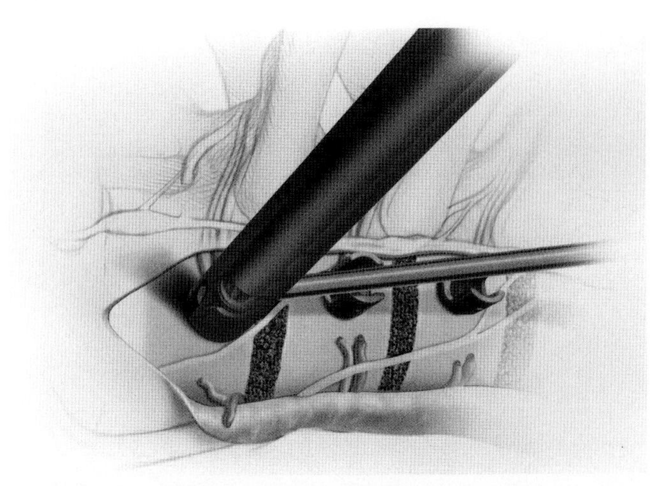

FIGURE 14–11 Schematic diagram of the rod as it is inserted into the most inferior screw, with the plug introduction tube over the screw. The window at the tip of the tube on the screw shows the plug inserted into the screw.

Rod Compression

Once the rod is in place and the plugs are provisionally inserted, compression between each screw is performed. The compressor is placed freely into the chest cavity and over the screw heads on the rod at the inferior end of the construct. Turning the driver clockwise to bring the two screws closer together performs compression. Segmental compression is sequentially performed from inferior to superior until all levels have been compressed (Fig. 14–12). A cable compressor is available as another option. The construct is visualized, the chest cavity is irrigated, and the lung is inflated under visualization of the endoscope to confirm that the entire lung is reinflated. A chest tube is placed through the inferior portal, and the incisions are closed in layers in standard fashion.

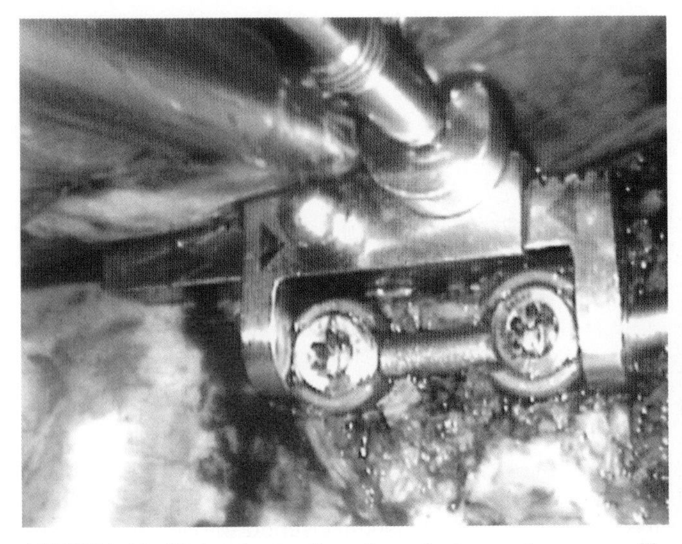

FIGURE 14–12 Intraoperative view via the endoscope, with the endoscopic compressor on the rod compressing two screws together.

Surgical Technique for Instrumentation, Correction, and Fusion of Primary Thoracolumbar Scoliosis

As the thoracic endoscopic technique evolved and our results began approaching that of the formal open technique with primary thoracic scoliosis, we proceeded to our next challenge[4]: to treat thoracolumbar scoliosis via a minimally invasive endoscopic approach. This endeavor, however, presents several new challenges that are not issues with the thoracic spine. The major challenges are endoscopically crossing the diaphragm and maintaining retroperitoneal exposure, especially after an opening has been made under the diaphragm. These goals need to be met, in addition to attaining lumbar lordosis and anterior column support.

General anesthesia is administered as in the thorascopic approach with a double lumen intubation. Once intubated, the patient is placed into the direct lateral decubitus position with the arms at 90/90. The hips and shoulders are then taped to the operating table. This will help to maintain the patient's correct positioning throughout the case. The C-arm is again used as in the thoracoscopic technique; however, each level to be instrumented is marked on the skin for reference (Fig. 14–13). Once the

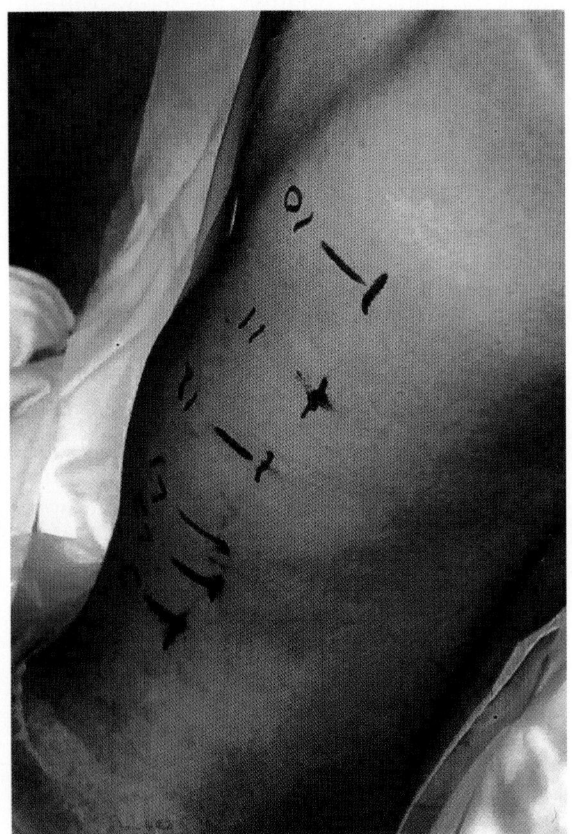

FIGURE 14–13 Photograph of a patient with skin markings for a T10–L3 minimally invasive instrumentation correction and fusion.

lung has been deflated, the proximal portal is inserted in line with the spine, positioned according to the amount of spinal rotation. Inserting the first portal at this level will help avoid injury to the diaphragm. Once the portal is made, digital inspection of the portal is performed to ensure that the lung is deflated and that no adhesions exist. The endoscope is then inserted into the chest, and additional portals are placed under direct visualization.

Three portals are needed in the thoracic cavity: a working portal, a second for the endoscope, and a third for retraction of the lung and diaphragm. Once the portals have been inserted and the scope introduced, the apex of the chest is visualized, and the ribs are counted caudally to the desired level. The hook bovie is placed on the pleura over a disk, and an opening is made. The hook is then inserted under the pleura, and the pleura is elevated and incised longitudinally in the midvertebral body, as in the thoracic technique.

The pleura is then dissected anteriorly off the anterior longitudinal ligament and posteriorly off the rib heads. A marker is placed into one of the disks to be removed, and a localization x-ray is obtained. The electrocautery is then used to incise the disk anulus. The disk is removed in standard fashion, using various endoscopic curettes, and pituitary, Cobb, and Kerrison rongeurs. Once the disk is completely removed, the anterior longitudinal ligament is thinned from within the disk with a pituitary rongeur. The ligament is thinned to a flexible remnant that is no longer structural, but will contain the bone graft. The disk and anulus are posterolaterally also completely removed.

Once the disk has been evacuated, the end plate is completely removed, and the disk space is inspected directly with the scope. The end plates are rasped to a homogeneous bleeding surface. The disk space is then packed with Surgicel to control end plate bleeding. All thoracic disks are removed in this fashion, as described in the thoracic technique.

The T12–L1 disk may also be removed from the thoracic cavity, depending on where the diaphragm inserts. If the diaphragm inserts below the T12–L1 disk space and the exposure of the disk does not require taking down any of the diaphragm, the disk must be removed from the thoracic approach. On the other hand, if the diaphragm inserts above the T12–L1 disk, the disk must be removed from the retroperitoneal approach below the diaphragm.

The scope, instruments, and portals are removed at this time. The anesthesiologist can be instructed to reinflate the lung, and the retroperitoneal approach is performed. The lumbar retroperitoneal incision is performed over the previously marked skin site via an eleventh rib approach. If the planned instrumentation is extending to the L2 level, then the skin mark should be placed over the L1–L2 disk space. This will allow for excellent access from the T12–L1 disk space to the L2 vertebral body. If the hardware is to extend to L3, the

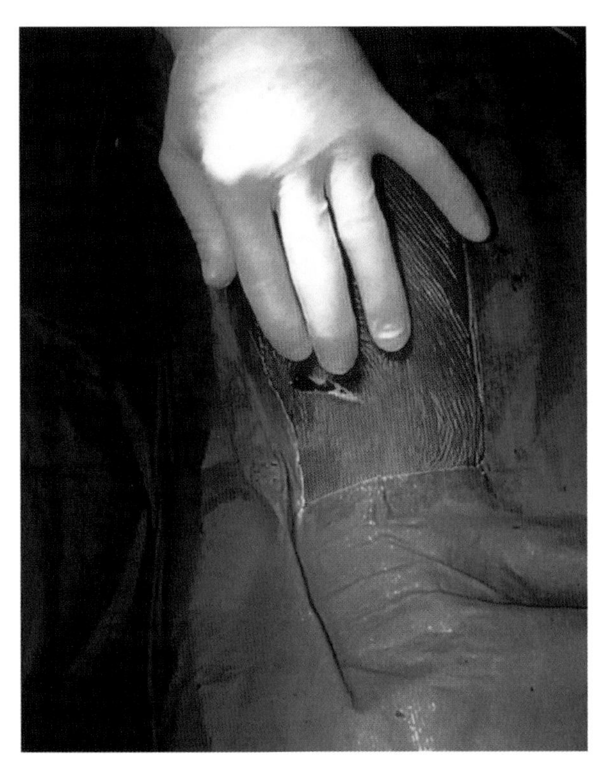

FIGURE 14–14 Photograph of the 4 cm skin incision for the retroperitoneal approach placed over the body of L2.

incision is placed directly over the center of the L2 vertebral body to allow access from the L1 vertebral body to the L3 vertebral body. If the hardware is to extend to L1, we can perform a retroperitoneal approach over the T12–L1 disk space; however, the approach to L1 is always attempted through the thoracic cavity first. To date, we have been able to approach L1 through the thoracic cavity on every attempt, although this may require extensive retraction of the diaphragm.

A 3 to 4 cm incision is performed over the predetermined location to expose the eleventh rib (Fig. 14–14). The eleventh rib is exposed by moving the incision as far anterior and posterior as possible (Fig. 14–15). Once the rib has been subperiosteally dissected, it is removed with the endoscopic rib cutter. This is performed by freeing the rib anteriorly from the soft tissue, placing the jaw of the rib cutter under the rib and the foot over the top, then sliding the rib cutter posteriorly along the rib as far as possible. Once this is done, the rib is amputated. Using this technique, virtually the entire rib can be harvested for bone graft (Fig. 14–16).

Dissection is carried through the muscle into the retroperitoneal space and onto the psoas. The peritoneum is then reflected off the psoas, spine, and diaphragm. Next, lighted Deaver retractors are inserted. The psoas is retracted posteriorly, and the disks and end plates are exposed and removed in the standard fashion. We have tried several different exposure techniques, and this approach appears to work the best. Other

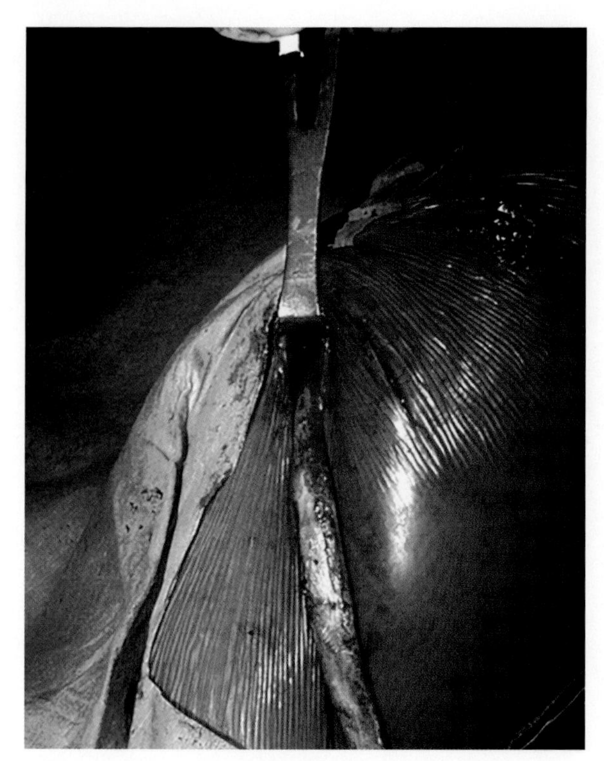

FIGURE 14–15 Photograph of the retroperitoneal incision with exposure of the eleventh rib.

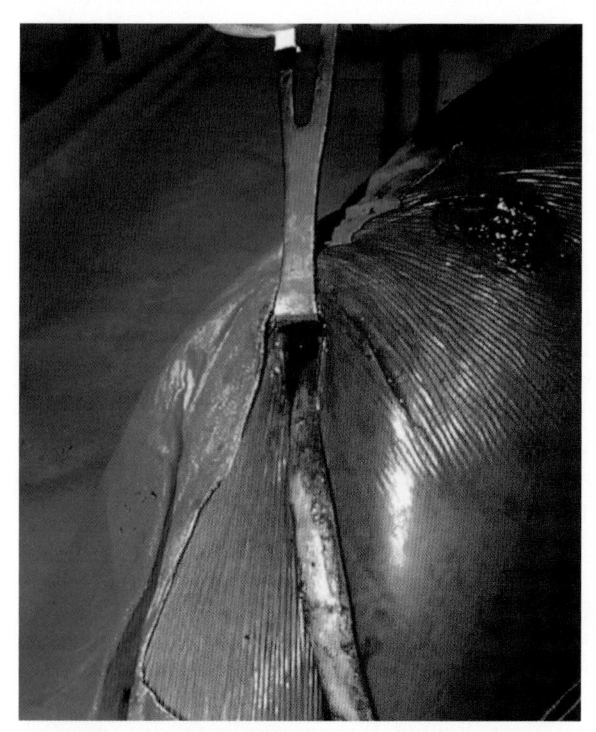

FIGURE 14–16 Photograph of the retroperitoneal incision. The eleventh rib has been amputated at its cartilaginous junction. With the endoscopic rib cutter, the rib can now be amputated at the rib head.

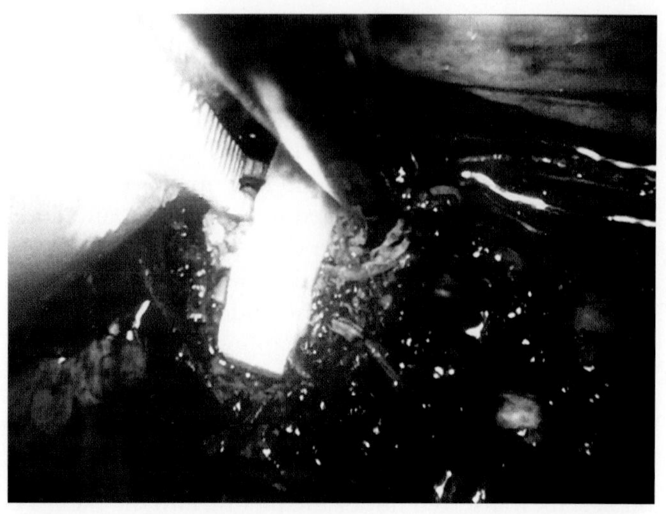

FIGURE 14–17 Intraoperative view of the retroperitoneal approach. A femoral ring filled with autograft is inserted into the L1–L2 disk space. To the left of the femoral ring is the diaphragm, and above the femoral ring is the peritoneum.

techniques have been problematic. The balloon technique can work, but the balloon can pop or can get in the way of the operative site. The laprolift can be bulky and obtrusive, and it can interfere with the C-arm. The CO_2 technique requires a closed system, and once the diaphragm has been crossed, the pneumoperitoneum and exposure are lost.

Once all the disks have been removed, more rib graft can be harvested from the thoracic portal sites, as described in the thoracic technique. After the graft has been obtained, the disk spaces from the lower thoracic through the lumbar are sized. Femoral ring allograft is cut and contoured into a tapered shape to produce lordosis. Once the femoral ring has been contoured, the center is packed with the morcellized rib graft and impacted into the disk space (Fig. 14–17). Morcellized graft is inserted into the disk space prior to placement of the femoral ring and then over the ring once in place. This is performed at each of the lumbar levels, decreasing the amount of taper of the grafts as they are placed proximally. At times, the lower thoracic vertebrae are smaller than the femoral rings. Humeral ring allograft can be used in these situations. An alternative to femoral or humeral allograft is cages. Both provide anterior column support and can be used to produce lordosis.

The C-arm is now placed into the operating field and positioned at the superior most vertebral body. It is imperative to have the C-arm parallel to the spine to give an accurate image. The undisturbed segmental vessels are grasped at the midvertebral body level and are ligated with the electrocautery. The vessels are located in the valley or middle of the vertebral body and serve as an anatomical guide for screw placement.

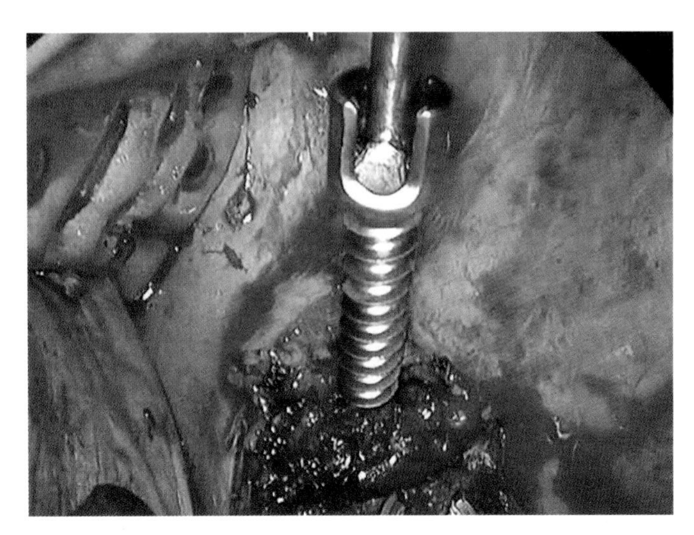

FIGURE 14–18 Intraoperative view through the endoscope showing a screw placed over the K-wire ready to be inserted into the vertebral body.

The body position and rotation are again checked. The K-wire guide is placed onto the vertebral body just anterior to the rib head. The position is checked with the C-arm to ensure that the wire is parallel to the end plates and in the center of the body. Next, the inclination of the guide is checked in the lateral plane by examining the chest wall and the rotation. The guide should be in a slight posterior to anterior inclination, directing the wire away from the spinal canal. A lateral C-arm image should be obtained if there is any doubt or concern.

Once the correct alignment of the guide has been attained, the K-wire is inserted into the appropriate cannula and drilled into the vertebral body parallel to the end plates. The position is confirmed with the C-arm as the wire is inserted. The guide is removed, and the tap is placed over the K-wire at the top of the guide. The wire is grasped with a clamp and held into position as the tap is inserted so the wire will not advance. The tap is slightly undersized, and only the near cortex is tapped. The appropriately sized screw is placed over the wire and advanced (Fig. 14–18).

The screw should penetrate the opposite cortex for bicortical fixation. The screws should be seated into the valley of the vertebral body. Using the rib heads as a reference for subsequent screw placement helps to ensure the screws are in line and yield proper spinal rotation. If each of the screws is placed in the same position of each vertebral body accounting for rotation, the screws will end in a V pattern and will aid in derotation of the spine during rod reduction. The sidewalls of the screws (saddles) are adjusted in line for receipt of the rod.

The screw heads need to be aligned so that the screws align in an arc. If a screw is inserted more than a few millimeters deeper than the rest of the screws, reduction of the rod into the screw head may be difficult. The C-arm image can clearly show depths as the screws are being inserted. Once all the screws have been placed, the Surgicel is removed from the upper thoracic disk spaces. The end plates are rerasped, and the graft is inserted. The graft is delivered to the disk space using the graft funnel and plunger. The disk space should be completely filled to the opposite side.

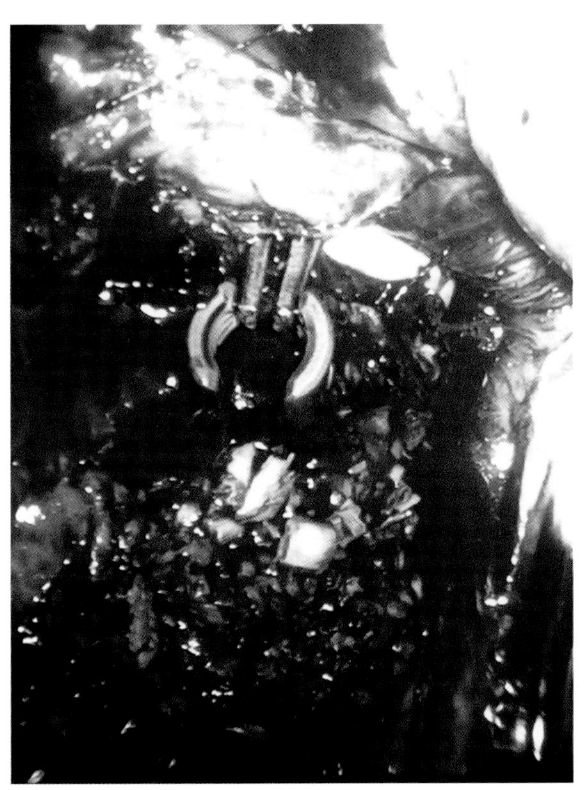

FIGURE 14–19 Intraoperative view through the endoscope showing the right-angle clamp under the diaphragm with the tips in the T12 screw.

All work has been performed on both sides of the diaphragm without its detachment until this point in the procedure. The diaphragm must now be crossed to obtain the rod length and perform the remainder of the procedure. With the endoscope in the chest cavity visualizing the diaphragm where it attaches to the spine, a right-angle clamp is inserted through the retroperitoneal incision. The right-angle clamp is used to make a small opening under the diaphragm at the center of the vertebral body (Fig. 14–19). The opening is made under direct endoscopic visualization and is only made large enough to permit the passage of the rod measurer, the rod, and the compressor arm.

The rod length is determined with the endoscopic rod measurer. The fixed ball at the end of the measuring device is placed into the saddle of the inferior screw. The ball at the end of the cable is then guided through the screws and the small opening under the diaphragm with a pituitary to the most superior screw and inserted into the saddle of the superior screw

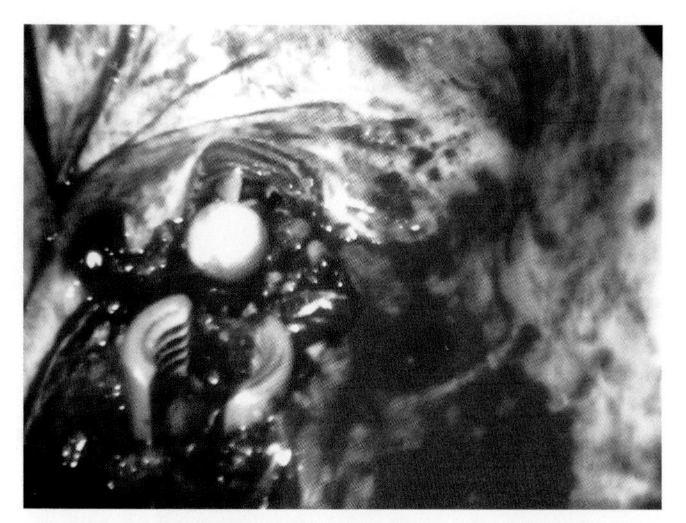

FIGURE 14–20 Intraoperative view through the endoscope showing the ball end of the endoscopic rod measurer coming through the small opening under the diaphragm.

(Fig. 14–20). The wire is then pulled tight, and a reading is taken from the scale. The 4.5 mm rod is cut to length and inserted into the chest cavity through the most inferior port, then manipulated superiorly until the rod is inside the chest cavity. The right-angle clamp is inserted into the retroperitoneal incision and under the diaphragm. The rod is placed into the jaws of the right-angle clamp and pulled into the retroperitoneal space (Fig. 14–21).

The rod is manipulated into the inferior screw flush with the saddle. Once the rod is in place, the plug introduction tube is placed over the screw to guide the plug and hold the rod in position. The plug inserter is placed through the plug introduction tube, inserted into the screw, and torqued. This is the only plug that is initially tightened completely. The rod is then sequentially reduced with the rod pushers. The plugs are inserted as the rod is reduced and provisionally tightened.

Compression between the screws is performed once the rod has been seated and all plugs inserted. The compressor is inserted through the retroperitoneal incision. The compressor fits over the screw heads on the rod, and compression is accomplished by turning the compressor driver clockwise and compressing the two screws together.

Compression is started at the inferior end of the construct with the most inferior screw fully tightened. Compression is sequentially performed from caudal to cranial. When the diaphragm is reached, the endoscope is reinserted into the chest cavity, and the long arm of the compressor is manipulated under the diaphragm and over the next screw head. Compression is performed at this level. The compressor is now removed and inserted into the chest cavity. Compression is sequentially performed superiorly until all the remaining levels have been compressed (Fig. 14–22). A chest tube is placed

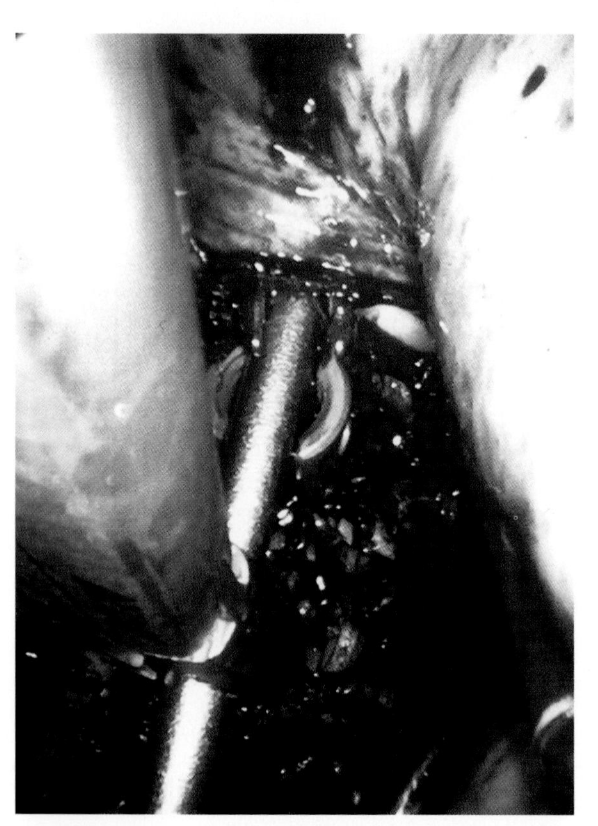

FIGURE 14–21 Intraoperative view through the endoscope showing the right-angle clamp under the diaphragm grasping the rod and pulling it into the retroperitoneal space.

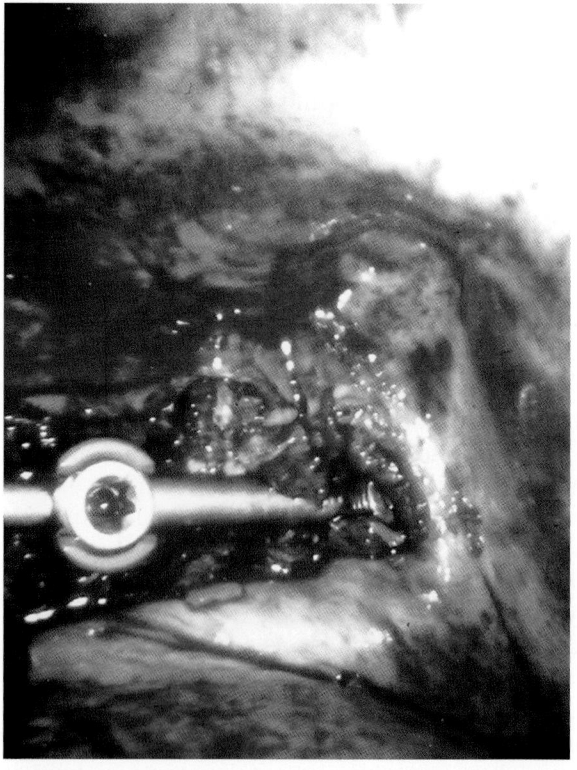

Figure 14–22 Intraoperative view through the endoscope demonstrating the construct going through the small opening under the diaphragm, as the diaphragm is tented over the construct.

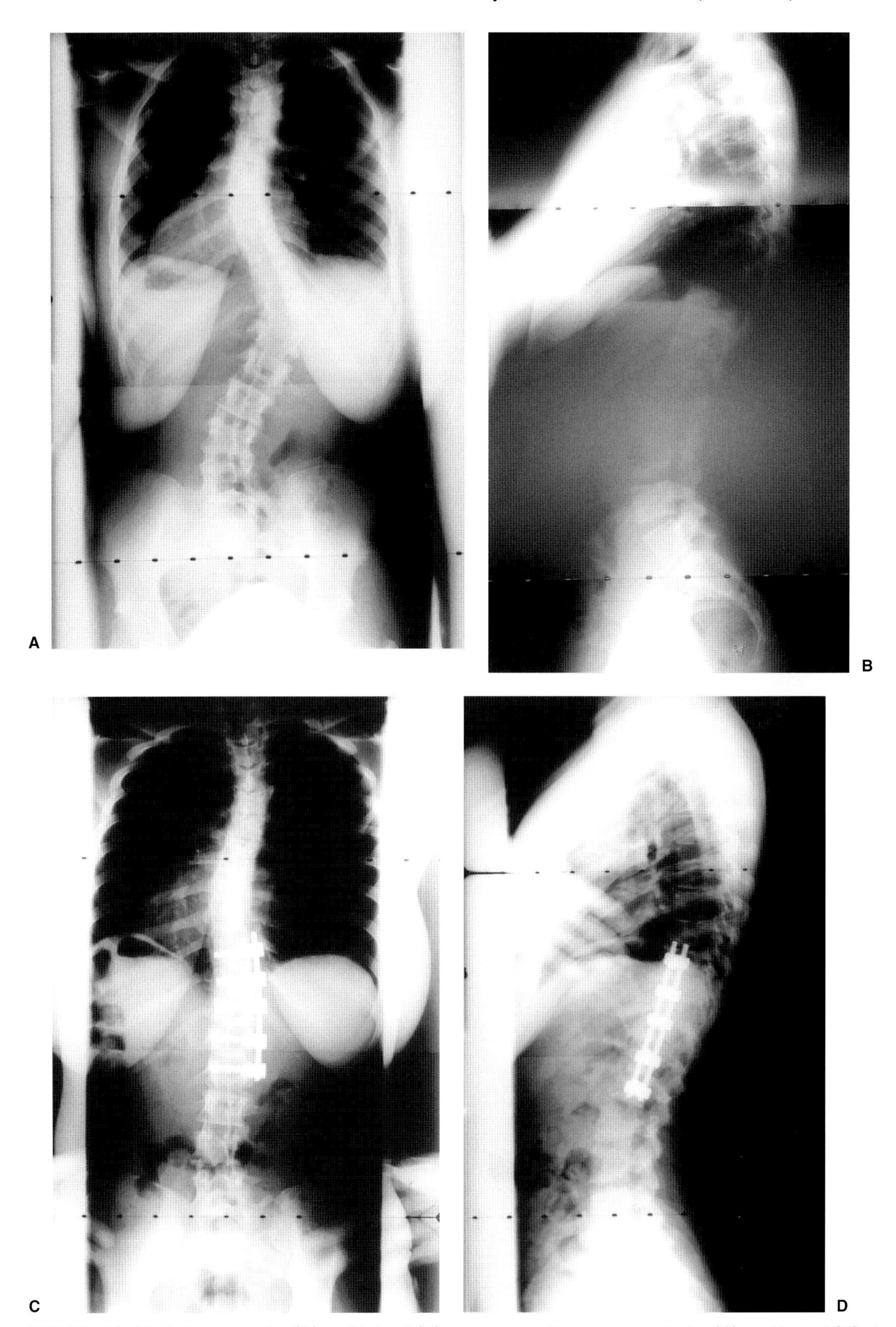

FIGURE 14–23 Anteroposterior **(A)** and lateral **(B)** preoperative x-rays of a 14-year-old female with a 26-degree T5–T10, 54-degree T10–L2, and 32-degree L2–L5 curve. Postoperative anteroposterior **(C)** and lateral **(D)** views of the same patient after a minimally invasive instrumentation, correction, and fusion with the new dual-head screws.

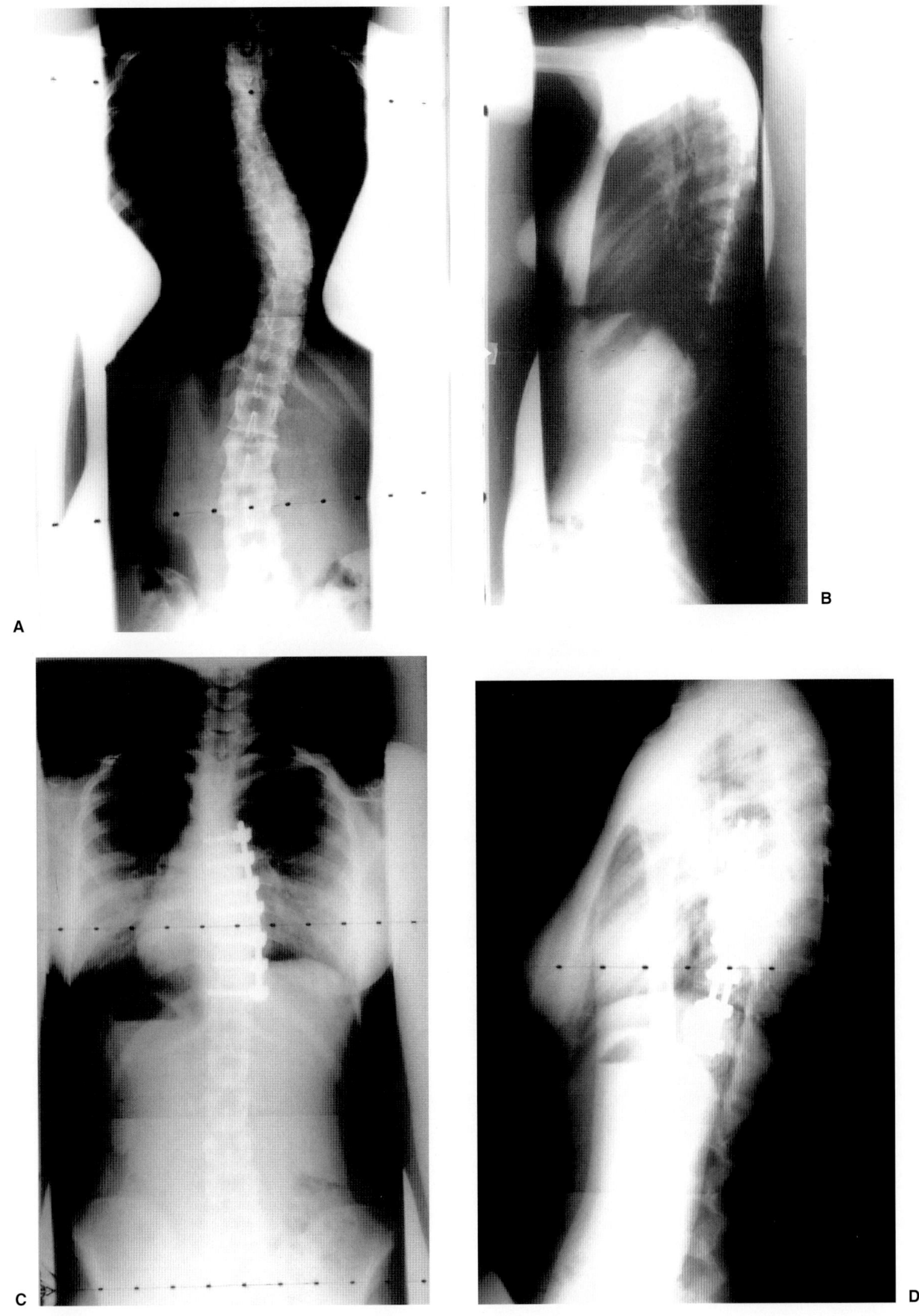

FIGURE 14–24 Anteroposterior **(A)** and lateral **(B)** preoperative x-rays of a 14-year-old female with a 48-degree thoracic and 25-degree lumbar curve. Postoperative anteroposterior **(C)** and lateral **(D)** views of the same patient after an endoscopic instrumentation, correction, and fusion with the new dual-head screws.

through the inferior portal, and the incisions are closed in layers in standard fashion.

Postoperative Care

Anteroposterior and lateral x-rays are obtained, and the patient is transferred to recovery. The patient stays in ICU overnight, and is then transferred to a regular floor. The patient is fitted for a custom thoracolumbosacral orthosis, which is worn for 3 months. The chest tube is removed when the drainage is less than 75 ml per shift, usually on postoperative day 2. The patient is ambulated the day the chest tube is removed and discharged when independent with ambulation, generally postoperative day 3. Patients are seen, x-rayed, and assessed at months 1, 3, 6, and 12 postoperatively.

Discussion

The development of the endoscopic technique of instrumentation, correction, and fusion of scoliosis has been an evolution, and the technique has undergone several modifications since our initial cases. The endoscopic treatment of thoracolumbar scoliosis has brought about a new set of challenges, many of which are explored in this chapter. As our preliminary work has shown, several basic principles must be adhered to, with the result that this minimally invasive approach does not necessarily equate to "minimal" or "less" surgery.

The key to successful fusion is a total diskectomy and complete end plate removal. Sagittal balance and anterior column support are critical in treating thoracolumbar scoliosis. This can be addressed with contoured femoral ring allograft or cages. We have used a 4.5 mm titanium rod in our initial series, with no rod complications noted to date.

Because of concern of rod size, however, especially with thoracolumbar scoliosis, we have developed a unique screw design: the dual-head screw. This distinctive design allows the flexibility of a single rod for easy endoscopic manipulation and for those curves that do not require such a powerful reduction. The first rod is inserted and the spine reduced, then the second rod is dropped into place. In those cases in which a greater reduction is required, both rods can be reduced simultaneously. In each case the end result is a two-rod construct, with the placement of only one screw. With this design we are able to place a 7.5 mm screw with a smaller staple into the upper thoracic vertebral body and an 8.5 mm screw and staple into the lower thoracic and lumbar spine. The result is the versatility of a somewhat flexible rod easily reduced endoscopically, with the benefit of a more rigid end construct with greater torsional stability. This screw design now allows a straightforward endoscopic alternative for the placement of a dual rod. With a dual rod–dual screw construct, the screws must be placed divergent, which is very difficult endoscopically, if not impossible. With the dual-head screw, however, the same central trajectory is used as with the standard single-screw placement. Other advantages of this screw design are the inherent stability each screw offers, acting like a cross-link, thus avoiding the difficulty and expense of endoscopically placing cross-links. The dual-head screw can be easily placed into smaller vertebral bodies, which cannot support a two-screw construct. Another benefit is the smaller size of the dual-head screw versus that of a dual screw–dual rod construct (Figs. 14–23, 14–24).

The preliminary results for the endoscopic treatment of thoracic and thoracolumbar scoliosis show promising trends. As decreasing surgical times continue to be accompanied by acceptable fusion rates and curve correction, investigation of this approach continues to proceed. The observed advantages for patients, including shorter hospitalizations and rehabilitation periods and decreased pain, strengthen the case for continued evaluation and follow-up of this technique.

REFERENCES

1. Regan JJ, Mack MJ, Picetti GD III. A comparison of VAT to open thoracotomy in thoracic spinal surgery. Paper presented at: Annual Meeting of the Scoliosis Research Society; September 18–23, 1993; Dublin, Ireland.
2. Picetti GD III. Video-assisted thoracoscopy (VATS) in the treatment of congenital hemivertebra. Paper presented at: Annual Meeting of the Spine Society of Australia; September 8,1996; Cairns, Australia.
3. Picetti GD III, O'Neal K, Estep M, et al. Correction and fusion of thoracic scoliosis using an endoscopic approach. Paper presented at: Annual Meeting of the Scoliosis Research Society; September 24, 1997; St. Louis, MO.
4. Picetti GD III, Ertl J, Bueff HU. Endoscopic instrumentation, correction and fusion of thoracic idiopathic scoliosis. *Spine.* 2001;1: 190–197.

15

Thoracoscopic Approach for a Deformity with Frontier Instrumentation

PETER O. NEWTON, RANDAL BETZ, DAVID CLEMENTS, AND ALVIN CRAWFORD

Thoracoscopic anterior scoliosis correction incorporates minimally invasive techniques with anterior thoracic instrumentation strategies for the correction and fusion of scoliosis. This approach, which is largely used for adolescent idiopathic scoliosis (AIS), avoids much of the morbidity associated with the traditional open anterior or posterior approaches. Anterior thoracic scoliosis correction is based on theories that AIS is generally associated with a hypokyphotic thoracic spine–relative anterior overgrowth, which leads to the rotational deformity and lateral deviation we see as scoliosis.[1] Anterior column overgrowth is thus treated with an anterior column shortening procedure. This is accomplished by disk excision and compressive anterior instrumentation of all the vertebrae of the measured curve. This has proven to be successful with the open approach[2] and is now possible (in select cases) via minimally invasive thoracoscopic methods.

The thoracoscopic approach, however, requires special attention to detail and is thought by some to be too demanding and/or tedious for widespread implementation. There is no doubt that the learning curve for this procedure is substantial,[3] but deliberate training and cautious adoption can result in excellent outcomes with reduced patient morbidity. The details of this chapter are meant to supplement such a training experience (not replace it), and it is hoped that the "tricks" as well as the "pitfalls" can be shared for the benefit of our patients. Although this represents current thoughts and techniques, surgery is always in evolution, one hopes in the direction that leads to true progress. Expect what we do today to be different tomorrow.

Indications

The procedure described in this chapter is primarily designed for idiopathic thoracic scoliosis with curves greater than 40 to 50 degrees (depending on maturity and truncal deformity), but less than 70 to 80 degrees. The curve pattern should be amenable to selective thoracic instrumentation between T4 and L1. This includes many Lenke I and King II or III curves. The size of the patient and sagittal profile are also important. The ideal size of the patient remains to be identified clearly, but it likely falls between 40 and 60 kg. Patients smaller than 40 kg provide additional challenges for secure vertebral body fixation, particularly at the proximal extent of the construct, where the size of the thoracic vertebrae may not be sufficient to hold a vertebral body screw. Patients who are too large may overstress a single rod construct to the point of fatigue failure before a solid arthrodesis occurs.

Contraindications

Excessive kyphosis is also problematic for these constructs. Anterior surgery is by its nature kyphogenic, and patients who begin with greater than 30 to 40 degrees of sagittal curvature (between T5 and T12) should be avoided to prevent excessive postoperative kyphosis. Rod failure should be expected if kyphosis correction is attempted with a single anterior rod system without substantial anterior column interbody support (which may be difficult to achieve in the upper thoracic spine due to soft end plates).

Other contraindications include those of thoracoscopic surgery in general. These include conditions that result in such intrathoracic pleural adhesions as prior ipsilateral thoracic surgery or infection. The patient must be able to tolerate single-lung ventilation. Collapse of the ipsilateral lung is critical to the safe visualization of the spine. Large curves greater than 80 degrees and those with substantial rigidity may be better dealt with by posterior or combined approaches.

Surgical Equipment

Thoracoscopic surgery is very much equipment dependent, the quality of which can have a significant impact on outcome. This requires high-quality endoscopes and three-chip camera video systems. A 10 mm diameter endoscope with angled viewing (0 to 45 degrees) is essential to visualize all of the aspects of the spine and implants. The equipment required can be broken down based on the various stages of the procedure: exposure, disk excision, instrumentation, and bone grafting.

Endoscopic exposure of the spine begins with single-lung ventilation. This can be accomplished by one of several methods, the most common of which uses a double-lumen endotracheal tube. After the ipsilateral lung is collapsed, thoracoscopic portals between the ribs allow access to the spine. The specialized equipment required to expose the spine includes an endoscopic retractor for the lung, peanut dissectors, a suction/irrigation device, and a harmonic scalpel. The harmonic scalpel is an ultrasonic device that can be used for cutting the pleura, coagulating the segmental vessels, and incising the anulus of the disk. By contrast, disk excision is largely dependent on mechanical tools typical to spine surgery, and including rongeurs, curettes, and mechanical end-plate shavers that have been modified in length and dimension to pass through 11.5 mm thoracoports. The tools required for placement of implants thoracoscopically are available in the Frontier anterior scoliosis set (DePuy-Acromed, Inc., Raynham, MA).

Image intensification with a C-arm is required to determine the intraoperative spinal level and is also important in assessing screw trajectory. Additional specific tools are utilized for iliac crest bone graft harvest typical to harvesting posterior iliac crest; however, this bone graft, after harvesting, is placed through a bone mill that morselizes the graft, allowing it to be delivered through a plunger system.

Operating Room Setup

The patient is positioned on a radiolucent table in the lateral position with an axillary roll. The surgeon and assistant may stand on either side of the patient, although we find it easier for surgeons to orient their mind's eye when the surgeon and assistant stand on the anterior side of the patient, with the endoscopic tower placed facing them on the posterior side of the patient. The harmonic scalpel generator, electrocautery generator, suction/irrigation, and cell saver are positioned at the head of the operating table on either side of the anesthesiologist.

Steps of the Surgical Procedure

One the critical initial steps of the procedure involves marking the patient to plan for the location of the thoracoscopic portals to allow proper screw orientation within each vertebra to be instrumented. With the patient in the direct lateral position, the image intensifier is used to mark a longitudinal line on the side of the patient that corresponds to the sagittal alignment of the spine. The midlateral position of the vertebra to be instrumented is marked on the lateral chest wall, and this typically approximates the posterior axillary line. With the image intensifier brought underneath the table for an anterorposterior projection, the orientation of each vertebra to be instrumented in the frontal plane is also marked on the posterior aspect of the patient (Fig. 15–1). The intersection of a line marking the frontal plane orientation of a vertebra and that line marking the midlateral portion of that vertebral body locates the ideal chest wall entry site to obtain an appropriate screw trajectory. Six to eight screws may be required in a typical scoliosis construct. This will therefore require a corresponding number of trajectories through the chest wall. Rather than making a skin incision for each screw trajectory, however, two or three screws can typically be placed through a single skin incision by

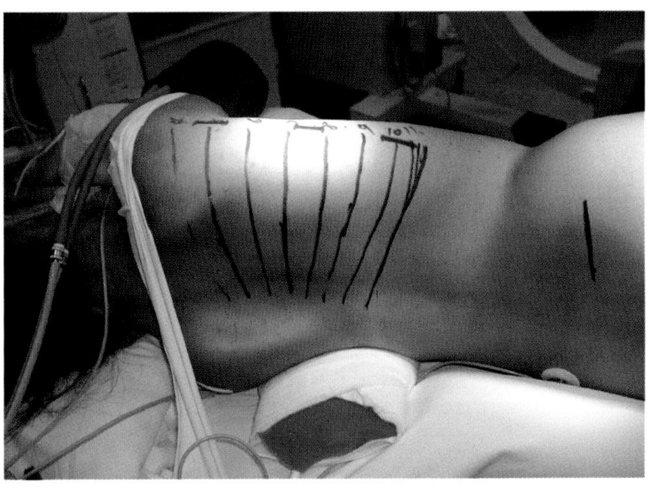

FIGURE 15–1 Posterior skin markings of the angulation of each vertebra to be instrumented.

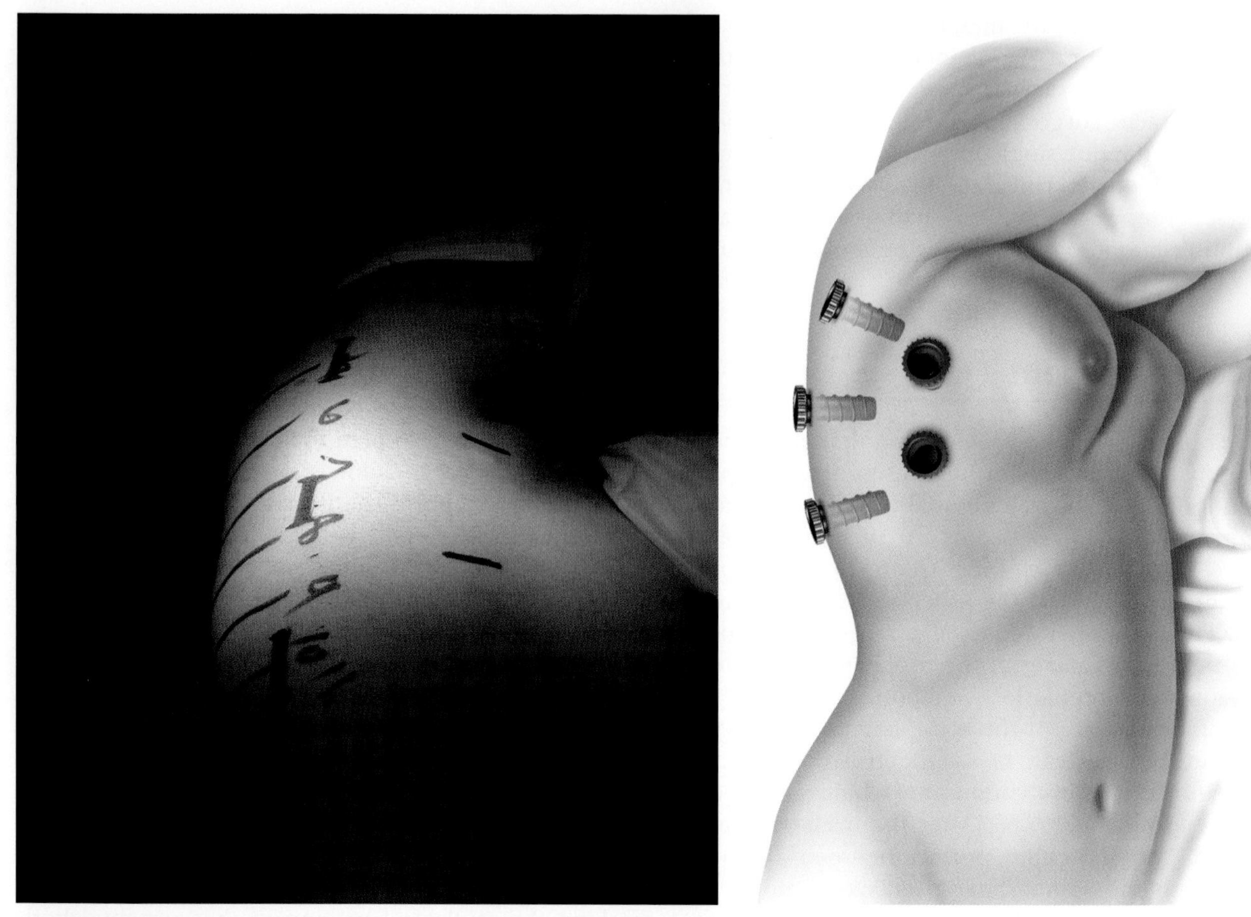

FIGURE 15–2 The planned anterior and posterior portals are marked on the chest. **(A)** Intraoperative photograph and **(B)** artist's depiction.

stretching the skin incision proximally and distally, above and below, the corresponding ribs. Using this strategy, typically three and occasionally four portals are required on the posterior axillary line, with two additional portals placed along the anterior axillary line (Fig. 15–2). The anterior portals are used for visualization of the spine as well as much of the dissection, diskectomy, and bone grafting work. The chest and iliac crest are widely prepped and draped, and the initial aspect of the surgery involves harvesting the posterior iliac crest bone. This graft is placed through a bone mill to create a soft, morcellized autogenous bone graft material.

The thoracoscopic approach to the spine is initiated with the two anterior axillary line portals. The 11.5 mm diameter rigid thoracoports are placed through 1.5 cm long incisions. Lung deflation is confirmed with direct visualization through the port. The third port to be placed is the inferior most posterior portal that will be used for both disk excision and screw insertion. If required or desired, the most inferior portal can be extended to create a small thoracotomy that will allow direct visualization through the wound. Some of the most challenging levels to be addressed thoracoscopically are those of the lower thoracic and thoracolumbar junction, and a small thoracotomy may substantially facilitate the treatment of these lower levels.

With these three portals established, a fan retractor is placed for lung retraction. This is frequently required during the initial stages of the operation because the atelectasis of the lung is not yet complete. The levels to be instrumented are determined by counting from the most proximal rib head, realizing that the first rib may be difficult to visualize and is most easily located by direct palpation with such an instrument as a peanut dissector. Radiographic confirmation with a K-wire is also required. The spine is exposed by longitudinal incision of the pleura ~5 mm anterior to the rib heads. The segmental vessels are coagulated and divided using the harmonic scalpel. If exposure to L1 is required, the insertion of the diaphragm over the T12–L1 disk will require incision as well. Circumferential exposure of the spine is achieved by stripping the pleura and segmental vessels off the anterior aspect of the spine, using a combination of blunt dissection and the harmonic scalpel. Gauze sponges packed in this interval between the aorta/esophagus and the spine substantially improve this exposure and allow the disk to be widely excised, particularly on the convex side, safely.

Disk excision is initiated with incision of the anulus and anterior longitudinal ligament using the harmonic scalpel. An upbiting rongeur is used to begin the diskectomy on the anterior and concave aspects of the disk space. The diskectomy then proceeds to the convex rib head. It is important to limit vertebral body bone bleeding, which impairs visualization into the depths of the disk. A nearly bloodless disk excision is possible in many AIS patients if the end plate cartilage is peeled off the vertebral body without biting into the bone of the vertebral body itself. An end plate reamer may be used once the disk is completely excised to confirm flexibility. Hemostasis is achieved following disk excision by packing the disk space with Surgicel. Disk excision proceeds in a proximal to distal fashion and requires adjustment of the portals and instruments placed through these portals to maintain ideal visualization into the depths of the disk space. The 45-degree angled endoscope is placed one portal proximal or distal to the portal used for disk excision, with the portal for disk excision being placed exactly in line with the disk. To achieve ideal access, it is frequently required to move the portal above or below a rib (using the same skin incision to do so).

With disk excision completed, reconstruction of the sagittal plane is performed, with structural allograft placed at levels inferior to T11. This structural grafting is typically in the form of a fibular ring cut to an appropriate height based on the preoperative sagittal alignment of the lower thoracic spine and thoracolumbar junction. The graft is placed directly through the posteroinferior skin incision, with the rigid port removed. Prior to final placement of the allograft, cancellous autografting is performed in the concave side of the disk space, with the allograft placed in the anterior aspect of the disk space. A true endoscopic disk space distractor is not used; however, direct pressure from an assistant to the posterior aspect of the spine is often sufficient to accomplish opening of the disk space for excision and grafting purposes.

Instrumentation

Insertion of the vertebral body screws requires two additional posterior axillary line portals (three total). The position has been planned previously with the image intensifier; however, before making a skin incision, it is confirmed by placing a K-wire through the chest wall at each proposed portal site. The image intensifier anteroposterior view is used to be sure the orientation of the K-wires is in line with the vertebra (parallel to the end plates) (Fig. 15–3). A longitudinal 2 cm skin incision is made, and with blunt dissection just anterior to the scapula through the musculature, the chest cavity is entered with Mayo scissors. A 15 mm rigid thoracoport is placed, and direct visualization down the port should line up with the lateral aspect of the superior vertebral body. Direct visualization is important to gain a three-dimensional orientation for the screw trajectory. The starting point for screw insertion is in the midvertebral body just anterior to the rib head. An awl and tap are used to establish the screw path. Screw length is determined by probing the tapped screw path and judging length from the calibrations on the probe. The screw should engage the far cortex, but it should not be excessively long. Screws are available in 2.5 mm increments to accommodate the variety of thoracic vertebral dimensions.

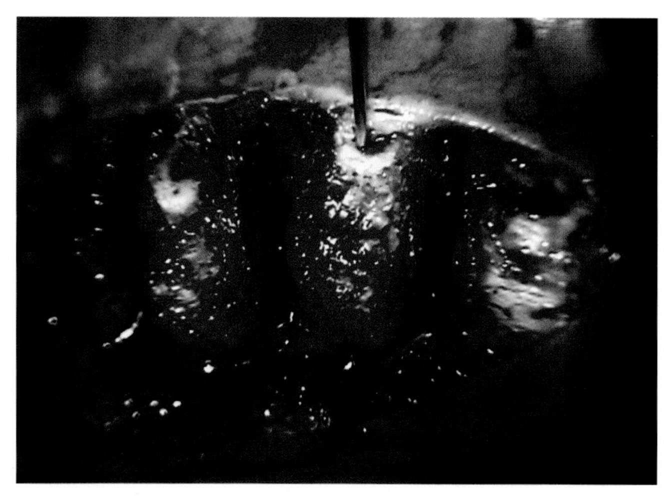

FIGURE 15–3 Appearance of the spine after diskectomy. The K-wire was placed through the chest at the planned site for the proximal posterior portal. The alignment of the K-wire was confirmed with the image intensifier before making the skin incision for this portal. The K-wire is in the T6 vertebra at the site for screw placement.

Subsequent screws are placed in similar fashion, moving the thoracoport distally one rib interspace at a time. Two or three screws can be placed through each skin incision. The alignment of each screw relative to the last is critical to the success of subsequent rod insertion (Fig. 15–4). Visualizing directly through the portals (both posterior and anterior) as well as with the endoscope and image intensifier ensures proper screw placement. The value of looking directly down the portal to judge screw placement cannot be overemphasized. After confirming screw position with the image intensifier, adjustment of the depths of the screws may be required. An incompletely inserted screw will make rod connection difficult in adjacent screws.

Rod length is determined based on direct measurement with a malleable calibrated template inserted through

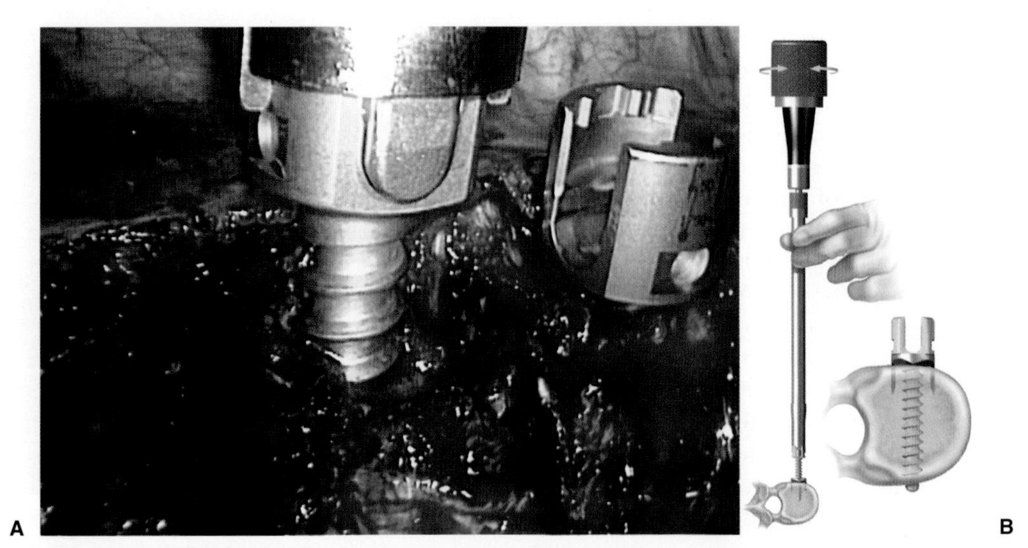

FIGURE 15–4 The screws are inserted to achieve bicortical purchase. **(A)** Intraoperative photograph and **(B)** artist's depiction.

the distal portal. Shortening of the spine by 1 to 1.5 cm should be anticipated due to compression. The rod is contoured to the desired degree of kyphosis and scoliosis based on the anticipated and desired postoperative alignment.

Just as screw insertion is initiated proximally, so is engagement of the rod, beginning with the most tenuous proximal screws. The hex-end rod holder maintains the orientation of the contoured rod (placed through the distal skin incision without a portal) as the proximal screws are engaged. A locking cap captures the rod and is tightened to fix the rod position (length and rotation). Subsequent screws are captured by cantilevering the rod into position (Fig. 15–5). As each screw cap is inserted, that level is bone grafted with the graft delivery tube. Morcellized autogenous graft (harvested from the posterior ilium or ribs) should fill the disk space prior to compression between the screws (Fig. 15–6). Compression is achieved with the endoscopic compressor placed directly through an anterior (proximal levels) or posterior (distal levels) skin incision. Compression of the proximal levels needs to be applied gently and with caution to prevent the screws from loosening in the bone (Fig. 15–7). More aggressive compression is applied to the apical levels if bone quality allows. Rod translation to the screws is greatly facilitated by the combination approximator/cap inserter tool. Through the distal incision the device is attached to one of the distal screws (usually the second one from the bottom) and used to push the rod into the more proximal screws sequentially (Fig. 15–8). The proximal caps are inserted with the grafting, compression, and the cap locking routine repeated at each level. The approximator may be required at the most distal level as well, with compression at this level applied across the structural graft (as well as additional morcellized autograft that was placed following diskectomy). Use of this structural graft prevents distal kyphosis as well as overcorrection in the coronal plane.

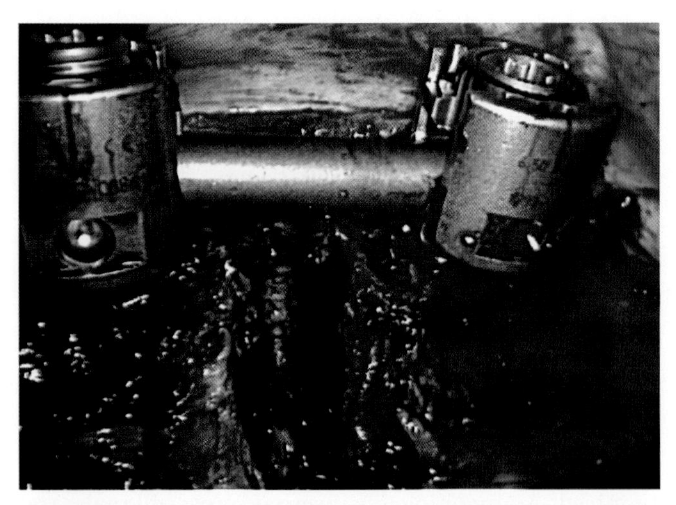

FIGURE 15–5 The rod has been locked to the proximal screw, with the cap engaged in the second screw (but with the set screw loose). This is the appearance just prior to bone grafting and compression.

Pleural closure completes the procedure and is accomplished with an endoscopic stitching device. A running closure covers the implants and maintains the bone graft in position postoperatively. A chest tube is required for several days postoperatively and is placed once the chest has been irrigated and loose debris removed. Lung reinflation is confirmed, and bronchial suctioning of the dependent lung is performed to reduce the incidence of postoperative atelectasis due to mucous plugs. Once the chest tube has been removed,

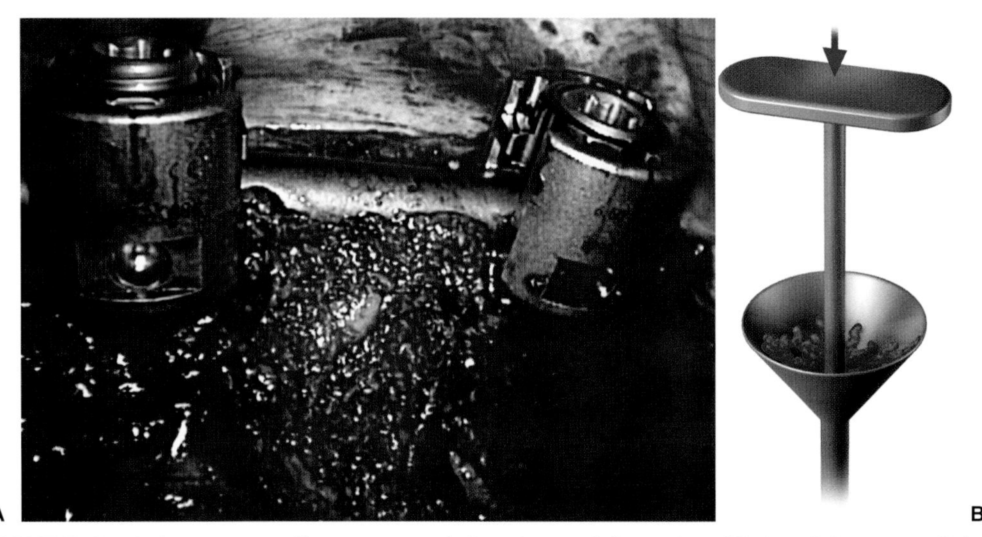

FIGURE 15–6 Autogenous iliac crest graft has been delivered to fill the disk space. **(A)** Intraoperative photograph and **(B)** artist's depiction.

a postoperative thoracolumbosacral orthosis (TLSO) is prescribed for 3 months that is to be worn when the patient is out of bed.

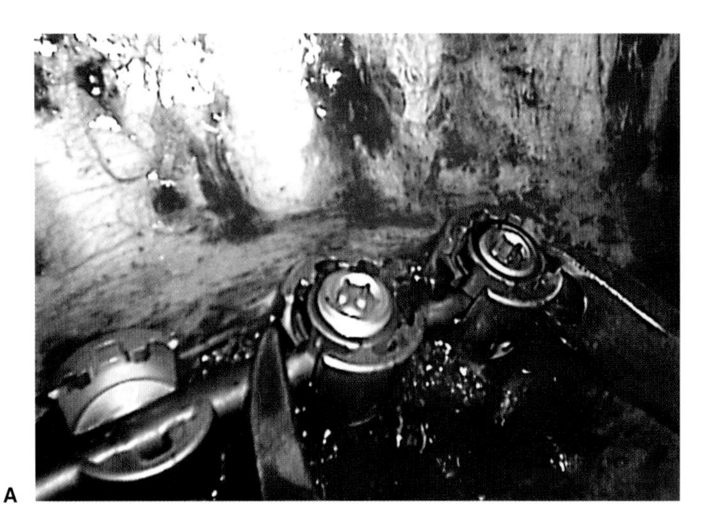

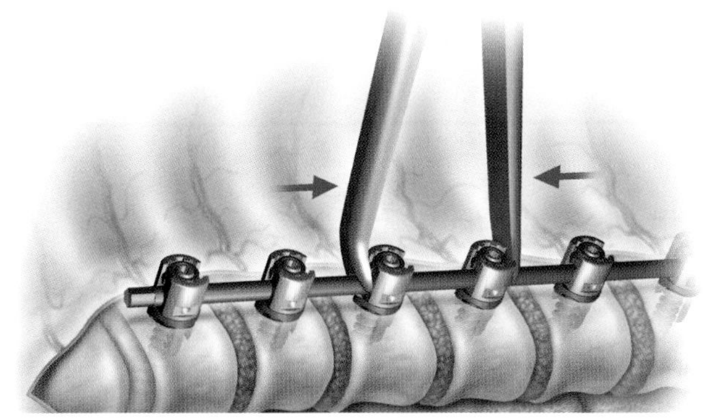

FIGURE 15–7 Segmental compression is applied with the endoscopic compressor. **(A)** Intraoperative photograph and **(B)** artist's depiction.

Complications and Avoidance

There are several times during this procedure that complications may develop and compromise the outcome. Minimizing and managing these challenges is key to the success of the procedure. The back-up plans include converting to an open approach and using posterior implants.

Many complications of a thoracoscopic procedure can be avoided if ideal visualization is maintained. This requires proper equipment (high-quality, angled optics), proper endoscope placement and camera orientation, limited bleeding, and appropriate retraction (lung, diaphragm, and great vessels). Bleeding during bony spinal surgery is unavoidable; however, it can be minimized, and doing so allows safe disk excision, particularly of the far-side anulus. Minimizing blood loss begins with deliberate use of the harmonic scalpel during exposure of the spine, coagulating all the small vessels along the spine as the circumferential stripping is performed. Bone bleeding can be addressed with wax applied with an Endo-peanut. Bleeding from the exposed bony end plate of the vertebral body is expected, but it can be substantially reduced if the technique of disk excision avoids early penetration of the cancellous bone.

Caudal exposure to T12 and L1 requires diaphragm retraction, which can be a challenge endoscopically. This is achieved with an angled fan retractor placed from the anterior proximal portal, pushing the diaphragm distally. To expose the L1 body, the diaphragm must be split for ~2 cm at its insertion. One option to facilitate this aspect of exposure is to perform a limited thoracotomy at the site of the inferior portal. A 5 to 7 cm incision allows standard retractors and rongeurs to be utilized at these more difficult distal levels.

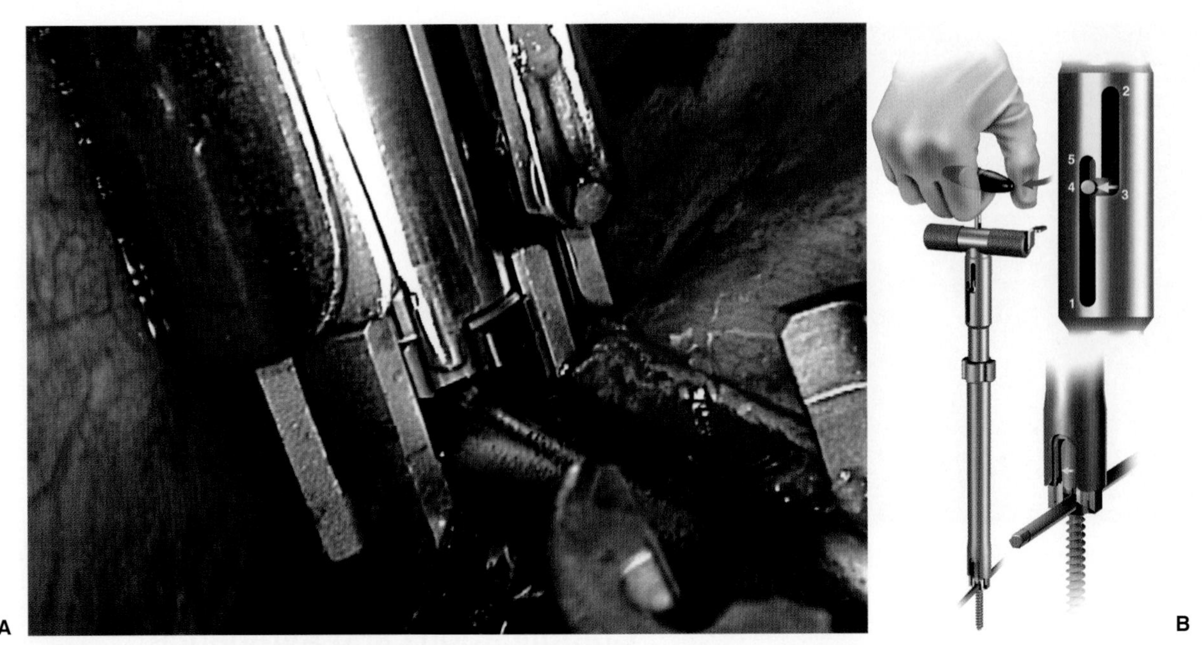

FIGURE 15–8 The cap inserter/approximator tool allows the rod to be cantilevered into the distal screws while applying the cap. **(A)** Intraoperative photograph and **(B)** artist's depiction.

Engaging the rod into the screws can be problematic when the screws are malpositioned. The screws should be placed in the midvertebral body and directly lateral. Employ every means possible to ensure absolutely this position for each screw. The most useful approach we use is looking directly through the rigid thoracoport. The orientation of the vertebral body can be seen with the Surgicel removed from the adjacent disk spaces, as can the position of the proximal screw that needs to be matched. The image intensifier can be used for confirmation, but nothing replaces the direct bird's-eye view through the port. A few extra minutes getting the screw position perfect will save hours of frustration at the time of rod insertion. Proper screw alignment does not guarantee simple engagement of every locking cap, although most of these issues are straightforward to deal with. If a cap will not turn and capture the screw head, stop and check the following. First, be sure that the set screw is not advanced through the end of the cap, preventing full cap insertion. If so, back out the set screw and reattempt. Second, be sure the rod is fully reduced into the screw head. This can be a problem if the screws are inserted to different depths—check and adjust based on the image intensifier view before rod insertion. Use the rod approximator to seat the rod fully. If the cap will not turn, resist the temptation of forcing the cap to engage the screw head. If it takes more than two fingers to click in the cap, stop and check all of the preceding items.

Many of the complications of open anterior thoracic instrumentation remain with the endoscopic approach and include implant-related problems (e.g., loss of proximal fixation and pseudarthrosis). Proximal fixation requires bicortical purchase with a cancellous designed screw. The diameter should be as large as possible without risking vertebral body fracture (5.5 or 6.5 mm diameter). In addition, a scoliosis bend in the upper section of the rod limits the force application to the proximal screws during rod cantilevering. This can also be accomplished by using a washer or staple under the proximal screw. It is also important to limit the compression applied at the proximal level because screw plow through the near cortex reduces the resistance to later axial screw pullout.

Pseudarthrosis prevention requires attention to detail during disk excision and grafting, as well as avoidance of high-risk patients. Single-rod constructs have a limited fatigue life that mandates early solid fusion. As such, the disk spaces must be filled with high-quality autogenous bone. A postoperative TLSO also seems prudent. Patient selection can limit this complication by avoiding large patients (i.e., less than 60–70 kg), smokers, and those with kyphosis (i.e., T5–T12 less than 30–40 degrees), all of which seem to be risk factors for rod failure with an anterior thoracic single-rod approach.

Case Illustration

A 15-year-old female, who was otherwise healthy, presented with a 58-degree right thoracic scoliosis (Fig. 15–9). The lumbar curve measured 33 degrees and

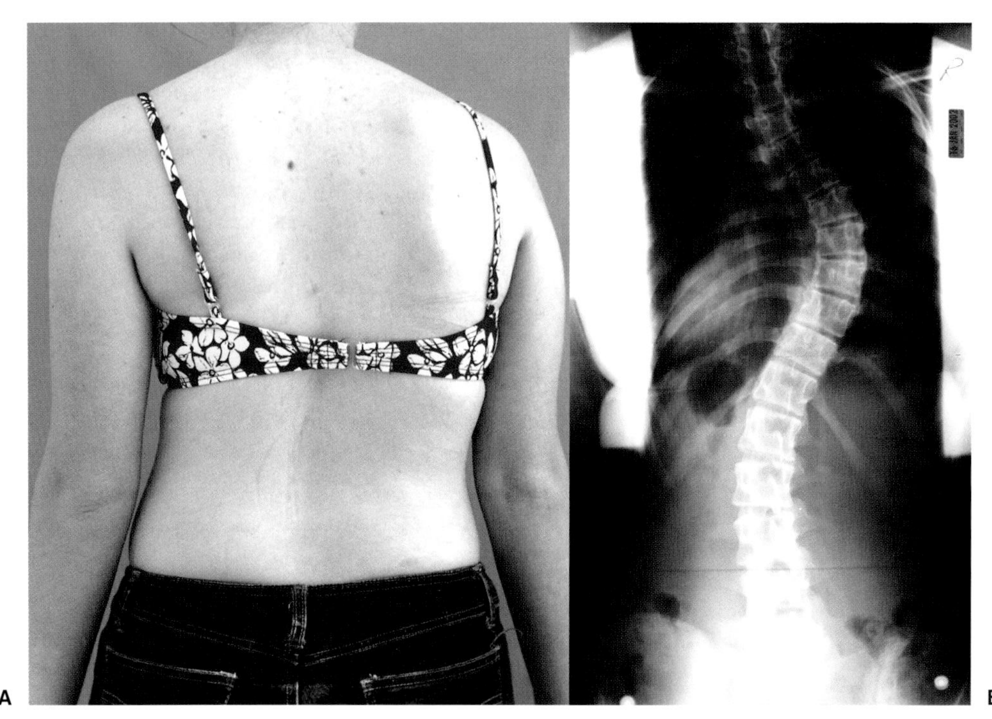

FIGURE 15–9 Clinical appearance **(A)** and preoperative posteroanterior radiograph **(B)** of a 15-year-old female with a 58-degree Lenke 1-A-N curve.

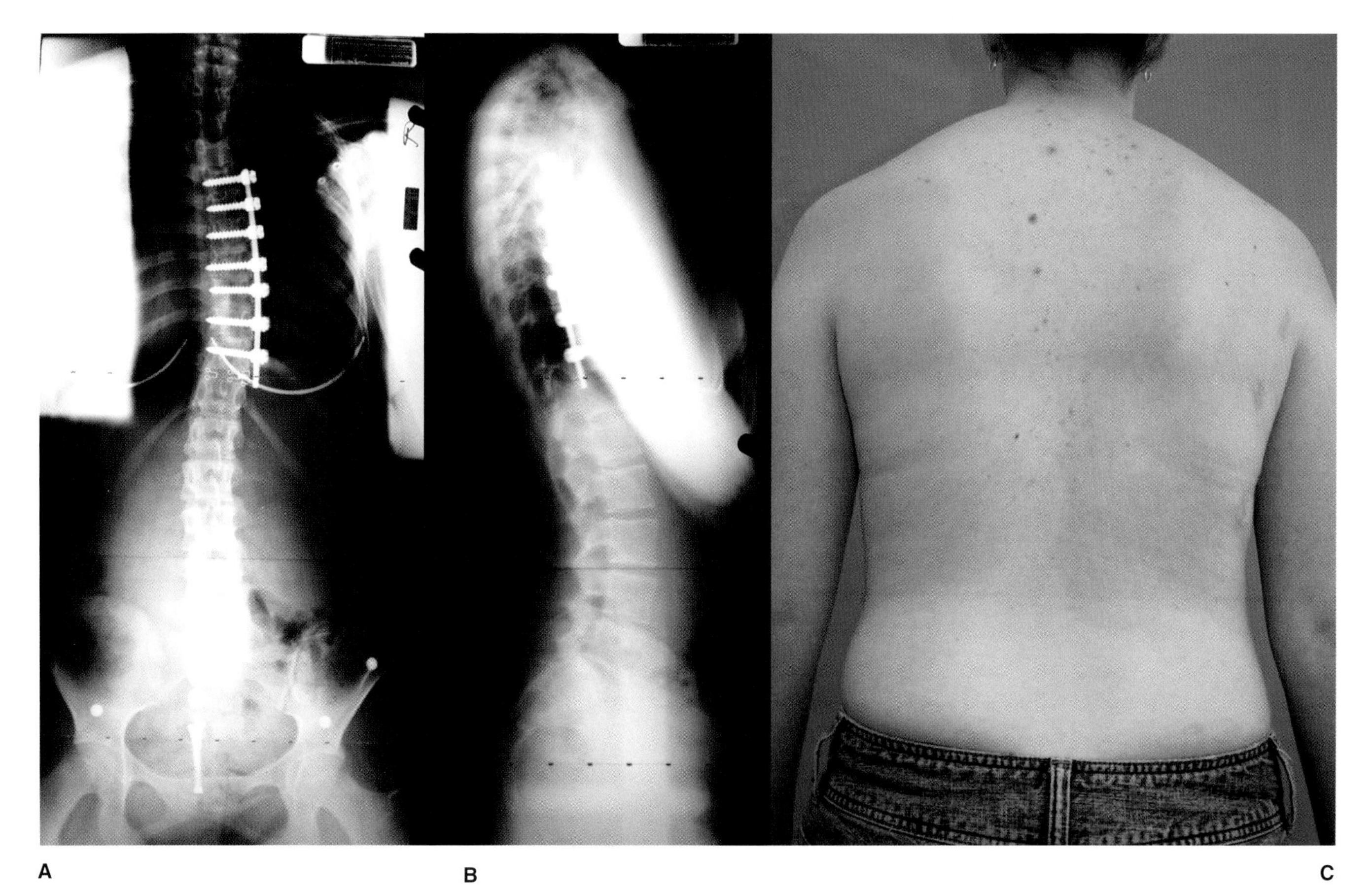

FIGURE 15–10 Postoperative appearance radiographically [posteroranterior **(A)** and lateral **(B)**] as well as clinically **(C)** of patient 6 months after procedure.

corrected on side bending to 7 degrees. The thoracic kyphosis between T5 and T12 measured 20 degrees, and the Lenke classification of this curve was considered to be a 1-A-N. The end vertebrae of the thoracic curve were T5 proximally and T11 distally. As such, these were the levels selected for anterior instrumentation and fusion. The patient underwent a thoracoscopic anterior spinal fusion with Frontier instrumentation placed between T5 and T11. A structural fibular allograft was placed at the T10–T11 disk space with all levels, including that level also grafted with autogenous morselized iliac crest bone. The operative time was 5 hours, with an estimated blood loss of 250 ml. The chest tube was removed on postoperative day 4, and the patient was discharged home on postoperative day 5. She wore a TLSO for 3 months postoperatively. Her radiographs and clinical appearance 6 months postoperatively suggest satisfactory correction and radiographic evidence of early arthrodesis (Fig. 15–10 A–C).

Thoracoscopic anterior spinal instrumentation for scoliosis correction is an evolving technology that holds promise. Minimally invasive deformity correction on par with open posterior methods is achievable in selected patients. The technique and indications continue to be defined, and further advancements should be anticipated. Large multicenter trials are in progress to evaluate the outcomes relative to open approaches in an attempt to confirm the speculated benefits of the limited exposure.

The learning curve for this technique is substantial, and the growth of the technique within the surgical community is appropriately modest at present. Mastering thoracoscopic spinal instrumentation takes time and should be initiated only after one becomes facile at thoracoscopic disk excision and open thoracic spinal instrumentation. Despite these concerns, there is a place for cautious optimism because this technique opens an avenue to potentially reduced morbidity for patients undergoing surgical correction of adolescent idiopathic scoliosis.

REFERENCES

1. Millner PA, Dickson RA. Idiopathic scoliosis: biomechanics and biology. *Eur Spine J.* 1996;5:362–373.
2. Betz RR, Harms J, Clements DH, et al. Comparison of anterior and posterior instrumentation for correction of adolescent thoracic idiopathic scoliosis. *Spine.* 1999;24:225–239.
3. Newton PO, Shea KG, Granlund KF. Defining the pediatric spinal thoracoscopy learning curve: sixty-five consecutive cases. *Spine.* 2000;25:1028–1035.

16

Combined Prone Position Thoracoscopic Anterior Release and Posterior Instrumentation for Deformity Surgery

ISADOR H. LIEBERMAN

In deformity surgery, anterior release and bone grafting of the thoracic spine is instrumental to maximizing correction, reducing the pseudoarthrosis rate, and preventing further progression of the deformity. Anterior releases were traditionally achieved with the patient in the lateral decubitus position through an open thoracotomy, after rib resection and spreading, on the convex side for scoliotic or on either side for kyphotic deformities. During the thoracotomy, the thoracic organs and tissues are exposed and manipulated and may become desiccated. As a consequence of thoracotomy, patients may develop a measurable reduction in pulmonary and shoulder girdle function and experience significant chronic incisional pain. Thoracotomy is clearly associated with distinct issues related to pain, cosmesis, and morbidity.

Video-assisted endoscopic transthoracic exposures to facilitate spinal releases, diskectomies, and osteotomies have been performed with the patient positioned in the lateral decubitus position, mimicking open thoracotomy.[1,2] By virtue of improved visualization (due to illumination and magnification of the operative site by the video system), less postoperative incisional pain (due to less muscle dissection and no rib spreading), and more cosmetically acceptable scars, these advances have reduced the thoracotomy-related consequences.

Prone position endoscopic transthoracic exposures have been used even more recently to facilitate deformity correction.[3] Although the lateral position affords the surgeon a more familiar anatomical alignment and approach, the prone position allows the mediastinal organs to fall away from the spine, obviating the need for retraction, and facilitates simultaneous anterior posterior procedures, eliminating the need for staged or subsequent surgeries.

Prior to embarking on any endoscopic exposure, the surgeon must be familiar with open anterior spinal anatomy and surgical techniques. The surgical procedure is the same, but the methods are different enough to challenge even the most experienced spinal surgeon. Whether using the lateral or prone position, the loss of depth perception and the necessity for triangulation may be familiar to a small joint arthroscopist, but the change in working distance and instrument excursion from 4 to 30 cm demands its own learning curve.

Indications

Many deformity patients, especially adults, are primarily concerned with aesthetic issues and elect to undergo surgery expecting a significant correction of their spinal deformity. Anterior spinal release, either open or endoscopic, is therefore indicated for curves with less than 50% correction on bending films, curves greater than 60 degrees in magnitude, and curves that require rebalancing into the stable zone in the coronal or sagittal plane. The contraindications to endoscopic anterior release include any preexisting lung parenchymal pathology, previous thoracotomy, previous empyema or pleurodesis, inability to tolerate single-lung ventilation, and a thoracic scoliotic curve greater than 75 degrees (i.e., in curves greater than 75 degrees, the chest cavity on the concave side and the rib interspaces are too small to accommodate the 10 mm diameter endoscopic portals and instruments). A further relative contraindication is a

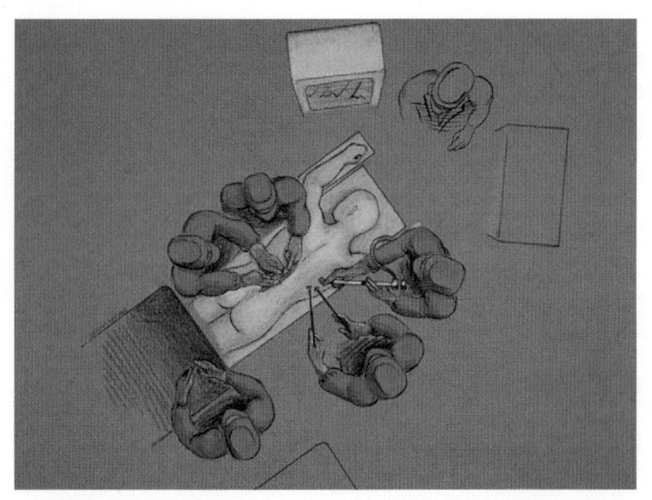

FIGURE 16–1 Operating room setup for prone position kyphosis correction.

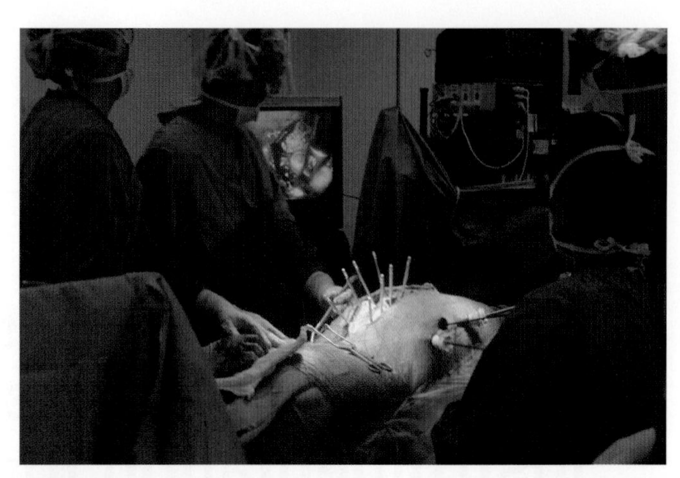

FIGURE 16–3 Operating room setup: patient positioned prone, posterior wound open, instruments in chest, simultaneous approach.

narrow anteroposterior chest diameter or significant vertebral rotation at the apex. These anatomic variants limit the working space in the chest cavity, and the rotation in particular may cause the mediastinal organs to obstruct exposure. These variables may be overcome by adding more working portals, but under these circumstances, it may be prudent to use a formal open thoracotomy.

Surgical Technique

In preparation for a prone position endoscopic exposure, the patient undergoes selective double-lumen endotracheal intubation. The patient is then positioned prone on a radiolucent spinal frame (Figs. 16–1, 16–2, 16–3). The function of the double-lumen tube is first checked in the supine position, then once again in the prone position. The patient must be continuously monitored throughout the case. The back is prepared and draped widely, extending beyond the anterior axillary line on each side. The spine is first exposed through a posterior midline incision to the tips of the transverse processes over the appropriate fusion levels. The appropriate lung is then deflated by clamping the lumen of the double-lumen tube. While waiting for the lung to deflate, bone graft can be harvested from the posterior iliac crest through a separate incision.

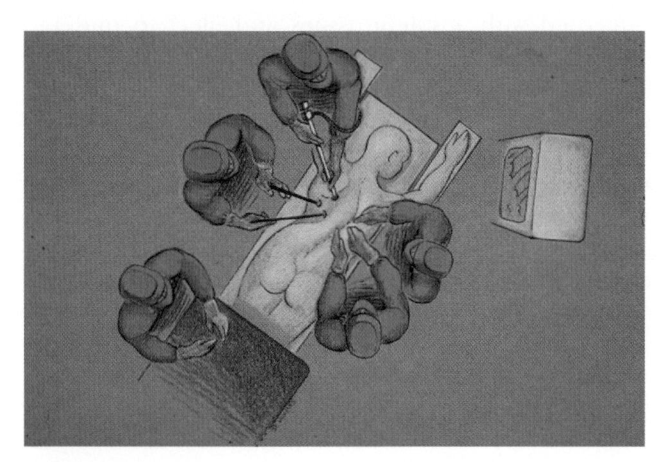

FIGURE 16–2 Operating room setup for prone position scoliosis correction.

For scoliosis correction, the spine can be exposed on the convexity or the concavity, depending on the clinical circumstances and the surgeon's preference. Release on the convexity may require more portals to gain parallel access to each disk space. In some curves, to release the structural tether, it may be difficult to gain access to the posterolateral corner on the concavity at the proximal and distal levels; however, if thoracoplasty is indicated, then only the convex approach is applicable. Working on the concavity, however, allows for fewer portals and provides direct access to the structural tether (posterolateral corner and costotransverse ligaments) over the entire curve. This concave approach does require more meticulous dissection of the aorta, which unfolds into the concavity of the curve. A theoretical vascular risk exists depending on which approach is selected. The aorta is a thick, resilient structure, less prone to injury, in contrast to the azygous system, with its large friable, tortuous veins that may prove more problematic.

For scoliosis cases, the first portal is created opposite the apex of the curve at the midaxillary line. For kyphosis correction, the spine can be approached from either chest at the surgeon's discretion. In these kyphosis cases, the first portal is created opposite the apex of the kyphosis at the midaxillary line. The first portal becomes the main working portal and is the only portal inserted blindly. It is inserted after blunt dissection with a Kelly forceps just over the top of the rib to avoid damage to the neurovascular bundle or deep structures. The 30-degree endoscope is then inserted and the chest cavity is explored. Two further

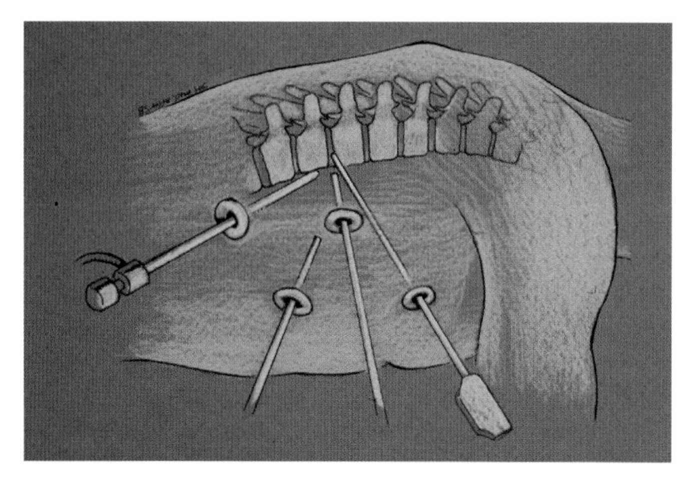

FIGURE 16–4 Portal placement: "V" shaped portal distribution with additioonal axillary portal.

working portals are created under direct video visualization at the posterior axillary line two interspaces cephalad and caudad to the endoscope portal. The remaining portals are inserted under direct view, with the lung protected. The pattern of portal placement can be either an L or V shape, depending on the chest wall morphology and the level of the spine to be approached (Fig. 16–4). The instruments and scope are interchanged between the portals to facilitate work at different levels. A fourth optional portal, two interspaces cephalad at the midaxillary line, can be used if necessary as a suction portal.

With the patient prone, the deflated lung and mediastinal structures fall out of view, requiring no retraction (Figs. 16–5A, 16–6A). The spinal levels are identified clinically by counting ribs and are confirmed with an anteroposterior radiograph. Multiple individual transverse pleural incisions are made directly over the disk spaces to be released (Figs. 16–5B, 16–6B). The segmental vessels are preserved, and the sympathetic chain is bluntly dissected out of harm's way. The anterior longitudinal ligament and anulus are incised with cautery. The nucleus pulposus is evacuated with rongeurs and curettes down to the bleeding subchondral bone end plates. For scoliosis cases, the posterolateral corner, costotransverse ligaments, and rib heads on the concave side are released under direct view to obtain optimal correction (Fig. 16–6C). The convex anulus, however, is left intact to act as a tether to prevent overdistraction and as a pivot point during the posterior correction. For kyphosis cases, the entire anulus is released. With transpedicular instrumentation in place, the disk spaces can be levered open to visualize the posterior longitudinal ligament to ensure complete evacuation of disk material (Fig. 16–5C).

During scoliosis cases, the aorta is mobilized with blunt dissection (Figs. 16–6A,B). It frequently lies in the acute angle between the rib head and the lateral vertebral body. Once mobilized, the aorta is protected during the preparation of the disk space with a small sponge and peanut retractor placed in the interval between the vertebral body and the aorta.

Bone graft, either structural tricortical crest or femoral allograft ring in kyphosis cases, or morcellized cancellous iliac crest graft in scoliosis cases, is inserted into the disk spaces with the bone holders or an extra long funnel. The endoscope is removed from the chest, and the portals are closed with a subcutaneous and running subcuticular stitch. A chest tube is inserted through the most convenient portal.

Timing the implantation of the posterior instrumentation and obtaining the correction are case specific. For cases of thoracic hyperkyphosis, it is typically easier and advantageous to expose the spine across the proposed levels through the posterior incision first, apply the implants, then enter the chest endoscopically to perform the releases. This allows the operating team to take advantage of the segmental instrumentation to lever open each level one at a time for complete and safe diskectomy. For cases of rigid scoliosis, performing the releases first and assessing segmental mobility may avoid disappointment if the releases are inadequate or the anatomy is not ideal. Doing the releases first allows the case to be converted more easily to a lateral thoracotomy by repositioning the patient before the posterior wound is opened.

Complications

The major concern of this endoscopic prone approach is unrecognized injury to the spinal cord, lungs, mediastinal organs, or major blood vessels. With good endoscopic technique, each disk space is directly visualized, and the evacuation of the nucleus is performed under direct view. The lungs and mediastinal organs are also in full view and with the prone position fall out of harm's way, eliminating the need for any retraction and minimizing iatrogenic injuries. Other minor concerns include intercostal neuralgias, infection, and wound breakdown. To minimize the risk of intercostal neuralgias, the portals are created under direct visualization from within the chest cavity, in a predetermined trajectory, with blunt dissection over the top of the appropriate rib. To date, there have been no major complications associated with the prone position endoscopic approach in more than 80 cases.

Postoperative Care

The postoperative care for these patients is identical to any anteroposterior deformity correction case. The patient is typically monitored in an intensive care or step-down setting for the first 24 hours. A chest tube is in place, with the drainage monitored and daily chest

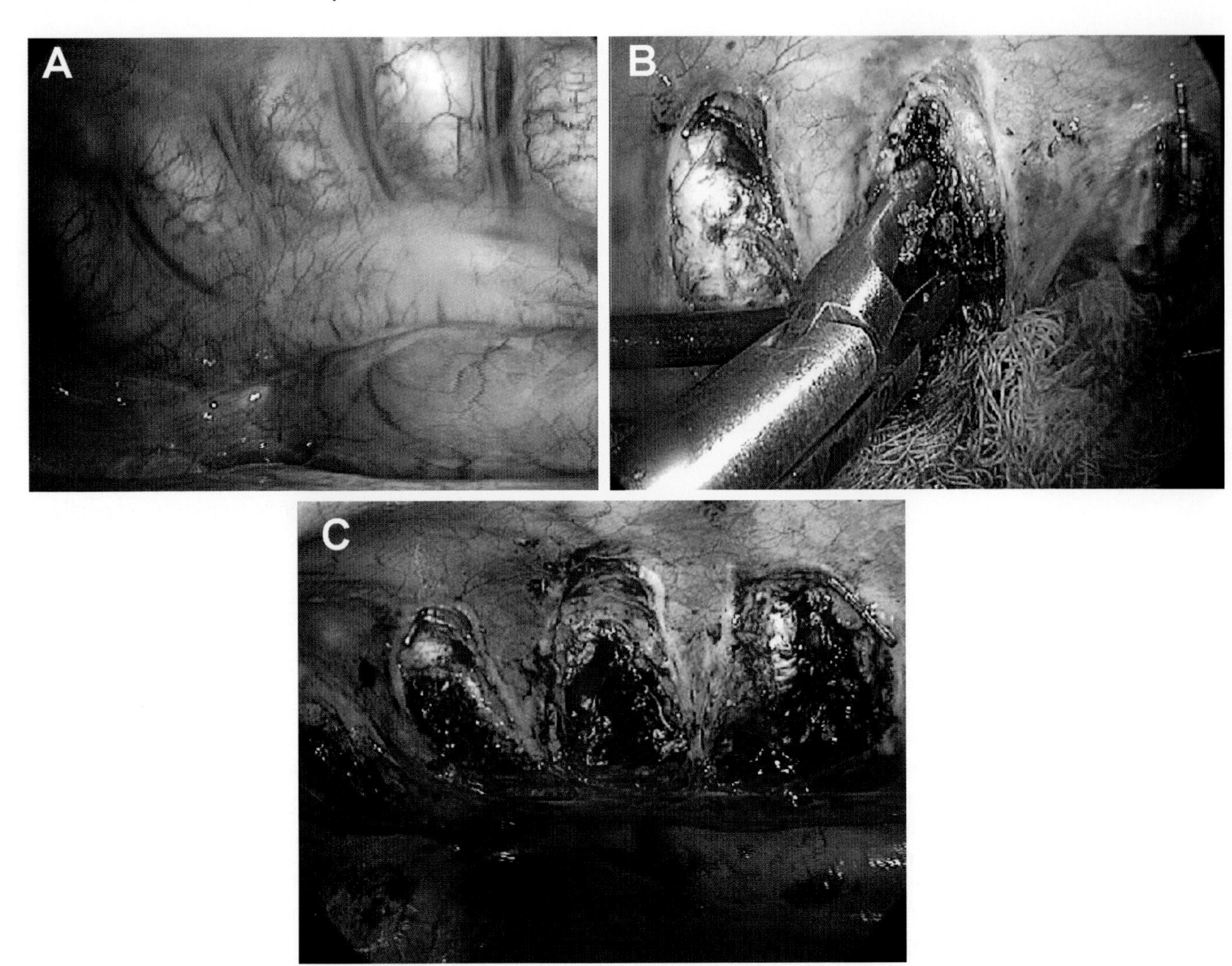

FIGURE 16–5 Endoscopic views of kyphosis correction. **(A)** Initial view, mediastinal organs fall out of harm's way. **(B)** Transverse pleural incisions and diskectomy. **(C)** Release circumferential to posterior longitudinal ligament.

x-rays performed. Drainage is typically scant, but if significant, once the drainage is less than 100 ml per shift, the tube is removed. The patient is encouraged to be out of bed the first morning after surgery, and chest physical therapy and incentive spirometry are initiated. The endoscopic portal incisions are inspected daily, and dressings are changed as necessary.

Outcomes

Many reports of transthoracic endoscopic techniques have now been published. Overall, the results have been predictable and satisfying for both surgeons and patients. The reported complication rate seems to be equivalent to similar traditional open procedures. The advantages of the endoscopic techniques in postoperative pain relief and preservation of pulmonary function have been realized. The operative time associated with the endoscopic procedure was initially reported as longer, yet as surgeons gained experience, the operative time has improved considerably. It now takes experienced endoscopic spinal surgeons ~20 minutes to place portals and expose the spine, and 10 to 15 minutes to release and bone graft each disk space. Comparisons of the extent of spinal correction in adult deformity to historical cohorts match or exceed the published curve corrections, and published animal studies conclude that the extent of diskectomy and quality of release are comparable to open techniques.

The obvious advantage of the endoscopic exposure is the cosmetically appealing incisions and easier recovery for patients (Fig. 16–7). Another advantage is the time saved associated with opening and closing a thoracotomy incision. The transthoracic prone position endoscopic approach as described here allows the surgeon the added opportunity to address anterior and posterior spinal pathology simultaneously. Time and cost will be saved by eliminating the need to reprep and redrape during staged

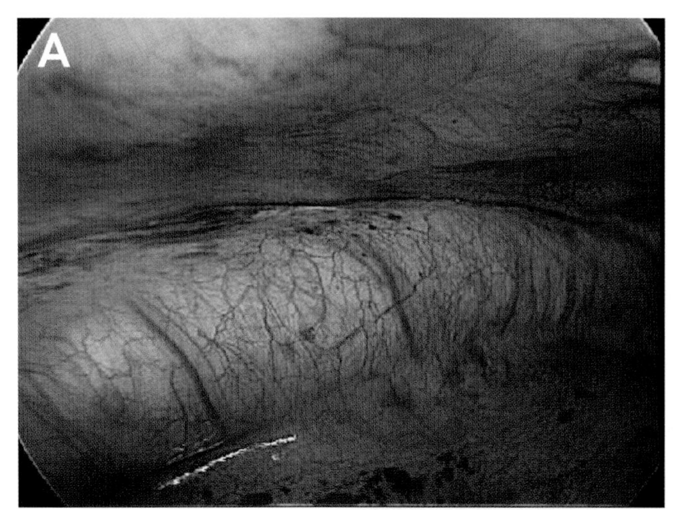

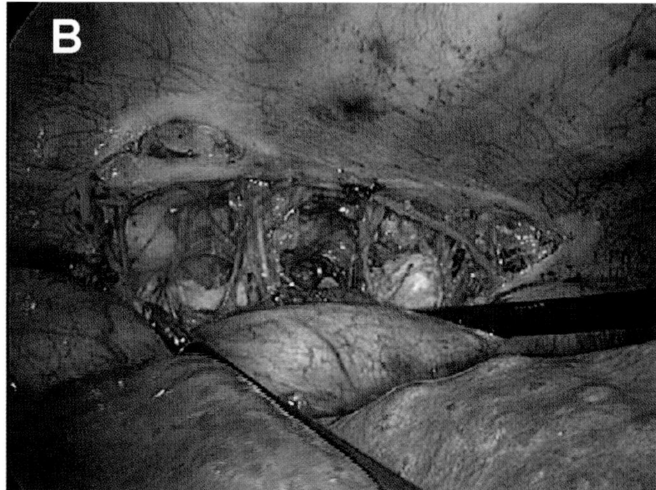

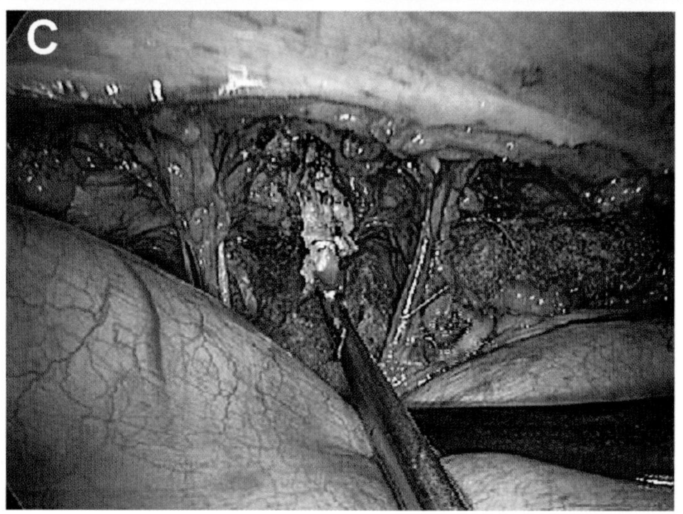

FIGURE 16–6 Endoscopic views of scoliosis correction. **(A)** Initial view of aorta unfolded into rib vertebra junction. **(B)** Longitudinal pleural incision. Preservation of segmental vessels. **(C)** Resection of annulus and evacuation of nucleus pulposus.

procedures. This technique can be used for other anteroposterior tumor or trauma spinal reconstructions.

Case Illustration

The following case exemplifies the benefits of a simultaneous posterior open, anterior endoscopic approach, which allowed for safe and expeditious access to the concavity of a progressive scoliotic curve in a revision situation, obviating the need for a staged procedure or approaching the curve through the previously scarred right thoracic cavity. This 13-year-old female presented with a progressive scoliosis (Fig. 16–8A) and underwent a posterior instrumentation and fusion (Fig. 16–8B). Within 4 months the curve progressed above the fusion (Fig. 16–8C), and she subsequently underwent a right-sided thoracoplasty. The thoracoplasty further exacerbated the curve progression, resulting in a rigid and unsightly deformity. The treatment options now included a staged procedure with further surgery through the previously operated areas or a simultaneous procedure with an endoscopic transthoracic approach from the left chest (concavity of the curve) to release the rigid curve at the same time as the posterior wound is reopened for revision and extension of the instrumentation. During this procedure the left arm was draped free to allow mobilization of the scapula and placement of high axillary ports (Fig. 16–8D,E). The left chest was virgin territory free of scarring, allowing the exposure of the respective levels to be released and bone grafted (Fig. 16–8F,G). The final correction was dramatic (Fig. 16–8H), and the entire procedure was successfully completed in one surgical setting.

Conclusion

Thoracoscopic combined anterior release and posterior instrumentation can be safely and effectively performed in the prone position, obviating the need for staged procedures in deformity correction in select

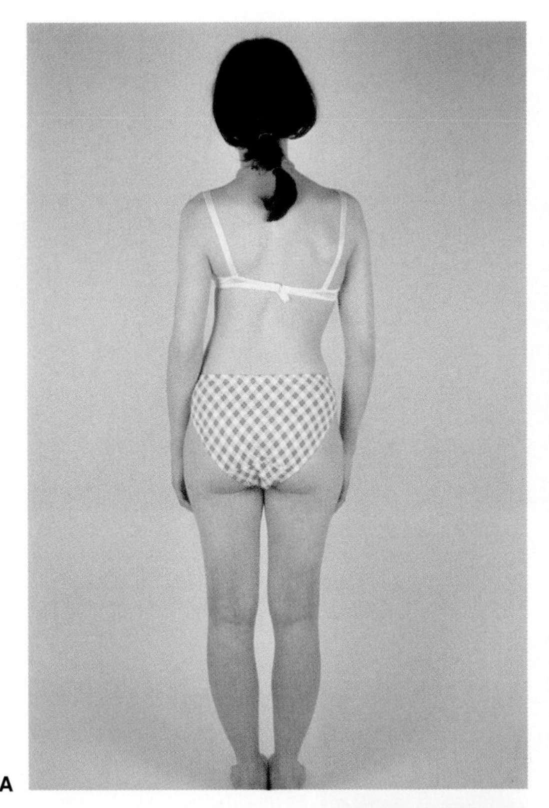

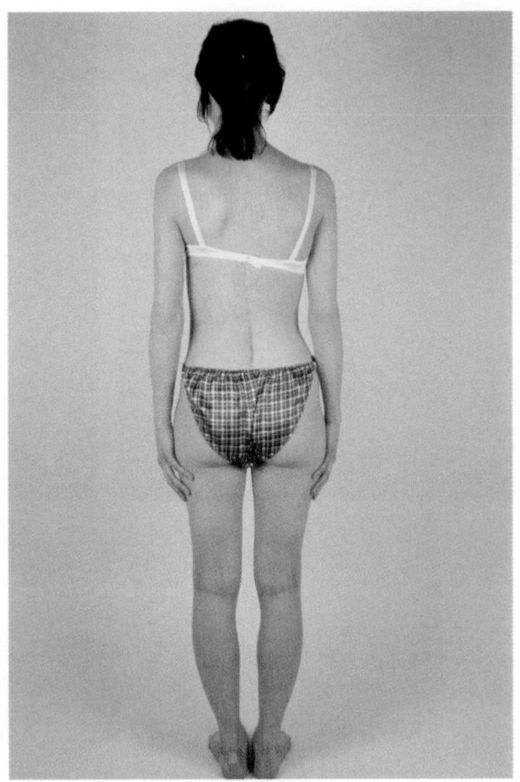

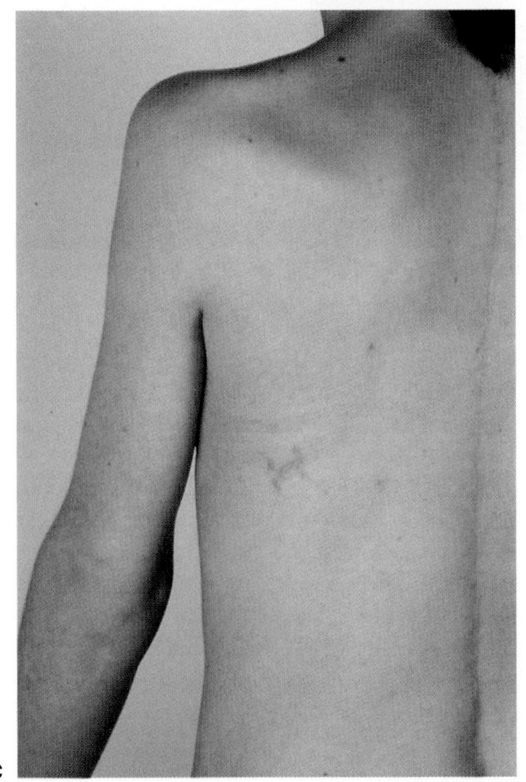

FIGURE 16–7 Correction and cosmetic result. **(A)** Preoperative photo. **(B)** Postoperative photo. **(C)** Close-up of scars of incisions used for endoscopic access.

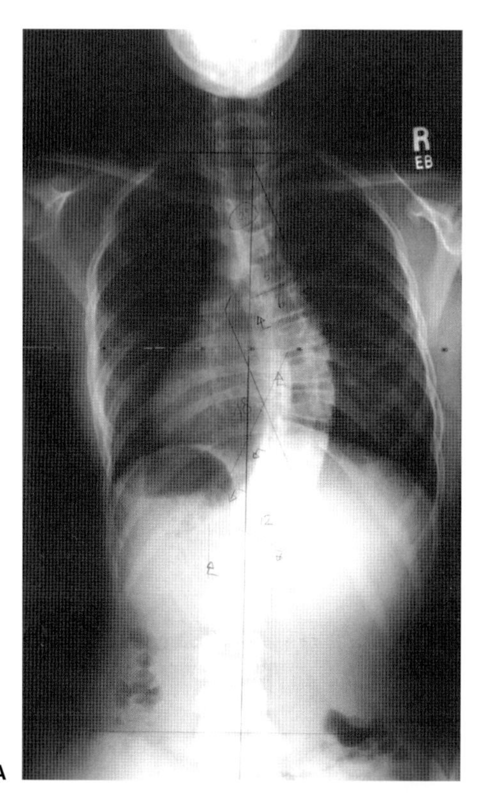

A

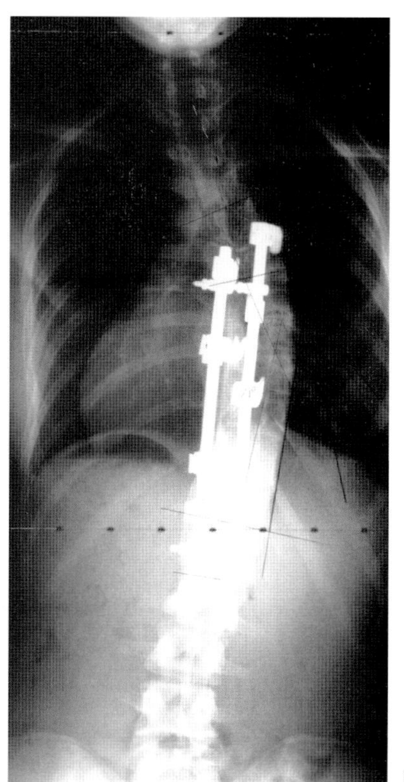

B

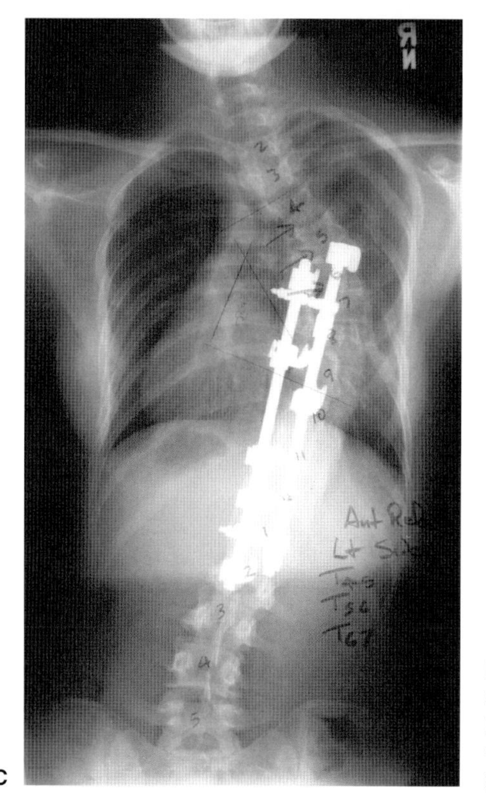

C

FIGURE 16–8 A 13-year-old female presented with progressive scoliosis. **(A)** Preoperative x-ray. She underwent a posterior instrumentation and fusion. **(B)** Postoperative x-ray. Within 4 months the curve progressed. **(C)** Postthoracoplasty progression.

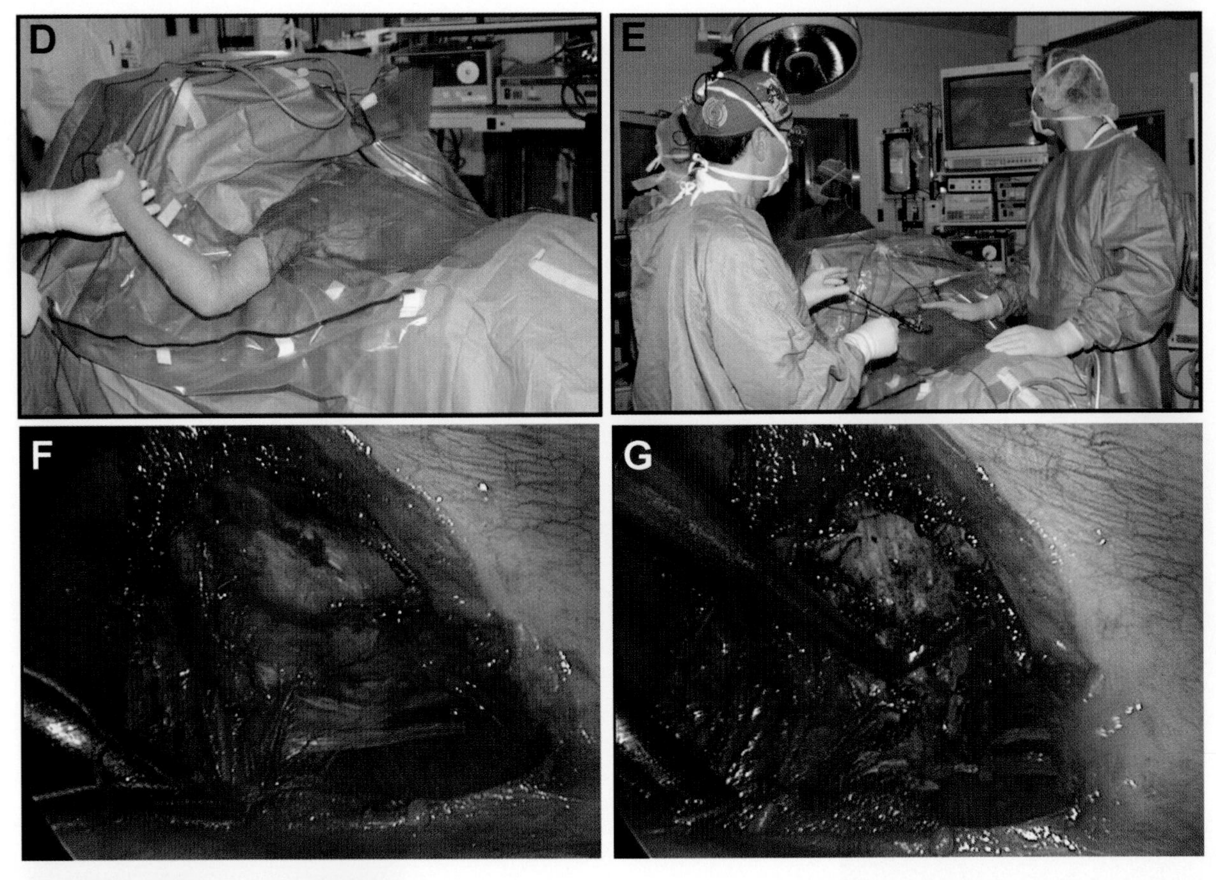

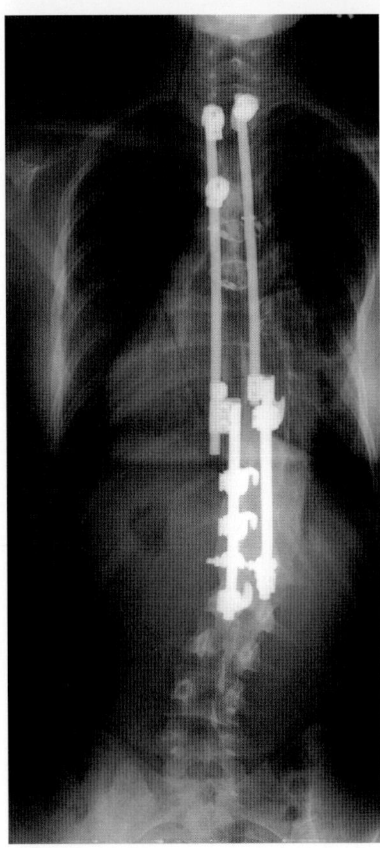

FIGURE 16–8 (*Continued*) She underwent a combined prone position thoracoscopic anterior release and posterior instrumentation. **(D)** Intraoperative setup. **(E)** Intraoperative technique. **(F)** Intraoperative view of prone approach to concave side. **(G)** Intraoperative view of disk excision for release. **(H)** X-ray showing the final correction.

patients. It avoids the risks and morbidity associated with staged procedures. Like most endoscopic techniques, it has a learning curve and requires familiarity of the thoracoscopic anatomy in the prone position.

REFERENCES

1. Lieberman IH, Salo PT, Orr RD, Kraetschmer BG. Prone position endoscopic transthoracic release with simultaneous posterior instrumentation for spinal deformity: a description of the technique. *Spine*. 2000;25:2251–2257.
2. McAfee PC, Regan JJ, Zdeblick T, et al. The incidence of complications in endoscopic anterior thoracolumbar spinal reconstructive surgery: a prospective multicenter study comprising the first 100 consecutive cases. *Spine*. 1995;20:1624–1632.
3. Newton PO, Wenger DR, Mubarak JS, Meyer RS. Anterior release and fusion in pediatric spinal deformity: a comparison of early outcome and cost of thoracoscopic and open thoracotomy approaches. *Spine*. 1997;22:1398–1406.
4. Newton PO, Cardelia JM, Farnsworth CL, et al. A biomechanical comparison of open and thoracoscopic anterior spinal release in a goat model. *Spine*. 1998;23:530–536.
5. Wall EJ, Bylski-Austrow DI, Shelton FJ, et al. Endoscopic diskectomy increases flexibility as effectively as open diskectomy. *Spine* 1998;23:9–16.

17

Thoracoscopic Decompression and Fixation (MACS-TL)

RAJU S. V. BALABHADRA, DANIEL H. KIM, MICHAEL POTULSKI, AND RUDOLF BEISSE

Thoracoscopic techniques have long been used by thoracic surgeons, who have had excellent experience and good results over the last decade. For spine surgeons, it represents a new procedure for treating spine problems through an anterior approach. The anterior approach in spine surgery has long been accepted for corpectomy, decompression, and stabilization. Unfortunately, a thoracotomy or thoracoabdominal approach is marked by high morbidity, with frequently occurring pain syndromes, relaxation of the abdominal wall, or neuralgia of the posterior segment nerves. Because the most common location of the thoracic spine fractures involve the thoracolumbar junction, this morbidity is again increased by the required diaphragm detachment.

The attempt to incorporate biomechanical advantages by using an anterior approach and to avoid the disadvantages of high morbidity by means of minimally invasive techniques has been addressed by various authors. It has expanded its application from metastatic spine disease and degenerative diseases to thoracolumbar spine trauma and deformity correction from any causes. The anatomically performed thoracic cavity allowed thoracoscopic access to the thoracic vertebrae T4-T12 without any major preparatory work. Even the rostral lumbar spine can be safely reached thoracoscopically by detaching the diaphragm. At the level of the second or third lumbar vertebra, further diaphragm detachment and proper retraction make it possible to expose the entire thoracolumbar transition for minimally invasive endoscopic procedures. This is made possible by an anatomical peculiarity of the pleural cavity and the diaphragmatic insertion, the lowest portion of which (i.e., the costodiaphragmatic recess) is projected onto the spine with perpendicular projection just on the base plate of the second vertebra (Fig. 17–1). Thus, the thoracic spine, as well as upper lumbar spine from T4 to L3, is accessible endoscopically using the thoracoscopic technique.

The goals of thoracoscopic surgery include neural decompression, restoration of normal curvature, and stability of the affected motion segment(s). This is usually achieved in a two-step procedure that includes posterior reduction and stabilization with a pedicle screw system if necessary in patients with significant deformity or three-column involvement. Anterior decompression of the spinal canal, reconstruction of the vertebra, and interbody fusion with autogenous bone graft (or bone-impacted cage) and screw plate fixation are performed through a thoracoscopic anterior approach, which can be extended into the retroperitoneal space down to L3 with thoracoscopic diaphragm detachments, if necessary.

Indications

As an alternative approach to thoracotomy or thoracoabdominal approach, the thoracoscopic technique can be used to perform thoracic corpectomy to decompress the spinal canal and to reconstruct and fixate the segments affected by destructive disease and trauma. The anterior thoracoscopic approach is indicated in the following situations (in combination with posterior instrumentation if needed):

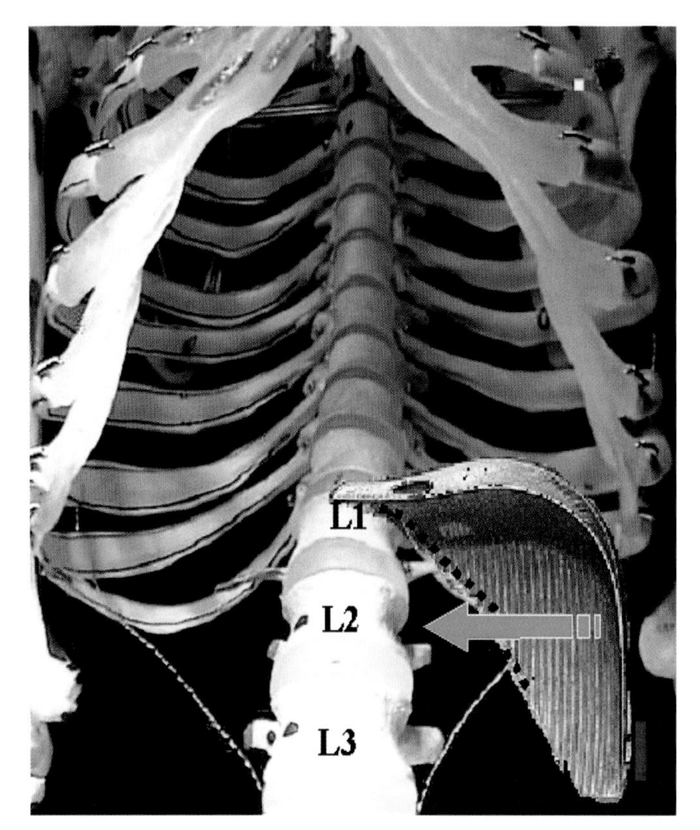

FIGURE 17–1 Extent of diaphragmatic opening by the thoracoscopic approach along the spine and ribs is marked for exposure of L2 vertebra. Note that the lowest point of the diaphragmatic insertion [i.e., the costodiaphragmatic recess (arrow)] projects onto the spine perpendicularly just above the base plate of L2. Thus, a minimal diaphragmatic opening (6–10 cm) allows instrumentation of L2 vertebra.

- Fractures of the thoracic spine located at the thoracolumbar junction from T4 to L3
- Fractures classified as A 1.2, A 1.3, A 2, A 3, B, and C according to the Association of Osteosynthesis (AO) classification[1] with significant curvature disturbance of 20 degrees and more in the sagittal or frontal plane
- Fractures of type B and C posterior instrumentation (mandatory; optional in other types)
- Posttraumatic, degenerative, or tumorous narrowing of the spinal canal
- Diskoligamentous segmental instability
- Posttraumatic deformities

Contraindications

The thoracoscopic approach is contraindicated in the following situations:

- Significant previous cardiopulmonary disease with restricted cardiopulmonary function
- Acute posttraumatic lung failure
- Significant disturbances of hemostasis

Instruments

The following instruments are necessary to perform endoscopic-assisted anterior approaches to the thoracic and lumbar spine:

- Routine surgical set for skin incision and preparation of the intercostal space
- Instruments for removal of bone graft from the iliac crest
- Video-endoscopy tower and endoscopes (Fig. 17–2A,B)
- Instruments for thorascopic dissection (Fig. 17–2C) of the prevertebral anatomic structures, as well as for resection of bone and ligaments, osteotomes, hooks for dissection, hook probes, sharp and blunt rongeurs, Kerrison rongeurs, curettes, graft holder, reamers, and mono- and bipolar probe. All thoracoscopic instruments are of suitable length and have large handles, making it possible to guide the instruments with both hands and to work safely and securely with them.
- Instruments for implant placements (modular anterior construct system for thoracolumbar spine, MACS-TL): Most currently available spinal implants for anterior thoracic instrumentation are developed for open surgery and thus had to be modified to make them compatible for endoscopic use. The MACS-TL system is designed for thoracoscopic use and thus greatly simplifies the instrumentation technique. Emphasis was placed on endoscopic insertion and intracorporeal assembly of the implants and free placement of screws and angular stability by using polyaxial screws. The use of targeting and centering sleeves guides self-centering of the assembly instruments (Fig. 17–3).
- Instrument preparation set: K-wires, cannulated punch/cortical drill for decortication
- Instrument insertion set: centralizer attachment, screw insertion assembly instrument, distraction ratchet, cannulated nut driver
- Implant set twin screw (MACS TL)
- Disposable instruments, lung retractor, clip applicator

Anesthesia

The procedure is performed with the patient under general anesthesia. Selected intubation with one-lung ventilation facilitates intrathoracic preparation. The positioning of the double-lumen tube is controlled by a bronchoscopic technique. A Foley catheter is placed, as well as central venous lines and an arterial line for continuous blood pressure monitoring.

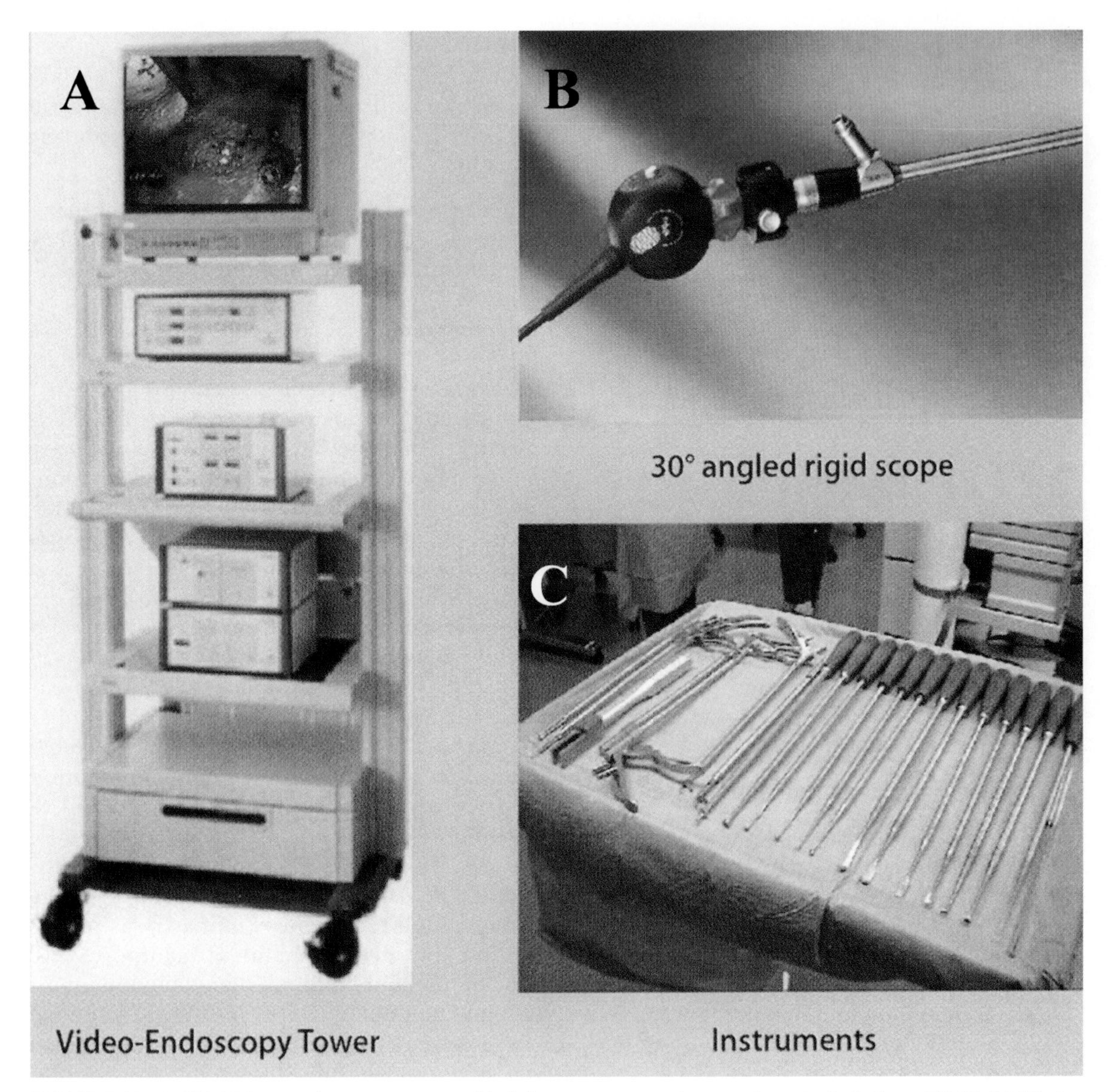

FIGURE 17–2 **(A)** Video-endoscopy tower with light source, monitor, and control station. **(B)** Right 30-degree-angled endoscope. **(C)** Thoracoscopic instruments set with varying sizes of osteotomes, curettes, rongeurs, and graspers.

Positioning

The patient is placed in a stable lateral position on the right side and fixed with a four-point support at the symphysis, sacrum, and scapula, as well as with arm rests (Fig. 17–4). A left-sided position is preferred for the treatment of fractures from T4 to T8. A right-sided position is preferred for the approach to the thoracolumbar junction (T9–L3). Care has to be taken that the upper arm is abducted and elevated in order not to disturb the placement and manipulation of the endoscope. Before the operation starts, the position and free tilt of the C-arm must be checked. Sterile draping extends from the middle of the sternum anterior to the spinous processes posterior, as well as from the axilla down to ~8 cm caudal to the iliac crest. Both monitors should be placed at the lower end of the operating table on opposite sides to enable free vision for the surgeon and the assistant. The operating room setup is shown in Figure 17–5. The surgeon and the camera operator stand behind the patient. The C-arm approach is between the surgeon and the camera operator. The assistant and the C-arm monitor are placed on the opposite side.

Surgical Technique

The surgical technique of thoracoscopic spine surgery has been described in detail by various authors.[2–4] Early

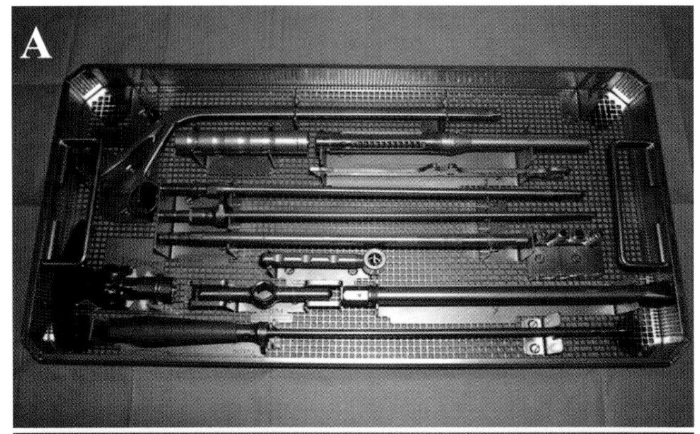

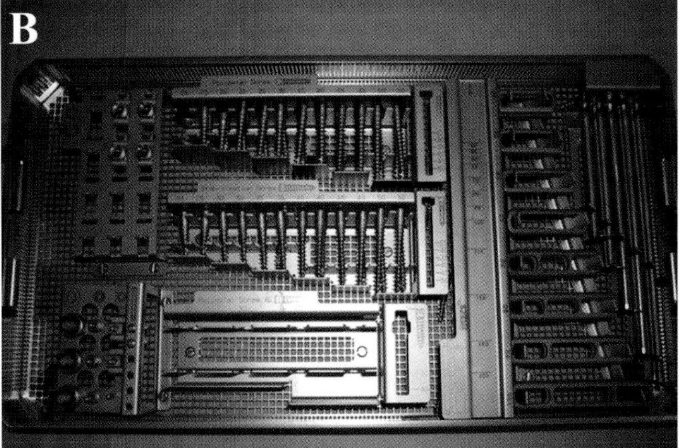

FIGURE 17–3 (A,B) MACS-TL (modular anterior construct system for thoracolumbar spine) instrumentation set.

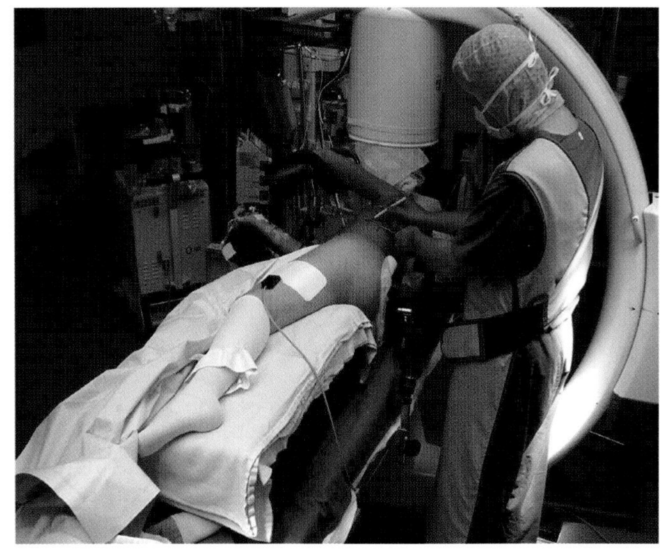

FIGURE 17–4 Operative photograph showing lateral positioning (on the right side) of the patient on a Jackson table.

on in our experience, we often reserved the thoracoscopic approach for thoracic fractures involving the T4 to T10 vertebrae. With increasing experience, we extended the indications to pathologies involving the thoracolumbar junction.

Localization

The target area (e.g., Ll fracture) is projected onto the skin level under fluoroscopic control (Fig. 17–6). The borders of the fractured vertebra are then marked on the skin. The working channel is centered over the target vertebra (12.5 mm). The optical channel (10 mm) is placed two or three intercostal spaces cranial to the target vertebra in the spinal axis. For fractures of the middle and upper thoracic spine, the optical channel is placed caudal to the target vertebra. The approach for suction/irrigation (5 mm) and retractor (10 mm) is placed ~5 to 10 cm anterior to the working and optical channel.

Placement of Portals

The position of the portals in relation to one another and to the operating site on the spine influences the entire course of the operation. The injured spinal section is therefore first projected exactly orthograde onto the lateral chest or abdominal wall using an image intensifier, then drawn onto the skin with a marker pen, indicating the line of the anterior and posterior edges as well as the end plates of the affected segments. The operating portal is the first position to be marked exactly over the target area; corresponding to this, the portal for the optical channel is drawn in over the spine, two or three intercostal spaces above the mark for the operating portal for thoracolumbar access, or underneath it for access to the central or upper thoracic spine (Figs. 17–7, 17–8). The portal for the suction and irrigation instrument is about four fingerbreadths from the operating portal in a ventral and cranial direction. The portal for the diaphragm or lung retractor should be placed as far as possible ventrally to avoid instruments coming into conflict. It is sometimes helpful to make two separate working portals, which are directed onto the vertebra to be fixed (above and below the affected segment).

The operation is started with the most cranial approach (optical channel). Small Langenbeck hooks are inserted through a 1.5 cm skin incision above the intercostal space.

The muscles of the thoracic wall are crossed in a blunt, muscle-splitting technique, and the intercostal space is opened by blunt dissection, thus exposing the pleura and creating an opening to enter the thoracic cavity, A 10 mm trocar is inserted, and one-lung ventilation is started. A

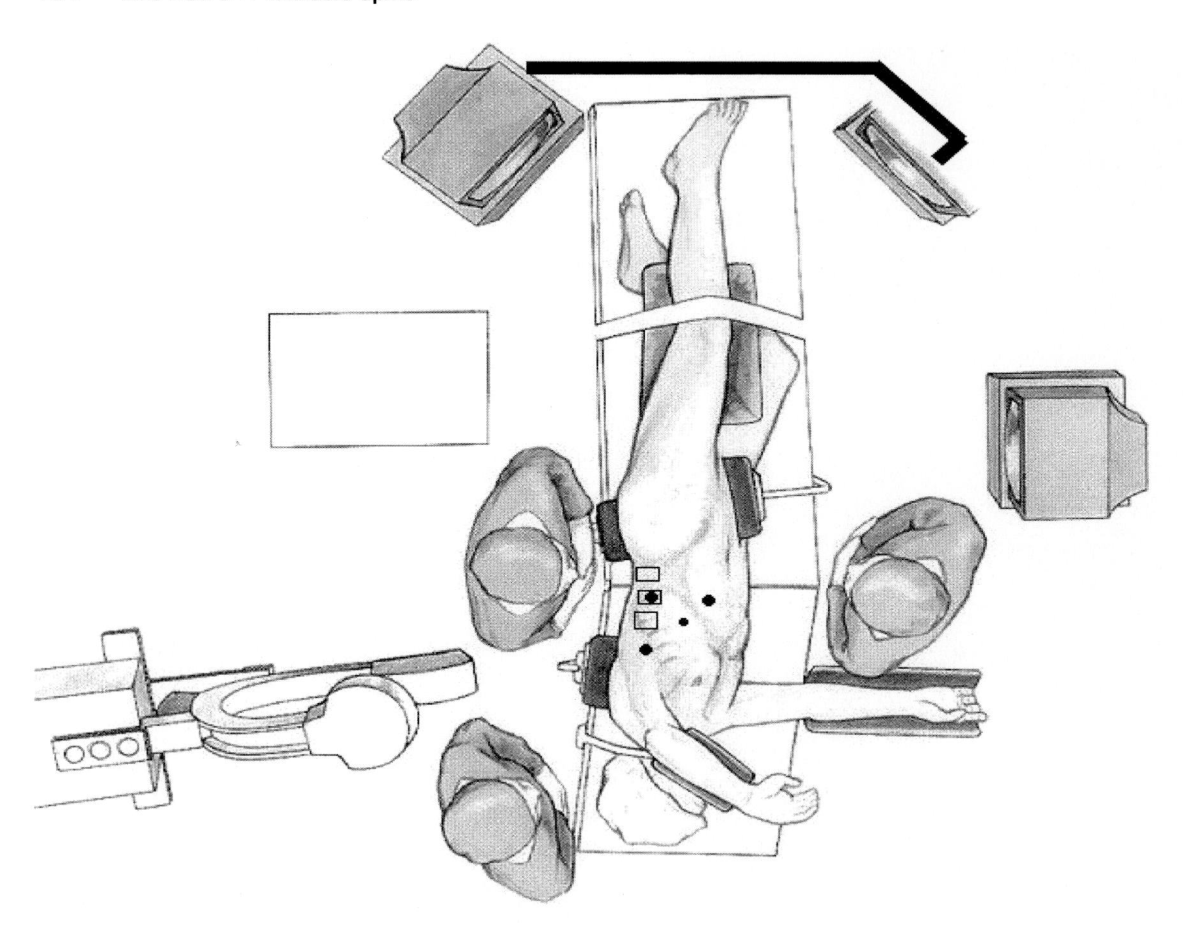

FIGURE 17–5 Operating room setup for thoracoscopic spine surgery. Note that the surgeon and the assistant holding the camera stand behind the patient, with the video and fluoroscopic monitor in front of them.

30-degree endoscope is inserted at a flat angle in the direction of the second trocar. Perforation of the thoracic wall to insert the second, third, and fourth trocars is performed under visual control through the scope, and the other trocars are inserted as shown.

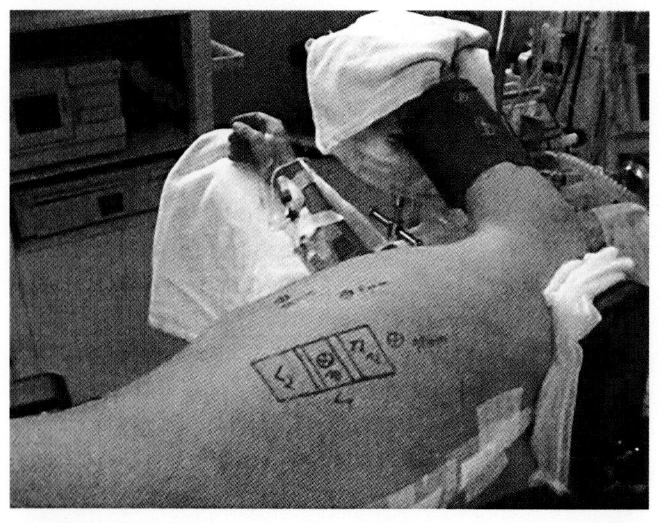

FIGURE 17–6 Localization. The target vertebra is projected and marked on the skin and marked under a fluoroscopic table.

Prevertebral Dissection and Diaphragm Detachment

The target area can now be exposed with the help of a fan retractor inserted through the anterior port. The retractor holds down the diaphragm and exposes the insertion of the diaphragm on the spine. Compared with extensive thoracolumbar exposures with total detachment of the diaphragm required for open surgery, the thoracoscopic approach to the thoracolumbar junction allows minimal diaphragmatic detachment. Thus, with a diaphragmatic opening of ~6 to 10 cm, the entire L2 vertebral body can be exposed (Fig. 17–9).

First, palpate the anterior circumference of the motion segment and the course of the aorta with a blunt probe. "Mark" the line of dissection for the diaphragm with monopolar cauterization. Next, incise the diaphragm using endoscissors. A rim of 1 cm should be left on the spine to facilitate closure of the diaphragm at the end of the procedure. The preferred incision runs along the spine and the ribs parallel to the diaphragmatic insertion and 1 to 2 cm away from it. The diaphragm is already thinner here than it is in the immediate area of insertion, and the remaining edge makes subsequent

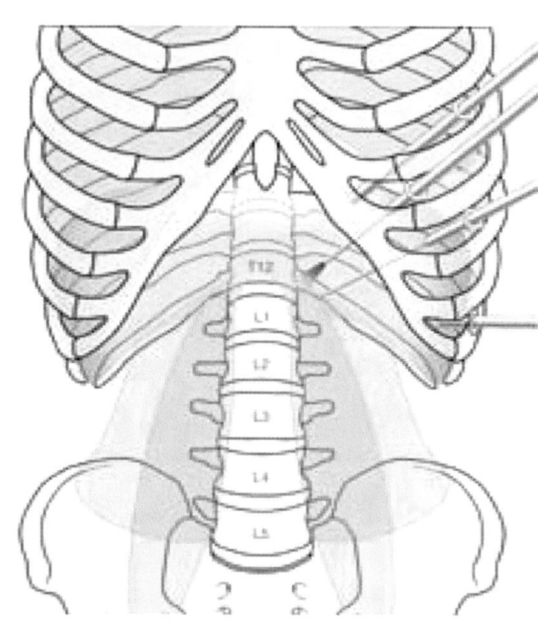

FIGURE 17–7 Diagram showing the placement for thoracoscopic portals for approaching the thoracolumbar junction.

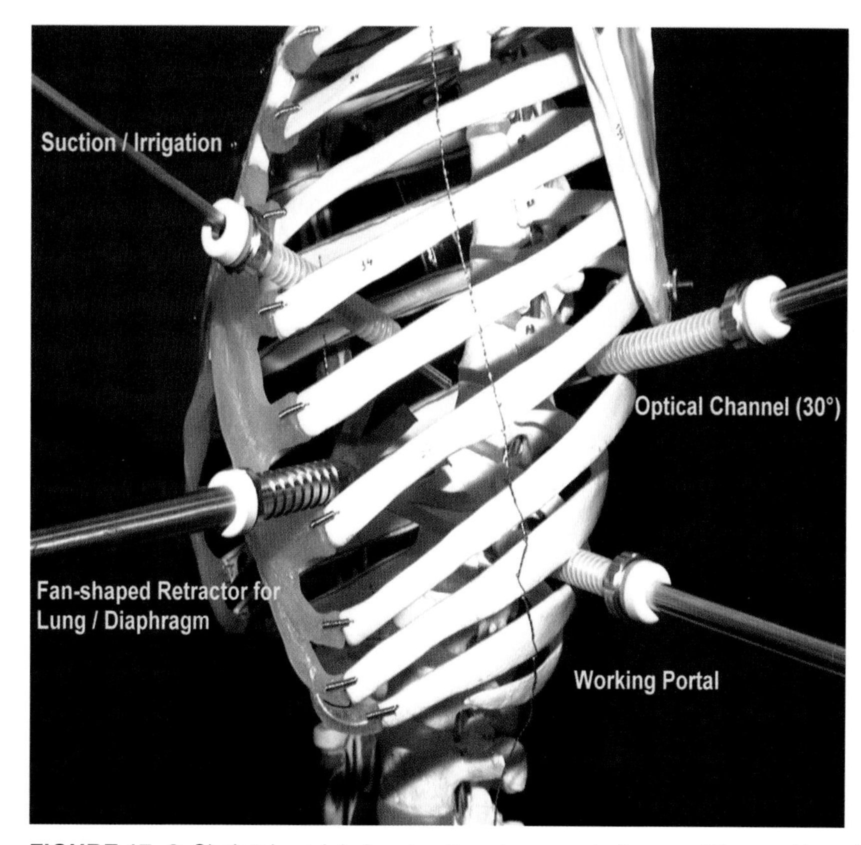

FIGURE 17–8 Skeletal model showing the placement of portals for thoracoscopy. The thoracoscope (10 mm) is placed two or three intercostal spaces cranial to the target vertebra. The working channel is placed over the target vertebra. Portals for suction/irrigation (5 mm) and retractor (10 mm) are placed ~5 to 10 cm anterior and cranial to the working portal.

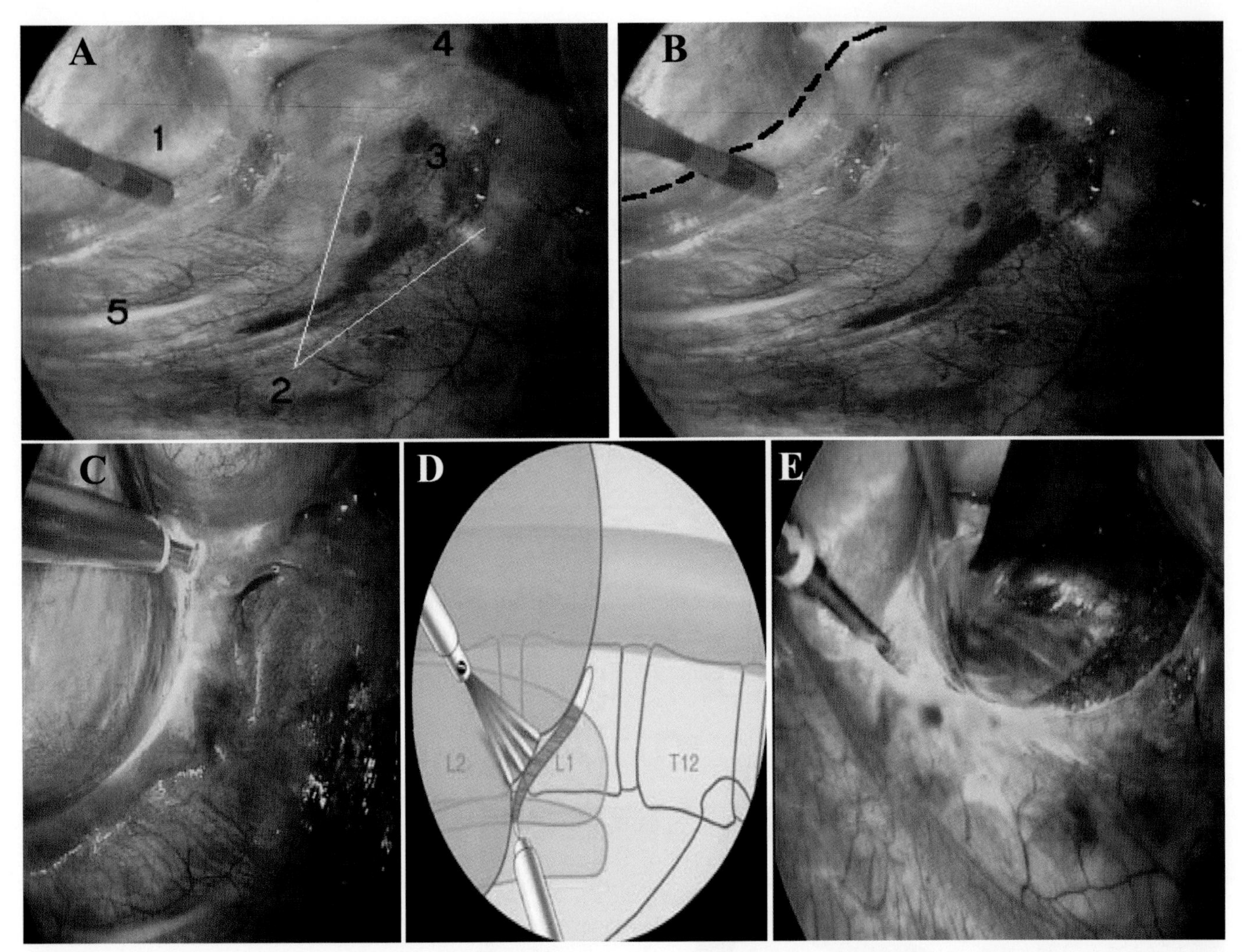

FIGURE 17–9 Operative steps in the thoracoscopic detachment of the diaphragm. **(A)** Thoracoscopic view showing the anatomy of the thoracolumbar junction [1, diaphragm; 2, vertebral bodies (T11 and T12); 3, segmental vessel; 4, aorta; 5, rib]. **(B)** Thoracoscopic view showing the line of diaphragmatic insertion. **(C)** Diaphragmatic opening with hook diathermy electrode. **(D)** Diagram showing the diaphragmatic opening with diathermy, with gentle retraction of the diaphragm with a fan retractor. **(E)** The fan retractor is introduced into the diaphragmatic opening, and retroperitoneal fat tissue is mobilized from the anterior surface of the psoas muscle. Later, the psoas muscle is gently dissected from the anterior aspect of the lumbar vertebrae.

suturing easier. Retroperitoneal fat tissue is now exposed and mobilized from the anterior surface of the psoas insertions. Carefully dissect the psoas muscle from the vertebral bodies in order not to damage the segmental blood vessels "hidden" underneath (Fig. 17–9). The retractor can now be placed into the diaphragmatic gap.

Screw Insertion Preparation

Insert a self-tapping screw under fluoroscopic control in the vertebra superior to the fractured one, as well as in the fractured vertebra. Next, insert the first screw of the MACS-TL system (Aesculap, Melsungen, Germany) into the caudal vertebral body. Open the cortical surface with a sharp trephine ~1 to 1.5 cm from the posterior border of the vertebral body infra- and supradjacent to the fracture.

K-Wire Insertion

Next, insert the K-wire in the distal cannulated end of the instrument, and connect it with the K-wire impactor. Position the K-wire under fluoroscopic control (Fig. 17–10).

The patient must be placed in a lateral position to expose the posterior edge of the corresponding vertebral body. It is important to confirm the perpendicular position of the patient to the beam.

If the instrument charged with the K-wire is well aligned, a dark inner point and a concentric ring will be observed, and the correct placement is ensured. If a line is observed on x-ray, the K-wire is not positioned parallel. Following alignment, the K-wire is impacted until it is stopped by the gray ring of the instrument (20 mm).

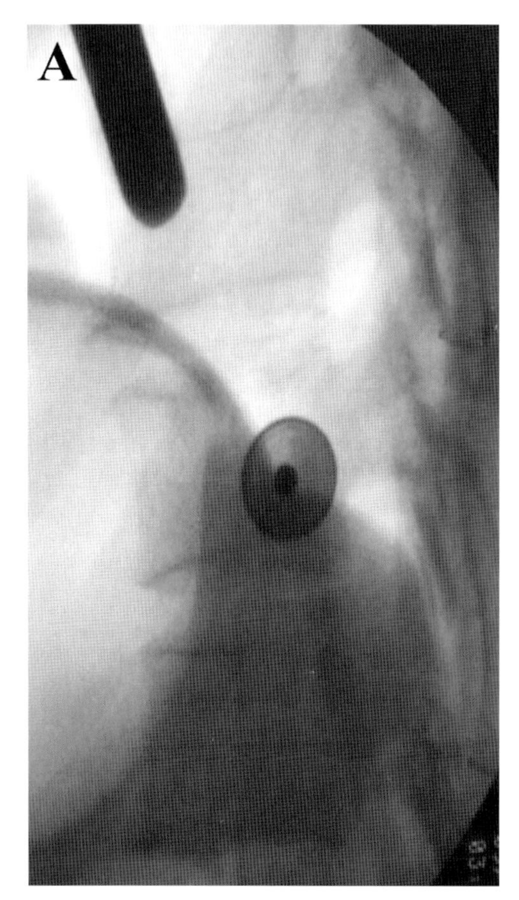
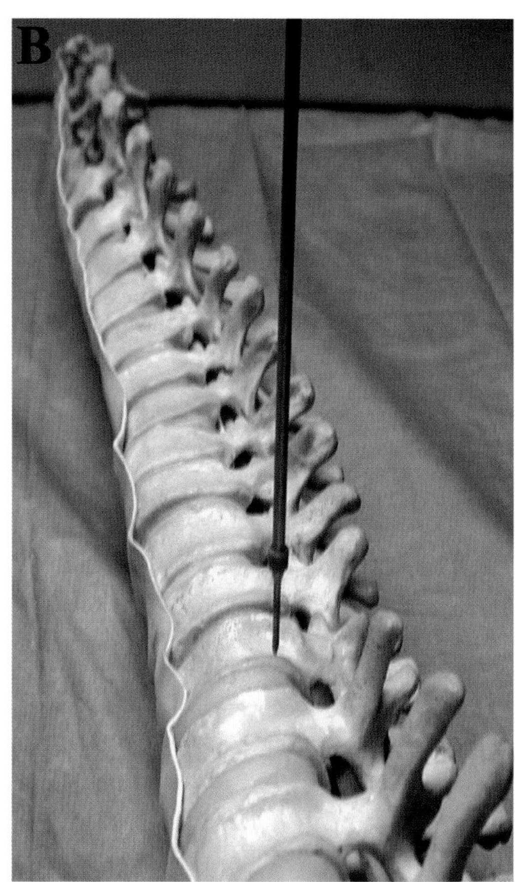

FIGURE 17–10 K-wire insertion. **(A)** X-ray views showing the placement of the K-wire impactor and K-wire, and **(B)** placement of K-wire in a saw bone model.

For safe screw implantation, the K-wire should be inserted ~10 mm away from the posterior edge of the vertebral body and 10 mm away from the end plate. Afterwards, release the K-wire by turning the knob of the impactor counterclockwise. The complete instrument can then be pulled back, with the K-wire remaining in place.

Decortication

A cannulated punch is used for a slight removal of cortical bone to prepare the entry hole for the polyaxial screw (Fig. 17–11).

Centralizer Attachment

The twin screws and the polyaxial clamp have to be preassembled before insertion. The centralizer has to be attached either to the polyaxial plate or to the twin screws. It then has to be screwed into the inner thread. This is accomplished by using the hex key for the centralizer. For rotational locking, the centralizer has two flanges, which correspond to the slots of the clamp. When fully seated, the centralizer should be snug but not overtightened (Fig. 17–12).

Assembly of Insertion Instrument

The handle must be connected to the proximal end, the external hex, of the insertion sleeve. The cannulated screwdriver has to be positioned through the insertion sleeve until it locks in position. The ratchet handle is connected to the cannulated screwdriver, and the ring of the Harris connector has to be pushed proximally. The assembled insertion instrument is then connected to the hexagonal end of the centralizer. The spring of the insertion sleeve snaps into the corresponding groove of the centralizer. The orientation of the polyaxial plate should correspond to the direction of the handle to ease the orientation, especially in endoscopic procedures. The polyaxial screw is put into a straight direction to attach the screwdriver (Fig. 17–13).

Screw Insertion

Next, place the polyaxial, posterior screw over the K-wire. The direction of the polyaxial clamp can be controlled by the handle. The clamp has to be oriented so that the hole for the anterior stabilization screw comes to lie anteriorly. After the initial turns of the screw into the vertebral body, the K-wire has to be removed to avoid the risk of tissue perforation by pushing the K-wire forward during screw insertion (Fig. 17–14).

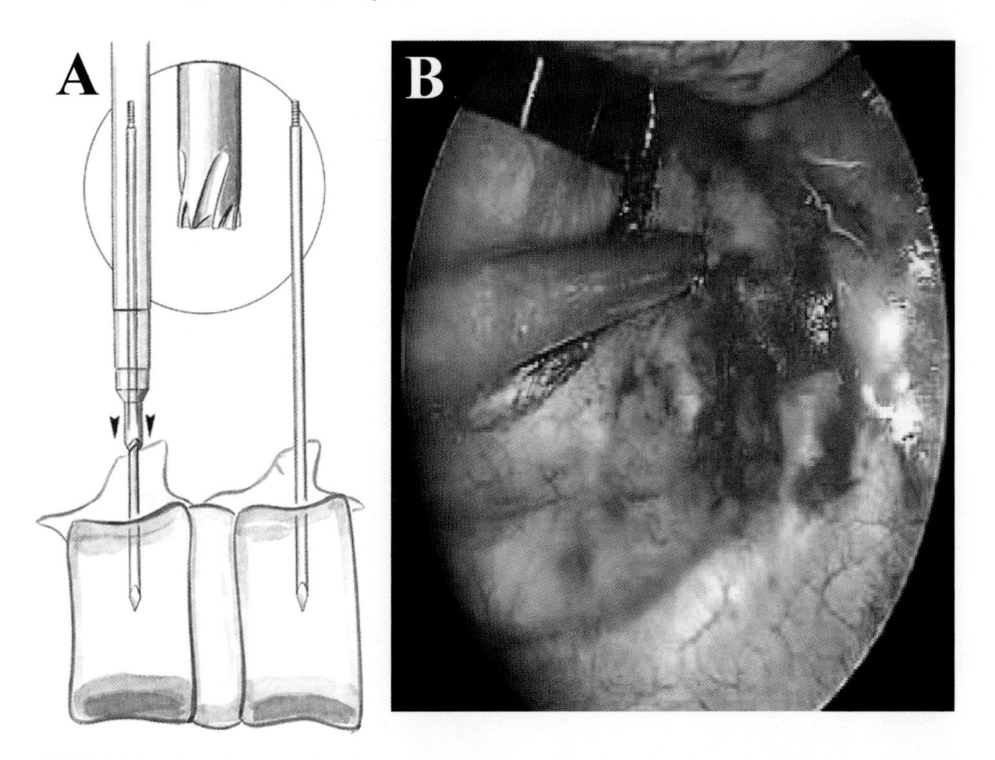

FIGURE 17–11 **(A)** Decortication to prepare for entry hole for the polyaxial screw. **(B)** Thoracoscopic view showing the decortication of the entry hole.

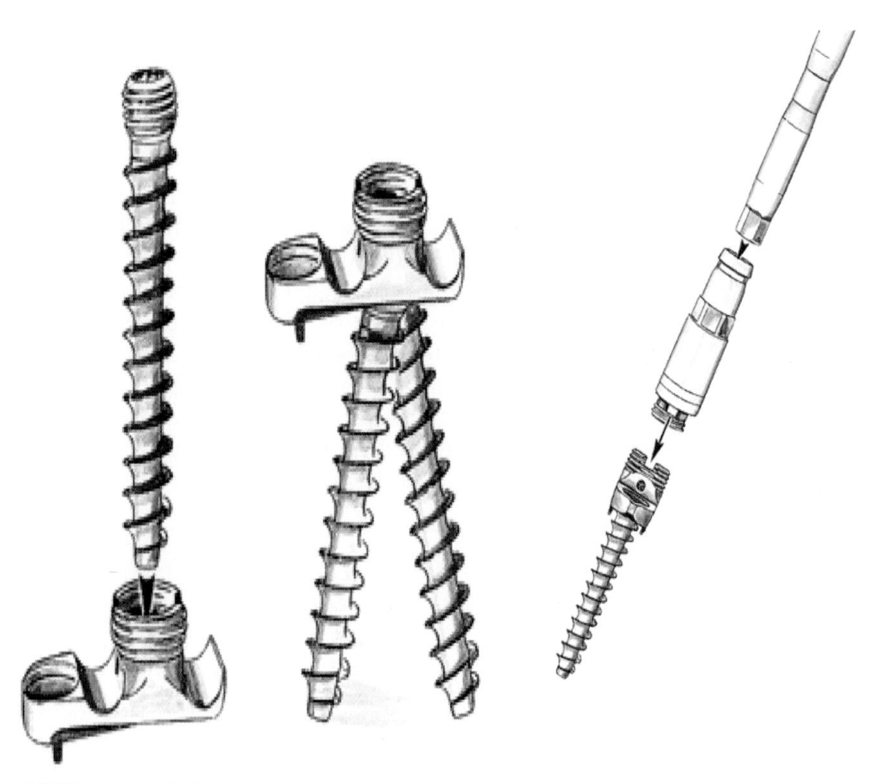

FIGURE 17–12 Centralizer attachment.

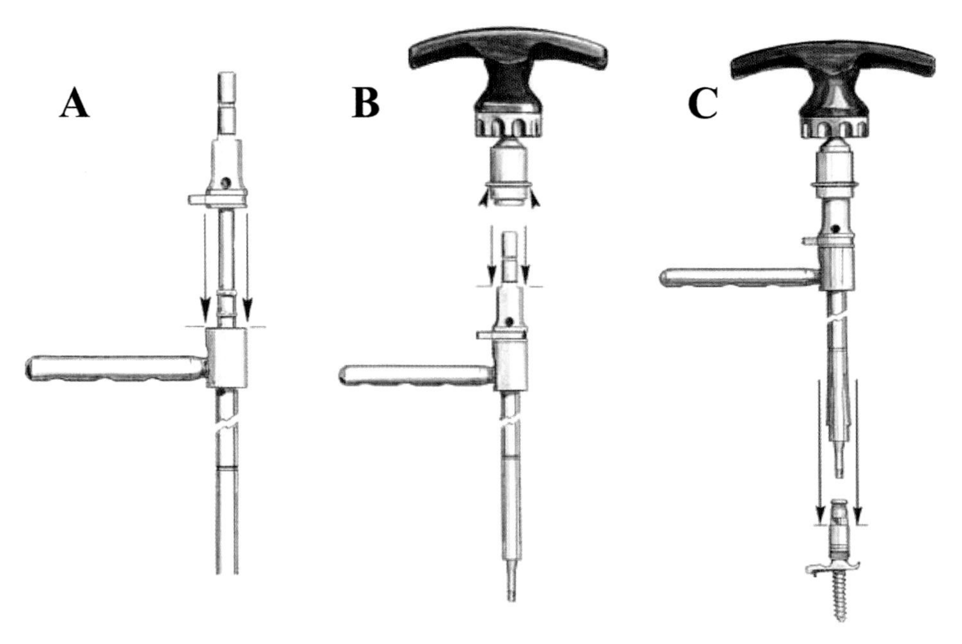

FIGURE 17–13 **(A–C)** Diagram showing the steps in the assembly of the insertion instrument.

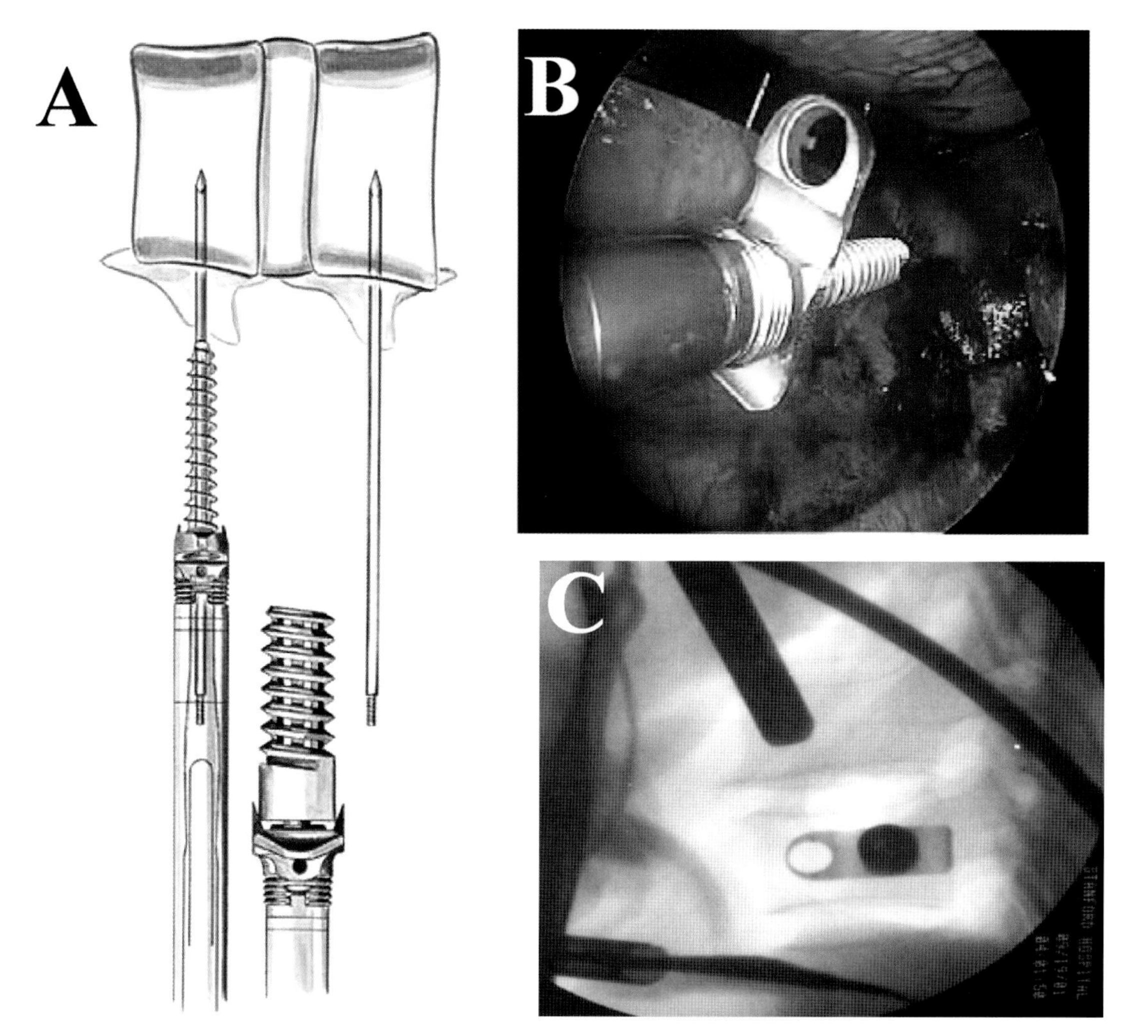

FIGURE 17–14 **(A)** Diagram showing the technique of screw insertion over the K-wire. **(B)** Endoscopic and **(C)** radiographic images of screw insertion.

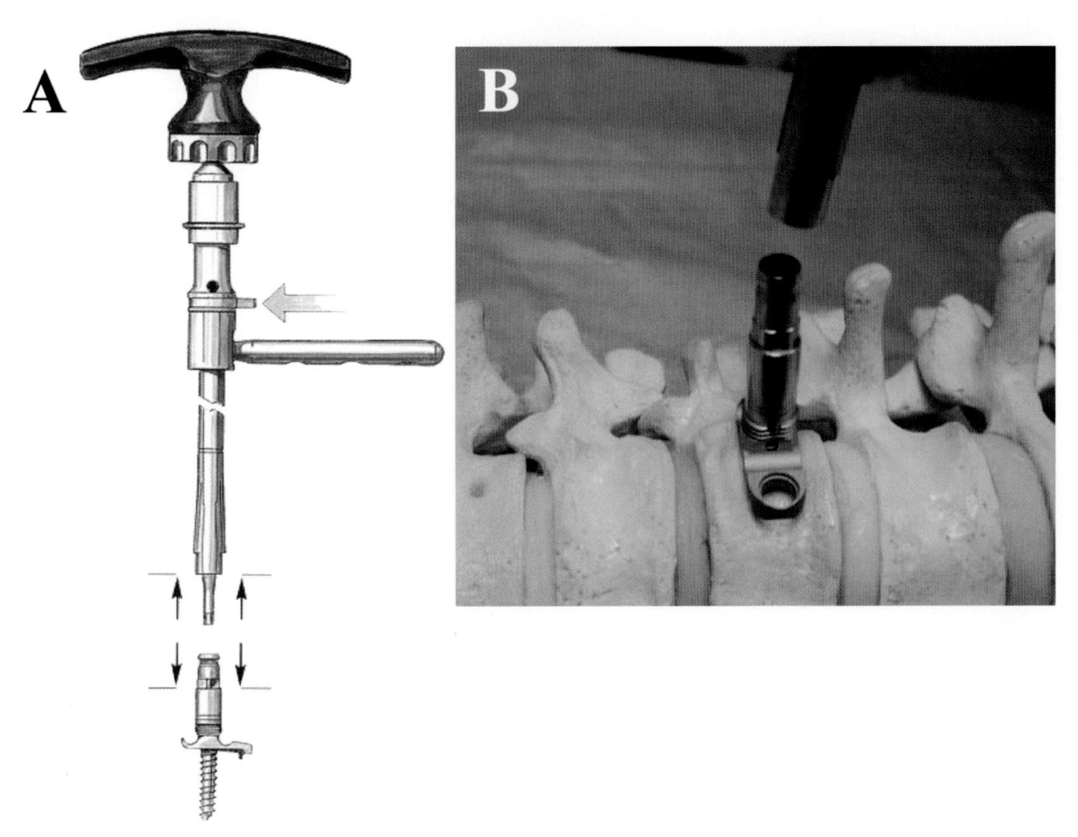

FIGURE 17–15 (A) Diagram showing insertion instrument removal. **(B)** Insertion instrument removal shown in a saw bone model.

K-Wire Removal

After partial insertion of the polyaxial screws, the K-wire has to be removed. Insert the removal instrument through the insertion instrument, and attach it to the K-wire by turning the removal instrument clockwise and screwing it onto the wire. The K-wire can then be pulled out through the cannulated instrument.

Insertion Instrument Removal

Push the slide of the insertion instrument, then release the instrument from the centralizer by pulling backward. The segmental vessels of the fractured vertebra are then mobilized, closed with vascular clips, and dissected (Fig. 17–15).

Distraction Maneuvers

After diskectomy or vertebrectomy and proper preparation of the graft bed, distraction can be applied to the vertebral bodies to insert a graft that is slightly larger than the prepared disk space and to achieve graft compression.

Place the distraction ratchet (Fig. 17–16) over the centralizers using holding forceps. According to the distance between the centralizers, choose the appropriate distraction bar. Before placing the ratchet onto the centralizers, unlock the bolt to allow the instrument to slide and be adjusted to the proper distance. After placing the distraction ratchets on the centralizers, engage the distraction forceps between the ratchet sleeves. Before applying the distraction forceps, lock the bolt.

Corpectomy and Decompression of the Spinal Canal

The extent of the planned partial vertebrectomy is defined with an osteotome.

First, open the disk spaces to define the borders. After resecting the intervertebral disk(s), carefully remove the fragmented parts of the vertebra with rongeurs. Radical removal of nonfractured parts of the vertebral body should be avoided. Resection close to the spinal canal is facilitated with the use of high-speed burrs. If decompression of the spinal canal is necessary, the lower border of the pedicle should first be identified with a blunt hook. The base of the pedicle should then be resected in a cranial direction with a Kerrison rongeur, and the thecal sac can be identified. Finally, the posterior fragment that occupies the spinal canal can be removed (Fig. 17–17).[2,3]

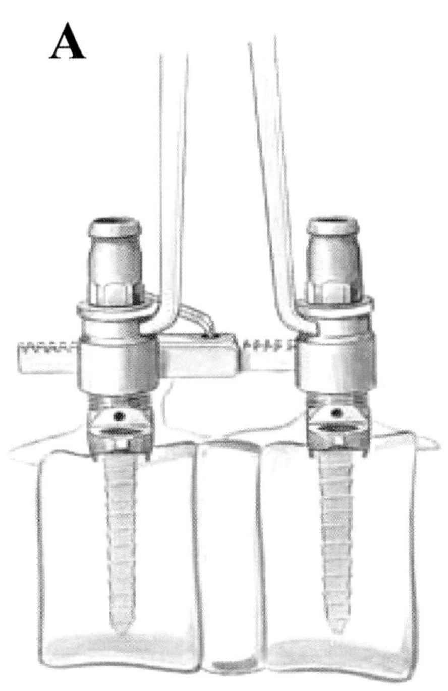

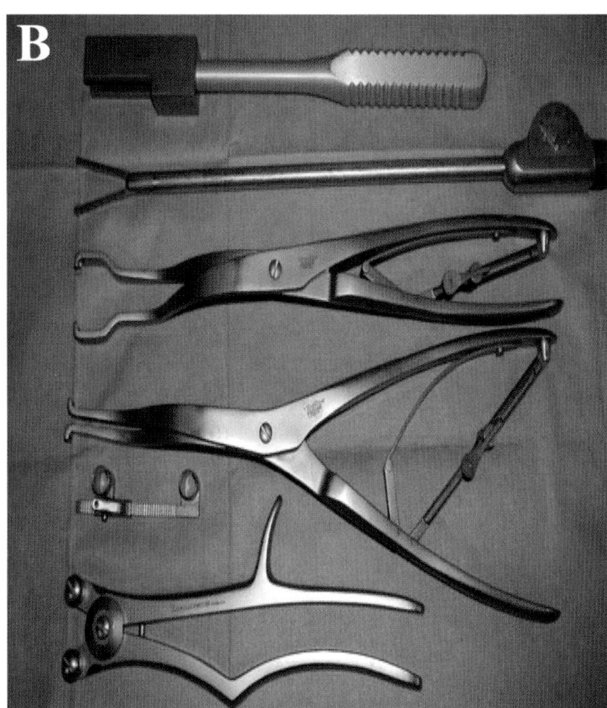

FIGURE 17–16 (A) Drawing showing the distraction maneuver using a distraction ratchet. **(B)** Various compression and distraction instrumentation and plate/rod benders used for MACS-TL instrumentation.

Bone Grafting/Cage Placement

Preparation of the graft bed is then completed, and the length and depth of the bone graft can be measured with a caliper. First, a tricortical bone is taken from the iliac crest. If the bone graft is longer than 2 cm, the iliac crest should be reconstructed. The bone graft should be prepared for insertion and mounted on a graft holder. The cortical bone is perforated with several burr holes to facilitate vascular ingrowth and new bone formation. Next, the working portal is removed, and a speculum is inserted. This allows the insertion of a bone graft up to 1.5 cm in length into the thoracic cavity. If the bone graft is longer, it is inserted without the use of a speculum, but with the help of Langenbeck hooks. In this case, the bone graft is mounted on the graft holder inside the thoracic cavity. Finally, insert the bone graft by press-fitting it into the graft bed. If slight reduction maneuvers are necessary, this can be achieved by manual pressure on the spinous processes of the involved segment, thus creating a segmental lordosis.

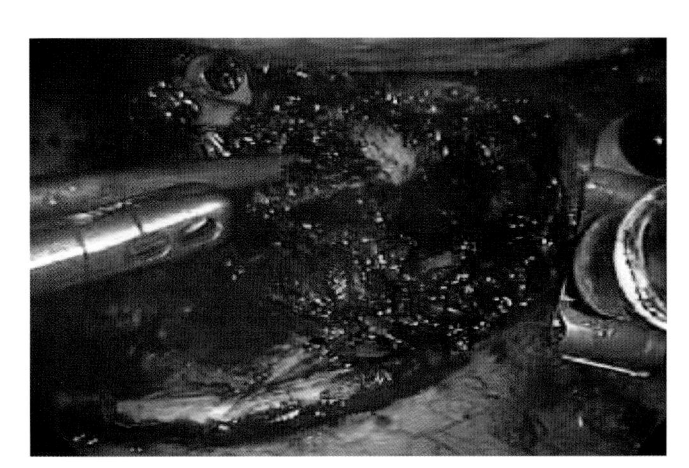

FIGURE 17–17 Thoracoscopic view showing corpectomy and decompression of the spinal canal.

Plate/Rod Placement

The distance between the polyaxial heads has to be measured. If plates are used, 30 mm must be added to select the proper plate length. The stabilization plate is then placed over the centralizer onto the polyaxial heads. The rounded side with the markings is on the upper side of the plate.

In cases of multisegmental assemblies, rod connection has to be chosen. Both rods have to be contoured in the same fashion. The anterior border of the polyaxial plate is slightly lower than the posterior. Thus, the posterior rod can be placed and temporarily closed by slightly tightening the nut to avoid rod loosening. A placement of the anterior rod is now still possible.

For both types of clamp, a degree of freedom should be preserved to allow angulation of the polyaxial heads. Final screw insertion is performed after the plates are placed and tightened with the fixation nuts (Fig. 17–18).

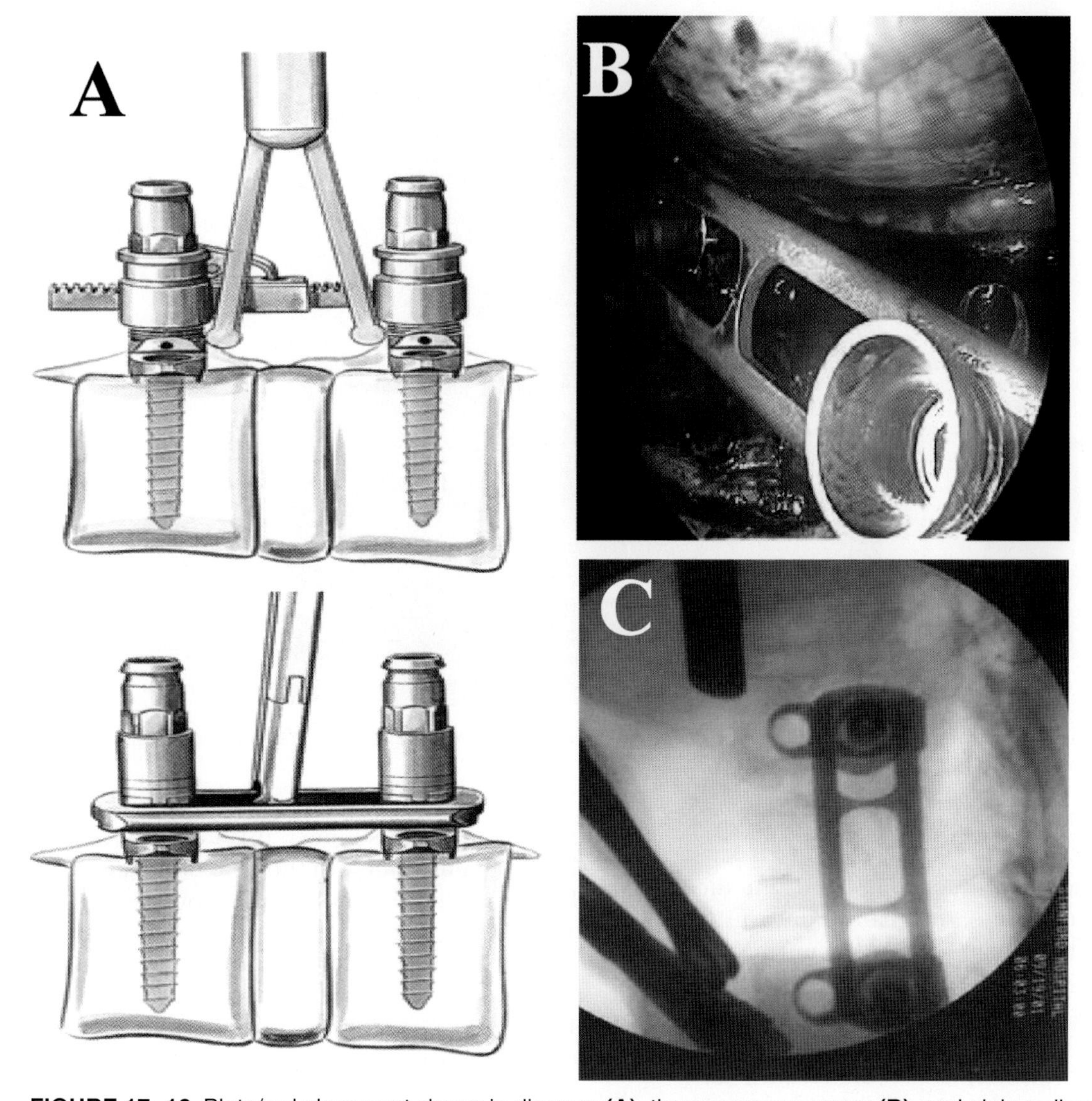

FIGURE 17–18 Plate/rod placement shown in diagram **(A)**, thoracoscopy surgery **(B)**, and plain radiograph **(C)**.

Final Fixation

Next, the insertion sleeve is attached on the centralizer. After the plate or rod is placed and the polyaxial plate is well aligned, the assembly can be closed by using a fixation nut. The nut should be placed with the smooth part against the stabilization plate. Using the cannulated nut driver, the nut can be placed over the centralizer. To apply countertorque during the tightening process of the nut, attach the handle to the insertion sleeve. Prefixation can be achieved using the nut driver with the countertorque handle. For final fixation, the torque wrench is applied to the nut driver, and countertorque is again applied by using the handle on the insertion sleeve. Thus, no torque is applied to the spine (Fig. 17–19).

Removal of the Centralizer

To remove the centralizer, attach the insertion sleeve with the handle and hex key to the centralizer. Remove the centralizer from the polyaxial clamp by turning the screwdriver counterclockwise (Fig. 17–20A).

Tightening of the Polyaxial Screws

Next, the assembly must be brought into final position directly onto the surface of the vertebral bodies. To achieve this, insert the screws until the plate is in direct contact with the bone (Fig. 17–20B).

Insertion of the Anterior Screw

The screw-guiding sleeve for the anterior stabilization screw has to be attached to the polyaxial clamp. To do so,

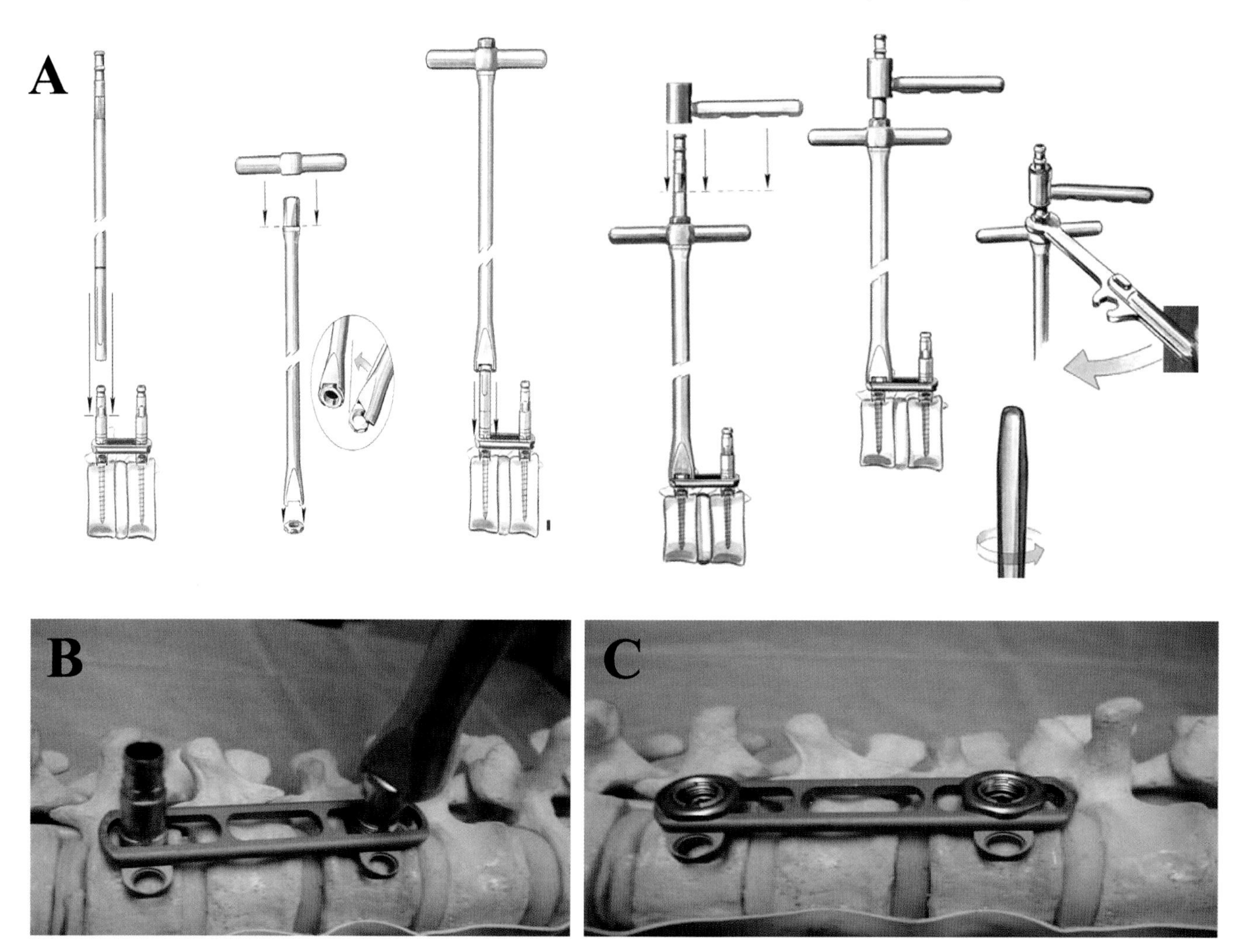

FIGURE 17–19 Illustrative diagrams **(A)** showing the final fixation of the polyaxial screw. Bone model **(B,C)** showing the final fixation of the screw.

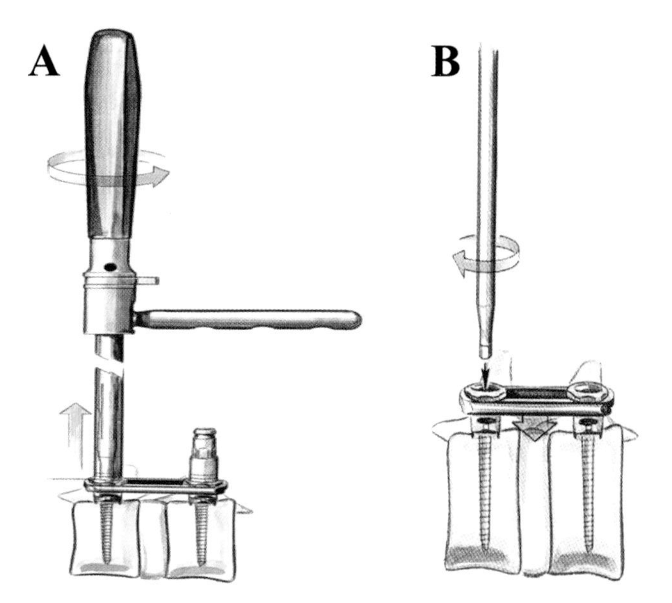

FIGURE 17–20 Diagram showing centralizer removal **(A)** and tightening **(B)** of the polyaxial screws.

insert the insertion sleeve with the handle and the hex key for the centralizer to the hexagonal end of the guiding instrument (same mechanism as for the centralizer). With the central punch, the cortex is then penetrated. After selecting the appropriate screw length, fix the anterior screw to the screwdriver with a retaining clip, then insert it through the guiding instrument into the vertebral body (Fig. 17–21). The guiding instrument can then be removed (same mechanism as removal of the centralizer).

Insertion of Locking Screws

To lock the polyaxial mechanism, attach the yellow locking screw to the screwdriver with a retaining clip. The instrument has to be positioned perpendicular to the plate/rod. Tighten the locking screw with a torque of 10 nm (Fig. 17–22). The torque wrench is applied to the screwdriver.

Closure

The retractor should be rearranged and the gap in the diaphragm closed with staples or adaptive sutures using

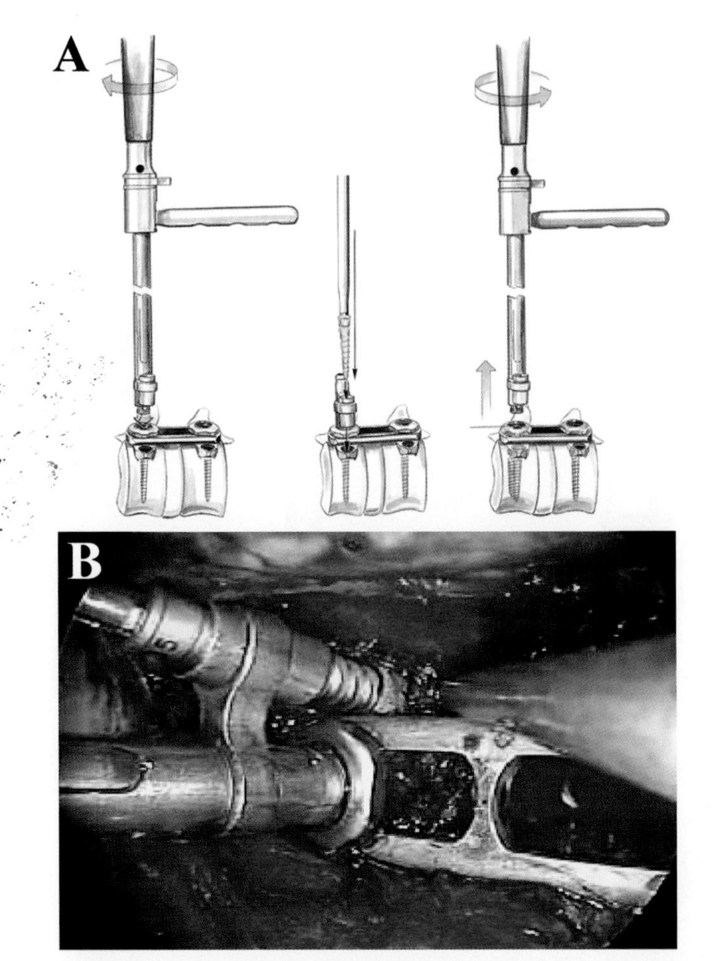

FIGURE 17–21 Diagram **(A)** and thoracoscopic view **(B)** showing insertion of the anterior screw.

the endoscopic technique (Fig. 17–23). Irrigate the thoracic cavity, remove any blood clots, and insert a chest tube with the end placed in the costodiaphragmatic recess. The portals can be closed with sutures after removal of the trocars (Fig. 17–24).

Postoperative Care

The patient is extubated immediately after the operation. Anteroposterior and lateral x-rays of the target area are performed postoperatively. In patients with chronic obstructive pulmonary disease, elderly patients, and patients with cardiovascular disease, artificial ventilation may be necessary for the first 24 hours after the operation. Low-dose, low-molecular-weight heparin is given for thromboembolic prophylaxis. The patient stays in the intensive care unit for 24 hours. Chest tubes can usually be removed on the first postoperative day. Mobilization and ventilation training start on the first postoperative day. Physiotherapy is started (1 hour/day) on the second postoperative day. From the third postoperative week, physiotherapy is intensified to 2 to 3 hours daily. Plain x-ray is obtained on the second postoperative day, after 9 weeks, as well as after 6 and 12 months. The patient is allowed to return to work after 12 to 16 weeks.

Results

The rate of conversion to the open procedure is less than 1% in our series of more than 400 cases. The average operating time of 2.5 to 3 hours, which can now be achieved for ventral treatment of fresh injuries, almost equals that for dorsal stabilization with transpedicular fusion and fixation. The average blood loss of 250 to 450 ml from the ventral endoscopic operation is less than that of a dorsal procedure. We observed a fusion of 90% with the MACS-TL system at 1-year radiological follow-up.

The essential advantages of the minimally invasive surgery on the spine include the reduction of postoperative pain, the related earlier recovery of function, and the reduction in duration and intensity of painkiller administered. The aesthetic and cosmetic results (Fig. 17–25) also speak in favor of the minimally invasive procedure, reducing the emotional damage caused among the predominantly young patient group by minimizing distressing scar formation. The impression that postoperative morbidity, as well as rehabilitation time, could be shortened by the endoscopic approach was shown in a clinical study comparing the results of 30 patients, following either open or endoscopic treatment. In the endoscopic group, the duration of application of analgesics was decreased by 31%, and the overall dosage of applied analgesics was decreased by 42%.[2] These results are supported by comparing our own results with those published by Faciszewski et al.[5] In this multicenter study[4] the complication rate of a total of 1223 open anterior approaches to the thoracic and lumbar spine were reported. The postoperative rate of pleural effusion, intercostal neuralgia, and pneumothorax was 14%, compared with 5.4% in our own series. The infection rate in the study was 0.57%, compared with 0.53% in ours.

Complications

The thoracoscopic procedure for corpectomy and instrumentation is relatively new, but the spectrum of complications is similar to that of open thoracotomy or thoracoabdominal approaches. The overall complication rate of the thoracoscopic technique is similar to or even less than the rate associated with postoperative functional recovery. In our series of more than 400 cases covering 5 years, such access-related complications as pleural effusion, pneumothorax, and intercostal neuralgia occurred in 5.4%. No hernia or relaxation of the diaphragm has been recorded. One transient injury of the L1 root occurred during thoracoscopic detachment of the diaphragm.

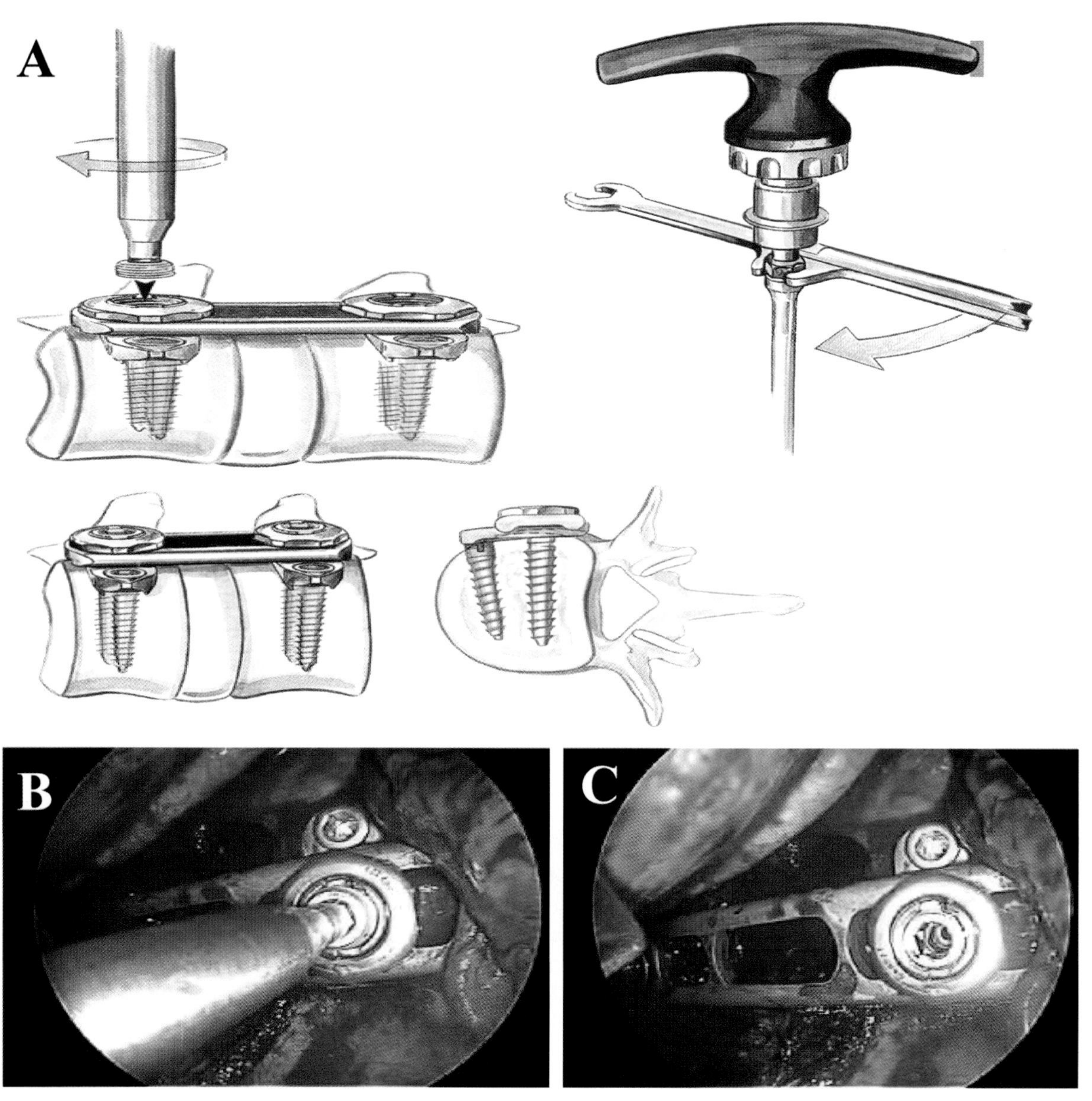

FIGURE 17–22 Diagrams **(A)** and thoracoscopic views **(B,C)** showing the insertion of locking screws.

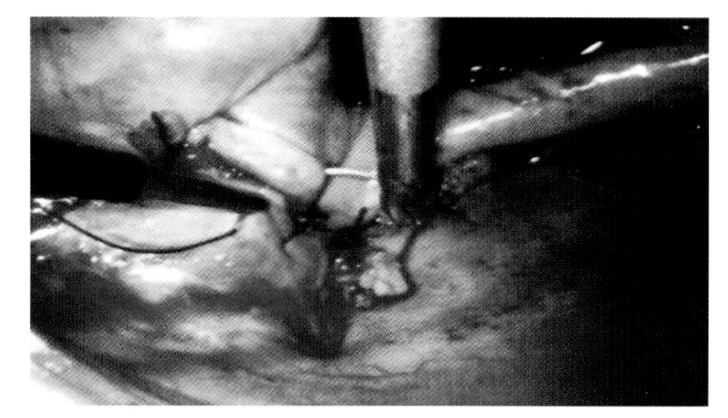

FIGURE 17–23 Thoracoscopic view showing repair of the diaphragm with adaptive sutures.

Injuries to major organs (lung or heart), the aorta, and vena cava are the most hazardous intraoperative complications. Distorted spine anatomy and insufficient preparation of the segmental vessels can result in accidental injury, bleeding, and loss of visual control. Other complications (e.g., dural tear, peritoneum opening, lung injury, and nerve injury by uncontrolled monopolar coagulation) can occur. Possible intraoperative complications are hemothorax, recurrent pleural effusion, intrathoracic adhesion, deep wound infection, and implant failure. Most of these complications occurred early in a series as a result of technical difficulties. With the use of the more endoscopically friendly MACS-TL implant, the complication rate has decreased gradually. Implant failure has been very rare in our

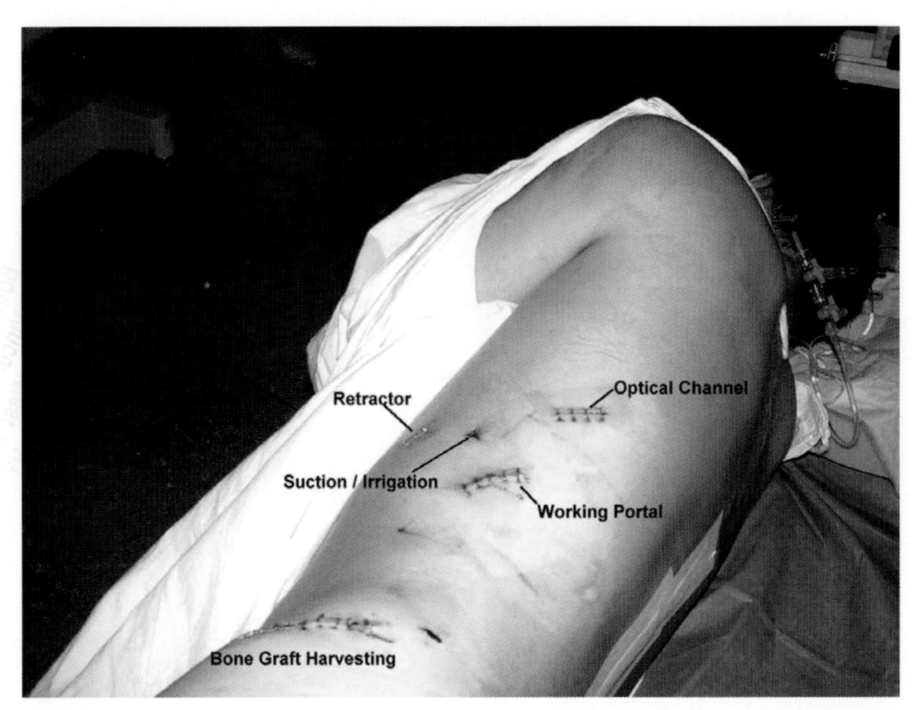

FIGURE 17–24 Closure of portal sites following thoracoscopic surgery and iliac bone graft harvesting.

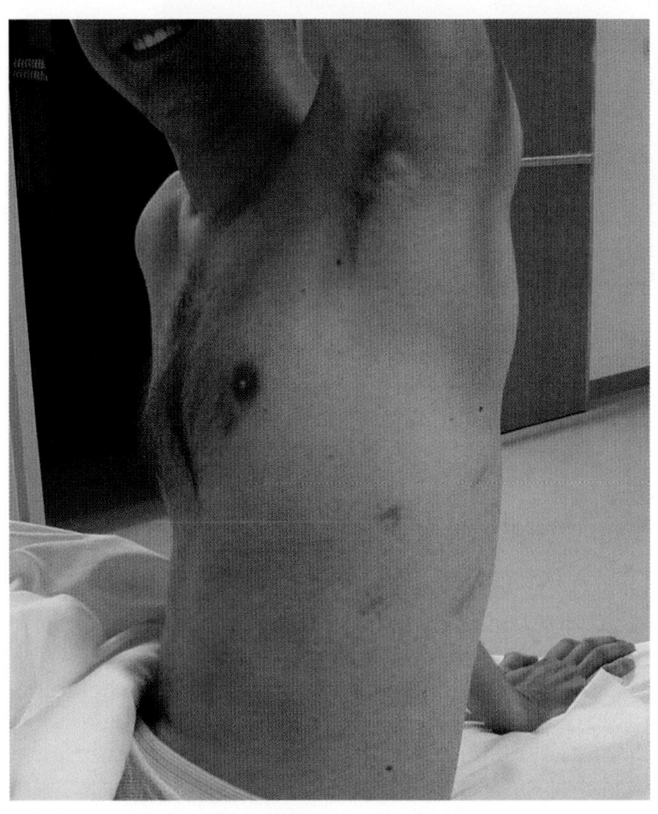

FIGURE 17–25 Postoperative scars following thoracoscopic surgery after 6 months, with excellent cosmetic result.

experience since introducing the MACS-TL system, which is suitable for endoscopic use and provides highly stable fixation. Implant loosening was caused in two patients by advanced osteoporosis. As the analysis of plain x-ray and CT images showed, the assembly of individual components held and did not alter over time, but the entire implant assembly shifted its position in vertebral bodies. Thus, if osteoporosis is suspected, extensive dorsal and shorter ventral fixation should be considered.

Some of these complications require thoracotomy or open revision, which abolishes all the advantages of minimally invasive procedures. In our series, four patients needed conversion to open surgery. This was necessary in two of the first five cases, in one case due to bleeding, and in the other due to technical difficulty. The third conversion was made due to leakage from the aorta. The fourth conversion was made due to upper thoracic injury. Thus, careful preoperative evaluation and meticulous manipulation are essential to prevent disastrous complications.

Technical Tips

To get desirable results with thoracoscopic surgery, every step should be done carefully to avoid complications. First of all, correct positioning of the patient and the C-arm is essential. Incorrect positioning of the patient or the C-arm may result in misplacement of the screws. Even current fluoronavigation systems may not help to avoid this problem when the correct position is not established properly. Selection of working portals upon correct positioning is also critical to insert screws correctly and to prevent instrument conflicts. Insufficient preparation of the segmental vessels can result in accidental injury, bleeding, and loss by uncontrolled monopolar coagulation. Thus, the use of monopolar cauterization should be cautious near segmental arteries as well as nerve roots. Insufficient preparation of the graft bed may lead to forceful impaction, with the risk of indirect injury to the dura and spinal nerves due to displacement of bone or disk fragments into the spinal canal or foramen. To prevent these complications, meticulous dissection with proper bleeding control is mandatory.

Future Developments

Current minimally invasive thoracoscopic spine surgery has been developed with improvement of endoscopic techniques and instrumentation. Future development of this procedure can be enhanced with the help of an image-guided system (IGS) and a surgical robotic arm. CT- and MRI-based navigation has several limitations, but fluoroscopic navigation can provide near-real-time imaging. The authors' initial experience using an IGS was impressive, especially in cases involving tumor deformity or trauma. This combination technique is also helpful in driving the screws for short-segment combined (anterior and posterior) fixation. Another potential possibility to improve the effectiveness of the thoracoscopic procedure is to utilize a surgical robotic arm. Surgical robotic procedures have already been developed for such things as cardiac bypass, but their application in spinal surgery is very limited, even with conventional spinal procedures. The operating theater for the thoracoscopic procedure is quite complex, with two video towers, endoscopic equipment, the C-arm fluoroscopic device, and numerous lines. Furthermore, two or three assistant surgeons are essential for proper retraction and endoscopic control. One or two articulated robotic arms, however, can be used for thoracoscopic procedures. For example, current cardiac bypass technique using robotic arms can be applied for diaphragmatic detachment and repair with little modification. Application of the robotic arm for suction/irrigation/retraction or the articulated arm for screw insertion/diskectomy can also be applied. These robotic arms can be controlled within the small endoscopic working space with voice activation or by using a foot pedal. Application of this technique can lessen the need for assistants, facilitate procedures, and improve surgical results with time saving. Refinement of these technologies can immensely benefit patients as well as surgeons.

Case Illustration

An 18-year-old female presented following a motor vehicle accident with weakness and numbness in the lower extremities. An examination revealed grade paraparesis and diminished sensations below the L2 dermatome. An x-ray (Fig. 17–26A) of the lumbar spine revealed a burst

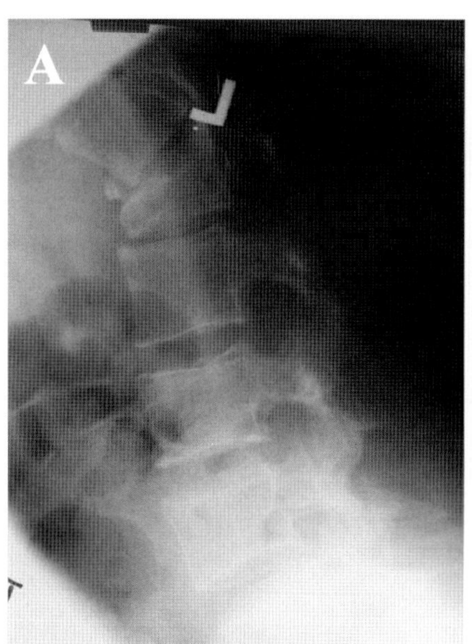

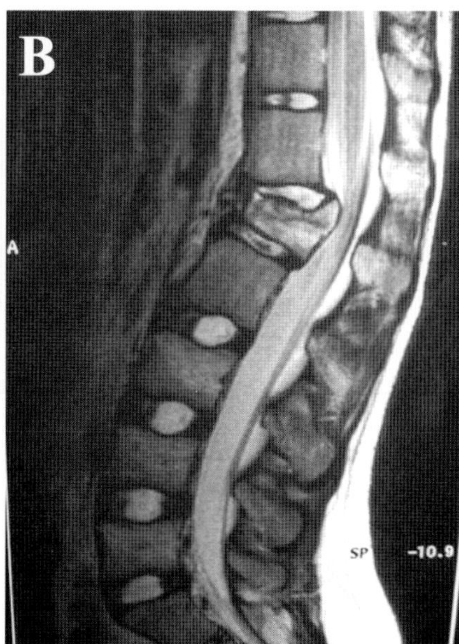

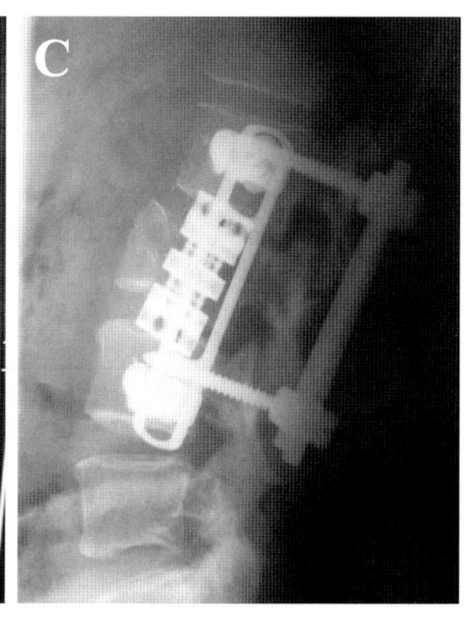

FIGURE 17–26 **(A)** Plain radiograph showing burst fracture of L1 vertebra. **(B)** MRI showing the burst fracture of L1 vertebra with severe compression of the spinal cord with the retropulsed bony fragments. **(C)** Postoperative radiographs following anterior thoracoscopic decompression, reconstruction of anterior column with distractable vertebral body reconstruction cage, and combined anterior (MACS-TL system) and posterior stabilization with excellent correction of deformity.

fracture of the L1 vertebra. MRI (Fig. 17–26B) revealed retropulsion of fracture fragments with severe compression of the spinal cord. The patient underwent a posterior stabilization with pedicle screws followed by thoracoscopic decompression of the L1 vertebral body reconstruction (VBR) with a distractable cage, and instrumentation with the MACS-TL system. Postoperative radiographs (Fig. 17–26C) showed excellent correction of the deformity. The patient was neurologically intact at 3 months' follow-up.

Thoracoscopic procedures for corpectomy and instrumentation are based on classic spinal surgery principles of repositioning, reconstruction, and retention of the anterior section of the spine. Thoracoscopic corpectomy and reconstruction have developed with this basic concept. This development was helped by a continuous improvement in instruments, which make it possible to perform even such subtle operations as anterior decompression of the spinal cord under endoscopic visualization.

Although thoracoscopic decompression and instrumentation are technically demanding, earlier functional recovery and better postoperative pain reduction can be achieved when compared with thoracotomy or the thoracoabdominal approach. To achieve good results with thoracoscopic procedures, the surgeon should get hands-on training in a laboratory before clinical implementation. This implies the necessity of training and influences the learning curve each surgeon has to master in adopting this technique. Thoracoscopic surgery can be performed safely, as reflected by lower complication rates and shorter operating times, which are at least comparable to open procedures.

REFERENCES

1. Magerl F, Aebi S, Gertzbein SD, Harms I, Nazarian S. A comprehensive classification of thoracic and lumbar injuries. *Eur Spine J.* 1994;3:184–201.
2. Beisse R, Potalski M, Temme C, Buhren V. Endoscopically controlled division of the diaphragm: a minimally invasive approach to ventral management of thoracolumbar fractures of the spine. *Unfallchirurg.* 1998;101:619–627.
3. Khoo LT, Beisse R, Potulski M. Thoracoscopic-assisted treatment of thoracic and lumbar fractures: a series of 371 consecutive cases. *Neurosurgery.* 2002;51(suppl 5):104–117.
4. Beisse R, Potulski M, Buhren V. Endoscopic techniques for the management of spinal trauma. *Eur J Trauma.* 2001;27:275–291.
5. Faciszewski T, Winter RB, Lonstein JE, Francis D, Johnson L. The surgical and medical perioperative complications of anterior spinal fusion surgery in the thoracic and lumbar spine in adults. *Spine.* 1995;20:1592–1599.

SECTION FOUR

Lumbar Spine

18

Posterolateral Selective Endoscopic Diskectomy: The YESS Technique

ANTHONY T. YEUNG AND CHRISTOPHER A. YEUNG

The intervertebral disk, an important supporting structure of the spinal column, is implicated as a major source of low back pain and sciatica.[1] The pathogenesis of disk degeneration and herniation is complex and multifactorial, but it was clearly outlined and documented by Wolfgang Rauschning's work illustrating the pathoanatomy of degenerative disk disease and degenerative conditions of the lumbar spine.[2] Most disk herniations are not the result of an acute event; rather, they are an accumulation of several insults to the spine that lead to degeneration, annular tears, and eventual disk herniation. There are several theories of disk degeneration, including mechanical, chemical, age-related, autoimmune, and genetic. Within the mechanical theory, the following types of abnormal loads have been proven experimentally to cause disk injury: torsion, compression, repetitive compressive loading in flexion,[3] hyperflexion,[4] and vibration.

Disk surgery has traditionally been reserved for disk herniations causing radiculopathy or nerve deficits due to mechanical compression on the spinal nerves. This is due to the inherent morbidity of the posterior surgical approach that must violate and alter the important function of the posterior spinal column. Open posterior diskectomy often includes or requires a midline incision, muscle and ligament stripping, prolonged muscle retraction, bone resection of the lamina and facet, and nerve root and dural tube retraction. This can cause instability and scarring around the sensitive nerve roots, even in a technically perfect operation. The morbidity of the standard posterior approach has therefore limited the use of surgery as an early treatment option in the cascade of disk degeneration and herniation. Thus, surgery was often not recommended for herniations without neurologic deficits, "small" herniations, central herniations, and annular tears. The dogma that "disk surgery is really decompressive nerve surgery" dominates the rationale for traditional microdiskectomy for herniated disks.

Minimally invasive surgical options that limit the inherent approach-related morbidity are possible with the posterolateral portal.[5–13] This approach to the disk is most challenging at the L5–S1 level due to the prominence of the iliac crest. Most L5–S1 disk spaces are accessible; however, entry into the disk may require foraminal decompression of the lateral facet.

The least invasive of all posterolateral intradiskal techniques is the injection of chymopapain, a treatment option validated by at least two large prospective, randomized double-blind studies and numerous cohort studies.[14] This treatment produced satisfactory results in many studies and came into widespread clinical use in the 1970s, but it lost popularity with reports of complications as severe as anaphylactic shock and transverse myelitis. Although these complications can now be virtually eliminated with preoperative antigen screening and diskography, the perceived risk has limited its continued use. More recent studies from experienced chymopapain users still tout chymopapain as a valuable adjunct to endoscopic disk surgery.[15]

The introduction of the operating microscope for diskectomy by Yasargil in 1967 and later by Williams encouraged smaller incisions for the standard posterior approach.[16,17] The transcanal microscope-assisted technique became the gold standard; however, it still requires retraction of the dural tube and nerve, periosteal stripping of the muscle and ligaments, hemilaminotomy,

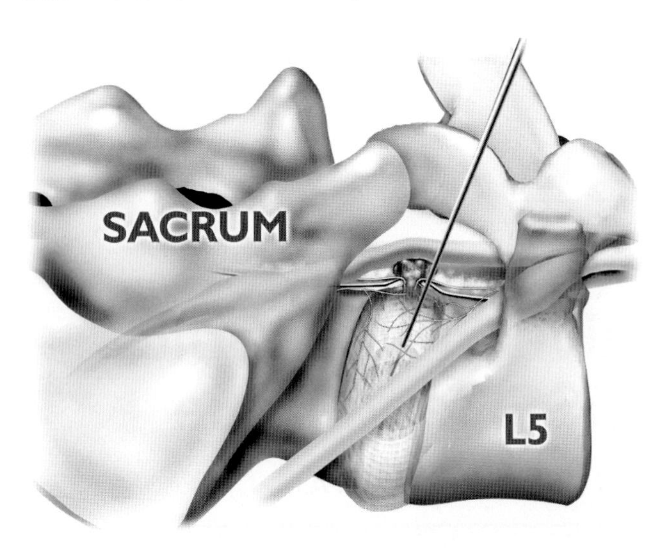

FIGURE 18–1 Kambin's triangular working zone is the site of surgical access for posterolateral endoscopic disketomy. It is defined as a right triangle over the dorsolateral disk. The hypotenuse is the exiting nerve root, the base (width) is the superior border of the caudal vertebra, and the height is the dura/traversing nerve root.

and regional or general anesthesia. Tubular retractors have recently been developed that can be used with either a microscope or an endoscope for this posterior transcanal approach.[18] This utilizes tissue dilation rather than cutting and minimizes the superficial tissue destruction, but it still requires the same amount of bone removal and neural manipulation as the standard microscopic posterior diskectomy.

The concept of indirect decompression of the spinal canal via a posterolateral, extracanal approach was introduced by Kambin in 1973 using a Craig cannula for limited nucleotomy in combination with a transcanal approach.[7,8] In 1975 Hijikata reported the first standalone nonvisualized posterolateral percutaneous central nucleotomy.[6]

Kambin went on to describe the safe triangular working zone (Kambin's triangle) (Fig. 18–1) and results of arthroscopic microdiskectomy, in which arthroscopic visualization of the herniation via the posterolateral approach was used for diskectomy of contained herniations.[5,7,8] Hermantin et al[5] reported satisfactory results from video-assisted arthroscopic microdiskectomy in 97% of patients, compared with 93% in traditional microdiskectomy with an average of 31 months' follow-up. The arthroscopic group had less narcotic use and less time off from work. The study was prospective and randomized, with 30 subjects in each group.

Mayer and Brock also showed promising results in a prospective randomized study comparing percutaneous diskectomy with microscopic diskectomy for contained or slight subligamentous herniations.[9] The percutaneous group showed comparable or superior results. Long-term disability, defined by return to work status, produced statistically significant differences. In the percutaneous group, 95% returned to their previous occupation, compared with 72.2% in the microdiskectomy group. Each group had 20 subjects.

Evolving methodology in the 1980s and early 1990s allowed for endoscopic lumbar nerve root decompression by a visualized, direct excision of contained and noncontained herniated disk fragments.[8,9,11,13]

Yeung[12] introduced a rigid rod-lens, flow-integrated, multichannel, wide-angle operating spinal endoscope in 1998 that allowed for even more flexibility accessing the disk and traversing and exiting nerve roots and the epidural space. The endoscope configuration offered significant visual improvement, and the complementary instrument system with specialized slotted and bevel-ended tubular access cannulas allowed for same-field viewing of the intradiskal space, annular wall, and epidural space. The Yeung Endoscopic Spine Surgery (YESS) technique allows for improved access to the posterior disk for visualized fragment resection, improved access to the undersurface of the superior articular facet for foraminoplasty, and protection of the neural structures by rotating the cannula.[12]

Indications

The following are indications for employment of the YESS technique:

- All lumbar disk herniations except migrated/sequestered fragments inaccessible through the foramen
- Annular tears
- Internal disk disruption (IDD), diagnosed with diskography producing concordant pain and radiographic abnormalities
- Foraminal stenosis
- Synovial cysts of the facet joint
- Diskitis

Perhaps the ideal lesion for posterolateral selective endoscopic diskectomy is the far lateral extraforaminal disk herniation. The exiting nerve is routinely visualized, and the cannula inserts directly at the herniation site. This approach requires less manipulation of the exiting nerve root than the paramedian posterior approach.

Any herniation contiguous with the disk space not sequestered and migrated is amenable to endoscopic disk excision. The timing of surgical treatment is similar to posterior transcanal diskectomy. The size and types of herniations chosen by the surgeon for endoscopic excision will depend on the skill and experience of the surgeon as well as the anatomic considerations in the patient relative to the location of the herniation. All contained disk herniations are certainly appropriate for endoscopic decompression. With experience, extruded herniations can be routinely addressed.

The posterolateral endoscopic approach only requires tissue dilation to accommodate a 7 mm working cannula. This tissue-sparing approach offers consideration for earlier surgical timing when approach-related risk:benefit ratios are factored in after patients fail conservative treatment and continue to have debilitating pain without neurologic deficit. Quality of life issues and functional issues associated with chronic diskogenic pain can be addressed with this minimally invasive surgical option; therefore, small disk herniations with predominant leg pain, central disk herniations with predominant back pain, IDD, and annular tears causing chemical sciatica are amenable to disk surgery by endoscopic means.

The diskectomy decompresses the disk, alleviating pressure on the anulus, and removes any unstable degenerated disk fragments that could herniate. Radiofrequency energy can be applied to the annular tears under direct visualization to contract the collagen and ablate ingrown granulation tissue, neoangiogenesis, and sensitized nociceptors. Interpositional nuclear tissue is frequently seen within the fibers of the annular tear, which prevents the tear from healing. This tissue can then be removed to allow the tear to heal.

Endoscopic foraminoplasty can readily be achieved with bone trephines/rasps and the side-firing holmium: yttrium aluminium garnet (YAG) laser.[19] The roof of the foramen is formed by the undersurface of the superior articular facet. This is easily visualized and accessed via the endoscope. The side-firing holmium: YAG laser and bone trephines strip the facet capsule and remove bone to enlarge the foraminal opening. Studies by Osman et al[20] have demonstrated that decompression through the foramen can be more effective than posterior decompression for foraminal stenosis. The posterior removal of one third of the medial facet produces more instability than posterolateral foraminal decompression.[20] Synovial cysts can also be visualized and removed.

Diskitis can be treated with posterolateral endoscopic diskectomy and debridement. Current methods rely on needle aspiration followed by prolonged antibiotic treatment. Needle aspirations are not as reliable as tissue samples from endoscopic debridement and are often negative even in the face of bacterial diskitis. Surgeons are often hesitant to perform open debridement because of the morbidity of the open approach, creation of dead space and devascularized tissue, and concern for spreading the infection in the spinal canal. Endoscopic excisional biopsy and thorough debridement via the posterolateral portal have provided almost immediate pain relief and a much more reliable tissue sample for laboratory analysis and culture. Because only tissue dilation is used, no dead space is created that would allow the infection to spread. Many patients with diskitis have co-morbidities, which make them poor open surgical candidates.

Surgical Equipment

The Yeung Endoscopic Spine Surgery (YESS) system (Richard Wolf GmbH, Knittlingen, Germany) consists of the following instruments (Fig. 18–2):

- Multichannel, 20-degree oval spinal endoscope with 2.7 mm working channel and integrated continuous irrigation (inflow and outflow) ports
- Multichannel, 70-degree oval spinal endoscope
- 7 mm working cannulas with various open slotted, beveled, and tapered ends
- Two-channel tissue dilator/obturator
- Specialized single- and double-action rongeurs for visualized fragmentectomy
- Larger straight and hinged rongeurs for diskectomy and targeted fragmentectomy
- Trephines for annulotomy and foraminoplasty
- Microrasps, curettes, and Penfield probes
- Annulotomy knife
- Flexible bipolar radiofrequency probe for hemostasis, thermal contraction of the annular collagen, and thermal ablation of the annular nociceptors (Ellman trigger-flex bipolar probe)

Adjunctive Equipment

Adjunctive equipment for the YESS technique includes the following:

- Straight and flexible suction-irrigation shavers for diskectomy (Endius MDS)
- Side-firing holmium:YAG laser (Trimedyne)
- Fluid pump for continuous irrigation
- Video-endoscopy tower

Operating Room Setup

Proper OR set up requires a radiolucent table with a hyperkyphotic frame, one C-arm, and a tower with the usual monitor for endoscopic viewing. The operating suite will ideally be equipped to record the procedure, including fluoroscopic images onto video and/or still images. Foot pedals controlling the radiofrequency probe, shaver, suction, C-arm, and laser should be ergonomically arranged. Required personnel include the anesthesiologist, scrub technician, circulator, C-arm

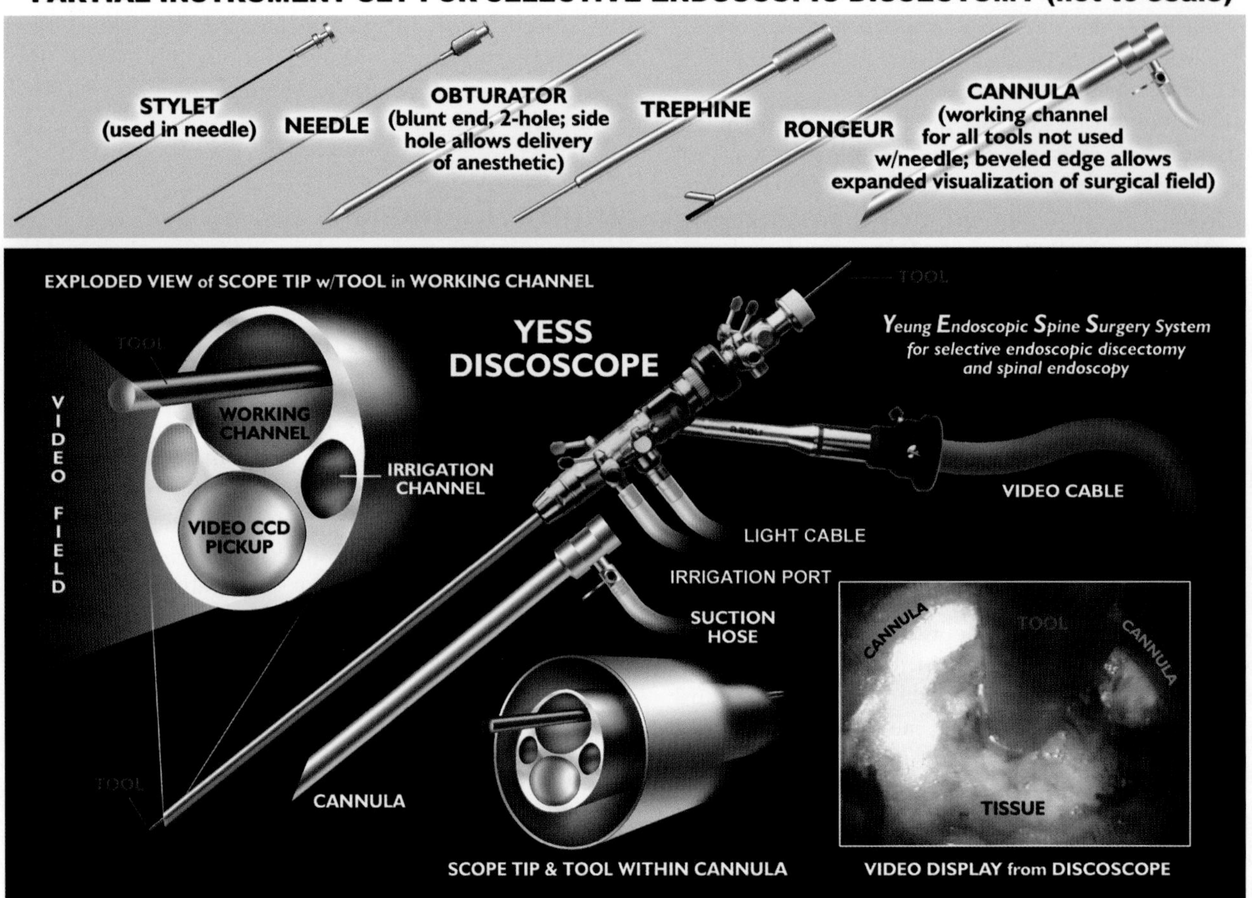

FIGURE 18–2 Partial instrument set for the Yeung Endoscopic Spine Surgery (YESS) technique.

technician, and a surgical assistant if a biportal approach is planned (Fig. 18–3).

The patient is placed prone on the radiolucent hyperkyphotic frame (Kambin frame, US Surgical), with the arms away from the side of the body. Care is taken to line up the patient with the C-arm to ensure a perfect posteroanterior and lateral view on the fluoroscopy. The spinous processes should be centered between the

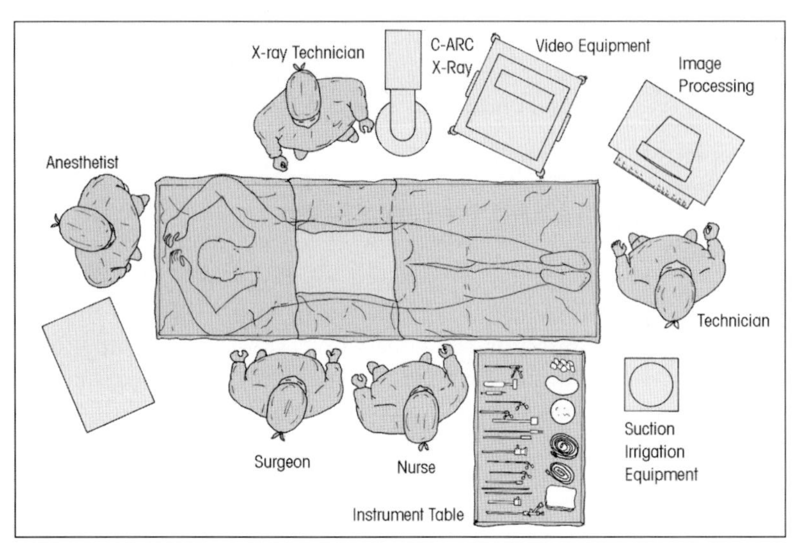

FIGURE 18–3 Proper operating room setup.

pedicles on the posteroanterior (PA) view and the end plates parallel on the lateral view. The surgical level must be centered to avoid parallax error. Anesthesia consists of 0.5% local lidocaine infiltration, supplemented by Versed and fentanyl for conscious sedation. The sedation is kept light enough to allow feedback if the patient experiences any painful nerve root irritation.

Surgical Technique

Protocol for Optimal Needle Placement

Utilizing a thin metal rod as a radiopaque marker and ruler, lines are drawn on the skin to mark surface topography for guidance in free-hand biplane C-arm needle placement. These surface markings help identify three key landmarks for needle placement: the anatomic disk center, the annular foraminal window (centered within the medial and lateral borders of the pedicles), and the skin window (needle entry point) (Fig. 18–4).

- Utilizing a metal rod as radiopaque marker and ruler, draw a longitudinal line over the spinous processes to mark the midline on the PA view.
- Draw a transverse line bisecting the targeted disk space to mark the transverse disk plane on the PA view. The intersection of these two lines marks the anatomic disk center.
- On the lateral fluoroscopic view, draw a line on the patient's side representing the disk inclination plane. This line determines the cephalad/caudal position of the needle entry point. When drawing this disk inclination line, the tip of the metal rod should be at the lateral anatomic disk center, and the rod should bisect and be parallel to the end plates.
- The distance from the rod tip to the plane of the posterior skin is measured by grasping the rod at the point where the posterior skin plane intersects it.
- This distance is then measured on the posterior skin from the midline along the transverse plane line.
- At the lateral extent of this measurement, a line parallel to the midline is drawn to intersect the disk inclination plane line. This intersection marks the skin entry point, or "skin window," for the needle.

The skin window's lateral location from the midline determines the trajectory angle into the foraminal annular window. Using the preceding method, a 45-degree trajectory to the disk should place the needle tip in the true anatomic disk center. This is good for a central nucleotomy to decompress the disk.

Because most of the pathology being treated is located posteriorly, however, placement in the posterior one third of the disk is optimal. Thus, one needs to "fudge" 1 to 2 cm laterally for the optimal skin window placement to access the posterior one third of the disk. This allows one to avoid the facet joint with a shallower needle trajectory (~30 degrees in the coronal plane) to the disk.

On the other hand, one can place the rod tip at the anterior portion of the disk when measuring the disk inclination plane on the lateral fluoroscopic view. This produces a longer measurement to the posterior skin plane, thus placing the skin window more lateral. This is the authors' preferred method. This coordinate system of finding the optimal anatomical landmarks for instrument placement will help decrease the steep learning curve for needle placement and eliminate the less accurate "down the tunnel" method favored by radiologists and pain management physicians.

The positive disk inclination plane of the L5–S1 disk is noteworthy. A steep positive inclination line (lordosis) will position the optimal skin window more cephalad from the transverse plane line, avoiding the high iliac crest. A flatly inclined L5–S1 disk will position the optimal skin window with the iliac crest obstructing the trajectory of the needle. The skin window will have to start more medial to avoid the iliac crest, and sometimes the lateral one fourth of the facet joint must be resected to allow for posterior needle placement in the disk.

The first neutrally aligned disk inclination plane is usually at L4–L5 or L3–L4. A neutrally aligned disk inclination plane is in the same plane as the transverse plane line; thus, the skin window is in line with the transverse plane line. A negatively inclined disk, often at L1–L2 and L2–L3, places the skin window caudal to the transverse plane line.

Needle Placement

Infiltrate the skin window and subcutaneous tissue with 0.5% lidocaine. Insert a 6-inch-long, 18-gauge needle from the skin window at a 25- to 30-degree angle from the coronal plane (reciprocal of 60–65 degrees from the parasagittal plane), anteromedially toward the anatomical disk center. Infiltrate the needle tract with 0.5% lidocaine as you are advancing the needle. The superficial portion of the needle trajectory is usually outside the C-arm viewing perimeter. Once the needle tip is visible within the C-arm viewing perimeter, tilt the C-arm beam parallel to the disk inclination plane (the Ferguson view). This allows one to visualize the advancing needle in the true disk inclination plane. Advance the needle toward the target foraminal annular window. If minor directional adjustments are necessary, use the plane of the needle bevel and hub pressure to navigate. At the first bony resistance or before the needle tip is advanced medial to the pedicle, turn the C-arm to the lateral projection. Do not advance the needle tip medial to the pedicle during the initial approach. Doing so risks inadvertent traversing nerve root and dural puncture.

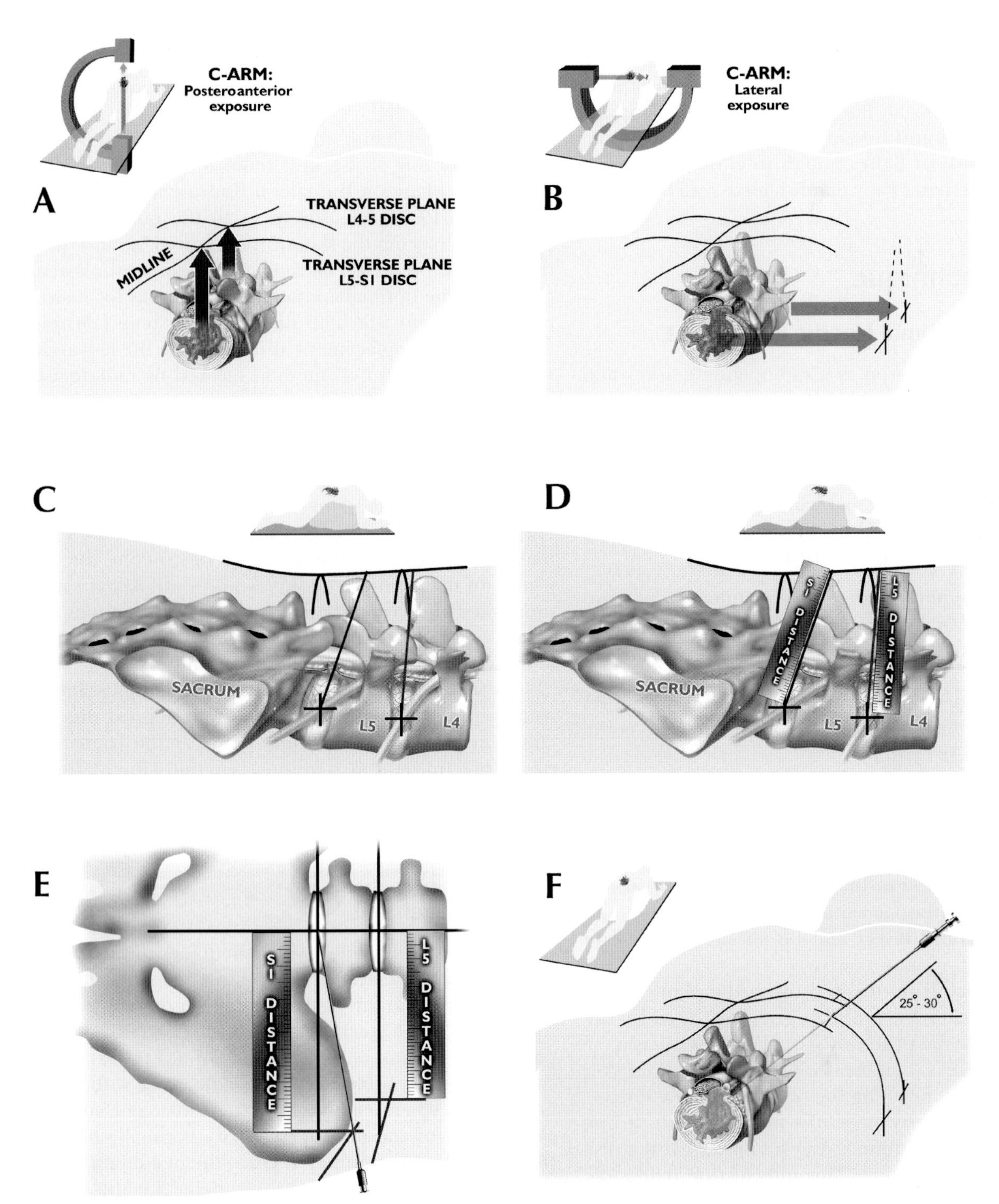

FIGURE 18–4 Protocol for optimal needle placement. **(A)** Posteroanterior (PA) fluoroscopic view enables topographic location of the midline and the transverse disk plane. The intersection of these lines is the PA anatomic disk center. **(B)** Lateral fluoroscopic view enables topographic location of the disk inclination plane. **(C)** The inclination plane of each target disk is drawn on the skin from the lateral disk center. **(D)** The distance from the lateral disk center to the posterior skin plane is measured along the inclination plane. **(E–F)** This same distance is measured from the midline along the transverse disk plane for each target disk. At the end of this measure a line parallel to the midline is drawn to intersect the disk inclination line. This is the skin entry point, or "skin window," for the needle.

The first bony resistance encountered most frequently is the lateral facet. Increase the trajectory angle to aim ventral to the facet, and continue the approach toward the foraminal annular window. Turning the needle bevel to face dorsal helps the needle tip skive off the undersurface of the facet. The C-arm lateral projection should confirm the needle tip's correct annular location. In the lateral view, the correct needle tip position should be just touching the posterior anulus surface. In the PA view, the needle tip should be centered in the foraminal annular window. The preceding two views of the C-arm confirm that the needle tip has engaged the safe zone, the center of the foraminal annular window.

While monitoring the PA view, advance the needle tip through the anulus to the midline (anatomical disk center). Next, check the lateral view. If the needle tip is in the center of the disk on the lateral view, you have a central needle placement, which is good for a central nucleotomy. The needle tip ideally will be in the posterior one third of the disk, indicating posterior needle placement. This is ideal for accessing most herniations.

Evocative Chromodiskography

Perform confirmatory contrast diskography at this time. The following contrast mixture is used: 9.0 ml of Isovue 300 with 1.0 ml of indigo-carmine dye. This combination of contrast ratio gives readily visible radiopacity on the diskography image, and intraoperative light blue chromatization of pathologic nucleus and annular fissures, which help guide the targeted fragmentectomy.

Chromodiskography is an integral part of PA selective endoscopic diskectomy. The indigo-carmine preferentially stains the acidic degenerated nucleus pulposus. This helps orient the surgeon to the endoscopic anatomy and selectively remove the herniated and unstable nucleus pulposus. The surgeon can follow the blue-stained tissue to the annular tears and the herniation tract.

The ability of diskography to evoke a concordant painful response is also helpful to confirm the disk as a pain generator. The literature on diskography is currently considered controversial. It is controversial partly because of the high interobserver variability by diskographers in reporting the patient's subjective pain as well as the ailing patient's inability to give a clear response, especially if pain response is altered by the use of analgesics or sedation during the procedure. The surgeon who is accomplished in endoscopic spine surgery should do the diskography to decrease the interobserver variability in interpreting the patient's response and thus better select for appropriate patients.

Instrument Placement

Insert a long, thin guidewire through the 18-gauge needle channel and into the disk. Remove the needle, and slide the bluntly tapered tissue dilating obturator over the guidewire until the tip of the obturator is firmly engaged in the annular window. An eccentric parallel channel in the obturator allows for four-quadrant annular infiltration, using small incremental volumes of 0.5% lidocaine in each quadrant, which is enough to anesthetize the anulus, but not the spinal nerves. Hold the obturator firmly against the annular window surface, and remove the guidewire. Infiltrate the full thickness of the anulus through the obturator's center channel using lidocaine.

The next step is the through-and-through fenestration of the annular window by advancing the bluntly tapered obturator with a mallet. Annular fenestration is the most painful step of the entire procedure. Advise the anesthesiologist to heighten the sedation level just prior to annular fenestration. Advance the obturator tip deep into the anulus, and confirm on the C-arm views. Now slide the beveled access cannula over the obturator toward the disk. Advance the cannula until the beveled tip is deep in the annular window. Remove the obturator, and insert the endoscope to get a view of the disk nucleus and anulus.

On the other hand, if you are worried about further extruding a large disk herniation, or if you want to inspect the outer annular fibers before fenestrating the anulus, you can engage the outer anulus with the blunt obturator. Next, advance the beveled cannula over the obturator to the anulus. Remove the obturator, and insert the endoscope. The outer annular fibers can be inspected to ensure that no neural structures are in the path of the cannula prior to the annulotomy. An annulotome or a cutting trephine can then be used for the annular fenestration under direct vision. Prominent disk tissue can be removed prior to entering the disk with the cannula.

The foraminal annular window is an easily identifiable C-arm and intraoperative anatomical landmark, and is the starting location for endoscopic disk excision. Through the endoscope, you may see various amounts of blue-stained nucleus pulposus. The general-purpose access cannula has a bevel hypotenuse of 12 mm and outside diameter of 7 mm. When the cannula is slightly retracted to the midstraddle position in relationship to the annular wall, the wide-angle scope visualizes the epidural space, annular wall, and intradiskal space in the same field.

Performing the Diskectomy

The basic endoscopic method to excise a noncontained paramedian extruded lumbar herniated disk via a

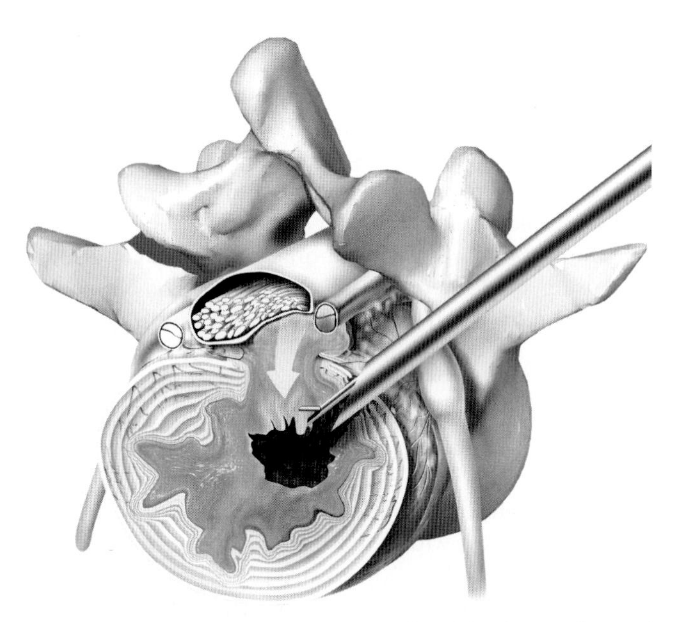

FIGURE 18–5 Uniportal technique for selective endoscopic diskectomy. Rongeurs are used for visualized fragmentectomy. The beveled cannula can be positioned to view the intradiskal cavity, annular wall, and epidural space in the same field of vision.

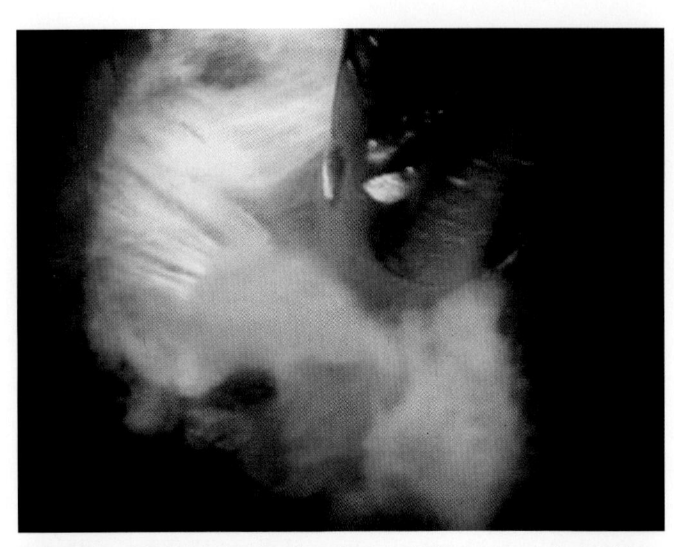

FIGURE 18–7 Endoscopic view of the removal of blue-stained herniated nucleus pulposus just underneath the traversing nerve root. Visualization of the traversing nerve root is blocked by the rongeur and disk fragment in this view. The attenuated unstained annular fibers can be seen dorsally and surrounding the blue-stained nucleus pulposus.

uniportal technique is described here. First, enlarge the annulotomy medially to the base of the herniation with a cutting forcep. The side-firing holmium:YAG laser can also be used to enlarge and widen the annulotomy. This is performed to release the annular fibers at the herniation site that may pinch off or prevent the extruded portion of the herniation from being extracted. A large amount of blue-stained nucleus is usually present directly under the herniation apex, which can be likened to the submerged portion of an iceberg. The nucleus here represents migrated and unstable nucleus. The endoscopic rongeurs are used to extract the blue-stained nucleus pulposus under direct visualization (Fig. 18–5). The larger straight and hinged rongeurs are used directly through the cannula after the endoscope is removed. Fluoroscopy and surgeon feel guide this step. By grabbing the base of the herniated fragment, one can usually extract the extruded portion of the herniation. Initial medialization and widening of the annulotomy reduce the prospect of breaking off the apex of the herniation. The traversing nerve root is readily visualized after removal of the extruded herniation (Figs. 18–6, 18–7, 18–8).

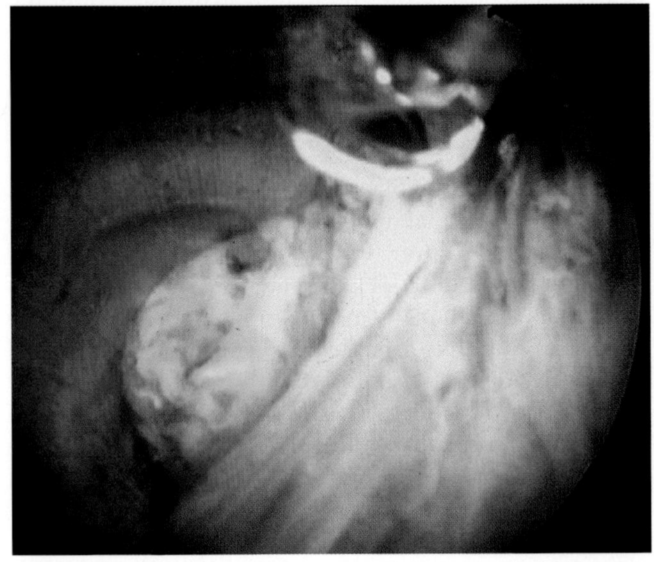

FIGURE 18–6 Endoscopic visualization of a right-sided foraminal L4–L5 herniated nucleus pulposus causing pressure on the inflamed exiting nerve root. The herniated nucleus is stained blue with indigo-carmine, which allows for improved targeted fragmentectomy. The top of the picture is dorsal, and the right is cephalad.

Next, perform bulk decompression by using a straight and flexible suction-irrigation shaver (Endius MDS). This step requires C-arm localization of the shaver head before power is activated to avoid nerve/dura injury and anterior annular penetration. The cavity thus created is called the working cavity. The debulking process serves two functions. First, it decompresses the disk, reducing the risk for further acute herniation. Second, it removes the unstable nucleus material to prevent future reherniation.

Inspect the working cavity. If a noncontained extruded disk fragment is still present, as indicated by the presence of blue-stained nucleus material posteriorly, then these fragments are teased into the working cavity with the endoscopic rongeurs and the flexible radiofrequency trigger-flex bipolar probe (Ellman) and removed. Creation

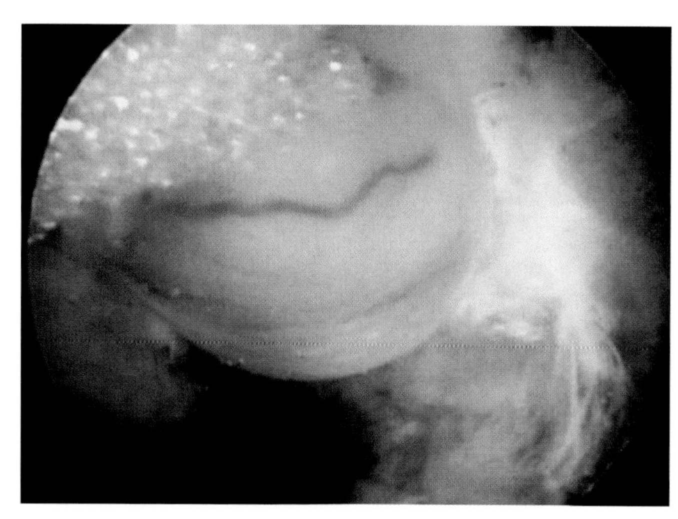

FIGURE 18–8 The same endoscopic view as Figure 18–7 after complete removal of the herniation. The traversing nerve root is clearly visualized and is no longer compressed.

of the working cavity allows the herniated disk tissue to follow the path of least resistance into the cavity. The flexible radiofrequency bipolar probe is used to contract and thicken the annular collagen at the herniation site. It is also used for hemostasis throughout the case.

The vast majority of herniations can be treated via the uniportal technique. For large central herniations, the disk sometimes needs to be approached from both sides (i.e., a biportal technique).

Complications and Avoidance

As with arthroscopic knee surgery, the risk of serious complications or injury is low, ~1 to 3% in our experience. As with any surgery, the usual risks of infection, nerve injury, dural tears, bleeding, and scar formation are always present. Dysesthesia, the most common postoperative complaint, occurs ~5 to 15% of the time, and is almost always transient. Its cause is still incompletely understood and may be related to nerve recovery, operating adjacent to the dorsal root ganglion of the exiting nerve, or a small hematoma adjacent to the ganglion of the exiting nerve because it can occur days or even weeks after surgery. Transient dysesthesia can occur even in cases where no adverse events were detected with continuous electromyography (EMG) and SEP neuromonitoring; therefore, it cannot be completely avoided. The symptoms are like a variant of complex regional pain syndrome (CRPS), but less severe, and without the skin changes that accompany CRPS. Dysesthesia is readily treated by transforaminal epidural blocks, rarely sympathetic blocks, and the use of Neurontin titrated up to 1800 to 3200 mg/day if needed.

Bowel injury or large vessel injury is extremely rare, but it is possible if the suction-irrigation shaver penetrates the contralateral anulus from an incompetent anulus or from a defect left after removing a disk herniation that has extruded through the annular wall. Careful intraoperative fluoroscopic localization and "feeling" the contralateral anulus with the instrument prior to activating it will help prevent the shaver from advancing past the contralateral annular wall.

Avoidance of complications is enhanced by the ability to visualize clearly normal and pathoanatomy, the use of local anesthesia and conscious sedation rather than general or spinal anesthesia, and the use of a standardized needle placement protocol. The entire procedure is usually accomplished with the patient remaining comfortable during the entire procedure and should be done without the patient feeling severe pain, except when expected (e.g., during evocative diskography, annular fenestration, or when instruments are manipulated past the exiting nerve). Local anesthesia using 0.5% lidocaine allows generous use of this dilute anesthetic for pain control and still allows the patient to feel pain when the nerve root is manipulated. Continuous EMG and SEP can also help monitor and prevent nerve irritation. This usually correlates well with patients' intraoperative feedback.

Discussion

Endoscopic spine surgery has a very high learning curve, but it is within the grasp of every endoscopic surgeon with proper training. As with any new procedure, the complication rate may be higher during the learning curve and may vary with each surgeon's skills and experience. The endoscopic technique is safer for the patient because he or she is conscious and able to provide immediate input to the surgeon when pain is generated. The surgeon's ability to perform the surgery without causing the patient undue pain will self-select for surgeons who can master the technique to the extent that the surgeon will prefer endoscopic over traditional surgery for the same condition. For most contained disk herniations and diskogenic pain, the experienced endoscopic spine surgeon will opt for the endoscopic approach as the treatment of choice.

Case Illustration

A 22-year-old male with a 2-year history of low back pain and intermittent right leg pain sustained an acute worsening of his right leg pain 12 days prior to evaluation. He proportionalized his pain to 5% back and 95% leg pain. He complained of a new onset of weakness, tingling, and constant numbness. The pain and numbness radiated down the posterolateral leg to the dorsum

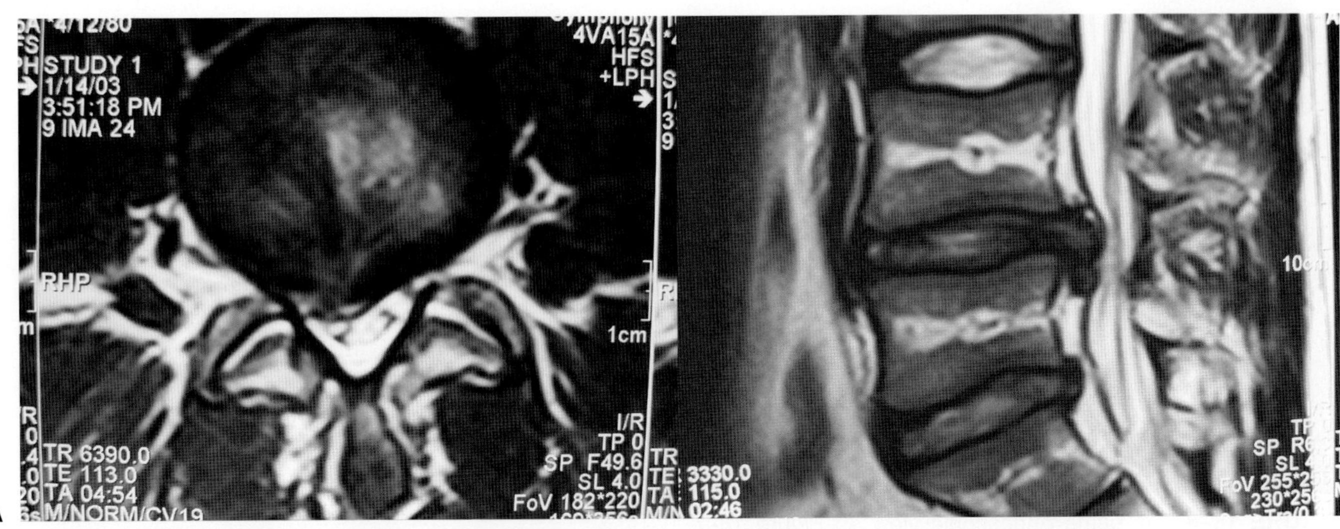

FIGURE 18–9 Preoperative axial **(A)** and sagittal **(B)** MRI revealed a large right paracentral/foraminal HNP causing compression on the exiting and traversing nerve roots. Other axial cuts showed migration caudally, but the fragment appeared confluent with the base of the herniation.

of the right foot. He was unable to bear weight on the right leg and was using a walking pole for support. He was unable to sleep supine and had to sleep in a recliner to minimize the pain. Sitting provided some relief. He denied bowel or bladder incontinence, but had constipation for the last 12 days. Physical exam revealed a limited lumbar extension to 10 degrees, tenderness in the right sciatic notch, positive straight leg raising (SLR) and Lasègue's tests, positive contralateral SLR, 2+ bilateral patella and Achilles deep tendon reflexes, decreased sensation to light touch over the dorsum of the foot and to a lesser extent the lateral border of the foot, and weakness. The right-sided weakness was graded as anterior tibialis, external hallucis longus (EHL), hip abductor, gastrocnemius soleus.

MRI revealed a large right paracentral/foraminal extruded herniated nucleus pulposus with slight caudal migration, causing compression of both the exiting and traversing nerve roots (Fig. 18–9). Surgery was recommended due to the acute onset and progressive neurologic deficits. After a full discussion of his risks, benefits, and alternatives, the patient elected to undergo outpatient selective endoscopic posterolateral diskectomy. The patient experienced better than 80% pain relief immediately postop. He had some mild dysesthetic burning over the L4 distribution that started a few days postop. This completely resolved by 4 weeks with the aid of Neurontin 300 mg TID. A postoperative MRI was ordered when the patient had acute worsening of his leg pain 11 days postop (Fig. 18–10). He said he "overdid it."

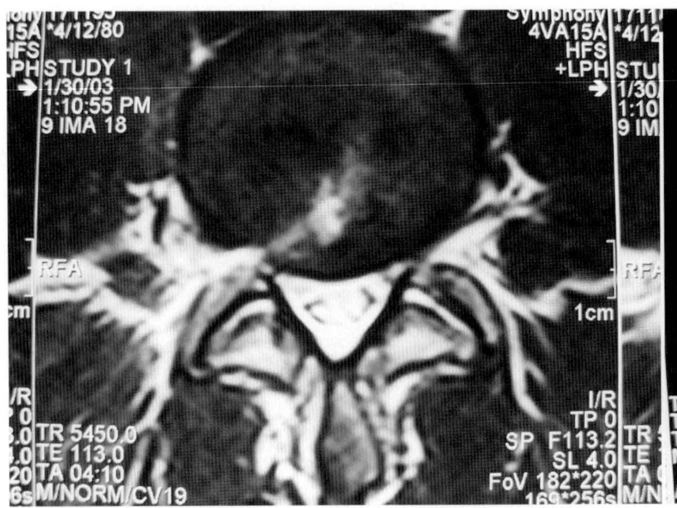

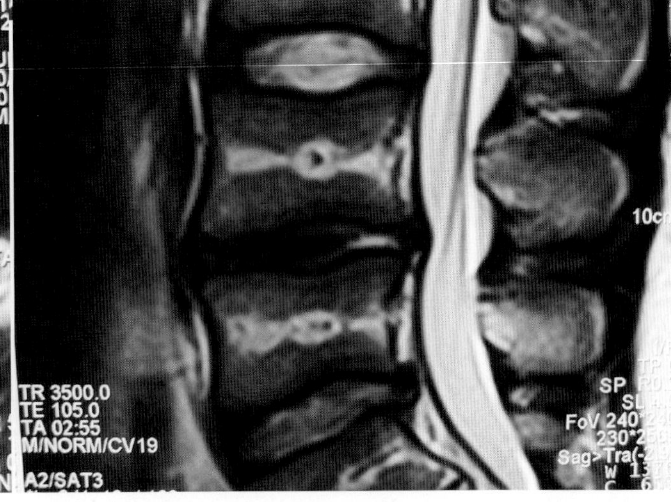

FIGURE 18–10 Postoperative MRI—**(A)** atrial and **(B)** sagittal—revealed excellent removal of the herniated disk and decompression of the nerve roots. The instrument trajectory can be seen within the disk as an area of higher signal on the T2-weighted image.

The patient's leg weakness was improving, but because some weakness was still present, we wanted to make sure he did not have a recurrent herniation. The MRI revealed excellent herniation removal without any retained fragments. The patient's acute pain resolved within 24 hours, and he had no pain at all by 4 weeks. His weakness continued to improve grading EHL, 5/5 hip abductor, 4+/5 anterior tibialis, and 5/5 gastrocnemius soleus at his last follow-up 8 months postoperatively.

Posterolateral endoscopic diskectomy provides excellent access to the epidural space from pedicle to pedicle, facilitating removal of extruded or migrated fragments, in addition to contained disks. The YESS technique is performed with tissue dilatation to accommodate a 7 mm working cannula. It avoids the significant trauma of muscle stripping, muscle retraction, bony resection, and nerve root retraction associated with standard open surgery. Because the patient is conscious throughout the procedure, it is safer than the open method by preventing nerve root injury.

REFERENCES

1. Bogduk N. The innervation of the intervertebral disc. In: Ghosh P, ed. *The Biology of the Intervertebral Disc*. Vol 1. Boca Raton, FL: CRC Press; 1988:135–149.
2. Boden S, Herzog R, Rauschning W, Rydevik B. Instructional course lecture #231: lumbar spine, the herniated disc. Paper presented at: Annual Meeting of the American Academy of Orthopedic Surgeons. Feb. 14, 1997, San Francisco, CA.
3. Adams MA, Hutton WC. Gradual disc prolapse. *Spine*. 1985;10: 524–531.
4. Adams MA, Hutton WC. Prolapsed intervertebral disc-hyperflexion injury. *Spine*. 1982;7:184–191.
5. Hermantin FU, Peters T, Quartararo L, Kambin P. A prospective, randomized study comparing the results of open discectomy with those of video-assisted arthroscopic microdiscectomy. *J Bone Joint Surg Am*. 1999;81:958–965.
6. Hijikata S. Percutaneous nucleotomy: a new concept technique and 12 years' experience. *Clin Orthop*. 1989;238:9–23.
7. Kambin P, Schaffer JL. Percutaneous lumbar discectomy: review of 100 patients and current practice. *Clin Orthop*. 1989;238:24–34.
8. Kambin P, O'Brien E, Zhou L, Schaffer JL. Arthroscopic microdiscectomy and selective fragmentectomy. *Clin Orthop*. 1998;347: 150–167.
9. Mayer HM, Brock M. Percutaneous endoscopic discectomy: surgical technique and preliminary results compared to microsurgical discectomy. *J Neurosurg*. 1993;78:216–225.
10. Onik G, Helms CA, Ginsberg L, Hooglund FT, Morris J. Percutaneous lumbar discectomy using a new aspiration probe. *Am J Roentgenol*. 1985;144:1137–1140.
11. Tsou PM, Yeung AT. Transforaminal endoscopic decompression for radiculopathy secondary to non-contained intracanal lumbar disc herniation. *Spine J*. 2002;2:41–48.
12. Yeung AT. The evolution of percutaneous spinal endoscopy and discectomy: state of art. *Mt Sinai J Med*. 2000;67:327–332.
13. Yeung AT, Tsou PM. Posterolateral endoscopic excision for lumbar disc herniation: the surgical technique, outcome and complications in 307 consecutive cases. *Spine*. 2002;27:722–731.
14. Gogan WJ, Fraser RD. Chymopapain: a 10-year, double blind study. *Spine*. 1992;17:388–394.
15. Van de Belt H, Franssen S, Deutman R. Repeat chemonucleolysis is safe and effective. *Clin Orthop*. 1999;363:121–125.
16. Yasargil MG. Microsurgical operation of herniated lumbar disc. In: Wullenweber R, Brock M, Hamer J, Klinger M, Spoerri O, eds. *Advances in Neurosurgery*. Vol 4. New York: Springer-Verlag; 1977: 81–94.
17. Williams RW. Microlumbar discectomy: a conservative surgical approach to the virgin herniated lumbar disc. *Spine*. 1978;3: 175–182.
18. Perez-Cruet MJ, Foley KT, Isaacs RE, et al. Microendoscopic lumbar discectomy: technical note. *Neurosurgery*. 2002;51(suppl 5): 129–136.
19. Knight MTN, Goswami AKD. Endoscopic laser foraminoplasty. In: Savitz MH, Chiu JC, Yeung AT, eds. *The Practice of Minimally Invasive Spinal Technique*. Richmond, VA. AAMISMS Education; 2000; 42:337–340.
20. Osman SG, Nibu K, Panjabi MM, Marsolais EB, Chaudhary R. Transforaminal and posterior decompressions of the lumbar spine: a comparative study of stability and intervertebral foramen area. *Spine*. 1997;22:1690–1695.

19

Endoscopic Lumbar Foraminoplasty

JOHN C. CHIU

With accumulated experience with endoscopically assisted mechanical and laser lumbar diskectomy,[1–18] the need for a more efficient method to decompress the lateral recess[19–26] and intervertebral neural foramen from very large or extruded disk protrusions, recurrent disks, scar tissue, and spondylitic spurs became evident. The most frequently seen lumbar spinal disk disease in the elderly is spinal and lateral foraminal stenosis.[24,26] Lateral stenosis may be congenital or degenerative when secondary to acute disk disease and spinal trauma. The classic wide posterior decompressive laminectomy with foraminotomy involves extensive muscle and soft tissue dissection for exposure, decompression, and resection of the posterior spinal elements. Despite varying degrees of success,[24] it is associated with significant iatrogenic trauma and failed back syndrome.[24,26] As a result, the search for a minimally invasive spinal surgery (MISS) technique began. This chapter will describe endoscopic lumbar foraminoplasty and diskectomy, including endoscopic laser foraminoplasty (ELF),[10] as reported by Dr. Martin T. N. Knight, with laser application, and minimally invasive transforaminal microdecompressive endoscopic assisted diskectomy and foraminoplasty (TF-MEAD), a new system of more aggressive mechanical instruments and laser application, developed at the California Center for Minimally Invasive Spine Surgery (C-MISS).

The pioneering work of Hijikata[1] with percutaneous manual diskectomy, Ascher[2] and Choy[3] with percutaneous laser diskectomy, and the application of endoscopy by Kambin[4] and others[27–32] resulted in monitored keyhole operations for removal of herniated lumbar disks. The use of endoscopy and laser, especially the holmium side-firing laser, allows removal of large protrusions and extruded disk fragments from the epidural space and stenotic foraminal decompression with ELF, which addresses one level and one side at a time.[10,29] This technique takes 90 to 120 minutes to complete using primarily the laser for foraminal decompression and diskectomy.[9]

Attention is now being directed to treatment of epidural scarring, lateral recess and foraminal stenosis, and advanced degenerative changes that are often bilateral and occur at multiple levels.[28] I have developed a more aggressive TF-MEAD system to address endoscopic transforaminal mechanical and laser microdecompressive diskectomy and foraminoplasty in a fast and effective manner for both unilateral single and bilateral multiple levels. These MISS procedures should now join the armamentarium of the spinal surgeon in treating advanced degenerative spinal stenosis and lateral foraminal stenosis.

Such procedures require the surgeon to be knowledgeable and competent in MISS, with a thorough knowledge of the procedure of endoscopic lumbar diskectomy and foraminoplasty, pathoanatomy of the neuroforamen and the spine, and the relationships of the lumbar exiting and traversing nerve roots, dorsal root ganglion, facet joint, disks, and vertebrae.

Indications

Endoscopic lumbar foraminoplasty is indicated in the following clinical situations[10,16]:

- Intractable low back pain with radiation down the leg (radicular pain)
- Symptoms of spinal neurogenic claudication

- Compressive and irritative radiculopathy with sensorimotor impairment
- Disk extrusion or sequestration with predominant back or leg pain
- Degeneration and settlement of the spine with predominant back pain, buttock pain, or leg pain
- Nonradicular low back pain persisting despite facet joint injection
- Lateral recess stenosis with dynamic compressive or noncompressive radiculopathy
- Prior failed conventional surgery with perineural scarring and failed back syndrome
- No improvement of symptoms after a minimum of 12 weeks of conservative therapy
- Spondylolytic spondylolisthesis
- Diagnostic imaging, MRI, CT, 3D CT, and CT myelogram that demonstrate disk herniation and/or extrusion or lateral recess stenosis
- Positive pre- or intraoperative diskogram and pain provocation test
- Positive electromyography
- Multiple lumbar disks/levels that can be treated at one sitting with TF-MEAD

Contraindications

The endoscopic lumbar foraminoplasty procedure is contraindicated[9,15] in the following clinical situations:

- Cauda equina syndrome
- Painless motor deficit
- Tumors
- Clinical findings that suggest pathology other than degenerative discogenic disease
- ELF does not treat multilevel or bilateral disks

Instruments and Preparations

These surgical instruments are necessary to perform endoscopic laser and/or lumbar foraminoplasty:

- Digital fluoroscopic equipment (C-arm) and monitor
- Radiolucent C-arm/fluoroscopic carbon-fiber surgical table
- Endoscopic tower equipped with digital video monitor, DVT/VHS recorder, light source, trichip digital camera, and photo printer system
- Panoramic Plus Discoscope, 0 degree, 2.2 mm working channel (Richard Wolf GmBH & Co., Knittlingen, Germany)
- Percutaneous fiberoptic foraminoscope, 0 degree, 6 mm OD, 3.9 mm working channel (Karl Storz, Tuttlingen, Germany) (Fig. 19–1A)
- Wide-angle posterolateral foraminoscope, 6 degree, 6 mm OD, 3 mm working channel (Karl Storz) (Figs. 19–1A, 19–2E)
- C-MISS TF-MEAD system instruments (Figs. 19–1B, 19–2B,D)
- Set of serial/progressive dilators, and cannulas in graduated sizes (3.5–5.8 mm); a set of progressive cannulas with duckbill extensions (with various lengths 5–10 mm on one side) (Fig. 19–1B)
- Aggressive toothed trephine set in graduated sizes
- 9.9 mm tubular retractor system with a gradual dilator set
- Wide-angle endoscopes, 0 and 30 degree, 4 mm OD (Karl Storz)
- Trephine, curette, grasper and spoon forceps, 2 mm rotating bone punch (rongeurs), rasp, and burr
- Lumbar diskectomy sets (2.5, 3.5, 4.7 mm) (Blackstone Medical, Inc., Springfield, MA) with various diskectomies (Fig. 19–1C)
- Endoscopic grasping and cutting forceps, probe, knife, scissors, diskectomy rongeurs, and curette (Fig. 19–1A,B)
- Holmium: YAG laser generator (Trimedyne, Irvine, CA)
- Holmium 550-μm laser bare fiber with flat-tip and right-angle (side-firing) probes with and without irrigating system of various sizes, and 2 mm side-firing irrigating laser probe (Fig. 19–1A)
- Steerable Spinescope (Karl Storz) (Fig. 19–2A,C) with 2.5 mm working fiberscope (for laser application with a flexible tip that can bend up to 90 degrees and rotate to reach 360 degrees)

Anesthesia

Knight's ELF procedure is done under neuroleptic (aware-state) analgesia in the prone position combined with local anesthesia. Patient feedback is essential in these cases when one works around the nerve.

TF-MEAD patients are treated in an operating room under local anesthesia and monitored conscious sedation. The anesthesiologist maintains mild sedation, but the patient is able to respond. Two grams Ancef and 8 mg dexamethasone are given intravenously at the start of anesthesia. Surface EEG (SNAP, Nicolet Biomedical, Madison, WI) monitoring provides added precision of anesthesia.

Patient Positioning

For TF-MEAD, if surgery is unilateral, the patient is placed in a lateral decubitus position (Fig. 19–3B,C),

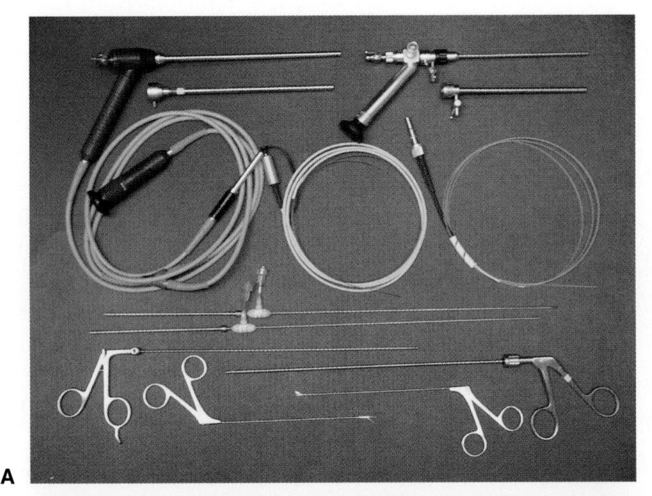

A

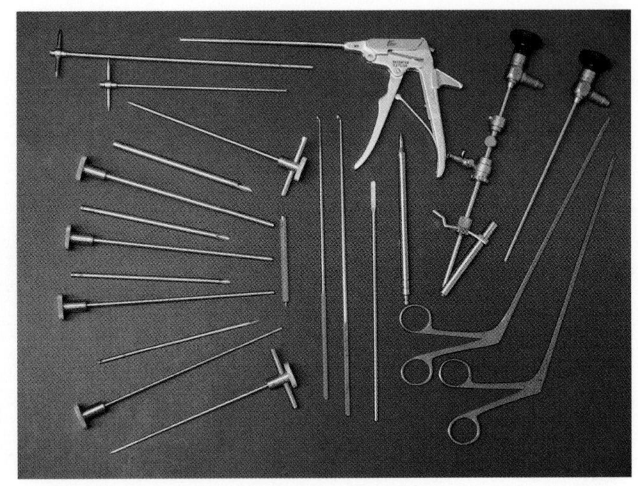

B

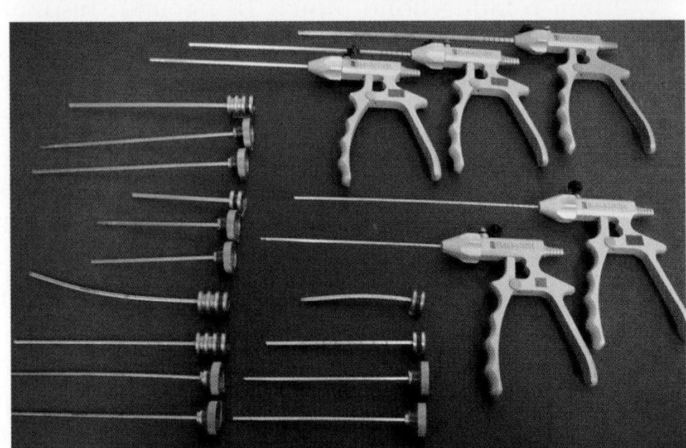

C

FIGURE 19–1 Surgical instruments for endoscopic lumbar foraminoplasty and diskectomy. **(A)** Percutaneous fiberoptic foraminoscope, 0 degrees, 6 mm OD, 3.9 mm working channel; posterolateral foraminoscope, 6 degrees, 6 mm OD working channel; bare holmium laser fiber, side-firing laser probe (Knight) (Trimedyne), and diskectomy forceps. **(B)** C-MISS TF-MEAD transforaminal decompressive system: endoscopes (0 and 30 degrees, 4 mm OD,) assisted tubular retractor, trephines, graduated duckbill cannulas, diskectomy rongeur, curette, and 2 mm bone punch. **(C)** Lumbar diskectomy set with dilators, working cannulas, trephines, and various discectomes.

with the painful leg up and both hips and knees in moderate flexion. If the patient has an increased medical risk (i.e., pulmonary, cardiac, morbid obesity, and other high-risk medical conditions), but requires a bilateral procedure, the decubitus position may be used first on one side, then, turning the patient over, on the other side to perform the bilateral procedure in one sitting. Bilateral operations are otherwise performed in the prone position on a radiolucent support similar to the Wilson frame (as for ELF). The arms are supported on arm boards over the head. When local anesthesia and mild sedation are used, the extremities, buttocks, and shoulders are secured and restrained from sudden motion with adhesive tape.

Localization

C-arm fluoroscopy is used to identify the lumbar levels relative to the sacrum. The midline, operative levels, and point of entry (operating portal) for surgery are marked on the skin with a marking pen (Figs. 19–3, 19–4A,B). The distance of the point of entry from the midline varies with the height and weight of the patient, but it is ~12 cm at the affected disk level for an average-size patient. Positioning of the instruments is checked throughout the procedure by fluoroscopy in two planes as often as needed (Figs. 19–5, 19–6B, 19–7B–D). At the involved nerve roots distribution, sterile needle electrodes are placed for continuous intraoperative neurophysiologic EMG monitoring.[29]

Surgical Technique for Endoscopic Laser Foraminoplasty

ELF[9,16,28,31] begins with spinal probing and diskography performed at the suspected level, which is clinically appropriate to the site of back or peripheral radiating pain or evidence of clinically related pathology. Knight has described diagnostic spinal probing plus provocative diskogram to identify any concordant pain-sensitive areas in the lateral recess and foraminal areas in a staged progression of the structures and scar tissue on the disk surface and around the nerve root, the facets, and the walls of the foramen. Symptoms reproduced by spinal probing and diskography determine the extent of the surgical exploration required for the

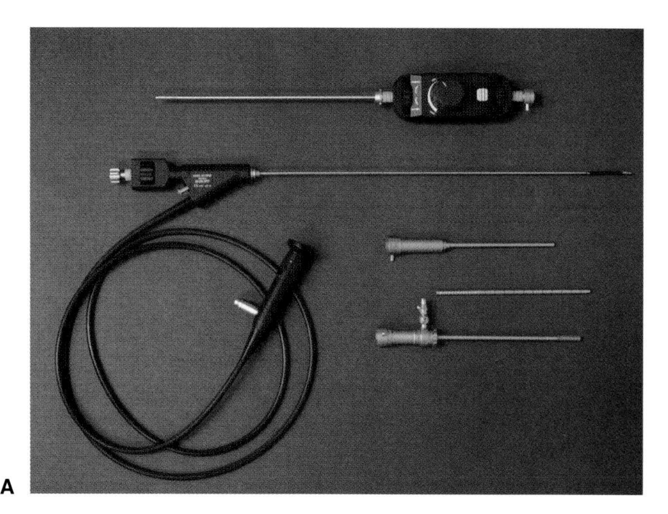

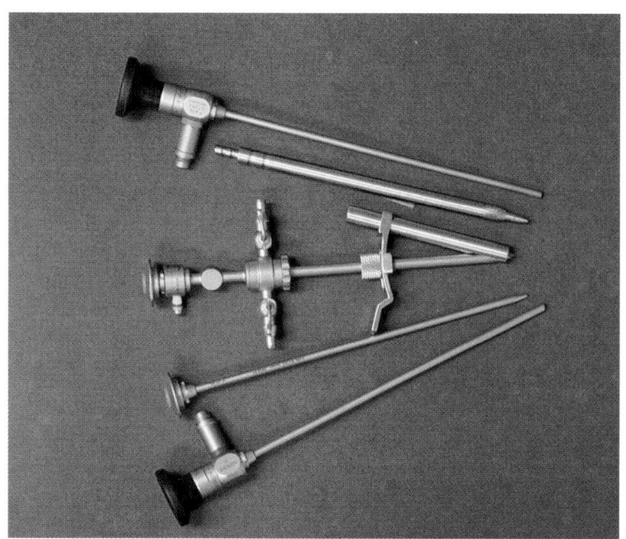

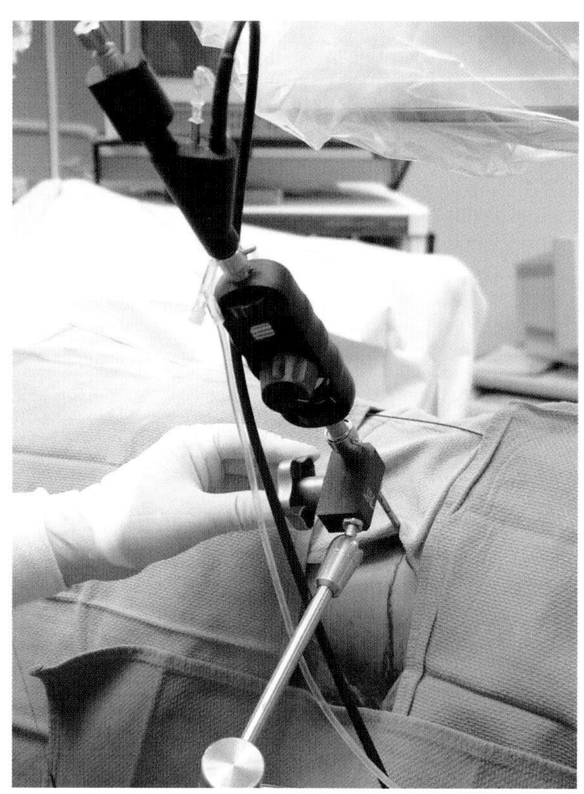

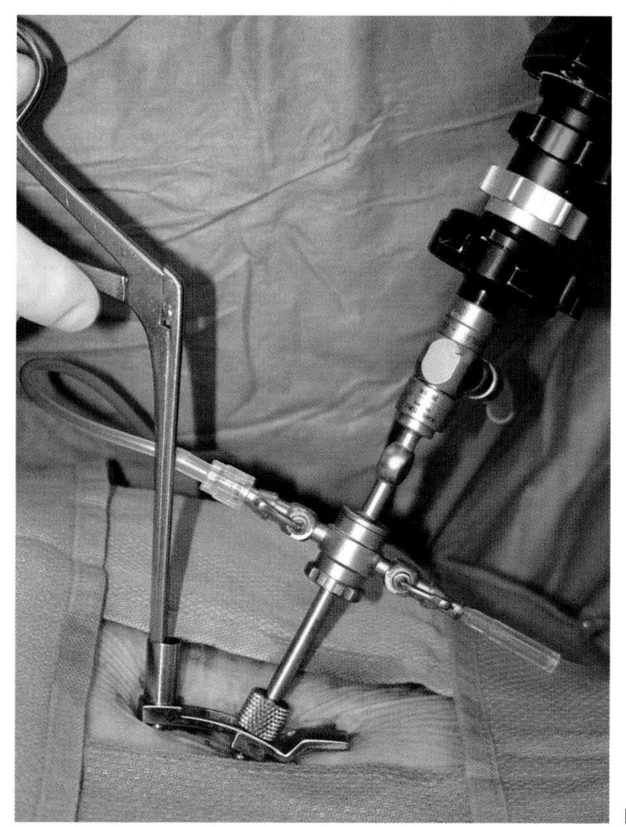

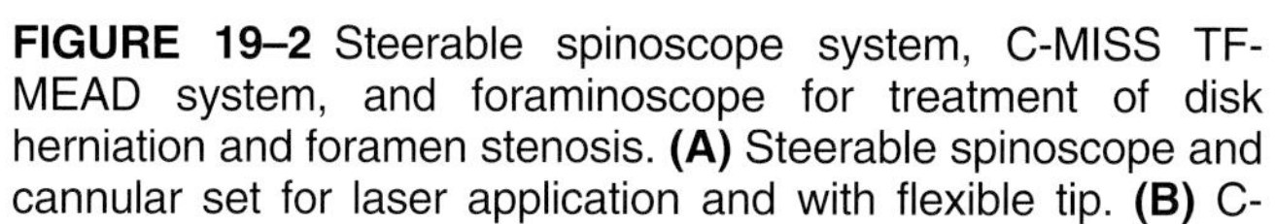

FIGURE 19–2 Steerable spinoscope system, C-MISS TF-MEAD system, and foraminoscope for treatment of disk herniation and foramen stenosis. **(A)** Steerable spinoscope and cannular set for laser application and with flexible tip. **(B)** C-MISS TF-MEAD system with a working channel 9.9 mm assisted by endoscopes (0 and 30 degrees, 4 mm OD). **(C)** Spinoscope surgical application for TF-MEAD. **(D)** Lumbar foraminoplasty with C-MISS TF-MEAD system in surgical application.

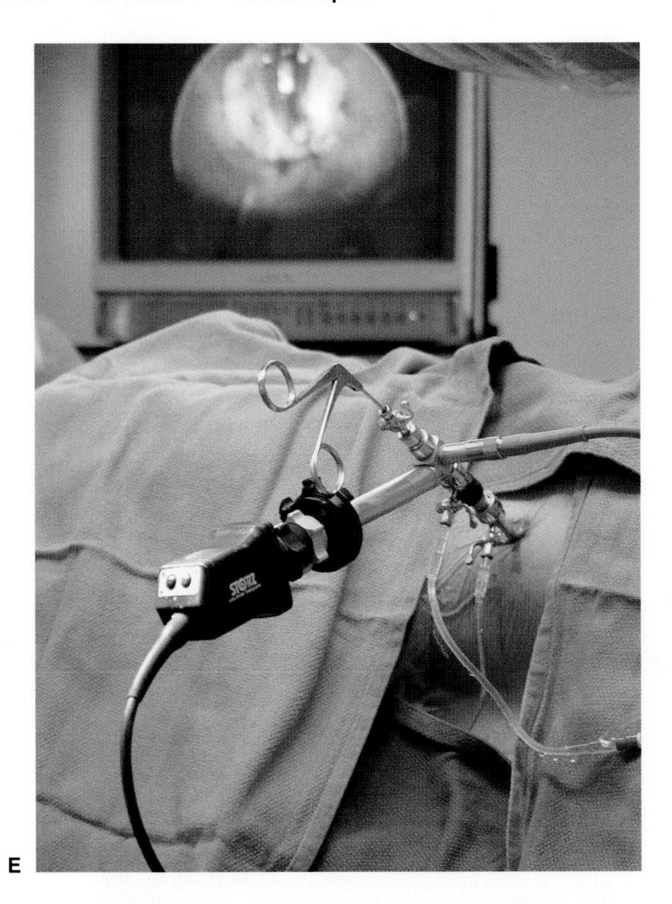

FIGURE 19–2 (*Continued*) **(E)** Posterolateral foraminoscopy with wide-angle 6-degree, 3 mm working channel operating foraminoscope.

ELF procedure (second stage of ELF procedure), including endoscopic diskectomy, neurolysis, undercutting of facets, osteophytectomy, and/or laser ablation of painful tissue and foraminoplasty (Figs. 19–4A,B, 19–6, 19–9A,D,E).

The diskography needle is replaced with a guidewire, and a 5 mm dilated tube is inserted into the exit root foramen. The procedure is performed under fluoroscopy. The trocar is then replaced with a working endoscopic channel (Richard Wolf). A side-firing 2 mm internal laser irrigation probe (Fig. 19–1A) is inserted through the endoscope (Trimedyne) to perform ELF (Figs. 19–6, 19–9A,D,E). The extraforaminal zone and margin of the foramen are cleared. The facet joint surfaces are cleaned and undercut to allow the endoscope to enter the epidural space. Vertebral body and facet joint osteophytes, ligamentum flavum and superior foraminal ligaments, and perineuro and epidural scarring are ablated and the facet joint undercut until the anulus and epidural space are visualized.

The exiting and traversing nerve roots are mobilized and decompressed medially and laterally until the functional axilla of the root at the apex of the safe working zone is displayed. The nerve is cleared of peripheral fibrosis. Clearance and undercutting are extended along the bone margin to the superior notch with resection of the superior foraminal ligament. Exploration is continued to the inferior pedicle, displacing the anulus and epidural space. Scarring is almost always associated with vascular bands. Inflamed soft tissue on the dorsum of the disk is exquisitely tender in some cases. Osteophytes along the ascending joint of the superior notch, the dorsum of the tibial margin, and the vertebral shoulder are ablated under endoscopic vision by laser. Thermal modulation in conjunction with undercutting of the facet may increase the cross-section of the area of foramen and provide decompression. Endoscopic laser diskectomy and epidural exploration and decompression complete the procedure.

Postoperative Care

The patient is discharged on the day following surgery. A muscle-balance physiotherapy regimen is recommended on the first day after discharge; later, the program is amplified with neural mobilization drills. Self-help drills are encouraged twice a day thereafter. A pain diary is maintained by the patient to identify the intensity and location of any residual pain.

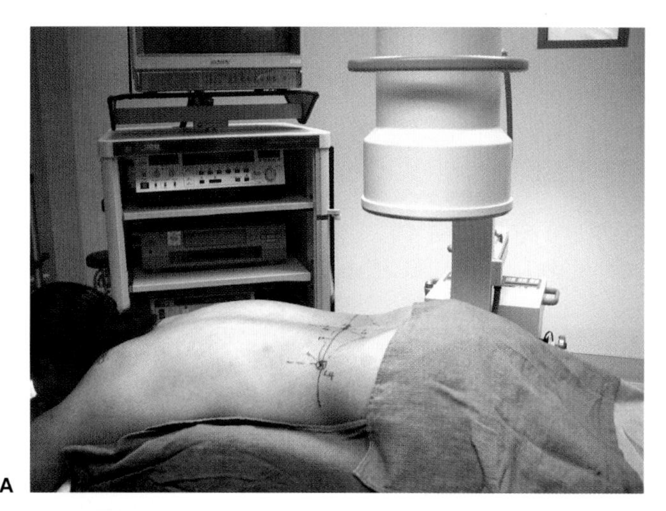

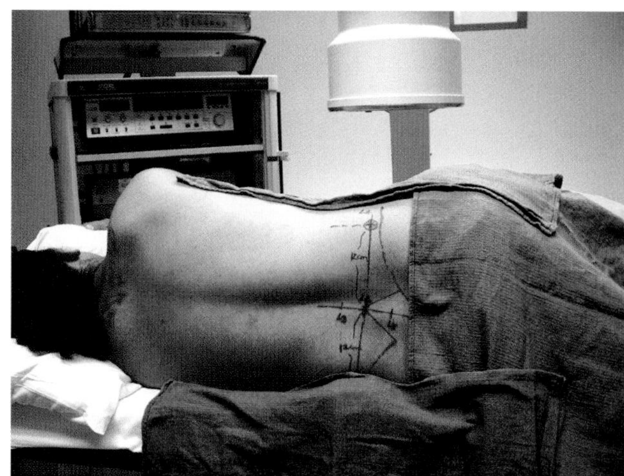

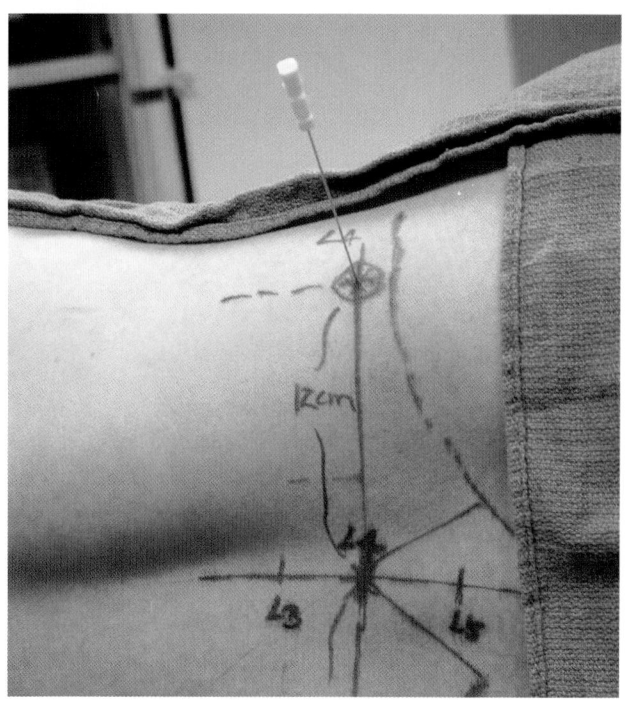

FIGURE 19–3 Patient positioning and localization. **(A)** Patient in prone position. **(B)** Patient in lateral decubitus position. **(C)** Localization: skin marking and placement of needle (portal).

Outcomes

Reported are a total of 958 ELF procedures performed on 716 patients who were evaluated at 6 and 12 weeks, 6 months, and yearly following the surgery, unless clinical symptoms required closer supervision. The outcome following ELF remains promising, with 61 to 70% of cases achieving 50% gain in their preoperative Oswestry Disability Index and visual analog pain score. There were 24 complications (1.6%), with diskitis in nine patients, dural tear in one, wound infections in one, foot drop in two, myocardial infarction in one, erectile dysfunction in one, and panic attack in one. Seven percent of patients worsened after the operation. About 3% of patients required subsequent open surgery.

Surgical Technique for Transforaminal Microdecompressive Endoscopic Assisted Diskectomy and Foraminoplasty

If a pain provocation test and diskogram were not done preoperatively, they are done at the outset. If the diskogram and pain provocation tests are confirmatory, surgery is performed (Figs. 19–2C–E, 19–4, 19–5, 19–7,

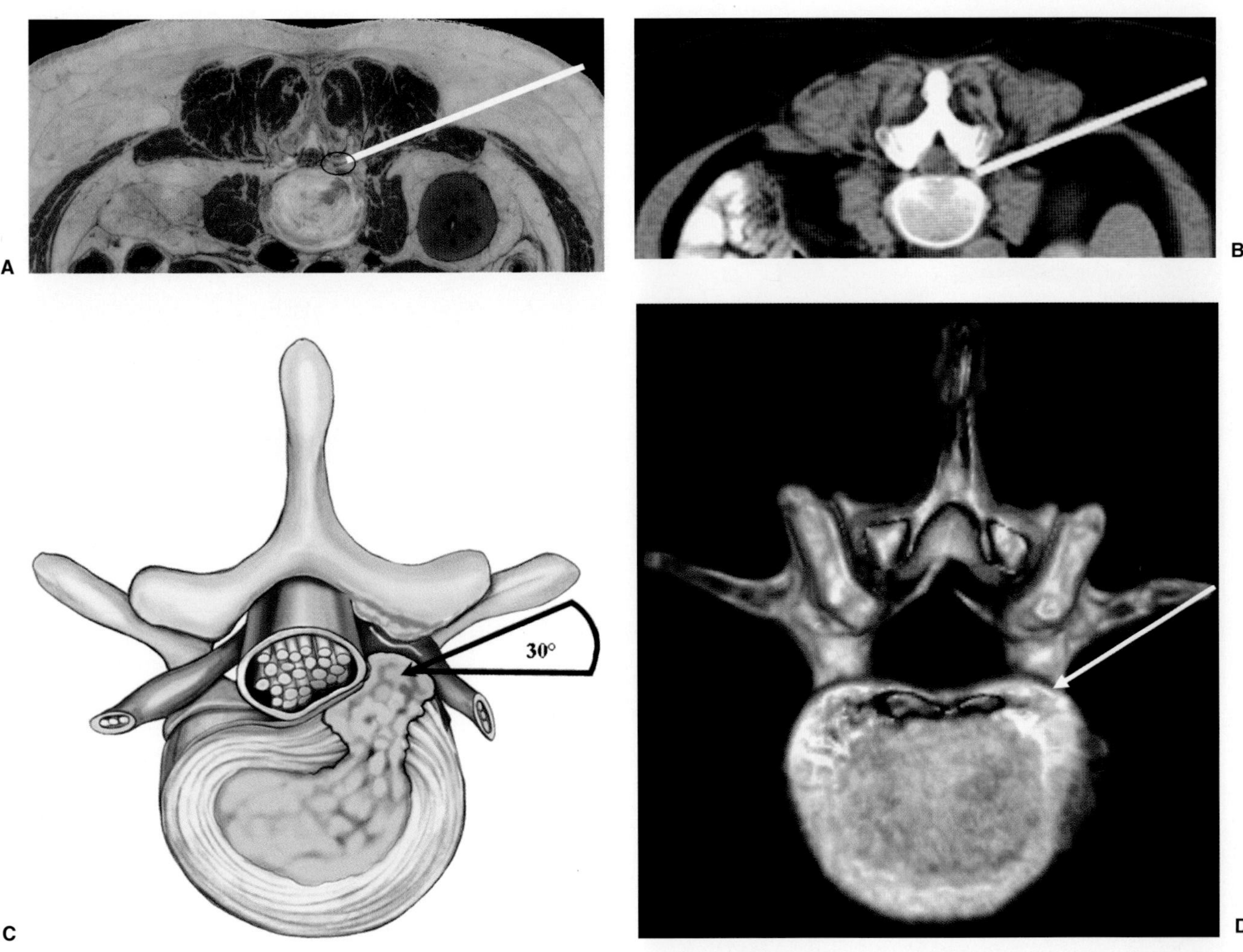

FIGURE 19–4 Safe surgical approach to neuroforamen for endoscopic lumbar foraminoplasty and diskectomy. **(A)** Posterolateral surgical approach to lumbar disk in cadaveric axial cryomicrotome. **(B)** Axial illustration of posterolateral lumbar surgical approach for needle placement into intervertebral foramen. **(C)** Posterolateral surgical approach on prone axial CT image at lumbar disk level. **(D)** Posterolateral surgical approach into the foramen on axial view of lumbar spine 3D CT image.

19–8, 19–9). An 18-gauge stylet is inserted and incrementally advanced under C-arm fluoroscopic guidance in two planes, at a 60-degree angle from the sagittal plane, targeting toward the center of the disk, through the safety zone, and into the desired interspace. All instrumentation is performed under C-arm fluoroscopic control and endoscopy. The usual procedure for MISS is followed.[15] The appropriate-size cannula and dilator are passed over the stylet to the anulus. Under fluoroscopy the extended side of this cannula is turned to face the nerve root in order to retract and protect it.

The cannula retractors have variously shaped extensions like a duckbill (with various lengths, 5 to 10 mm on one side; Figs. 19–1B, 19–5E,F) to retract and protect the nerve root once the cannula is inserted through the foramen into the epidural space and the extension is oriented properly toward the root. The larger, more aggressively toothed trephines (Fig. 19–5B) are then inserted and rotated to cut through anulus, disk protrusion, spur, or spondylitic bar. The cannula is large enough to admit a slim punch (rongeur), spinal disk forceps or pituitary forceps, and full-size curettes to aid decompression of the foramen and the lateral recess (Fig. 19–5C–F). An endoscope can be passed through it instead of the endoscope's sheath to facilitate mechanical and laser decompression, foraminoplasty, and diskectomy. The endoscope is useful in TF-MEAD surgery for decompression in the lateral recess and periforaminal area. Biting forceps, discectome, and holmium laser with continuous irrigation are used consecutively to perform intradiscal diskectomy; lower energy nonablative laser is applied for shrinking and tightening of the disk (laser thermodiskoplasty).[16,17]

The decompression area can be enlarged with a larger cannula retractor/trephine set. A small amount of bleeding usually can be controlled with cold saline

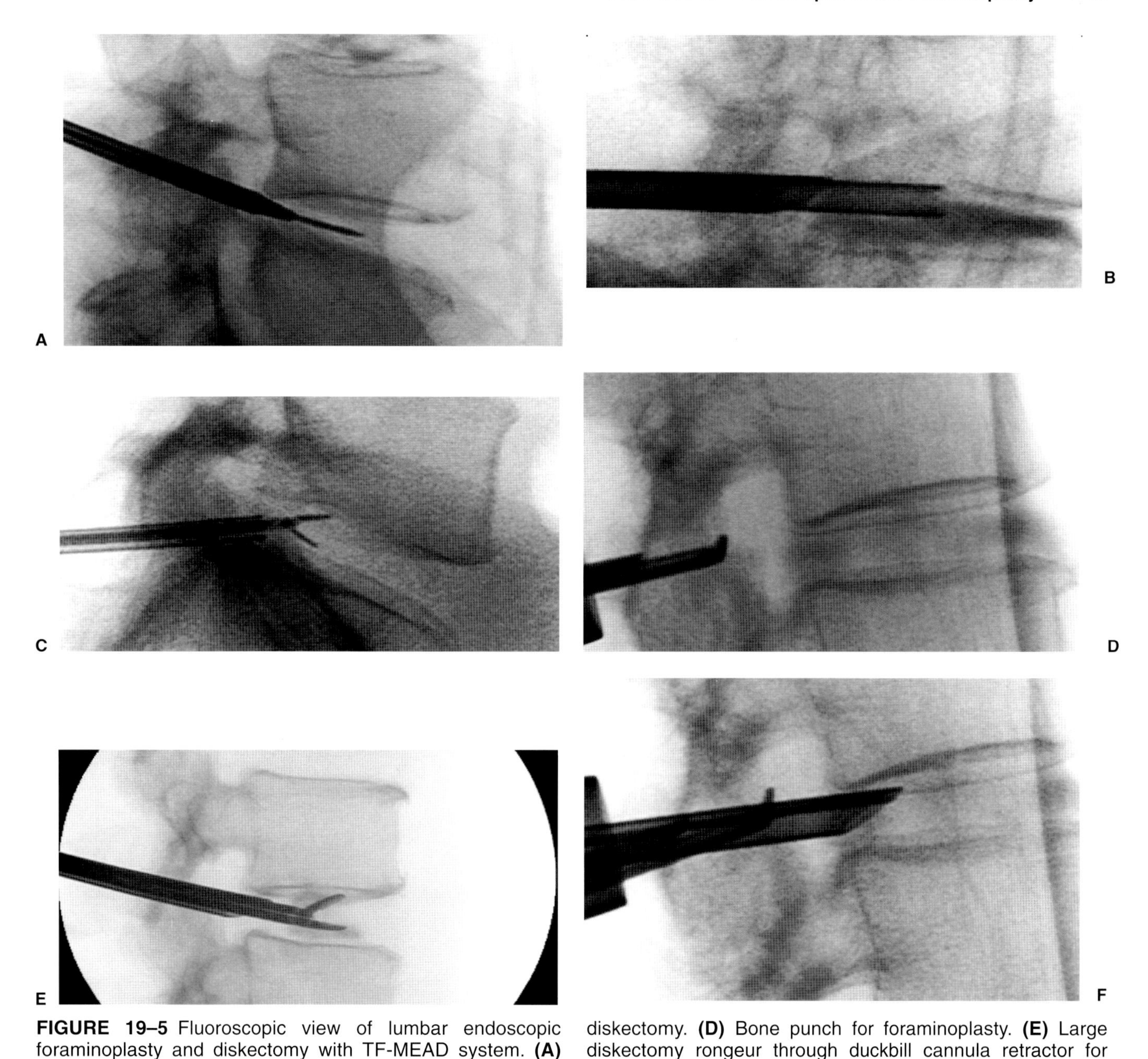

FIGURE 19–5 Fluoroscopic view of lumbar endoscopic foraminoplasty and diskectomy with TF-MEAD system. **(A)** Stylet and dilator in disk space. **(B)** Trephine for disk and osteophyte decompression. **(C)** Diskectomy forceps/rongeur for diskectomy. **(D)** Bone punch for foraminoplasty. **(E)** Large diskectomy rongeur through duckbill cannula retractor for diskectomy. **(F)** Duckbill cannula and bone punch in action through TF-MEAD tubular retractor for foraminoplasty.

irrigation and rarely requires hemostasis by laser or bipolar coagulation. Holmium:YAG laser with a side-firing probe or 550-μm holmium laser bare fiber (Fig. 19–1A) is used to ablate the disk and to shrink and contract the disk, reducing the profile of protrusion and hardening the disk tissue (i.e., laser thermodiskoplasty). Disk removal is aided by a rocking excursion of the cannula in a 25-degree arc, a "fan sweep maneuver"[16,18] from side to side, that creates an inverted oval cone-shaped area of removed disk totaling up to 50 degrees. Laser thermodiskoplasty can also cause sinovertebral neurolysis or denervation. The diskectomies is again used to remove charred debris.

The disk space and neural foramen can be directly visualized and examined by endoscopy to confirm adequate disk decompression and to perform further decompression if necessary. If the foramen is compromised, the depth of insertion of the endoscope is adjusted, the nerve root is again protected by the duckbill extension, and spurs are removed with curettes, bone

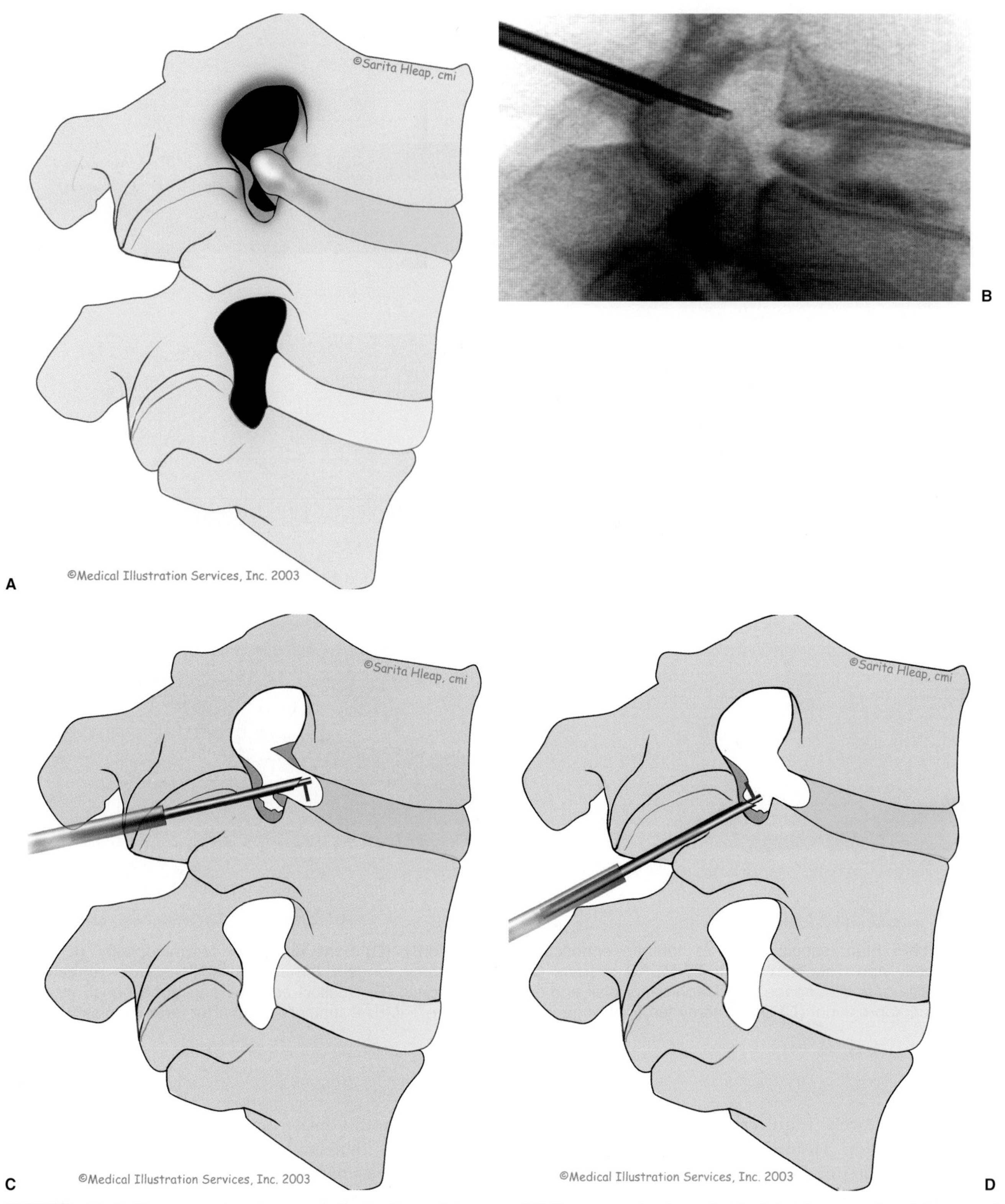

FIGURE 19–6 Fluoroscopic view and illustration of laser side-firing probe for lumbar laser foraminoplasty (Knight). **(A)** Illustration of lateral spinal stenosis secondary to disk protrusion, shoulder osteophytes, and facet hypertrophy. **(B)** Fluoroscopic view of side-firing laser probe at foramen for lumbar facet decompression. **(C)** Illustration of lumbar laser diskectomy. **(D)** Illustration of lumbar laser foraminoplasty for facet hypertrophy.

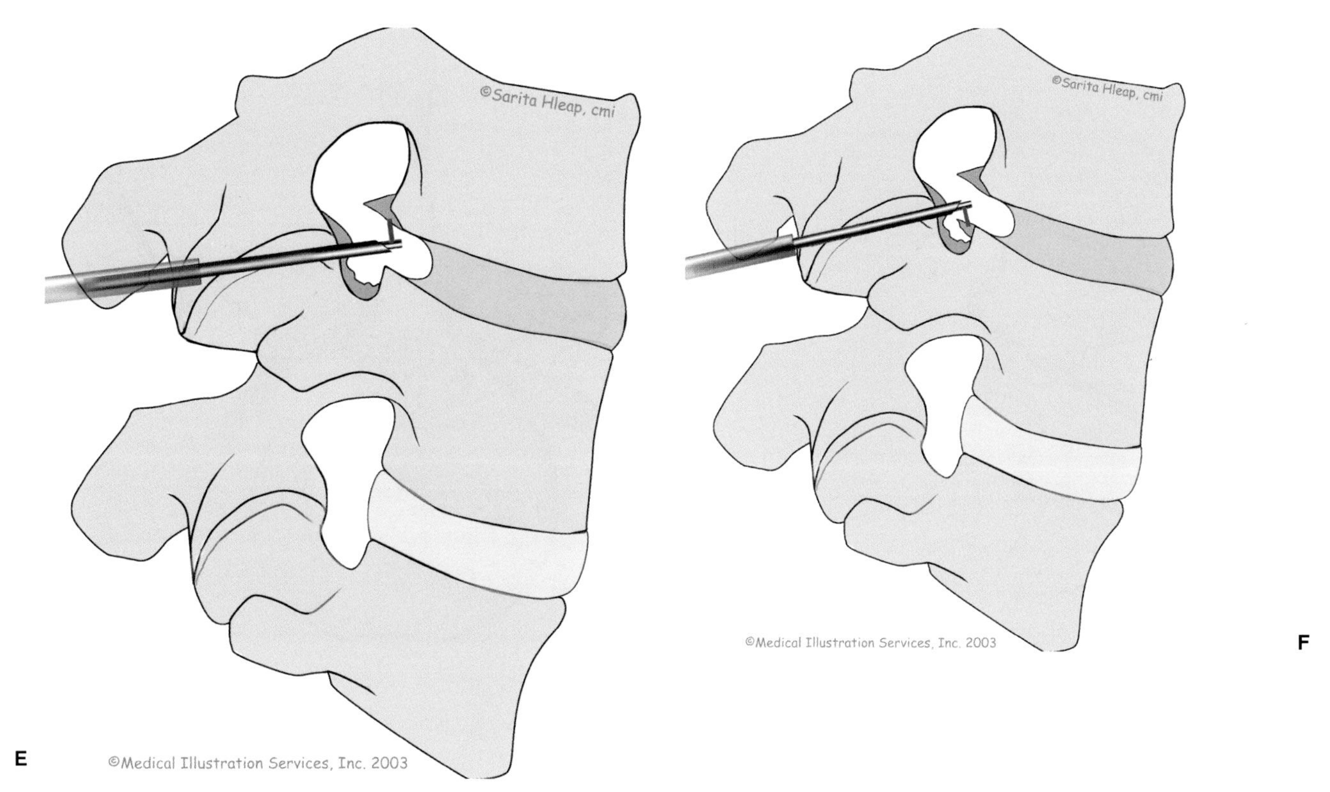

FIGURE 19–6 (*Continued*) **(E)** Illustration of lumbar laser foraminoplasty for upper shoulder osteophyte. **(F)** Illustration of lumbar laser foraminoplasty for lower shoulder osteophyte.

punches (rongeurs), and Kerrison rongeurs that can be passed through the large cannula for decompressive foraminoplasty, or laser application. An endoscopically assisted larger 9.9 mm tubular retractor system (Figs. 19–1B, 19–2B,D, 19–5B,C,E) has been added to facilitate foraminoplasty (Figs. 19–1B, 19–2B,D, 19–5B,C,E).

The steerable Spinescope (Karl Storz) can also be used to perform intradiscal lumbar laser diskectomy and laser foraminoplasty (Figs. 19–2A,C, 19–7, 19–9B). The Spinescope is fixed in a holding device, which allows the surgeon to guide and steer very precisely a flexible fiberscope and a working channel for a laser fiber of 0.6 mm diameter to the pathologic part of the disk and the intra- and periforaminal tissue. The laser fiber can be advanced or retracted millimeter by milllimeter inside the disk under direct vision with the fiberoptic endoscopic system, within a given distance. Also, the tip of the applicator/laser fiber can be navigated and angulated from 0 to 90 degrees with fine adjustment and rotated through 360 degrees in all directions.

After removing all instruments, 0.25% Marcaine is injected intradermally and into the incision and the paraspinal muscles along the path of the cannulation to prolong analgesia. A bandage is applied at the incision sites.

Postoperative Care

Ambulation begins immediately after recovery, and the patient is usually discharged 1 hour after surgery. The patient may shower the following day. Applying an ice pack is helpful. NSAIDs are prescribed, and mild analgesics and muscle relaxants are recommended as needed. Patients typically return to usual activities in 10 days to 3 weeks, provided heavy labor and prolonged sitting are not involved.

Outcome

At C-MISS, the first 60 consecutive cases of the 180-plus cases treated with TF-MEAD to date (since year 2000) included 31 males and 29 females. Thirty-six (60%) had surgery at one level, 24 (40%) at two or more levels, eight bilaterally. All patients had complained of chronic low back pain with radicular pain, usually unilateral, and in eight instances, bilateral. Physical examination, as well as positive MRI and/or CT, EMG, and intraoperative or preoperative diskograms appropriate to the symptomatic levels, confirmed the diagnosis and levels. All had failed to

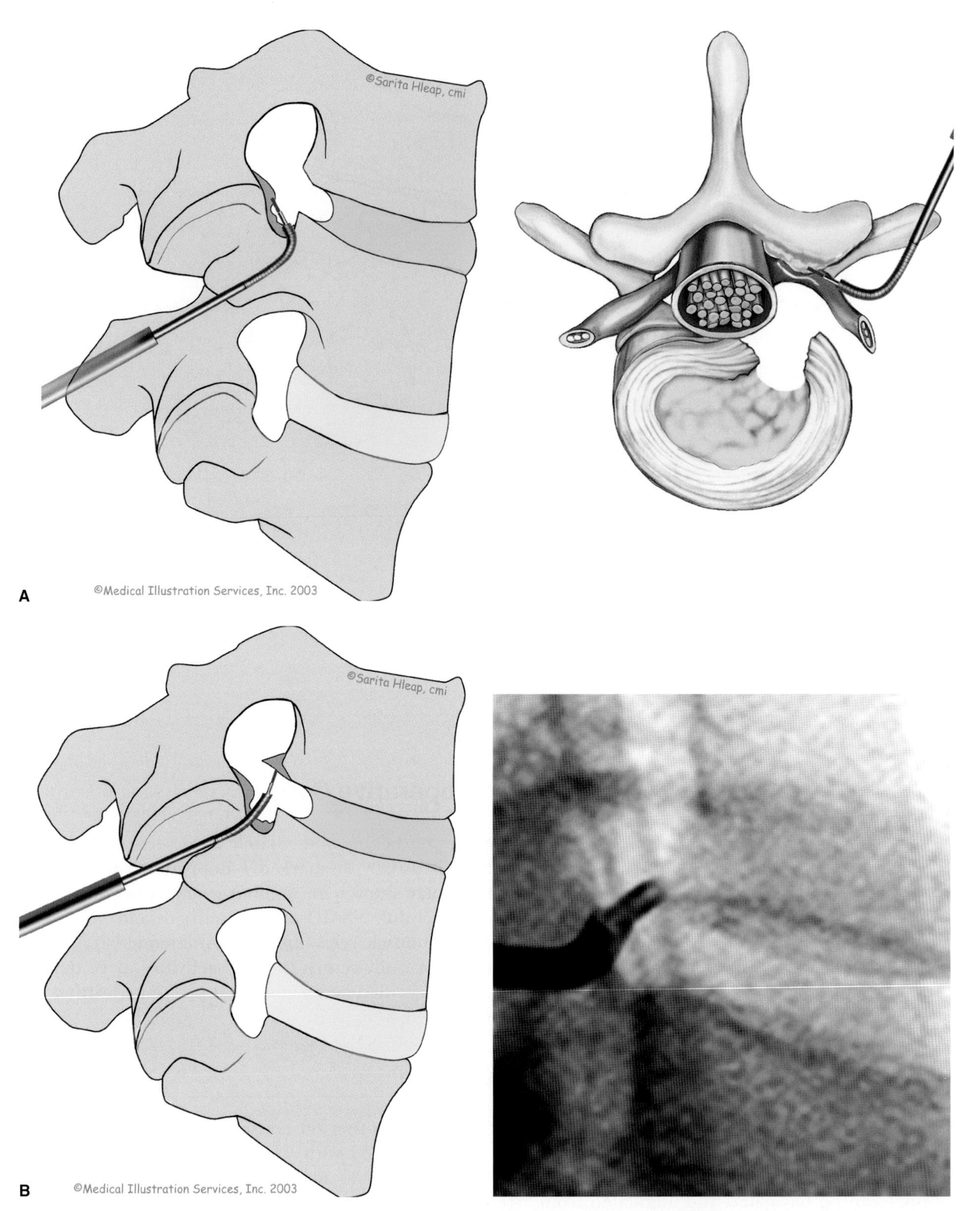

FIGURE 19–7 Fluoroscopic view and illustration of laser side-firing probe in action for lumbar laser foraminoplasty with steerable spinescope. **(A)** Illustrations of lumbar laser foraminoplasty with spinescope for facet hypertrophy (lateral and axial views). **(B)** Illustration and fluoroscopic lateral views of lumbar laser foraminoplasty with spinescope for upper shoulder osteophyte.

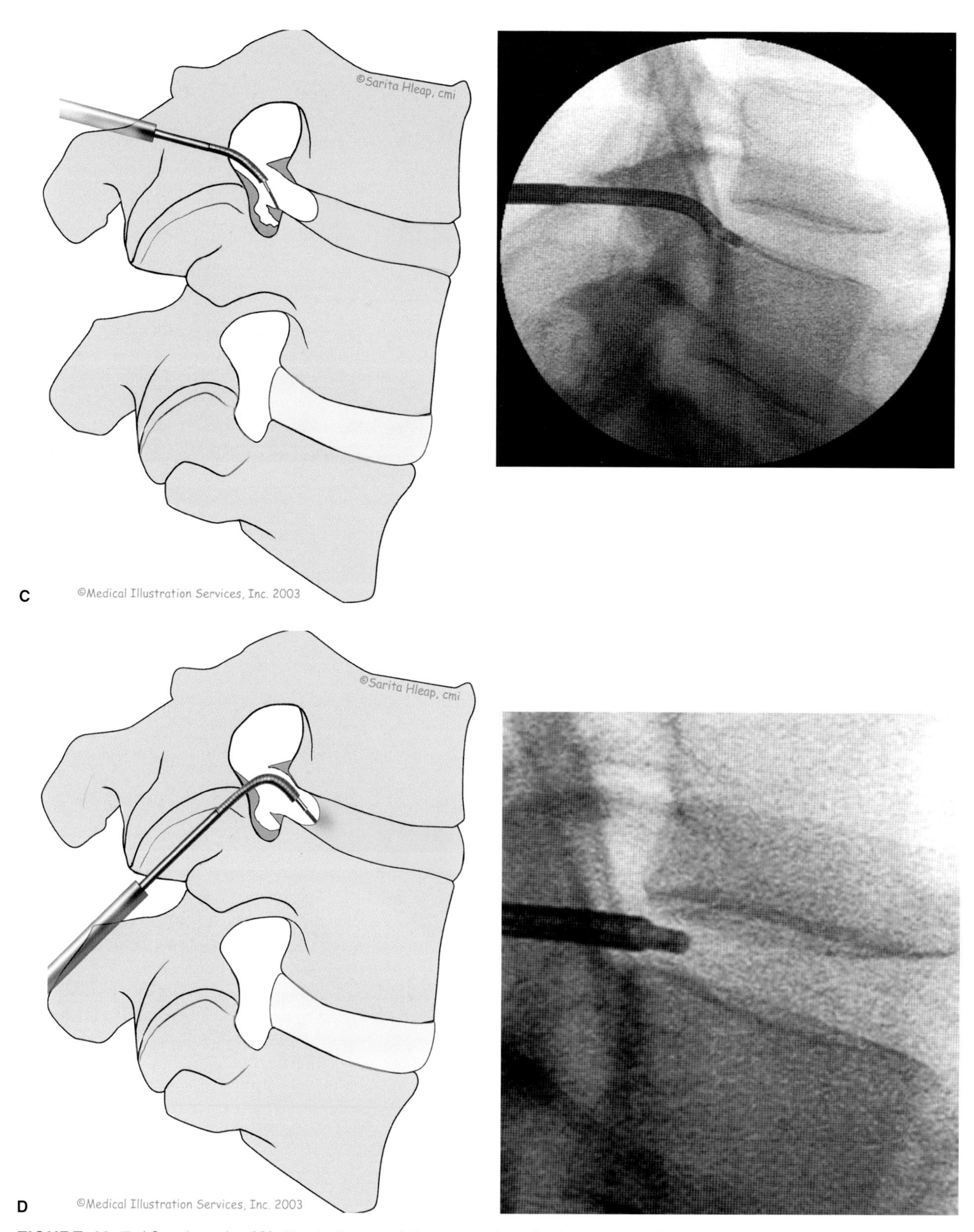

FIGURE 19–7 (*Continued*) **(C)** Illustration and fluoroscopic lateral views of lumbar laser foraminoplasty with spinescope for lower shoulder osteophyte. **(D)** Illustration and fluoroscopic lateral views of lumbar laser diskectomy with spinescope.

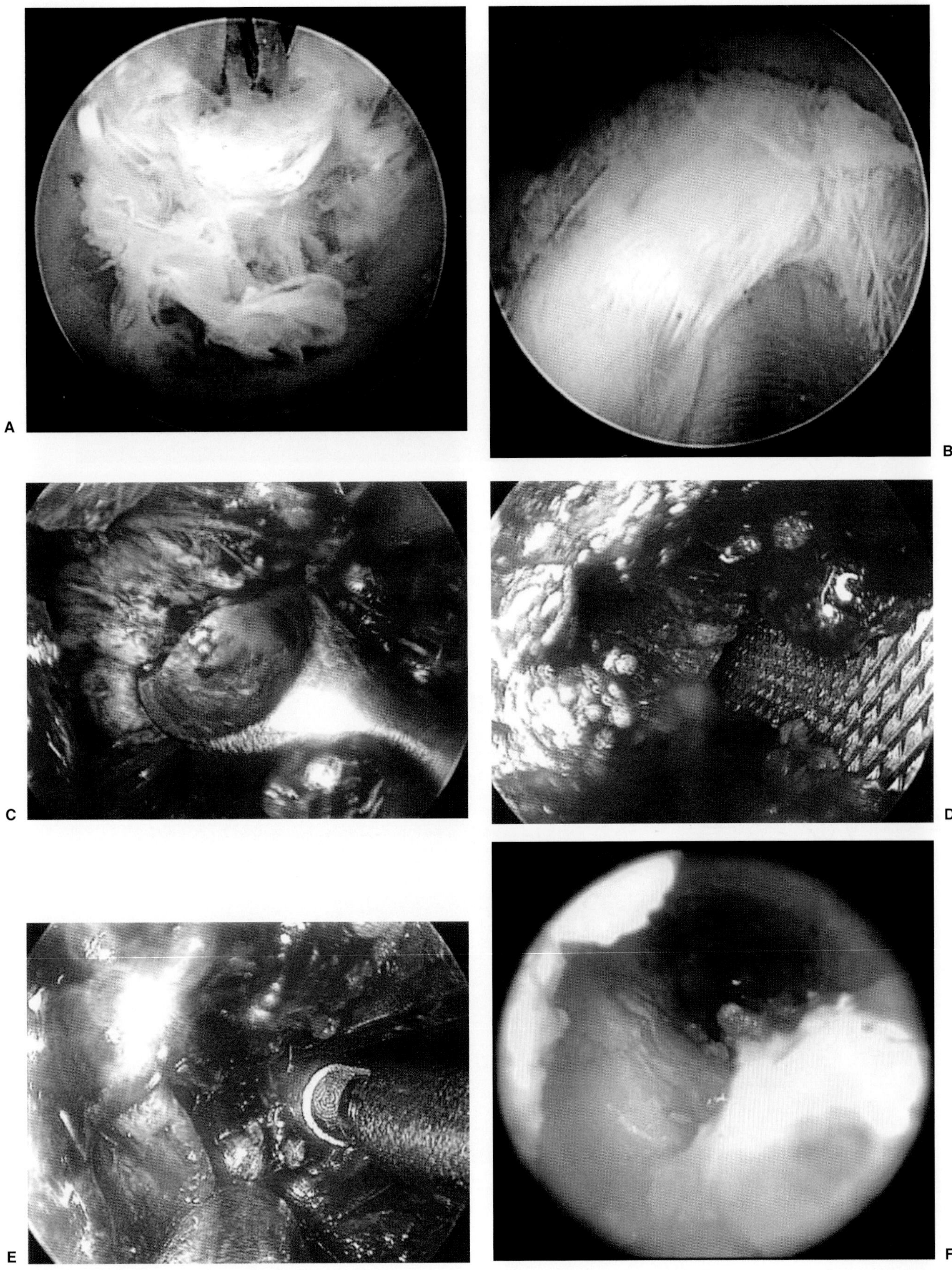

FIGURE 19–8 Endoscopic view of lumbar mechanical decompressive foraminoplasty and diskectomy. **(A)** Disk removal with cutter forceps. **(B)** Disk decompression below the nerve. **(C)** Curette for osteophytic decompression. **(D)** Rasp for osteophytic decompression. **(E)** Bone punch/rongeur for foraminal decompression. **(F)** Disk and foramen appearance post foraminoplasty.

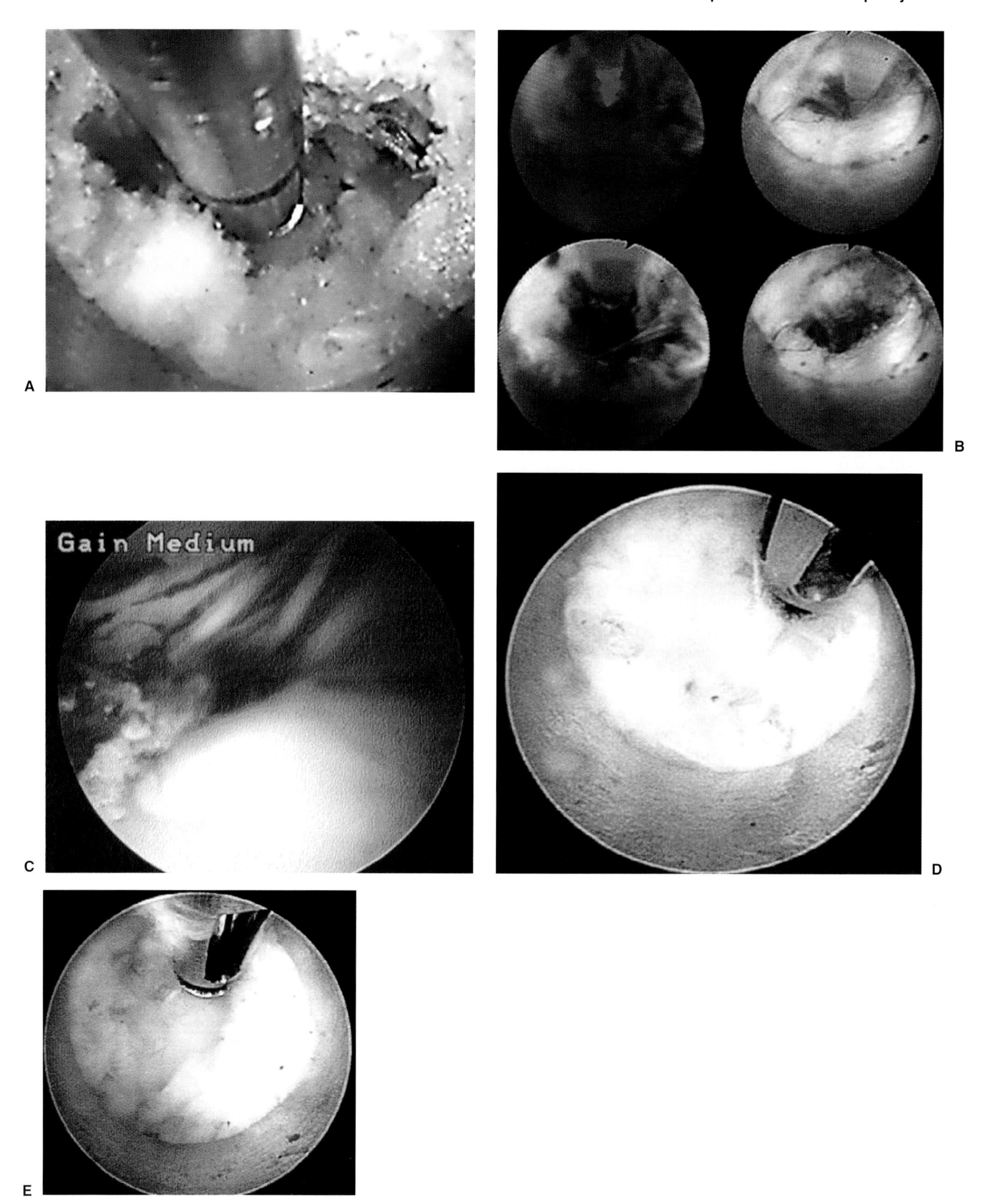

FIGURE 19–9 Endoscopic views of lumbar laser foraminoplasty, disk decompression, and laser thermodiskoplasty. **(A)** Side-firing laser probe in action for disk decompression and foraminoplasty. **(B)** Disk defect after decompression and laser thermodiskoplasty with bare laser fiber. **(C)** Lumbar nerve root above the disk after disk decompression and foraminoplasty. **(D)** Disk before laser thermodiskoplasty. **(E)** Disk shrinkage after laser thermodiskoplasty.

TABLE 19–1 Laser Setting for Lumbar Laser Thermodiskoplasty*

Stage	Watts	Joules
First	15	1500
Second	10	500

*Laser energy used (at 10 Hz) 5 seconds on and 5 seconds off for TF-MEAD.

improve after at least 12 weeks of conservative therapy. There were no significant intraoperative or postoperative complications. Fifty-three patients (88.33%) had a good or excellent result (McNabb criteria). Six had some continuing complaints but were improved overall. One did not significantly benefit from the procedure. Most patients found this procedure extremely gratifying.

Discussion

The TF-MEAD, with mechanical and laser applications using newly devised, more aggressive instruments, allows wider and more complete removal of larger disks and decompressive foraminoplasty at bilateral and multiple levels in one sitting. It has proven to be safe and effective. To become competent and avoid complications, the TF-MEAD or ELF surgeon must have a thorough knowledge of the surgical anatomy and the procedures, and specific surgical training with hands-on experience in a laboratory and working closely with an endoscopic surgeon expert at these procedures through the steep surgical learning curve.

Advantages

With endoscopic lumbar foraminoplasty, decompression of the lateral recess and foramen is accomplished at a single sitting and can be at multiple levels or bilateral. Other advantages are:

- Same-day outpatient procedure
- Less traumatic, both physically and psychologically
- Small incision and less scarring
- Zero mortality
- Minimal blood loss and little or no epidural bleeding
- No dissection of muscle, bone, ligaments, or manipulation of the dural sac or nerve roots
- Does not promote further instability of spinal segments or adjacent segment recurrent disks
- Commonly done under local anesthesia; no general anesthesia necessary
- Multiple level diskectomy feasible and well tolerated[28]
- Least challenging to medically high-risk patients and the obese
- Exercise programs can begin the same day as surgery
- No significant incidence of infection
- Direct endoscopic visualization and confirmation of the adequacy of decompression
- Minimal use of analgesics postoperatively
- Earlier return to usual activities, including work
- Costs less than conventional lumbar surgery

Disadvantages

Disadvantages of endoscopic lumbar foraminoplasty include:

- More than grade I spondylolisthesis
- Acute traumatic or neoplastic conditions
- ELF unisegmental and unilateral
- ELF requires overnight stay

Complications and Avoidance

A thorough knowledge of the endoscopic lumbar foraminoplasty and diskectomy procedures and surgical anatomy of the lumbar spine and intervertebral foramen, careful selection of patients and preoperative surgical planning with appropriate diagnostic evaluations, and meticulous intraoperative technique facilitate the ELF and TF-MEAD procedures and prevent potential complications. All potential complications of open lumbar disk surgery are possible, but they are much less frequent in endoscopic lumbar foraminoplasty.[26,28,31]

- Inadequate decompression of disk material: Minimized by using such multiple modalities and instruments as forceps, discectome, and laser application both to vaporize tissue and to perform thermodiskoplasty (shrinking and hardening the disk with laser energy at a lower level).
- Neural injury: Rare with MISS. Nerve root injury, although possible, can be avoided with the warning provided by continuous intraoperative neurophysiologic monitoring (EMG/NCV)[31] and direct endoscopic visualization. Operating strictly within the safe zone or triangle minimizes the root's exposure to injury. Sympathetic nerve injury is extremely remote because the procedure is largely intradiscal or in the foramen. Use of local anesthesia with a verbally responsive patient also provides a further warning system.
- Ganglion (dorsal root) injury: One of the commoner complications reported in posterolateral lumbar percutaneous approaches to the foramen is dysesthesia (the incidence of transient dysesthesia has been reported as high as 25% transient at one center but usually less than 2 to 3%, and permanent less than 1%)[31] in the leg on the operated side.

Careful technique guided by close endoscopic and C-arm fluoroscopic monitoring and knowledge of the surgical anatomy of the lumbar nerve root, dorsal root ganglion, and foramen minimize this complication.

- Operating on wrong level: A major complication of disk surgery at any level of the spine is operating at the wrong level. Proper use of digital C-arm fluoroscopy for correct anatomical localization avoids operating at the wrong disk level. Routine pain provocation test and diskogram give additional verification of the proper level.
- Infection: Avoided by careful sterile technique, the much smaller incisional area, the absence of

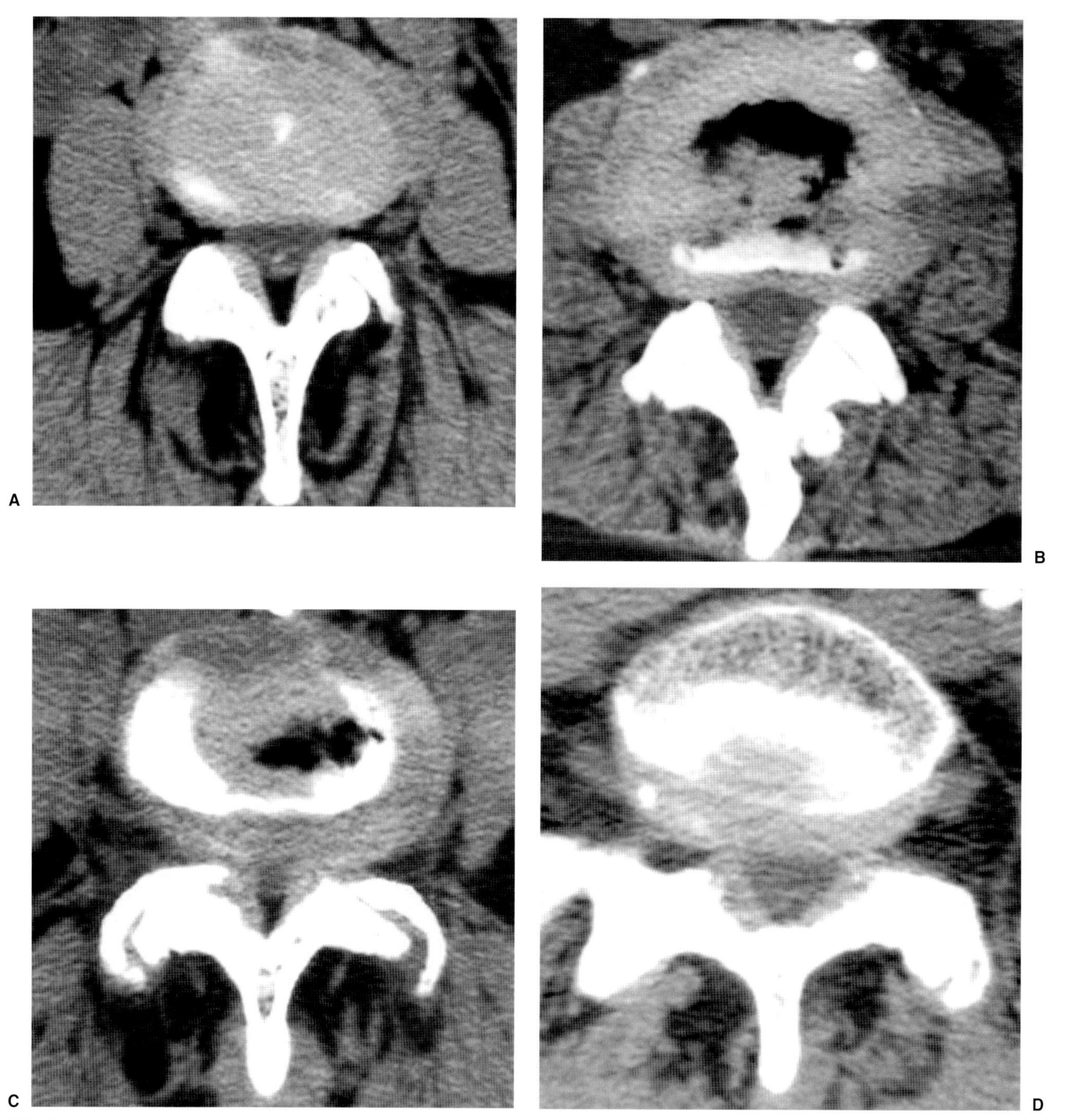

FIGURE 19–10 Axial CT images demonstrating severe bilateral lumbar foraminal stenosis secondary to posterior circumferential disk bulge/protrusion and facet osteophytic hypertrophy at **(A)** L1–L2, **(B)** L3–L4, **(C)** L4–L5, and **(D)** L5–S1.

prolonged retraction of soft tissues, and the use of prophylactic antibiotics IV intraoperatively.

- Diskitis: Prophylactic antibiotics, continuous irrigation of the interspace throughout the procedure, and the introduction of instruments through a cannula without contact with the skin tissues help minimize the incidence of infectious diskitis.
- Aseptic diskitis can be prevented by aiming the laser beam in a "bowtie" fashion to avoid damaging the end plates (at 6 and 12 o'clock).
- Hematoma (subcutaneous and deep): May occur with MISS (reported in the early literature), but is minimized by careful technique; by not prescribing anticoagulants, aspirin, or NSAIDs within a week prior to surgery; by doing a basic clotting screening preoperatively; by application of gentle digital pressure or placing a full IV bag over the operative site for the first 5 minutes after surgery; and by application of an ice bag thereafter.
- Vascular injuries: They are extremely rare when care is taken to remain within the disk space with stylets and cannulas. The aorta, vena cava, femoral arteries, and veins are best avoided by accurate placement of all instruments. No vascular injury has been reported with lumbar MISS since the early experience with similar procedures.
- Bowel and ureteral injuries: Ureteral injuries have not been reported with MISS. Bowel perforation was reported in the early experience, but was not reported in a multicenter study[31] of more than 26,860 cases.
- Cerebrospinal fluid leak or dural injury: Dural injury has not occurred in any sense other than as evidenced by spinal headache and presumed CSF leakage. The incidence of only transient leakage in the multicenter study[32] was less than 1%, and none required surgery to repair a dural tear. Spinal headache has responded to simple blood patches.
- Excessive sedation: Avoided by surface EEG monitoring, providing more precise estimation of the depth of anesthesia; reduces amount of anesthetics and prevents excessive or insufficient sedation. Operations under local anesthesia with conscious sedation allow the patient's responsiveness to be directly tested.
- Soft tissue injuries due to prolonged forceful retraction as occurs in many open disk operations are not an issue with TF-MEAD or ELF.

Case Illustration

An 80-year-old man was evaluated for complaints of progressive low back and right, more than left, lower extremity pain with numbness and tingling of both legs intermittently for 3 to 4 years, with neurogenic claudication after walking for one or two blocks in both lower extremities. After evaluation in his home country, he was treated with analgesics and an anti-inflammatory medication for arthritis of the spine, along with pain injectional therapy. He had paraspinal muscle spasm and tenderness with limited range of motion of the back. Deep tendon reflexes were decreased for right knee and both ankle jerks; strength and gait were normal. Straight leg raising was 70 degrees on the right and 75 degrees on the left. Pain and touch sensation were impaired on the dorsal and lateral aspect of the right foot and ankle. EMG showed bilateral L5 and S1 radiculopathy; CT image demonstrated disk defects of 3 mm at L1–L2, 4 to 5 mm at L3–L4, L4–L5, and L5–S1 with bilateral foraminal stenosis (Fig. 19–10). He had facet joint hypertrophy and intervertebral spurring. The patient was positive on provocative diskogram at all four levels. Outpatient TF-MEAD surgery was performed at four levels bilaterally. The patient was ambulatory postoperatively, with relief of all leg pain and numbness.

Endoscopic lumbar decompressive diskectomy and foraminoplasty (including ELF and TF-MEAD) has replaced open decompressive lumbar surgery for lateral spinal stenosis and disk herniation in this group of treated patients and has proven to be safe, less traumatic, easier, and efficacious, with significant economic savings. Both ELF and TF-MEAD are minimally invasive techniques that decrease intraoperative and postoperative complications significantly by using endoscopic surgical techniques.

ELF is a technically demanding procedure that requires 90 to 120 minutes to affect once the learning curve has been surmounted. It is intended for and ideally applied to the treatment of unilateral and unisegmental pathology; however, the complication rate of ELF has been significantly lower than conventional spinal surgery. With this procedure, MISS is no longer confined to percutaneous endoscopic diskectomy but also deals with effective decompression of lateral spinal stenosis, lateral recess, and foraminal large extruded herniated disks effectively.

TF-MEAD combines more aggressive mechanical decompression and laser application effectively to treat spinal pathology at multiple levels and bilaterally. Many elderly patients (even octogenarians and beyond) suffering symptoms caused by lateral spinal stenosis and disk problems can be successfully treated. The results of this operation can be extremely gratifying for both the patient and the surgeon.

These procedures require a knowledgeable and competent surgeon with a thorough appreciation of the surgical anatomy. A minimally invasive spine surgeon must have specific surgical training with hands-on experience in the laboratory and, most importantly, must spend time working through the steep surgical learning curve with an endoscopic spinal surgeon expert at this procedure.

REFERENCES

1. Hijikata S. Percutaneous nucleotomy: a new concept technique and 12 years' experience. *Clin Orthop.* 1989;238:9–23.
2. Ascher PW. Application of the laser in neurosurgery. *Laser Surg Med.* 1986;2:91–97.
3. Choy DS. Percutaneous laser disc decompression (PLDD): twelve years' experience with 752 procedures in 518 patients. *J Clin Laser Med Surg.* 1998;16:325–331.
4. Kambin P, Saliffer PL. Percutaneous lumbar discectomy: reviewing 100 patients and current practice. *Clin Orthop.* 1989;238:24–34.
5. Onik G, Maroon J, Davis G. Automated percutaneous discectomy: a prospective multi-institutional study. *Neurosurgery.* 1990;26:228–233.
6. Schreiber A, Suezawa Y, Leu HJ. Does percutaneous nucleotomy with discoscopy replace conventional discectomy? Eight years of experience and results in treatment of herniated lumbar disc. *Clin Orthop.* 1989;238:35–42.
7. Mayer HM, Brock M. Percutaneous endoscopic discectomy: surgical technique and preliminary results compared to microsurgical discectomy. *J Neurosurg.* 1993;78:216–225.
8. Savitz MH, Chiu JC, Yeung AT. History of minimalism in spinal medicine and surgery. In: Savitz MH, Chiu JC, Yeung AD, eds. *The Practice of Minimally Invasive Spinal Technique.* Richmond, VA: AAMISMS Education; 2000:1–12.
9. Jaikumar S, Kim DH, Kam A. History of minimally invasive spine surgery. *Neurosurgery.* 2002;51(suppl 2):1–14.
10. Knight M, Goswami A, Patko J, Buxton N. Endoscopic foraminoplasty: an independent prospective evaluation. In: Gerber BE, Knight M, Seibert WE, eds. *Laser in the Musculoskeletal System.* New York: Springer-Verlag; 2001:320–329.
11. Savitz MH. Same day microsurgical arthroscopic lateral approach laser assisted (SMALL) fluoroscopic discectomy. *J Neurosurg.* 1994; 80:1039–1045.
12. Jaikumar S, Kim DH, Kam A. Minimally invasive spine instrumentation. *Neurosurgery.* 2002;51(suppl 2):15–22.
13. Perez-Cruet M, Fessler R, Perin N. Review: complications of minimally invasive spinal surgery. *Neurosurgery.* 2002;51(suppl 2):26–36.
14. Destandau J. Endoscopically assisted microdiscectomy. In: Savitz MH, Chiu JC, Yeung AD, eds. *The Practice of Minimally Invasive Spinal Technique.* Richmond, VA: AAMISMS Education; 2000:187–192.
15. Chiu J, Clifford T, Princenthal R. The new frontier of minimally invasive spine surgery through computer assisted technology. In: Lemke HU, Vannier MN, Invamura RD, eds. *Computer Assisted Radiology and Surgery, CARS 2002.* New York: Springer-Verlag; 2002: 233–237.
16. Chiu J, Clifford T. Microdecompressive percutaneous discectomy: spinal discectomy with new laser thermodiskoplasty for non extruded herniated nucleus pulposus. *Surg Technol Int.* 2000;8: 343–351.
17. Chiu JC, Hansraj K, Akiyama C, Greenspan M. Percutaneous (endoscopic) decompressive discectomy for non-extruded cervical herniated nucleus pulposus. *Surg Technol Int.* 1997;6:405–411.
18. Chiu JC, Clifford T, Greenspan M. Percutaneous microdecompressive endoscopic cervical discectomy with laser thermodiskoplasty. *Mt Sinai J Med.* 2000;67:278–282.
19. Malis LI. Instrumentation and techniques in microsurgery. *Clin Neurosurg.* 1979;26:626–636.
20. Lin PM. Internal decompression for multiple levels of lumbar spinal stenosis: a technical note. *Neurosurgery.* 1982;11:546–549.
21. Caspar W, Campbell B, Barbier C, Kretschmmer R, Gottfried Y. The Caspar microsurgical discectomy and comparison with a conventional standard lumbar disc procedure. *Neurosurgery.* 1991; 28:78–87.
22. Kambin P, Casey K, O'Brien E, Zhou I. Transforaminal arthroscopic decompression of lateral recess stenosis *J Neurosurg.* 1996;84:462–467.
23. Atlas SJ, Keller RB, Robson D, Deyo RA, Singer DE. Surgical and nonsurgical management of lumbar spinal stenosis: four-year outcomes from the Maine lumbar spine study. *Spine.* 2000;25:556–562.
24. Katz JN, Stucki G, Lipson SJ, Fossel AH, Grobler LJ, Weinstein J. Predictors of surgical outcome in degenerative lumbar spinal stenosis. *Spine.* 1999;24:2229–2233.
25. Haag M. Transforaminal endoscopic microdiscectomy: indications and short-term to intermediate-term results. *Orthopade.* 1999;28: 615–621.
26. Khoo L, Fessler R. Microendoscopic decompressive laminotomy for the treatment of lumbar stenosis. *Neurosurgery.* 2002;51(suppl 2): 146–154.
27. Yeung AT, Tsou PM. Posterior lateral endoscopic excision for lumbar disc herniation: surgical technique, outcome, and complications. *Spine.* 2002;27:722–731.
28. Chiu JC, Clifford T. Multiple herniated discs at single and multiple spinal segments treated with endoscopic microdecompressive surgery. *J Minim Invasive Spinal Tech.* 2001;1:15–19.
29. Knight M, Goswami A. Endoscopic laser foraminoplasty. In: Savitz MH, Chiu JC, Yeung AD. eds. *The Practice of Minimally Invasive Spinal Technique.* Richmond, VA: AAMISMS Education; 2000:337–340.
30. Clifford T, Chiu JC, Rogers G. Neurophysiological monitoring of peripheral nerve function during endoscopic laser discectomy *J Minim Invasive Spinal Tech.* 2001;1:54–57.
31. Chiu JC, Clifford T, Savitz M, et al. Multicenter study of percutaneous endoscopic discectomy (lumbar, cervical and thoracic). *J Minim Invasive Spinal Tech.* 2001;1:33–37.
32. Clifford TJ, Chiu JC, Batterjee KA. Transpinal approach for endoscopic discectomy at L5–S1. *J Minim Invasive Spinal Tech.* 2001; 1:68–69.

20

Lumbar Microendoscopic Laminoforaminotomy and Diskectomy

PAUL SANTIAGO AND RICHARD G. FESSLER

Lumbar radiculopathy is one of the most common problems encountered by the practicing spine surgeon. The source of the pathology is often entrapment of an exiting nerve root at the level of the neural foramen or disk space.[1–4] In such cases, surgical intervention should be aimed at decompression of the exiting nerve root; however, iatrogenic injury to the surrounding structures is common and, in some cases, may precipitate further degenerative change. Lumbar diskectomy and foraminotomy are the most common approaches to lesions of this region.[5,6] Although this approach is unilateral and limits exposure only to the affected level, the approach results in injury to the midline muscular and ligamentous structures. Furthermore, the pathology is encountered laterally as opposed to medially. We will describe in this chapter an endoscopy-based modification of the microdiskectomy/foraminotomy technique that preserves the midline structures, provides a lateral approach to the neural foramen, and results in minimal muscular injury.[7–9]

Indications

Patients in our series complained of predominantly unilateral radicular symptoms, although in cases of large, central disks bilateral symptoms may be present. Standard preoperative imaging should start with anteroposterior (AP), lateral, flexion, and extension views of the lumbar spine. Patients with abnormal motion or greater than grade I spondylolisthesis should be considered for lumbar fusion. Further imaging should include an MRI of the lumbar spine. Patients with a history of previous surgery should also undergo MRI with and without gadolinium to distinguish recurrent disk herniation from scarring of the nerve root. In cases where the anatomy is unclear, lumbar myelography with postmyelography CT scanning remains the gold standard, albeit invasive, study. Myelography can be particularly useful in the assessment of pathology involving the neural foramen. Imaging should reveal disk herniation with impingement upon the adjacent nerve root as it traverses the neural foramen. In cases of large, rostrally displaced disk fragments, the nerve root can be compressed as it passes beneath the pedicle to exit through the neural foramen. Far lateral disk herniations may entrap the exiting nerve root within the foramen. In cases of degenerative facet disease, the adjacent nerve root may be compressed dorsally by hypertrophy of the facet complex as the nerve root crosses the medial aspect of the neural foramen to exit below the inferior pedicle. Patients with a history of multiple recurrences should be considered for lumbar fusion. Patients should have a complete medical work-up prior to surgery and meet the criteria for general anesthesia. The majority of our patients are treated as outpatients. Age is not a significant criterion; the senior author (RF) has performed the procedure successfully on patients in their 90s. Depending on their level of independence in the community and their home situation, elderly patients have been kept in the hospital overnight for observation. Obese patients in particular benefit from the use of the tubular retraction system (see later). Using standard microdiskectomy techniques, obese patients require an incision two to four times the standard length to provide adequate exposure. Using our technique, the same incision can be used for obese and nonobese patients.

Surgical Equipment/Operating Room Setup

A tubular retractor system is required. The only commercially available system currently is the MetRx system (Medtronic Sofamor Danek, Memphis, TN). This system provides both the dilators, retractors, and clamps required for the procedure as well as extra-long, antiglare coated instruments (Fig. 20–1A–C). Endoscopic diskectomy provides better visualization of the surgical anatomy over that provided by conventional microscopy. As such, a 30-degree angled endoscope and video tower are required (Fig. 20–1D). The coupler provided with the MetRx kit allows for the use of a variety of different endoscopes with either the 16 or 18 mm working channel. C-arm fluoroscopy is mandatory.

The patient is transported to the operating room while awake. General endotracheal tube anesthesia is administered while the patient is supine on a hospital stretcher. Perioperative antibiosis consists of a first-generation cephalosporin or vancomycin/clindamycin in penicillin-allergic patients. Intraoperative EMG-SSEP monitoring is generally not used. A Foley catheter is not inserted because operative time is ~45 to 60 minutes per level. Once the patient has been released by anesthesia for positioning, he or she is turned from the supine to the prone position onto an awaiting Wilson frame. The patient should be positioned such that the level of interest is centered on the apex of the frame. This position results in distraction of the laminae and facets at this level, aiding in exposure of the nerve root and foramen. For obese patients and in cases where a Wilson frame is unavailable, chest and pelvic rolls may also be used. Care should be taken to ensure that the patient's neck is in a neutral position and that the eyes are free of any pressure. Pressure points should be examined and adequately padded.

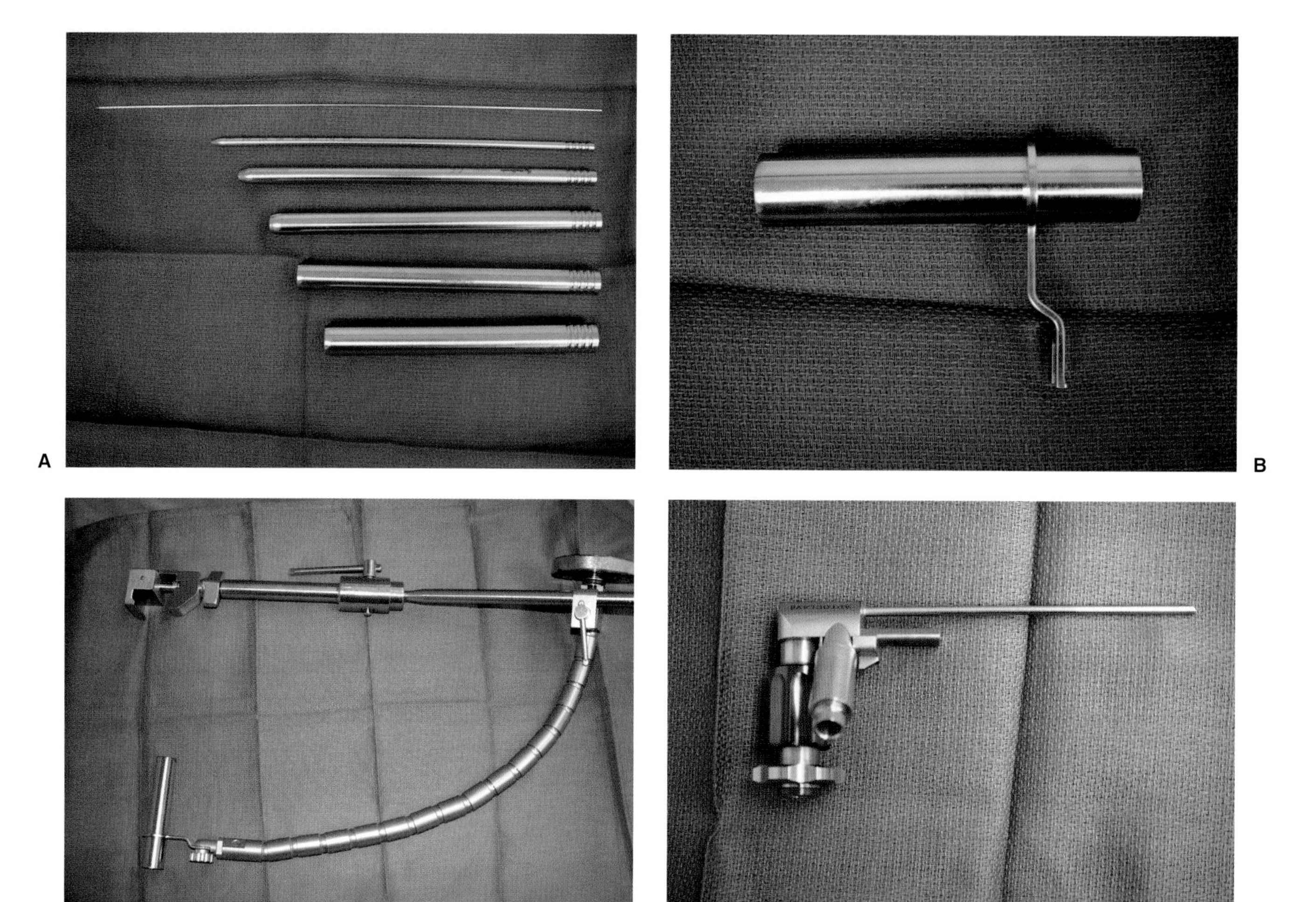

FIGURE 20–1 Surgical equipment. **(A)** Dilators. **(B)** An 18 mm working channel. **(C)** Table clamp with flexible arm. **(D)** A 30-degree angled endoscope.

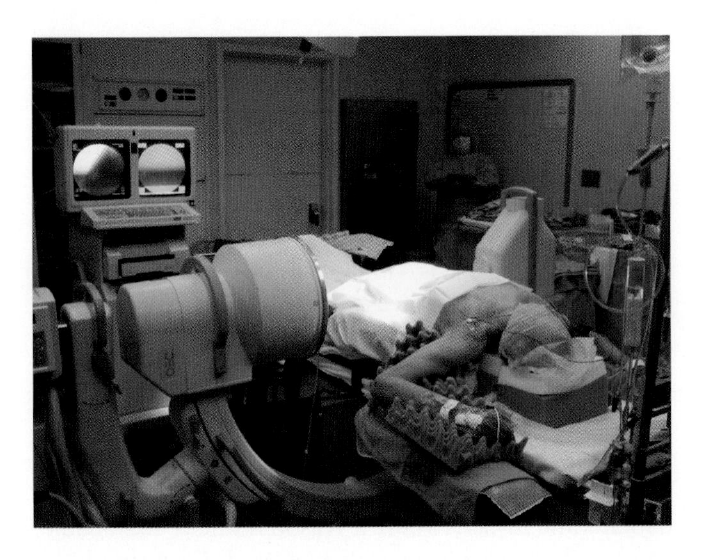

FIGURE 20–2 Room setup for a microendoscopic case. The patient is positioned prone on a Wilson frame. The C-arm is brought in from the contralateral side. The video tower is placed directly across from the patient. The C-arm monitor is placed at the foot of the operating table.

Surgical Technique

Once the patient has been properly positioned, the fluoroscope is wheeled into place. To avoid later confusion, a true lateral C-arm image must be obtained, adjusting the patient and C-arm as needed. It is also important to study a preoperative AP image of the spine to confirm the number of lumbar vertebrae because this can be quite difficult intraoperatively. Based on this review, the sacrum is used as the starting point for counting. Once the desired disk space has been identified, a long Steinmann pin can be placed along the patient's flank, directly overlying the disk space. This should cross the more dorsally located facet complex. With this as a guide, a point 1.5 cm off the midline should then be marked on the patient's skin ipsilateral to the desired approach. If done correctly, this point should lie superficial to the facet complex at the previously identified disk space.

The skin should then be prepped and draped in the standard sterile fashion. The C-arm should be draped sterilely into the field. As opposed to the standard microdiskectomy technique, the C-arm is used throughout the procedure, and as such, the surgeons and OR staff should wear safety aprons throughout the case. The operative site is then infiltrated with local anesthetic containing epinephrine. The assistant can simultaneously secure the clamp and snake retractor to the operative table. The clamp and retractor should be placed at approximately the level of the hip, contralateral to the operative site. The endoscopy tower and C-arm base are similarly placed directly across from the surgeon. If a microscope is to be used in lieu of endoscopy, the microscope base can be brought in from the ipsilateral side to avoid the C-arm base. It is usually easiest to position the C-arm monitor at the foot of the operating table (Fig. 20–2).

An 11-blade scalpel is used to make a small stab incision in the skin as previously marked. The stainless steel guide pin provided with the tubular retractors should then be passed through the stab incision and soft tissues onto the underlying bone. Fluoroscopy should be used to confirm the location of the guide pin. The safest approach is to direct the guide pin perpendicular to the entry point. This will often result in contact with the transverse process rather than the facet complex. It is preferable to be lateral to the facet complex rather than medial, where there is risk of entering the interlaminar space and injuring the contents of the spinal canal. The guide pin can then be directed medially to dock on the facet complex and centered on the disk space (Fig. 20–3A,B). A second stab wound can be made if the first proves to be inadequate. Once the appropriate trajectory has been found, the incision can be lengthened to 2 cm. The first dilator is then passed over the guide pin. Fluoroscopy is used to confirm that the dilator is docked on the facet complex. To avoid entering the spinal canal, the guide pin is removed, and the first dilator is left in place. The remaining dilators are then passed sequentially. Fluoroscopy is used to ensure maintenance of the desired trajectory. The dilators should be passed with a twisting motion to split the dorsal lumbar fascia. The underlying musculature is split along its fibers rather than torn. It is important to confirm that the dilators are resting against bone, minimizing the amount of tissue that needs to be removed later (Fig. 20–3B-F). Again under fluoroscopic guidance, the working channel is passed over the final dilator and angled slightly medially. The working space can be dilated to 16 or 18 mm for endoscopic applications and up to 22 mm for use with the microscope. We find 18 mm to be ideal for lumbar applications.

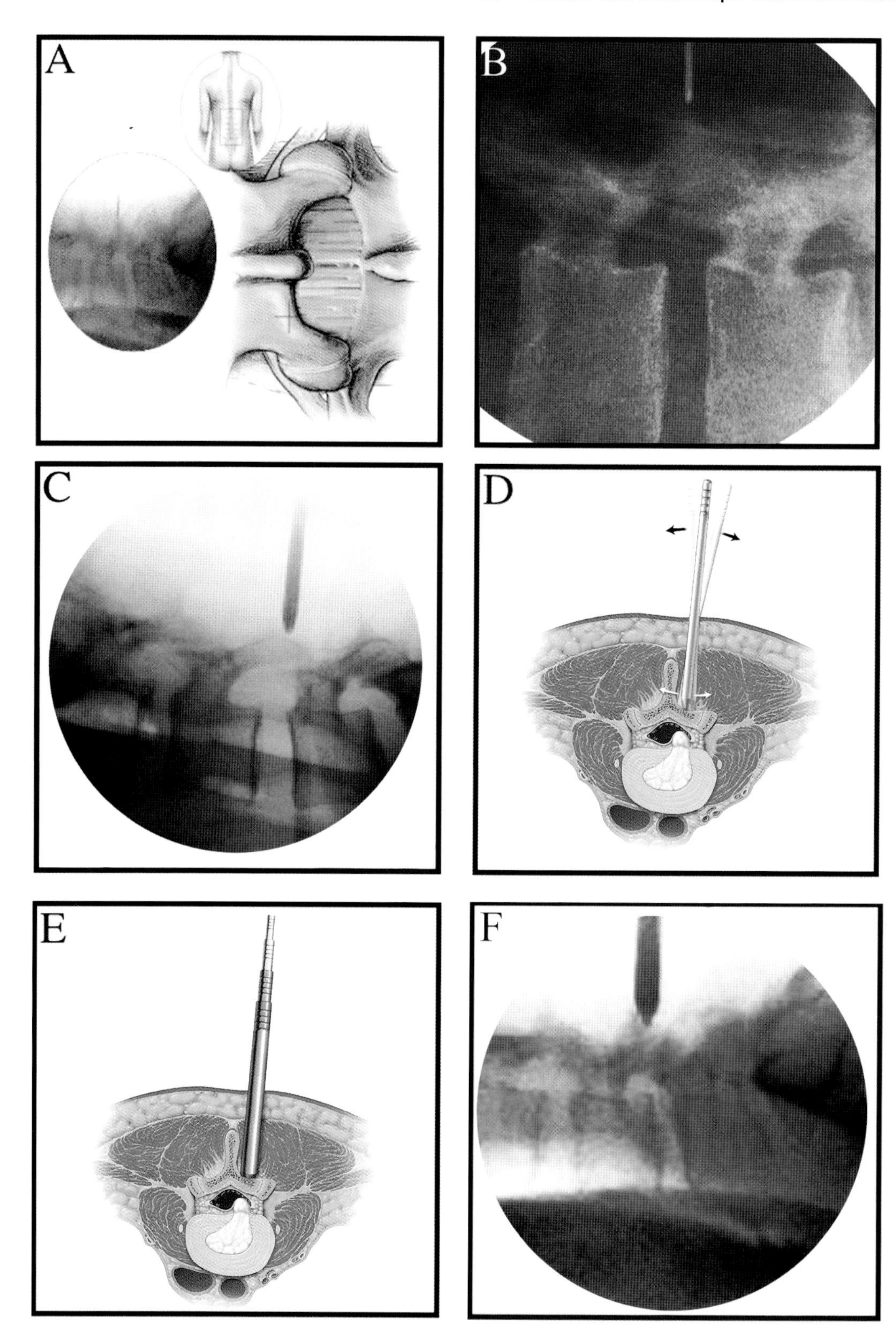

FIGURE 20–3 (A) The *cross* marks the target for the guide pin on the facet complex. **(B)** Guide pin docked on the facet complex over the disk space. **(C)** First dilator passed over guide pin. **(D)** The dilators can be arced to ensure ideal placement. **(E)** Serial dilation of the soft tissues. **(F)** C-arm image prior to passage of working channel.

The endoscope is then attached to the working channel (Fig. 20–4A). A radiopaque sucker is then passed into the working channel, and the location of the working channel is confirmed on fluoroscopy (Fig. 20–4B). Care should be taken to attach the endoscope as high up on the working channel as possible to avoid damage to the endoscope when using monopolar cautery. Monopolar cautery is then used to divide the residual muscular attachments to the underlying bone. It is important to ensure that cautery is used only when working on bone. It is safest to begin work laterally on the facet complex and then work medially, taking care to identify the interlaminar space. The muscle should be detached completely along the circumference of the tube prior to attempting removal of the muscle. Failure to do so can result in excessive bleeding and pulling more muscle into the field beneath the edges of the working channel. The "cut" setting on the cautery appears to be more effective than the "coagulation" setting during initial exposure. Once the muscle has been cleared, a straight current can be used to remove any residual soft tissue and to identify the interlaminar space and the inferior edge of the lamina.

The working channel should be directed medially to identify the junction of the spinous process and lamina (Fig. 20–4C). It is usually necessary to use cautery to remove additional tissue. A straight curette should then be used to detach the ligamentum flavum medially from the overlying lamina (Fig. 20–5). It is safest to define this plane medially and then to work laterally. A curved curette can be passed under the lamina to detach the ligamentum flavum from the undersurface of the lamina. Fluoroscopy should be used to confirm the location under the lamina dorsal to the desired disk space. Once an adequate plane has been established, 3 and 4 mm Kerrison punches should be used to perform a laminotomy. For the purposes of a foraminotomy or diskectomy, work should be aimed laterally. An angled curette is useful to define the plane and to prevent injury to the underlying dura and nerve roots. In general, the laminotomy should extend the length of the neural foramen, from pedicle to pedicle. At the junction of the lamina and facet complex it is usually necessary to use a high-speed drill to perform a medial facetectomy (Fig. 20–6). The facetectomy should continue until an angled curette passes easily into the neural foramen. Again, fluoroscopy is used to confirm the extent of the laminotomy and foraminotomy. It can be helpful when working laterally to reposition the working channel laterally. Bony bleeding is easily addressed using bone wax. In most cases, the bony opening exposes the ligament superficial to the shoulder and lateral margin of the nerve root as it passes along the foramen.

With the bony opening completed, attention is then turned toward removal of the ligamentum flavum. A Penfield number 4 is used to make an opening in the ligament along the rostral-most aspect of the laminotomy (the ligamentum is often thinnest at this point). If another opening has been made elsewhere, it can be used. A curved curette is then used to establish a plane between the dura and ligament and can be used to detach the ligament from the bone along the edges of the laminotomy (Fig. 20–7A). Right-angle rather than angled punches are useful for removal of the ligamentum. The ligament should be resected along the lateral border of the nerve root.

In cases of disk herniation, the nerve root may be distorted, and it may be necessary carefully to resect more of the medial facet to visualize the shoulder of the nerve root adequately (Fig. 20–7B). In cases of foraminal disease only, a ball-tip probe should be passed into the foramen to confirm adequacy of decompression. A spatula or blunt hook can be used to explore the ventral aspect of the dura for an occult disk herniation. Acute disk herniations are handled in a fashion similar to standard microdiskectomy. A Penfield number 4 is used to explore the axilla and shoulder of the nerve root. If the disk is found to herniate through the axilla and prevent mobilization of the nerve root medially, the axilla should be decompressed first. A combination nerve root retractor/sucker is used to retract the thecal sac medially (Fig. 20–7C). It is often necessary at this point to position the working channel laterally to retract the thecal sac medially. A suction retractor can then be used to protect the nerve root. Epidural veins are coagulated as necessary, the anulus is incised, and the disk fragment is removed (Fig. 20–7D). Once the axilla has been decompressed, the retractors should be positioned lateral to the shoulder of the nerve root, and the nerve root and shoulder pulled medially. Further diskectomy should then be performed in the standard fashion (Fig. 20–7E). Because a 30-degree endoscope is used for the procedure, the endoscope can be directed medially to help with decompression of more medially located disks, a maneuver not possible with the operating microscope (Fig. 20–7F). After completion of the diskectomy, the wound is irrigated with copious amounts of antibiotic saline. Hemostasis should be confirmed, and, if necessary, a small piece of thrombin-soaked Gelfoam may be left behind. If the nerve root appears swollen, Gelfoam soaked in 40 mg methylprednisolone acetate (Depo-Medrol, Pharmacia & Upjohn Co., Kalamazoo, MI) may also be used.

The snake retractor is then loosened, and the working channel with attached endoscope is slowly

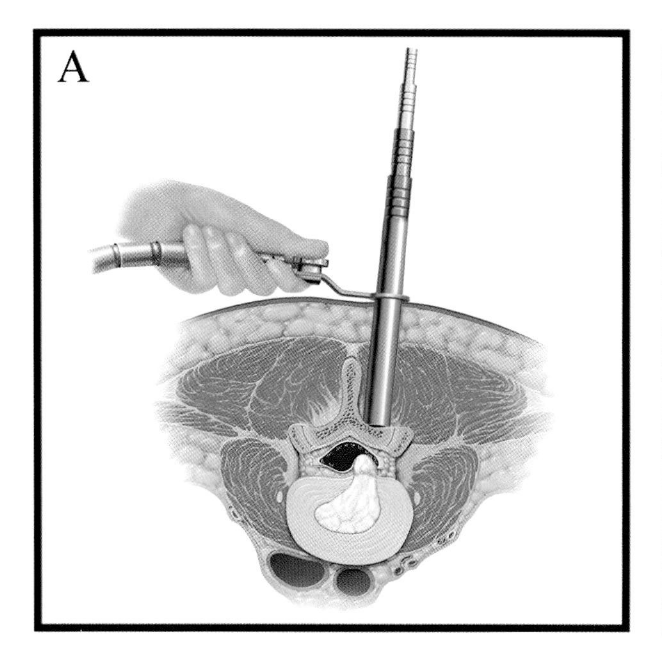

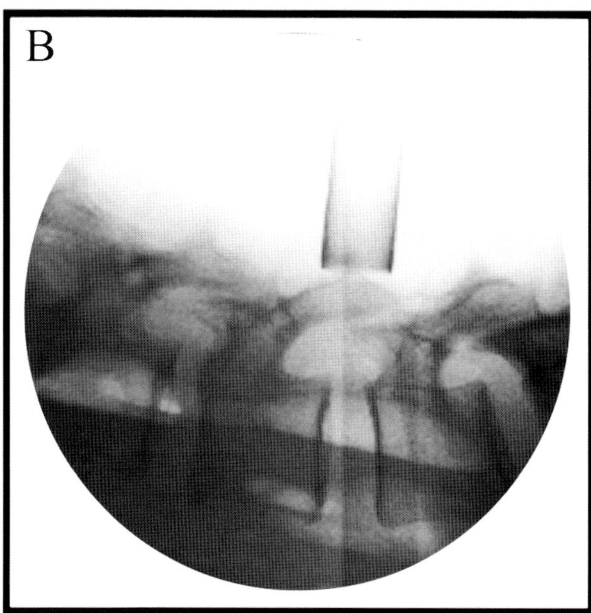

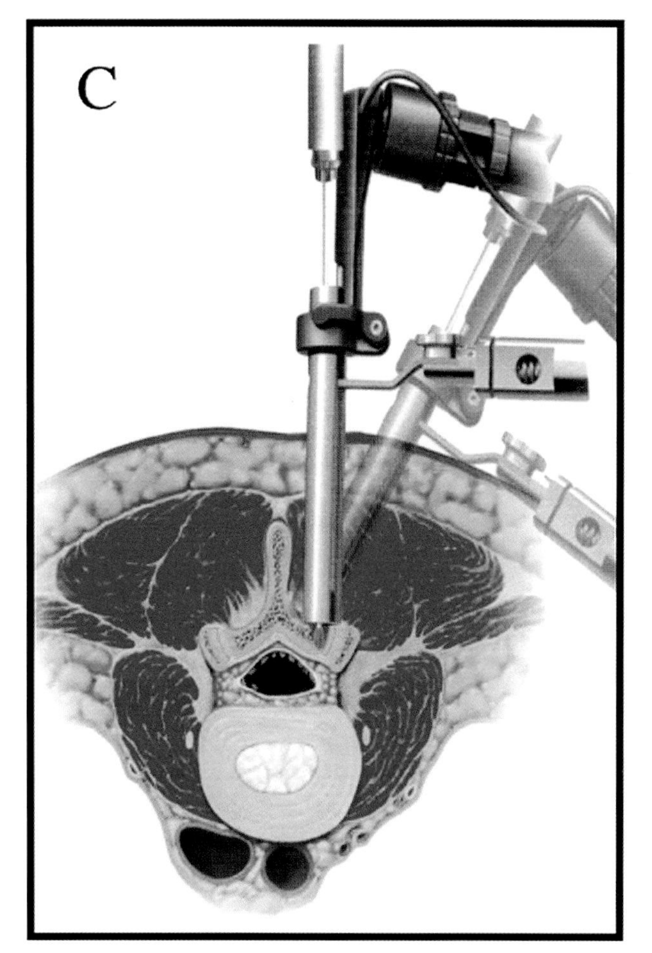

FIGURE 20–4 (A) The working channel is passed over the final dilator and secured to the table clamp. **(B)** Ideal placement of working channel over the disk space. **(C)** The endoscope is attached and angled medially.

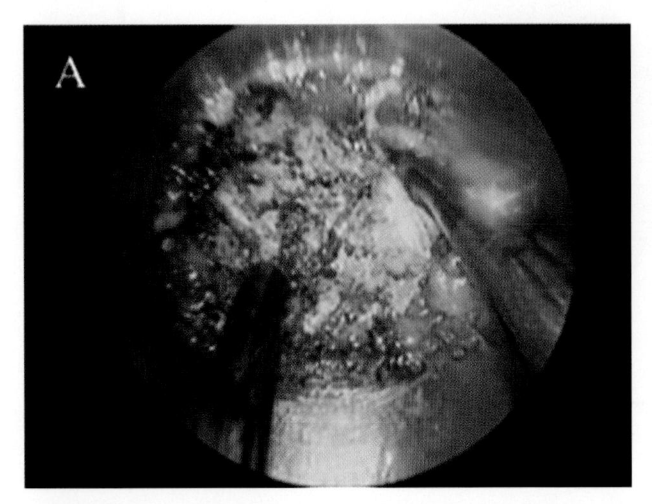

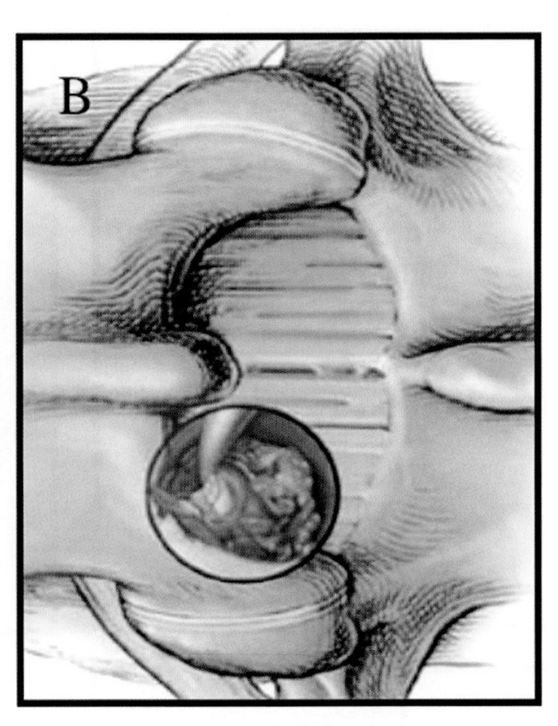

FIGURE 20–5 (A) After dissection of the muscular attachments from the lamina using electrocautery, a curette is used to clear the soft tissue from the edge of the lamina and establish a plane between the lamina and the ligamentum flavum. **(B)** Artist's representation of the soft tissue clearance.

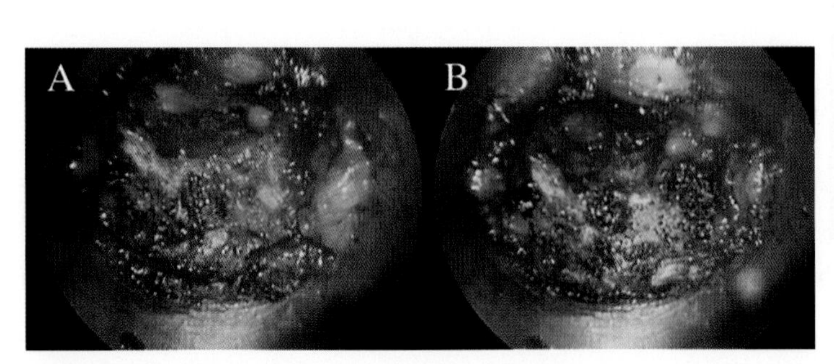

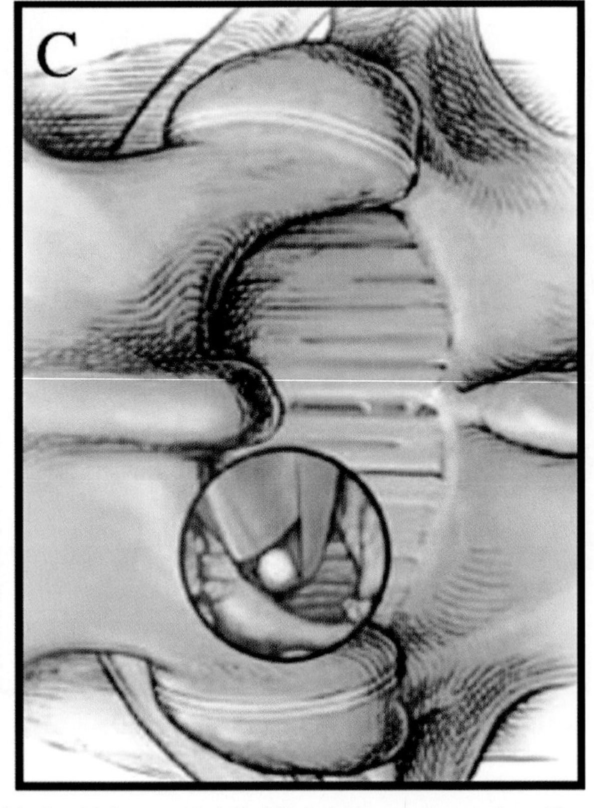

FIGURE 20–6 (A) Starting medially, a punch is used to perform a hemilaminotomy. **(B)** The hemilaminotomy extends laterally. A partial medial facetectomy is also performed with the aid of a high-speed drill. **(C)** Artist's representation. Note that the ligamentum flavum is kept intact to protect the underlying dura and a hemilaminectomy with Karrison punch.

removed. Muscle bleeders tamponaded by the retractor are thus easily identified and coagulated. The wound should again be irrigated. The dorsal lumbar fascia is then closed, the subcutaneous tissues are approximated, and the skin is closed with interrupted subcuticular stitches. The wound is dressed with cyanoacrylate (Fig. 20–8). The patient is then turned over to the anesthesia team.

In most cases, patients are monitored for 2 to 4 hours and discharged to home after demonstrating adequate pain relief, lack of nausea/vomiting, ambulation, and baseline bladder function. In patients in whom there is no contraindication (i.e., impaired renal function, reactive airway disease, NSAID allergy, etc.), a single IV/IM dose of ketorolac has proven useful in the management of postoperative pain. Patients are allowed to shower on the day after surgery. Lifting is restricted to less than 10 lbs (4.54 kg) for 6 weeks after surgery.

Because our technique allows for a lateral approach to the disk space, microendoscopy is particularly useful in the management of recurrent disk herniation. In this sit-

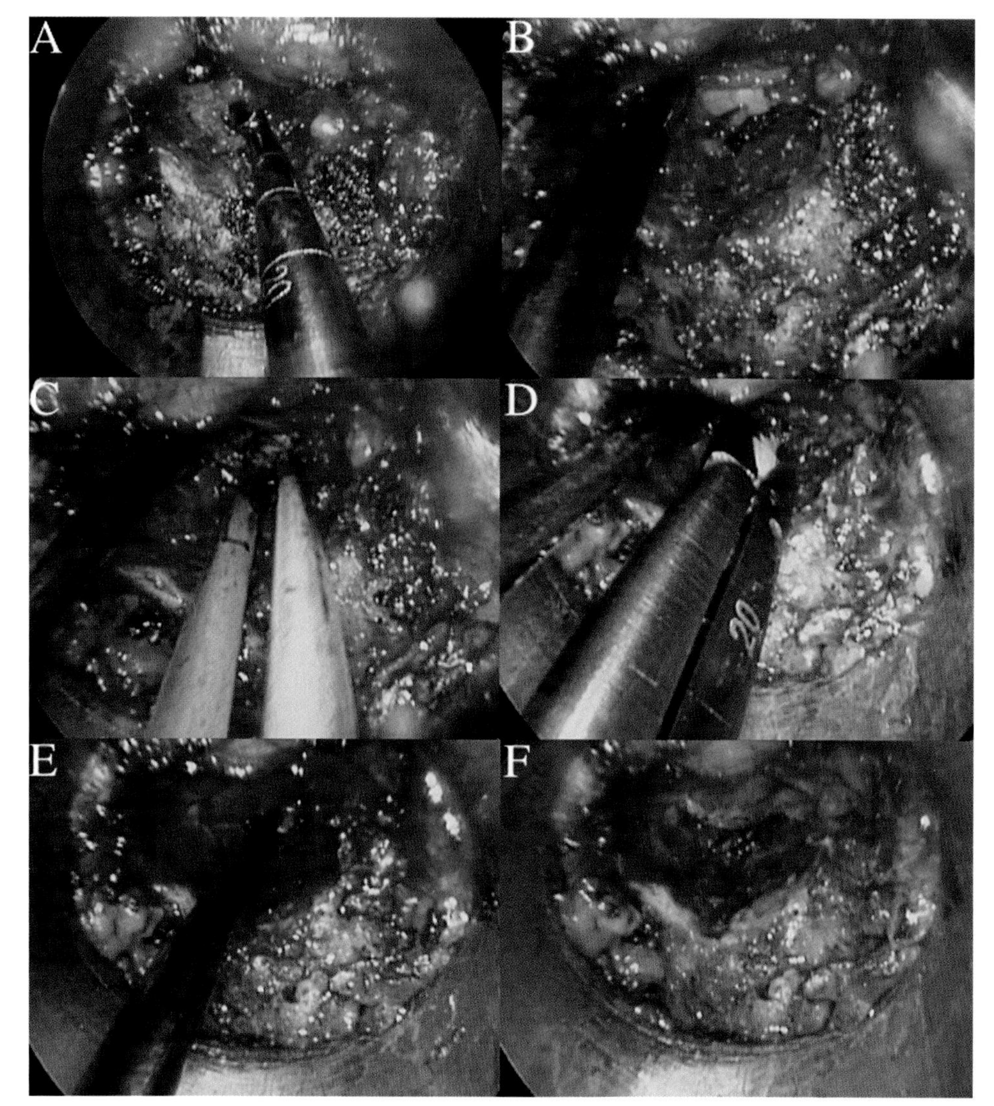

FIGURE 20–7 **(A)** An angled curette is used to establish a plane between the dura and the ligamentum flavum. Kerrison punches are then used to resect the ligament. **(B)** The exposed nerve root distorted by the ventrally placed disk is then visualized. **(C)** A suction retractor is used to retract the nerve root and the thecal sac medially. Bipolar cautery is used to control epidural bleeding. **(D)** The anulus is divided with a scalpel, and the disk fragment is removed with a pituitary rongeur. **(E)** The disk space is explored for further disk fragments. **(F)** With the herniated disk removed, the nerve and its relation to the thecal sac are clearly visualized.

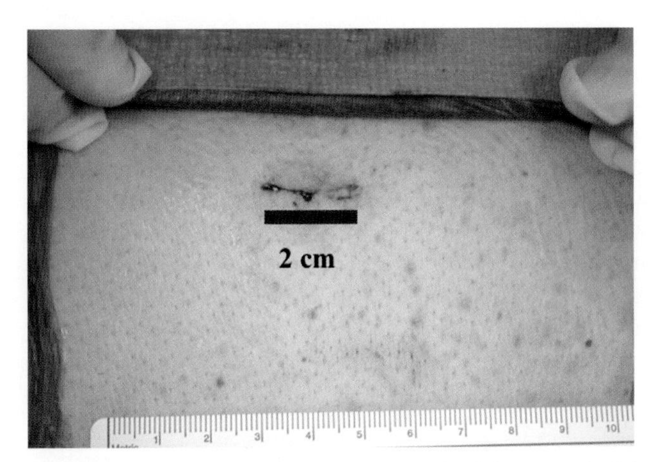

FIGURE 20–8 Standard microendoscopic diskectomy incision. The wound is dressed with cyanoacrylate.

uation, care is again taken to localize the facet complex from lateral to medial. Soft tissue resection begins laterally, and curettage is used medially. The edge of the neural foramen is defined with a curette, and a medial facetectomy is performed with the high-speed drill and Kerrison punches. The majority of the scar remains attached to the midline. Once the lateral edge of the nerve root is identified, the surgeon continues as with the standard procedure.

Patients are discharged with a 2-week supply of oral narcotics (oxycodone/acetaminophen or hydrocodone/ acetaminophen every 4 to 6 hours as needed) and stool softeners. We have also found that the addition of baclofen 10 mg PO tid for 30 days is quite effective in the management of postoperative muscular spasm and pain. Patients are seen in follow-up by our nurse practitioner at 7 to 10 days for a wound check and pain medication adjustment as needed. Six weeks of physical therapy commences 1 week postoperatively. Most patients are off narcotics by the fourth postoperative week. Patients are again seen in follow-up at 6 weeks and discharged from our clinic if no further issues remain.

Potential Complications and Avoidance

Vascular and intra-abdominal injury is a potential complication of the microendoscopic diskectomy procedure during localization and diskectomy. During localization it is important to use fluoroscopy to confirm the depth of the guide pin. The tip of the guide pin should be kept dorsal to the transverse process. The goal is to dock on the facet complex firmly. During the diskectomy portion of the procedure, fluoroscopy can be used to confirm the depth of the instruments within the disk, ensuring that the ventral aspect of the anulus fibrosus is not violated, risking injury to the vascular structures of the retroperitoneum and bowel.

In a previously reported series, the incidence of durotomy was ~3 to 5%.[10] During localization, care should be taken to ensure that the guide pin is firmly docked on the facet complex. Directing the guide pin perpendicular to the skin and not medially protects against entering the interlaminar space, which is especially important in recurrent disk herniations, when a laminar defect is present. Removal of the guide pin after passage of the first dilator prevents migration of the pin during passage of the larger dilators. Establishment of the plane between the lamina and the ligamentum flavum medially prior to the laminotomy helps to prevent accidental durotomy. If a small durotomy does occur, we have been successful in using a small piece of Gelfoam and 24 hours of supine bed rest. Larger durotomies have been repaired primarily with 48 to 72 hours of lumbar drainage. Delayed pseudomeningocele has been encountered in only one patient.[10]

Acute radiculopathy has been encountered in patients with large disk herniations, requiring aggressive mobilization of the nerve root. In these patients, a rapid methylprednisolone taper has proven useful. Although quite painful, the symptoms usually resolve within 7 to 10 days.

Persistence of symptoms at the 6-week follow-up, despite physical therapy and a steroid taper, are managed with a repeat MRI. In the absence of a gross recurrence, epidural steroid injections can be attempted for pain control. If a small-to-moderately sized disk herniation is obvious, repeat exploration, and decompression can be attempted.

Case Illustration

A 60-year-old female presented with a 6-month history of right-sided sciatica, radiating to the dorsum of her right foot. There were no sensory or motor deficits detected on physical examination. Imaging revealed a large right-sided disk herniation at the L4–L5 level (Fig. 20–9). Bed rest and physical therapy failed to result in lasting symptomatic improvement. The patient underwent right-sided L4–L5 microendoscopic diskectomy. There were no complications. The patient was seen at 1 week for a wound check and at 4 weeks for postoperative evaluation. Except for a few episodes of mild sciatica associated with heavy activity, the patient's symptoms were completely resolved.

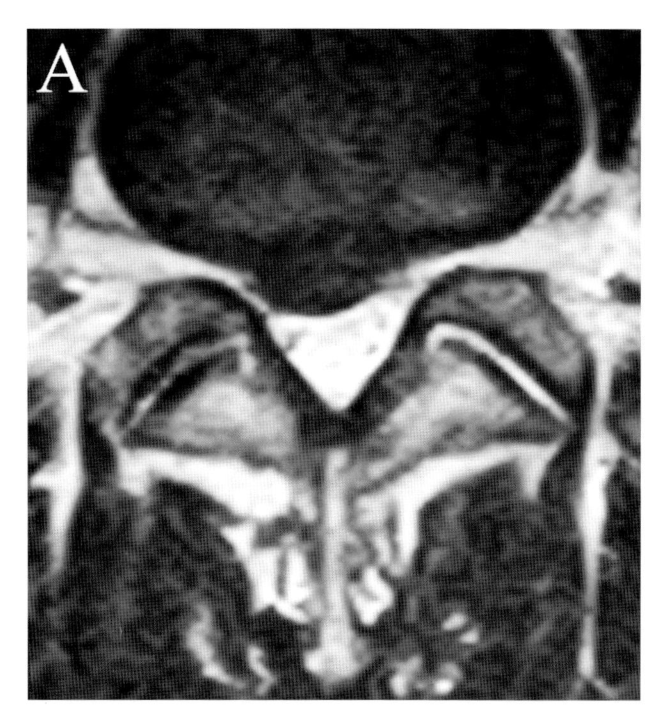

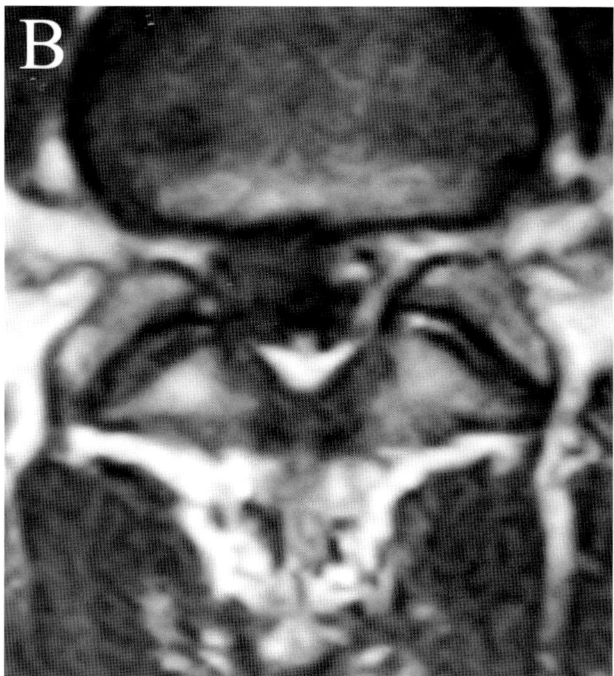

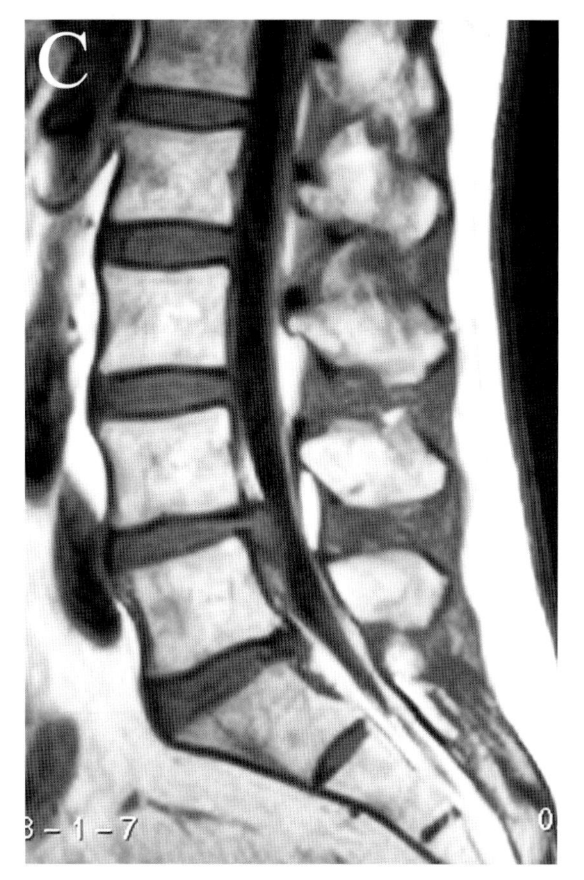

FIGURE 20–9 (A) T1-weighted MRI, revealing a right-sided herniated nucleus pulposus at L4–L5 displacing the L5 nerve root. **(B)** T2-weighted MRI of the same disk herniation in A. **(C)** Sagittal T1-weighted MRI further demonstrating the herniated nucleus pulposus at L4–L5.

REFERENCES

1. Silvers HR, Lewisa PJ, Suddaby LS, Asch HL, Clabeaux DE, Blumenson LE. Day surgery for cervical microdiscectomy: is it safe and effective? *J Spinal Disord.* 1996;9:287–293.
2. Rutkow IM. Orthopaedic operations in the United States, 1979 through 1983. *J Bone Joint Surg Am.* 1986;68:716–719.
3. Hoffman RM, Wheeler KJ, Deyo RA. Surgery for herniated lumbar discs: a literature synthesis. *J Gen Intern Med.* 1993;8:487–496.
4. Dvorak J, Gauchat MH, Valach L. The outcome of surgery for lumbar disc herniation, I: A 4–17 years' follow-up with emphasis on somatic aspects. *Spine.* 1988;13:1418–1422.
5. Javedan S, Sonntag VK. Lumbar disc herniation: microsurgical approach. *Neurosurgery.* 2003;52:160–162.
6. Mixter WJ, Barr JS. Rupture of the intervertebral disc with involvement of the spinal canal. *N Engl J Med.* 1934;211:210–215.
7. Foley KT, Smith MM. Microendoscopic discectomy. *Tech Neurosurg.* 1997;3:301–307.
8. Perez-Cruet MJ, Foley KT, Isaacs RE, et al. Microendoscopic lumbar discectomy: technical note. *Neurosurgery.* 2002;51(suppl 5): 129–136.
9. Perez-Cruet MJ, Smith MM, Foley KT. Microendoscopic lumbar discectomy. In: Perez-Cruet MJ, Fessler RG, eds. *Outpatient Spinal Surgery.* St. Louis: Quality Medical Publishing; 2002:171–183.
10. Perez-Cruet MJ, Fessler RG, Perin NI. Review: complications of minimally invasive spinal surgery. *Neurosurgery.* 2002;51(suppl 5): 26–36.

21

Paraspinal Endoscopic Laminectomy and Diskectomy

JEAN DESTANDAU

There is no doubt that the future of surgery lies in the development of minimally invasive techniques, and that spinal surgery does not escape this rule. This belief prompted the development by the author of special instrumentation to facilitate posterior endoscopic surgery,[1] first for prolapsed lumbar disks, and then for lumbar spinal canal stenosis. This instrumentation was custom-designed in 1993 to resolve two key difficulties presented by endoscopic surgery for disk herniation in the lumbar region. First, the instrument creates a working space mechanically rather than by the use of a fluid under pressure, which was unacceptable given the danger that such pressure would represent for the neural elements. Second, the angle between the working channel and the optics channel provides the triangulation necessary to keep the extremity of the instruments constantly in view to facilitate the operation. Prototypes of the device were used until 1998, when standard instrumentation (Karl Storz GmbH & Co., Tuttlingen, Germany) became available.

Indications

The posterior endoscopic approach of the spine can be used in all types of lumbar disk herniations, including lateral or recurrent disk herniations, lumbar spinal stenosis (central or lateral), and soft lateral cervical and thoracic disk prolapses.

Contraindications

This endoscopic approach is contraindicated in cases of calcified midline thoracic herniations.

Instruments

The Endospine (Karl Storz) consists of a small speculum provided with an inserter that penetrates the superficial layers, bringing the speculum into contact with the lamina. The inserter is then removed, and the surgeon slides a device into the speculum housing three tubes, one for the endoscope (4 mm in diameter), another for the suction cannula (4 mm in diameter), and the largest for the surgical instruments (9 mm in diameter) (Fig. 21–1). The first two are parallel, whereas the third is at an angle of 12 degrees to them; thus, the tubes generally converge in the plane of the posterior longitudinal ligament. This angulation enables the surgeon to keep the ends of the instruments in view at all times and to use the suction cannula as a second instrument. The system also includes a nerve root retractor that can be pushed into the spinal canal and used to retract the nerve root medially, thus clearing the operative field of any fragile structure.

Surgical Technique

The intervention is typically performed under general anesthesia, with the patient in the knee-chest position on the operating table. The surgical technique itself is classic and begins with a posterior approach to the spinal canal between the muscles and the lamina.

Marking the Point of Entry

With the aid of a special device with two arms (Karl Storz), the point of entry and the direction of approach

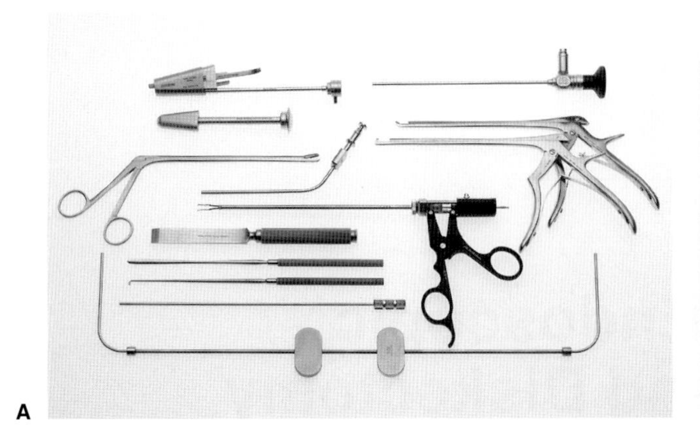

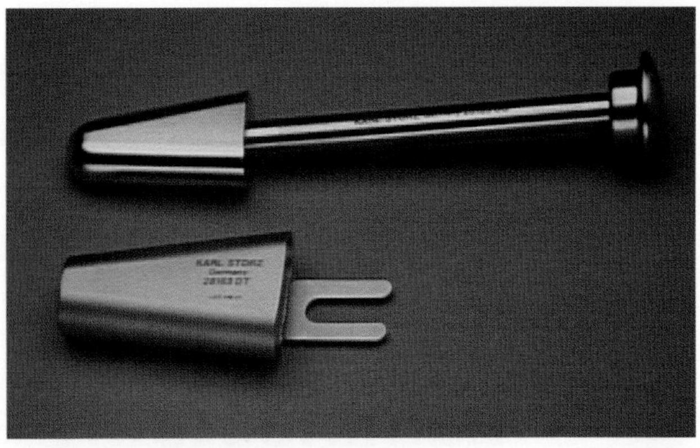

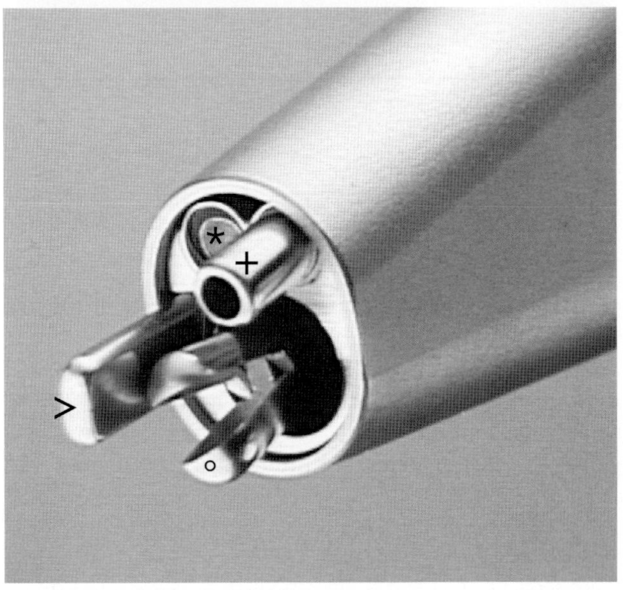

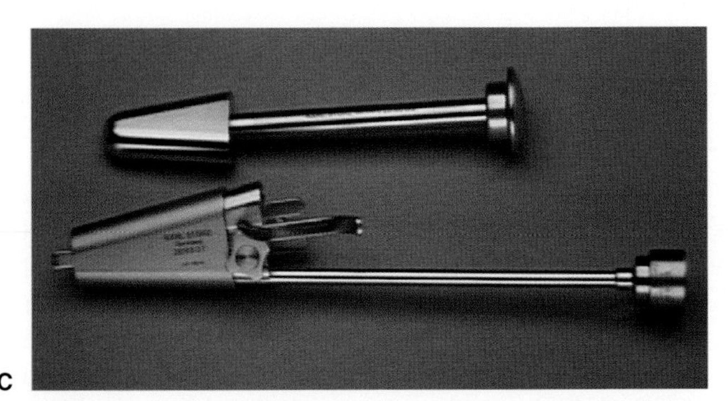
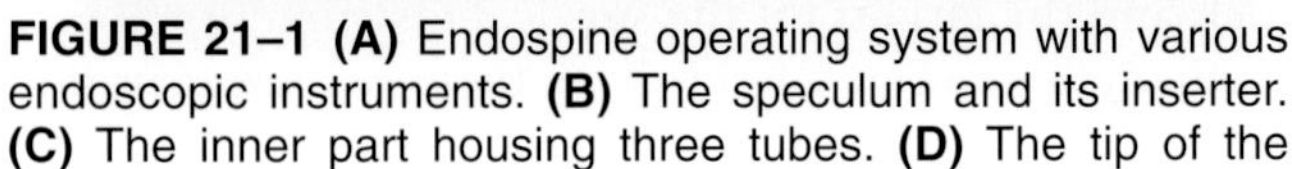

FIGURE 21–1 (A) Endospine operating system with various endoscopic instruments. **(B)** The speculum and its inserter. **(C)** The inner part housing three tubes. **(D)** The tip of the system, with the suction (+), the endoscope (*), a pituitary forceps (°), and the nerve-root retractor (>) indicated.

to the disk space are determined under fluoroscopic control (Fig. 21–2).

Skin Incision and Approach

At the mark left on the skin, the surgeon makes a 15 to 20 mm incision. The aponeurosis is sectioned with dissecting scissors. The underlying paravertebral muscles are progressively retracted. Bipolar coagulation is used to stop any bleeding. Through the access, a 12 mm osteotome is inserted down to the lamina.

Dilation of the Soft Tissues with the Operating Cone

The operating cone with its cap is inserted down to the lamina. The cap is then removed. Any soft tissue bulging into the operating cone is excised.

Preparation of the Tool Sheath

The tool sheath is then placed in the operating cone and attached to it with a screw. The suction cannula and endoscope are inserted into their respective channels. The use of a 0-degree endoscope provides a clear, undeformed view of the operative field. The extremities of the surgical instruments are always visible. This constant visibility reduces the danger of damaging the neural elements. All of the following steps in the procedure are video assisted.

Bony Resection

Part of the superior lamina and articular process are resected to expose the lateral edge of the dural sheath and nerve root. This bony resection facilitates access to the herniated disk without excessive traction of the root

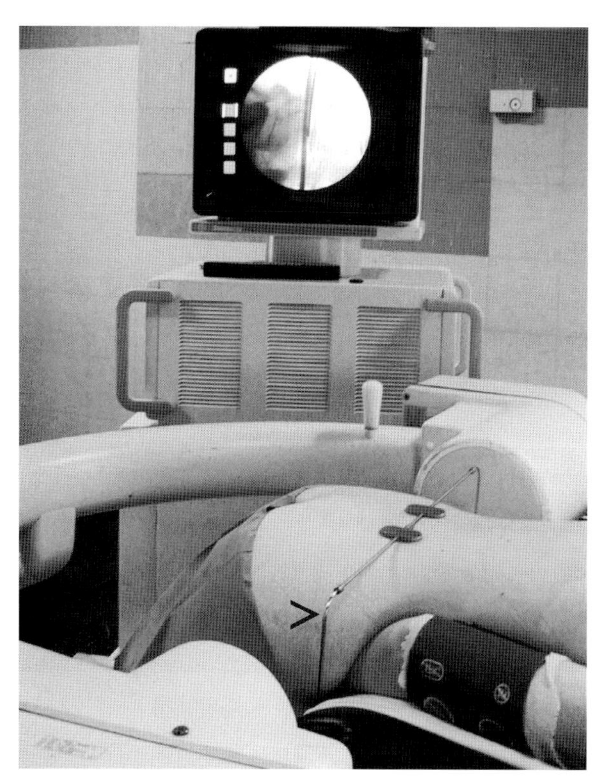

FIGURE 21–2 Fluoroscopic control with a special device (>) to determine the point of entry and the direction of the approach to the disk.

and, above all, avoids damage to another root that might be fused to the root that one expects to find.

Resection of the Ligamentum Flavum

After bone removal, the surgeon can attain the cephalad insertion of the ligamentum flavum, which is then excised with a Kerrison rongeur. Some surgeons may prefer to incise the ligamentum flavum with a scalpel.

Dissection of the Nerve Root and Resection of the Disk Herniation

Once the nerve root has been well identified, the surgeon isolates it with the nerve retractor at greater magnification. Epidural veins are cauterized, if necessary. The built-in root retractor permits retraction of the nerve root and access to the disk herniation without endangering the neural structures (Fig. 21–3). In certain cases, microdiskectomy is then performed, removing loose fragments of the nucleus.

Closure

The instrumentation is removed as a single unit. This feature provides video control for hemostasis of the

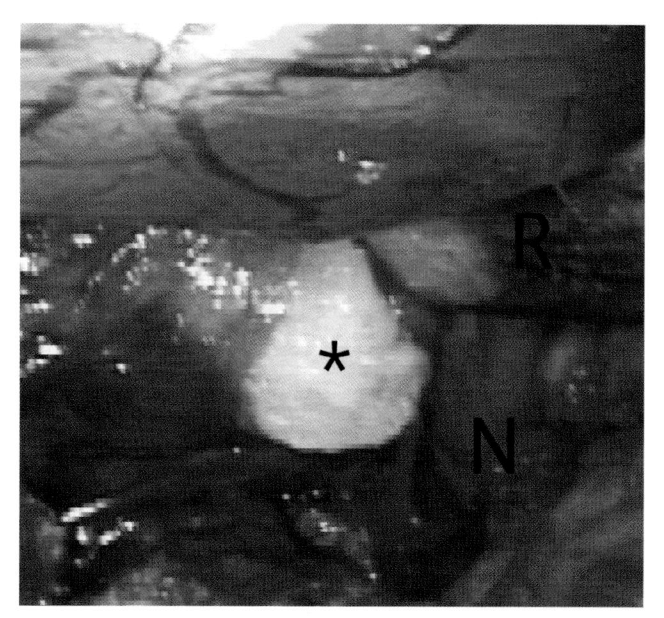

FIGURE 21–3 Use of the nerve-root (N) retractor (R) in a left L4–L5 herniation (*). Cranial is at the left side of the image, and midline is at the top.

muscles during withdrawal. After the aponeurosis is sutured, the skin is reapproximated with a dermal suture, and a special waterproof bandage is applied.

Postoperative Care

The patient is returned to the upright position immediately after the operation. A muscle relaxant is given systematically. Without delay, rehabilitation is begun to mobilize the lumbar spine and relax the paravertebral muscles. The waterproof bandage permits the patient to bathe or take a shower normally. The resumption of previous activities, including sports, is encouraged as soon as possible. No restriction in activity is recommended to the patient.

Surgical Technique in Foraminal Herniations

After localization of the operative zone with an image intensifier, a small longitudinal incision is made over the spinous process.[2] The muscles are detached. The underlying window is found, then one follows the lamina rostrally and laterally to find the lateral, arched edge of the isthmus. This edge is resected more or less according to the placement of the disk herniation in the foramen. The intertransverse ligament and its projections are resected, revealing the root. Dissection then shows the herniated disk (Fig. 21–4). In most cases, only the herniated fragment is excised. No drainage is left in place at closure.

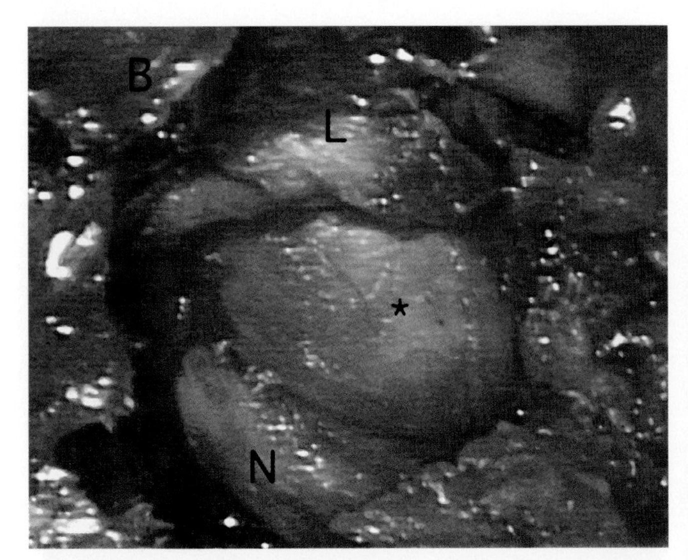

FIGURE 21–4 Left foraminal L3–L4 herniation (*). Lateral part of the isthmus (B) and ligamentum (L) have been resected. The nerve root (N) is pushed laterally by the hernia. Cranial is at the left side of the image, and midline is at the top.

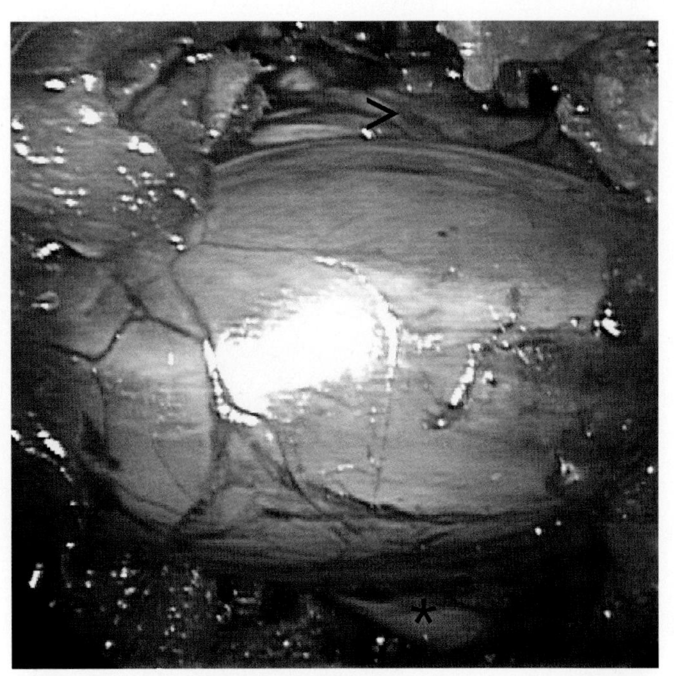

FIGURE 21–5 Lumbar spinal stenosis. Both left (*) and right (>) L5 nerve roots are exposed. Cranial is at the left side of the image.

Surgical Technique in Lumbar Spinal Stenosis

A unilateral approach is made, usually on the left side. A part of the lamina, articular process, and ligamentum flavum are resected to expose the dural sac and the nerve-root. A part of the posterior arch of the two vertebrae is then removed, and the posterior part of the dural sac is followed toward its contralateral limit at the upper part of the space. The ligamentum flavum and articular process are then partly resected from upward to downward to expose the contralateral nerve root (Fig. 21–5).[3]

Complications

The following are complications that are possible with the paraspinal endoscopic approach:

- *Dural tears:* Dura was torn in 1.6% of the cases. All of these cases healed after simple packing with Surgicel. In 0.5% of patients with the dural tear the nerve root was damaged, and there were sensory deficits in 0.2%.
- *Infectious complications:* Deep infectious complications are less frequent with the endoscopic technique.[4] Nevertheless, spondylodiskitis occurred in 0.3% of cases and resolved without sequelae within 6 months.
- *Recurrences:* In a study of 1562 patients, 54 recurrences were noted, of which 44 underwent repeat surgery. This 3.5% rate is low, but the average follow-up time was only 21 months.

Advantages of the Endoscopic Technique

Limiting the extent of the operative path minimizes muscle lesions and postoperative pain and facilitates rapid resumption of activities. Patients appreciate the cosmetic advantage of the endoscopic procedure (smaller incision).

Transporting the surgeon's field of vision directly into the operative site enhances the delineation of structures, more than compensating for the absence of three-dimensional perception. The endoscopic view also facilitates both the hemostasis of deep structures as well as that of the muscles, thus contributing to postoperative comfort. Furthermore, the relatively wide angle of vision enlarges the field of intraoperative exploration. This extension of exploratory limits is particularly helpful in cases of foraminal disk herniation, in which the difference between the view provided by conventional minimally invasive techniques and the present video-assisted technique is striking and widens the indications of this foraminal approach to intracanalar herniations that have migrated rostrally in the axilla of the nerve root. This paramedial endoscopic technique can also be applied in monosegmental stenosis of the lumbar canal, in which case the wide field of view permits decompression of the dural sheath and roots on both sides through a unilateral access.

This endoscopic approach to the lumbar spine is a minimally invasive procedure that provides a safe and effective alternative to standard microdiskectomy and spinal stenosis. The technique can be mastered after a short learning curve. Its results are as good as those of microdiskectomy because the surgical technique is the same, but the postoperative comfort is better and patients can resume their previous activities very quickly after surgery.

REFERENCES

1. Destandau J. A special device for endoscopic surgery of lumbar disc herniation. *Neurol Res.* 1999;21:39–42.
2. Destandau J. Chirurgie endoscopique des hernies discales foraminales lombaires. In: Le Huec JC, Husson JL ed. *Chirurgie endoscopique et mini-invasive du rachis.* Montpellier, France: Sauramps Medical; 1999:279–284.
3. Destandau J. Chirurgie endoscopique du canal lombaire étroit segmentaire: àa propos de 30 cas. *Rachis.* 2001;13:315.
4. Destandau J. Chirurgie endoscopique et antibioprophylaxie: intérêt dans la prévention des spondylodiscites post-opératoires. *Rachis.* 2000;12:321–323.

22

Endoscopic Pedicle Screw Instrumentation and Decompression

KEE D. KIM AND MARK W. HAWK

Standard posterolateral lumbar fusion requires extensive myoligamentous dissection and retraction. The paraspinal muscle injury associated with open surgery is often grossly visible by the ischemic discoloration of the paraspinal musculature after a lengthy procedure.[1–6] Histologic findings include denervation and reinnervation changes that lead to early aging of the musculature.[1–6] In addition, the postoperative pain and blood loss involved with open lumbar fusion are often significant.

Atavi endoscopic instrumentation developed by Endius (Plainville, MA) allows the surgeon to perform up to a two-level posterolateral spinal fusion with limited myoligamentous disruption and muscle retraction. Instead of a midline incision with extensive lateral dissection, a more direct approach along the plane of the pedicle is used via bilateral paramedian incisions.[7] With less myoligamentous dissection, intraoperative blood loss and muscle injury are reduced. With the use of a patented flexible tubular retractor system, retraction injury to the surrounding musculature is minimized. Our preliminary study indicates that the intramuscular pressure adjacent to the tubular retractor is ~30 to 40 torr less than that with the use of a standard rigid retractor. If necessary, decompression may be performed through the same tubular retractor, and the ability to deliver an interbody fusion device endoscopically in the near future should make this system even more versatile.

In this chapter, we describe the Atavi endoscopic system and the surgical technique used to achieve the same posterolateral fusion as the standard open technique, but with a much smaller incision. The Atavi endoscopic lumbar decompression technique is also briefly described. It is important to emphasize that the technique given here is familiar to spine surgeons, with the exception of the Atavi endoscopic instrumentation, which is designed for use through a small working port.

Indications

Indications for endoscopic posterolateral fusion are similar to the standard open technique, with the exception that endoscopic fusion is limited to one or two levels. Some of the current indications include the following:

- Degenerative disk disease
- Grade I spondylolisthesis
- Supplementation of anterior lumbar interbody fusion
- Pseudoarthrosis from anterior stand-alone lumbar interbody fusion
- Lumbar spinal stenosis requiring fusion after decompression

When initially attempting the endoscopic technique, patients who have had previous surgery at the same level should be avoided. The anatomic landmarks seen through an endoscopic procedure are more limited compared with those visualized in open procedures. Patients with previous microdiskectomy and limited laminectomy, however, do not pose a special challenge. Any posterolateral fusion that may be difficult with an open technique (e.g., grade II or higher spondylolisthesis) should not be attempted until sufficient endoscopic fusion experience is achieved with more simple cases.

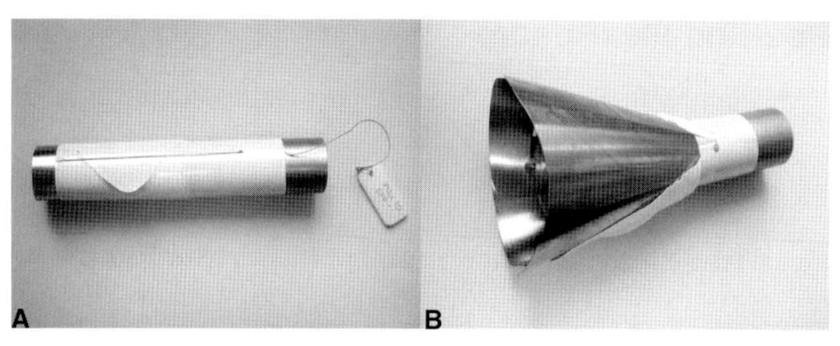

FIGURE 22–1 Smaller FlexPosure (maximum diameter of 40 mm) before **(A)** and after **(B)** deployment.

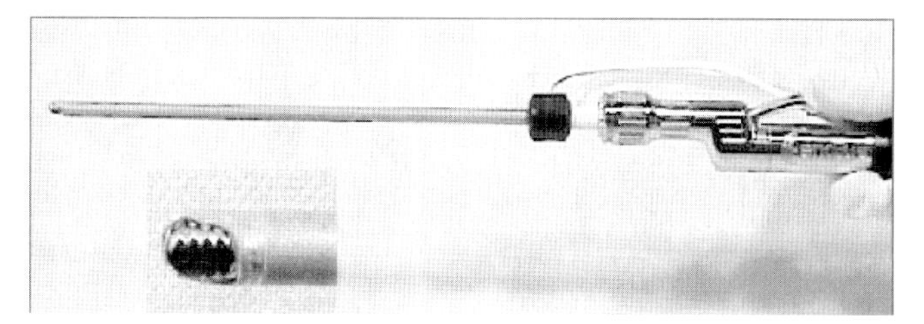

FIGURE 22–3 Microdebrider system with bipolar sheath and side port suction.

Surgical Equipment/Instrumentation

As in any endoscopic procedure, the Atavi instrumentation allows the surgeon to establish access, provide visualization, and perform surgery through an endoport.

Establish Access

- *Guidewire and series of dilators:* Five to 20 mm diameter dilators in 5 mm increments are available.
- *FlexPosure endoretractor* (Fig. 22–1): The FlexPosure is a 24 mm diameter cylindrical tube with a pivot in the center. When deployed, the distal part of the tube opens in a conical fashion to a maximum diameter of 40 or 63 mm, depending on whether or not the small or large FlexPosure is used. In general, the smaller-sized FlexPosure is adequate for a single-level fusion and decompression.
- *FlexPosure spreader:* The spreader is used initially to open the distal skirt of the FlexPosure. Because the FlexPosure is not rigid, the skirt may close partially during the procedure. During the surgical procedure, the spreader is then used to expand or redirect the skirt.

Provide Visualization

- *Vacuum-controlled FlexArm* (Fig. 22–2): This mechanical arm with multiple articulating joints is mounted to the operating table. It holds the FlexPosure endoretractor, scope, and camera in a steady position for surgery.
- *Camera, light guide, and 30-degree scope:* A bright light source with a three-chip camera provides a clear and crisp picture on the video monitor.
- *Video monitor*
- *Standard fluoroscopy*

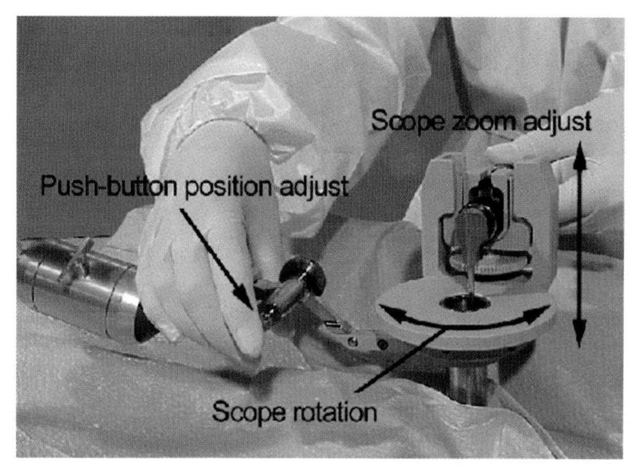

FIGURE 22–2 FlexArm with camera, light guide, and scope attachment.

Perform Surgery

- *Microdebrider system (MDS) with bipolar coagulator* (Fig. 22–3): This single instrument allows the surgeon to debride and coagulate without changing to another instrument.
- *Suction/irrigator:* This suction instrument has an additional lumen connected to a sterile saline bag to provide irrigation. Blood and smoke may be suctioned, and the surgical field may be irrigated to provide adequate visualization.
- *Endo instruments:* The Atavi instrumentation tray has all the standard instruments necessary for posterolateral fusion adapted for use through an endoscopic port. A separate tray with a variety of curettes and rongeurs may be requested if decompression is planned.
- *Implants:* Top-loading polyaxial self-tapping pedicle screw/rod implants (TiTLE system, Endius) are available in a variety of sizes. Screw/plate implants (TriFix system, Endius) are also available for single-level fusions.

Operative Setup/Patient Positioning

Request one of the larger operating rooms because more equipment is required in endoscopic cases. A careful operative setup prior to skin incision will decrease mistakes and improve efficiency throughout the case.

The patient is placed prone on a radiolucent operating table, with the anesthesia equipment at the head of the table. The C-arm is placed caudad to the arm boards and cephalad to the surgeon. Positioning the endoscopic video tower at the foot of the bed will allow the surgeon and the assistant to perform the surgery without having to turn in an awkward position. For the same reason, the fluoro video monitor should be stationed across from the surgeon or at the foot of the table. The MDS and electrosurgical generators are placed in an unobtrusive location.

Surgical Technique

Determine Incision Site

- Check the patient to ensure that the trunk is not rotated or unevenly positioned on the table.
- Mark the midline using the anteroposterior fluoroscopic view.
- Delineate the cephalocaudad line of the incision by using an AP Ferguson view to mark the transverse lines through the middle of the superior and inferior pedicles of interest on each side.
- Determine the paramedian line of incision by using oblique views to mark vertical lines over the middle of the pedicles of interest. Oblique angles are set to look down the barrel of the pedicle and may vary from 10 to 25 degrees, depending on the level to be fused. The angle may also be estimated from preoperative CT or MRI.
- Mark bilateral vertical skin incision lines to be used over the previously marked paramedian lines. The lines should extend 1.25 to 1.5 inches (3.20 to 3.85 cm) in length, depending on whether one- or two-level fusion is to be performed. They should also be centered between the horizontal cephalocaudad lines previously drawn. For the purpose of illustration, an L4 to S1 posterolateral fusion will be described.

Sequentially Dilate Soft Tissue

- Mount the FlexPosure retractor arm to the side of the bed.
- Prep and drape the patient.
- Make an incision over the marked vertical paramedian line. Extend the incision through the lumbodorsal fascia.
- Place an index finger through the lumbodorsal fascia, and palpate the bony landmarks. Medially angle the index finger and feel the transverse process, sacral ala, and facet joint.
- Position a dilator over the L5 transverse process and lateral to the pars interarticularis.
- Confirm proper position with AP Ferguson and lateral fluoroscopic views.
- After the first dilator is placed, place the next size dilator and remove the first. Repeat this process until the largest dilator has been placed. With the distal end of the dilator, gently scrape the soft tissue over the transverse process, sacral ala, and facet joint to expand the working space circumferentially.

Position FlexPosure

- Place the FlexPosure over the largest dilator, with the deployment string facing medially.
- Reconfirm the proper position of the FlexPosure using AP and lateral fluoroscopic views. On the AP view, the FlexPosure should be over the transverse process and pars interarticularis of L5; on the lateral view, it should be directly in line with the L5 pedicle and above the transverse process.
- Remove all dilators.
- Pull the FlexPosure deployment string upward while pushing FlexPosure against the bony surface to minimize the amount of soft tissue creeping under the skirt. Pulling the deployment string separates the distal cover of the FlexPosure to allow the skirt of the FlexPosure to open.
- Insert the FlexPosure expander all the way down to the stop tabs, and maximally expand the skirt.
- Gently rock the FlexPosure until the cephalad aspect of the FlexPosure skirt is above the L4 transverse process and the caudal aspect of the FlexPosure is over the sacral ala.

Secure FlexPosure

- Slide the saucer-shaped mount clamp over the FlexPosure.
- Attach the scope retractor mount assembly to the distal end of the FlexArm.
- Dock the scope retractor mount assembly to the mount clamp. A vacuum-release button is used to move the mechanical arm so that the FlexArm holds the FlexPosure in a secure position.

Establish Visualization

- Slide the camera, light guide, and scope assembly into the scope retractor mount (Fig. 22–4).
- Ratchet the scope assembly laterally so that the 30-degree scope is pointing medially.
- Use a probe to correlate superior, inferior, lateral, and medial aspects of the surgical field with the view seen on the video monitor.

Prepare Surgical Site

- Palpate the transverse process, sacral ala, and facet with a radiopaque instrument, and confirm with fluoroscopic views. Tactile feedback and a direct view down the FlexPosure are helpful to establish good anatomic orientation.
- Debride and coagulate the soft tissue with the MDS over the entry point for the pedicle screws, and extend laterally over the fusion surface. Take caution to

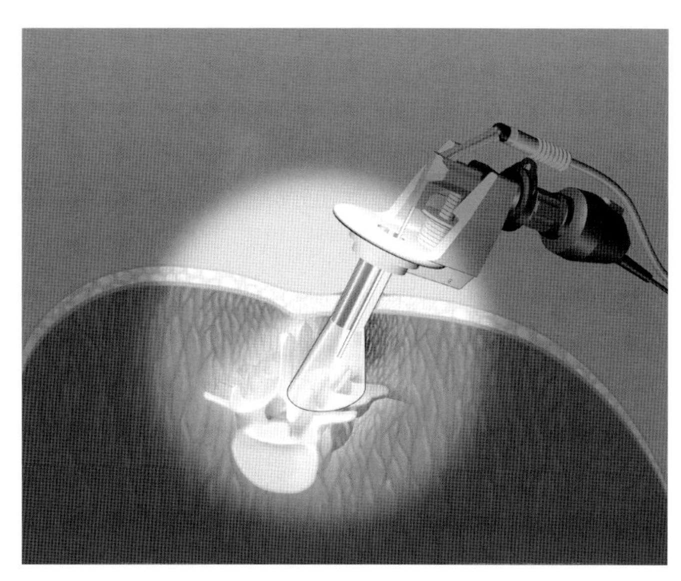

FIGURE 22–4 FlexArm securely holds FlexPosure and scope mount, allowing the surgeon free use of both hands.

avoid the segmental artery at the intersection of the pars with the inferior edge of the transverse process.

- Pivot the FlexPosure tube over the skirt to visualize the entire surgical site.
- Decorticate the fusion surface using the high-speed drill. To minimize bleeding, this step may be deferred until the pedicles are prepared for placement of the screws.

Placement of Pedicle Screws

- Use a high-speed drill to clear the space around the entry point for the pedicle screw head.
- Place an awl at the entry point of the L4 or S1 pedicle. Use AP and lateral fluoroscopic views to adjust the position of the awl (Fig. 22–5).
- Gently tunnel the pilot hole down the pedicle with the pedicle probe. Verify with fluoroscopic views, and sound the pedicle wall to ensure that it has not been violated.
- Tap the pilot hole, and place the pedicle screw.
- Repeat the steps for other levels. Place the L5 pedicle screw last and in line with L4 and S1 screws to allow easier placement of the rod. Screw heads at L4 and S1 are anchor points to prevent the FlexPosure skirt from closing.

Assemble the Construct

- Align the tulip head of the pedicle screws with an endoCobb dissector. The tulip head of the pedicle screws allows for several degrees of freedom and facilitates rod placement.
- Slide the appropriate-length rod over the tulip head of the screws. A rod holder may be used to adjust the position of the rod. If a curved rod is chosen, use a marking pen to distinguish the lordotic side.
- After the Marksman guide is snugly positioned over the L5 screw tulip head, insert and hand-tighten the cap screw. Use a torque wrench for final tightening while using the Marksman guide to provide countertorque. In two-level fusions, the middle pedicle screw is secured to the rod first.
- The cephalad and caudad screw caps are similarly placed and tightened. If compression or distraction is desired, an endoscopic compressor/distractor may be used. This instrument maintains a compression or distraction force while the loose cap screw is being tightened. For mild reduction of spondylolisthesis, the Spondy reduction driver may be used to pull a pedicle screw toward the rod before the pedicle screw nut screw is tightened.

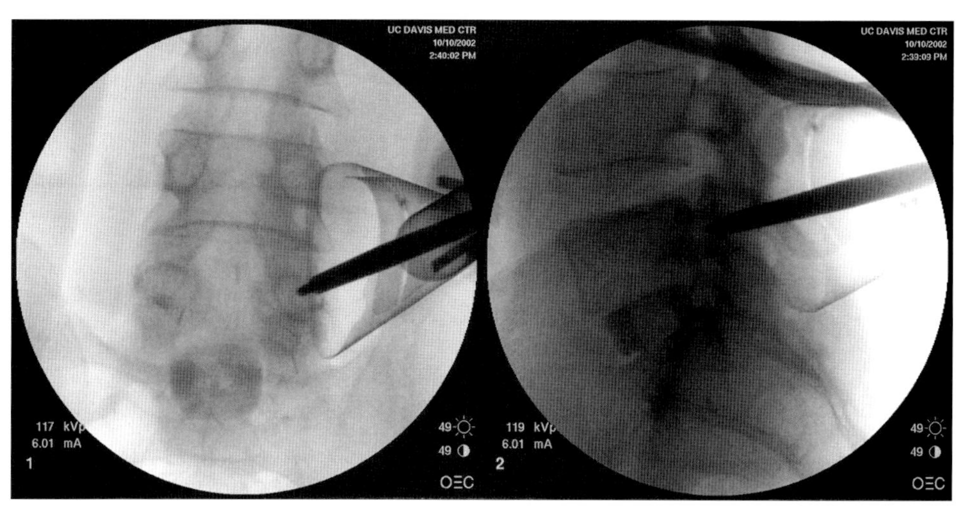

FIGURE 22–5 Anteroposterior **(A)** and lateral **(B)** fluoroscopic views confirm that the tip of the awl is in the pedicle and in good position. FlexPosure used in this case has a 40 mm maximum diameter.

Bone Graft Placement and Wound Closure

- Pack bone graft over the fusion surface.
- Obtain final hemostasis, and remove the FlexPosure by turning in a clockwise fashion. The muscle and fascia will close over the space previously occupied by the FlexPosure.
- Close fascia and skin in a standard manner. Because of the small size of the incision, this step takes only a couple of minutes.

Lumbar Decompression

If decompression is desired in addition to the posterolateral fusion, the same steps are taken, except that the endoscopic decompression is performed before the pedicle screws are placed.

- Place pedicle markers after the pilot holes for the pedicle screws are prepared. They serve as useful landmarks and are less obtrusive than the pedicle screws.
- Direct the FlexPosure skirt medially against the spinous process (Fig. 22–6). This may be aided by using the spreader to open the skirt in a mediolateral direction.
- Debride and coagulate the soft tissue over the facet and lamina with the MDS to expose the bony surface to be resected. An AP fluoroscopic view may be helpful in confirming the correct site prior to decompression.
- Thin down the bony surface, and delineate the border to be decompressed with a high-speed drill. Because an instrumented posterolateral fusion will be performed, aggressive bony resection including facetectomy may be performed.

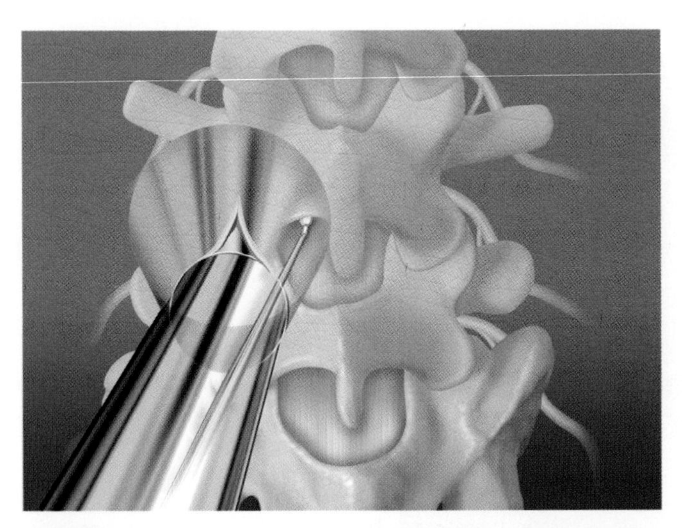

FIGURE 22–6 Palpate, dissect, and confirm with an instrument prior to bony resection. Limited depth perception requires careful use of instruments during decompression.

- Detach the ligamentum flavum of the cephalad lamina and perform a laminotomy with Kerrison rongeurs. A ligamentum flavum elevator, chisel, and different Kerrison rongeurs are available for use.
- Confirm that adequate decompression is achieved using a Woodsen elevator and, if necessary, with AP/lateral fluoroscopic views.
- Redirect the FlexPosure laterally to remove pedicle markers and place pedicle screws.
- Complete the rest of the procedure as described previously.

Complications and Avoidance

- Although the three-chip camera gives an excellent view of the surgical site, it does not provide a three-dimensional perspective; therefore, in portions of the surgery that require good depth perception, viewing directly down the FlexPosure may be necessary.
- *Bleeding:* Dissect very gently until the FlexPosure with the scope mount is positioned. If bleeding occurs before visualization is established, hemostasis will be difficult to achieve.
- *Nerve root injury:* A sharp instrument placed deep to the intertransverse ligament may damage the nerve root. Instead of using a guidewire that may inadvertently penetrate and injure a nerve root, use the 5 or 10 mm dilator to establish initial access.
- *Pedicle screw misplacement:* Always confirm with fluoroscopic views if there is any question about the position of the awl/probe/tap or pedicle screws.
- *Durotomy:* Dissect to define and visualize the thecal sac better prior to using a Kerrison rongeur to avoid inadvertent durotomy. If a durotomy with a CSF leak occurs, converting to an open procedure may be the only way to achieve a watertight dural closure. Another, less preferred, option is to cover the defect with Surgicel, followed by fibrin glue. To decrease the chance of developing a pseudomeningocele, a lumbar intrathecal drain may be placed just cephalad to the site of the leak.

Illustrative Cases

Case 1. Spondylolisthesis with Foraminal Stenosis

A 65-year-old woman presented with low back and left leg pain lasting for more than 10 years. Her pain was refractory to repeated nonsurgical therapy and was compromising her activities of daily living. Preoperative

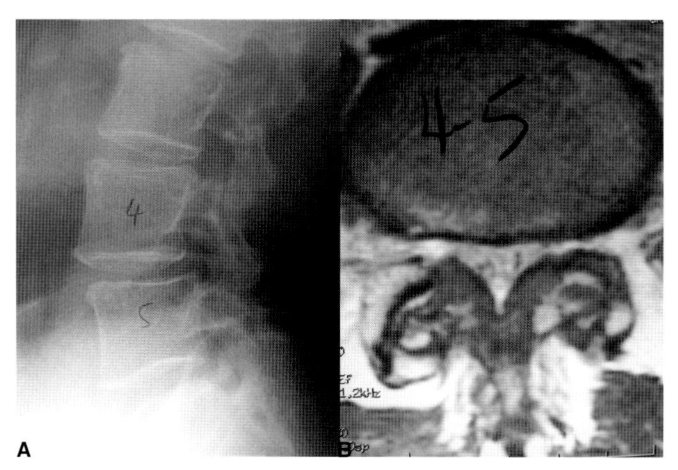

FIGURE 22–7 Lumbar lateral x-ray **(A)** and axial T2-weighted MRI **(B)** at the level of L4–L5 disk.

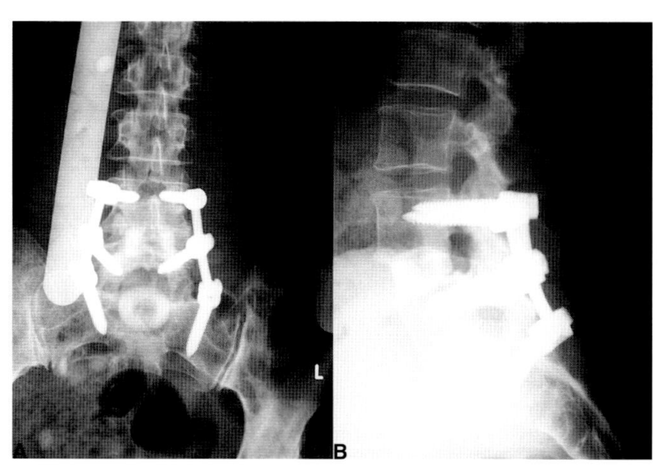

FIGURE 22–9 Immediate postoperative anteroposterior **(A)** and lateral **(B)** x-ray.

lumbar plain films and MRI showed grade I L4–L5 degenerative spondylolisthesis with foraminal stenosis (Fig. 22–7). The patient underwent an L4–L5 anterior interbody arthrodesis with femoral ring allograft, followed by endoscopic L4–L5 posterior instrumentation and left L4–L5 foraminotomy (Fig. 22–8). She had good relief of low back and left leg pain postoperatively.

Case 2. Degenerative Disk Disease

A 56-year-old woman reported the severity of her chronic low back and bilateral leg pain to be 10 out of 10 on the visual analogue scale. On lumbar plain films and MRI, she had mild degenerative changes at L4–L5 and L5–S1. Because her pain was not getting better with analgesics, epidural steroid injections, and physical therapy, lumbar diskogram was performed. She had a positive diskogram at L4–L5 and L5–S1, reproducing her baseline symptoms. The patient underwent L4–L5 and L5–S1 anterior lumbar arthrodesis with femoral ring allograft supplemented with posterior endoscopic instrumented fusion (Fig. 22–9). She reported more pain postoperatively from the abdominal incision than the lumbar incisions (Fig. 22–10). She had near complete relief of her preoperative symptoms 1 month after surgery.

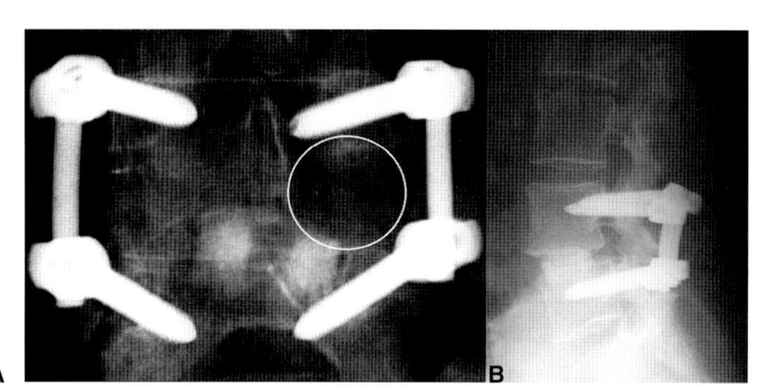

FIGURE 22–8 Anteroposterior **(A)** and lateral **(B)** postoperative x-ray. Although not easily visualized (the area within the circle), the left L4–L5 decompression is demarcated on the AP x-ray by its lucency compared with the right side.

Acknowledgment

We would like to thank Dorie DeCosta and Bruce Dilts for assisting with the manuscript and Endius for providing some of the illustrations.

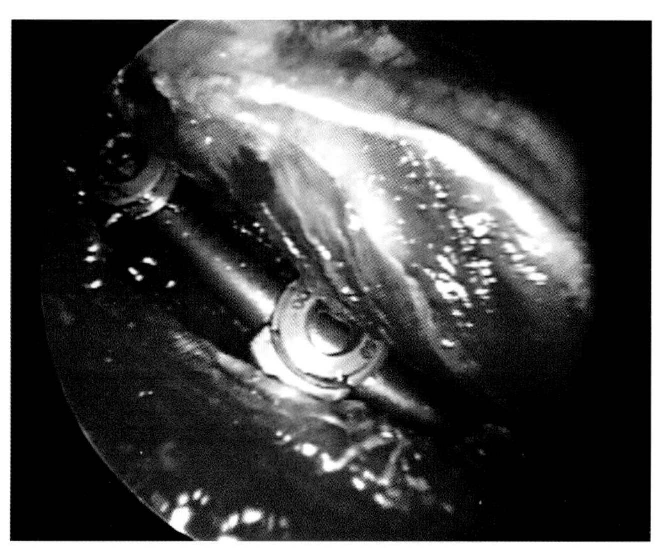

FIGURE 22–10 Intraoperative endoscopic view as the FlexPosure is being removed. Note the lack of ischemic discoloration involving the paraspinal musculature commonly encountered with open cases.

REFERENCES

1. Gejo R, Matsui H, Kawaguchi Y, et al. Serial changes in trunk muscle performance after posterior lumbar surgery. *Spine.* 1999; 24:1023–1028.
2. Hultman G, Nordin M, Saraste H, et al. Body composition, endurance, strength, cross-sectional area and density of MM erector spinae in men with and without low back pain. *J Spinal Disord.* 1993;6:114–123.
3. Mayer TG, Smith SS, Keeley J, et al. Quantification of lumbar function, II: Sagittal plane trunk strength in chronic low-back pain patients. *Spine.* 1985;10:765–772.
4. Roy SH, De Luca CJ, Casavant DA. Lumbar muscle fatigue and chronic lower back pain. *Spine.* 1989;14:992–1001.
5. Suzuki N, Endo S. A quantitative study of trunk muscle strength and fatigue in the low-back-pain syndrome. *Spine.* 1983;8: 69–74.
6. Takemasa R, Yamamoto H, Tani T. Trunk muscle strength in and effect of trunk muscle exercises for patient with chronic low back pain: the differences in patients with and without organic lumbar lesions. *Spine.* 1995;20:2522–2530.
7. Wiltse LL, Bateman JG, Hutchinson RH, Nelson WE. The paraspinal sacrospinalis-splitting approach to the lumbar spine. *J Bone Joint Surg Am.* 1968;50:919–926.

23

Endoscopic/Percutaneous Lumbar Pedicle Screw Fixation

KEVIN T. FOLEY AND LANGSTON T. HOLLY

Pedicle screw fixation has become a widely accepted method for spinal stabilization. This technique provides rigid, three-column stability and can be used in the surgical management of a wide range of spinal disorders. One of the disadvantages of traditional pedicle screw placement, however, is that it requires extensive soft tissue dissection to expose the anatomical landmarks and achieve the proper trajectory for screw insertion. The tissue trauma that occurs during the surgical exposure can be considerable and is at least partially responsible for the significant cost and lengthy hospital stays associated with instrumented lumbar fusion.[1] In addition, the morbidity associated with these procedures has become an increasing concern for many surgeons. In part, this morbidity is related to the significant iatrogenic muscle and soft tissue injury that occurs during routine lumbar fusion exposures.

Multiple authors have documented the harmful effects of the extensive muscle dissection and retraction that normally occur during lumbar procedures.[2–8] Kawaguchi et al[2,3] analyzed the effects of retractor blade pressure on the paraspinous muscles during lumbar surgery. They determined that elevated serum levels of creatine phosphokinase MM isoenzyme, an indicator of muscle injury, is directly related to the retraction pressure and duration. These findings support the work by Gejo et al,[4] who examined postoperative MRIs and trunk muscle strength in 80 patients who previously had lumbar surgery. They concluded that the damage to the lumbar musculature was directly related to the time of retraction during surgery. Furthermore, the incidence of low back pain was significantly increased in patients who had long muscle retraction times. Styf and Willen[5] determined that retractor blades may actually increase intramuscular pressure to levels of ischemia. Mayer et al[6] evaluated trunk muscle strength in patients who had previous lumbar surgery and found that patients who had undergone fusion procedures were significantly weaker than those who had undergone diskectomy. Rantanen et al[7] concluded that patients with poor outcomes after lumbar surgery were more likely too have persistent pathologic changes in their paraspinal muscles.

In this chapter we will describe a technique and instrumentation designed by the senior author (KTF) for minimally invasive posterior fixation of the lumbar spine by using percutaneous screws and rods (Sextant; Medtronic Sofamor Danek, Memphis, TN). Paraspinous tissue trauma is greatly minimized without sacrificing the quality of the spinal fixation. Although percutaneous lumbar pedicle screw insertion has previously been reported, a minimally invasive approach to inserting a longitudinal connector for these screws has proven more challenging. The Sextant system allows for the straightforward placement of lumbar pedicle screws and rods through percutaneous stab wounds. The screws and rods are placed in an anatomical position similar to that achieved by an analogous open surgical approach.

Minimally Invasive Lumbar Interbody Fusion

A tubular retractor system was first developed for microdiskectomy in 1994 by Foley and Smith[9]; its basic concept is the foundation on which several contemporary approaches to minimally invasive posterior lumbar fusion are based. The system consists of a series of concentric dilators and thin-walled tubular retractors of variable length. The spine is accessed via serial dilation of the natural cleavage plane between muscle fascicles, instead of a more traumatic muscle-stripping approach. The use of a tubular retractor, rather than blades, allows the retractor itself to be thin-walled (0.9 mm), even when the wound is quite deep. In addition, unlike blades, the tube circumferentially defines a surgical corridor through the paraspinous tissues. This helps prevent muscle from intruding into the exposure. All of the midline supporting musculoligamentous structures are left intact with this technique. An appropriately sized working channel is created that permits spinal decompression and fusion. Surgery can be performed using the operating microscope, loupes, an endoscope, or a combination of techniques, depending on the preference of the surgeon. The tubular retractor approach can be utilized for minimally invasive lumbar fusion via posterolateral onlay posterolateral interbody fusion (PLIF) or transforaminal lumbar interbody fusion (TLIF).

Sextant Percutaneous Pedicle Screw and Rod Fixation

This section will describe the technique for Sextant percutaneous pedicle screw and rod fixation. Of course, the percutaneous instrumentation is always performed in conjunction with fusion. The fusion may be done anteriorly (standard, mini-open, or laparoscopic anterior lumbar interbody fusion, ALIF). If so, then the patient is merely turned to the prone position after the ALIF (same operative setting), and the percutaneous screws and rods are inserted. Each screw is placed through a 14 to 15 mm incision. Because of the lumbar lordosis, the small incisions for screw placement at L5–S1 typically overlap; thus, both screws are placed through the same 1-inch (2.56 cm) incision. If the patient requires a concomitant posterior decompression, or if there is no indication (or a contraindication) for an ALIF, posterior and posterolateral approaches to fusion are performed in conjunction with Sextant fixation. We typically perform these in minimally invasive fashion using a 22 mm diameter tubular retractor. This tubular retractor, which derives from the microendoscopic diskectomy technique, can be inserted through a 1-inch (2.56 cm) paramedian incision and relies on the same muscle-splitting principle that is used with the Sextant system. We have used this approach for instrumented PLIF and TLIF. Once the fusion has been performed through the tubular retractor, the retractor is removed, and the Sextant instrumentation is inserted through the same 1-inch (2.56 cm) incision. Single-level posterior and posterolateral fusion and pedicle screw instrumentation can therefore be performed through bilateral, paramedian 1-inch (2.56 cm) incisions. Sextant fixation has also been successfully applied to two-level fusion and fixation.

Patient Position

- The patient is in the prone position.
- A radiolucent table and padded bolsters support the clavicle, anterior chest wall, and iliac crest.
- The hips are neutral or slightly extended, maintaining or improving the lumbar lordosis.
- The upper extremities are padded and placed laterally on arm boards with less than 90 degrees of shoulder abduction to prevent brachial plexus injury.
- Avoid compression along the medial side of the elbow to prevent ulnar nerve injury.
- The head should rest gently on a donut or foam cutout that allows a neutral neck position and prevents any pressure points from developing on the face.
- Prior to prepping and draping the patient, a C-arm fluoroscopy unit is used to ensure that the appropriate spinal anatomy is visible.
- On anteroposterior images the pedicles should be oval-shaped and have crisp, dark outer cortical margins. The position of the spinous process should appear to bisect the interval between the two pedicles symmetrically at each level of interest.
- The lateral images should reveal sharp vertebral body end plates and a single pedicle.
- The fluoroscope is draped into the operative field in preparation for surgery.

PLIF Using the METRx and Tangent Technique

- Operative interspace is determined with the fluoroscope and a 22-gauge spinal needle (Fig. 23–1).

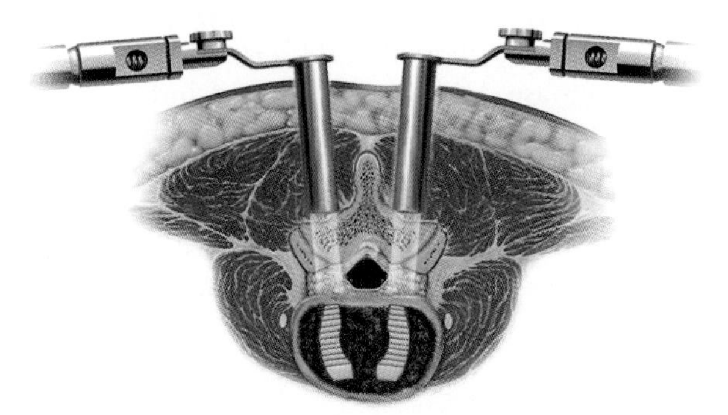

FIGURE 23–1 PLIF using the METRx and Tangent system.

- Two 1-inch (2.56 cm) incisions are made at this level, ~25 mm to either side of the midline, and carried only into the subcutaneous tissue.
- The METRx Microdiskectomy Surgical Technique (Medtronic Sofamor Danek) instruments are used.
- A guidewire is inserted through the small incision and penetrates the underlying fascia.
- A cannulated soft tissue dilator is passed over the guidewire, directed toward the inferior aspect of the superior lamina.
- Once the dilator penetrates the fascia, the guidewire is removed, and the dilator is advanced to the lamina.
- Sequentially larger dilators are passed over the first dilator down to the lamina.
- Markings on the sides of the dilators indicate the depth from the skin surface. A 22 mm tubular retractor of appropriate length is chosen and advanced over the final dilator.
- After the retractor has been locked in position using the articulated, table-mounted retractor arm, the dilators are removed.
- The underlying anatomy is visualized with the operating microscope, an endoscope, or surgical loupes.
- Residual soft tissue is cleared from the laminar surface, exposing the lamina and the ligamentum flavum.
- A second tubular retractor is placed in an identical fashion through the contralateral incision.
- Laminotomies are performed bilaterally through the tubular retractors, using rongeurs and/or a high-speed drill. The ligamentum flavum is removed, exposing the dural sac and the traversing nerve root.
- Bilateral diskectomies are then performed, using the Tangent Posterior Impacted Instrument Set (Medtronic Sofamor Danek).
- Interspace height is restored using sequentially larger interbody distractors inserted via the tubular retractors. The final distractor is left in place on the contralateral side.
- The appropriate-sized box chisel is then used to mortise the end plates on the ipsilateral side. The box chisel is removed, the interspace is packed with morcellized autograft bone, and a Tangent machined allograft is impacted into the interspace (Fig. 23–2).
- On the contralateral side, the distractor is removed, the interspace is mortised, and a second Tangent allograft is inserted along with additional autograft bone.
- The tubular retractors are then removed, and segmental fixation with the Sextant pedicle screw and rod system is performed.

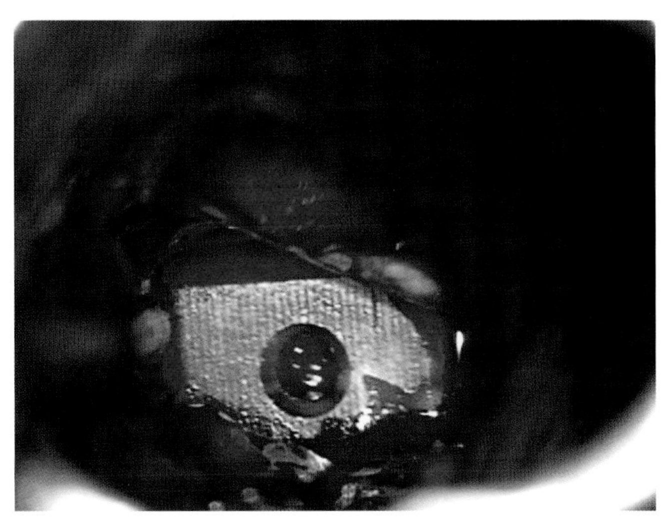

FIGURE 23–2 Placement of the Tangent interbody bone graft as seen through a METRx tubular retractor system.

Sextant Screw and Rod Placement Technique

The Sextant screws are inserted through the same 1-inch (2.56 cm) incisions that were used for the tubular retractors. The pedicles are localized with anteroposterior and lateral fluoroscopy. The FluoroNav Virtual Fluoroscopy System (Medtronic Sofamor Danek) can be utilized as an alternative.

- An 11-gauge bone biopsy needle is inserted until its tip reaches the junction of the facet and transverse process (Fig. 23–3A).
- Lateral fluoroscopy should show the needle at the top of the pedicle cylinder, aligned with and bisecting the pedicle. Anteroposterior fluoroscopy should show the tip to be located at the lateral margin of the pedicle cylinder (Fig. 23–3B).
- Using a medially directed trajectory, the needle is then carefully advanced into the pedicle by tapping the base of the needle with a mallet.
- The needle will pass through the cancellous bone toward the base of the pedicle on the lateral image (Fig. 23–3C).
- As the needle reaches the pedicle–vertebral body junction, the tip should be positioned in the center of the pedicle on the anteroposterior image.
- If the needle reaches the center of the pedicle on the anteroposterior image when first entering the pedicle, the trajectory is too medial, and there is a significant risk of entering the spinal canal.
- Once the needle has safely entered the vertebral body, the inner trocar is removed, and the K-wire is placed into the needle. A power driver is used to pass the wire through the pedicle under serial anteroposterior and lateral fluoroscopic guidance (Fig. 23–4).

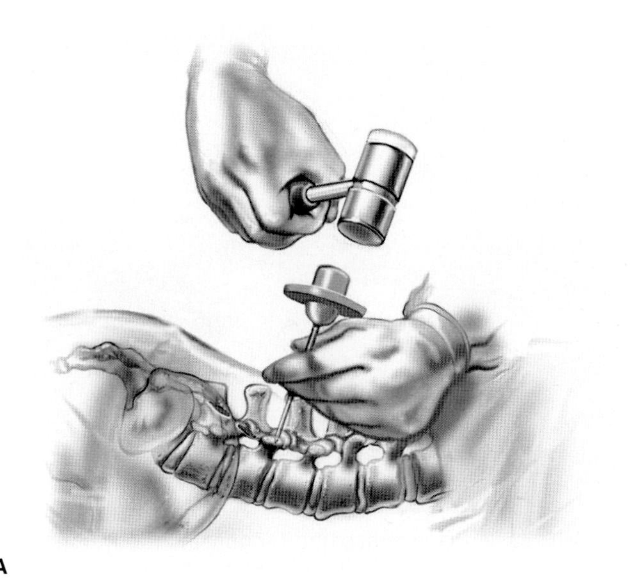

A

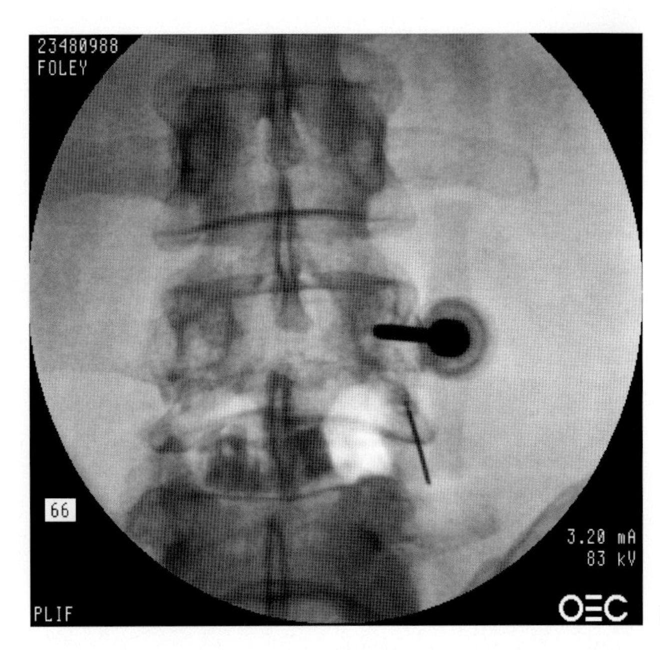

B

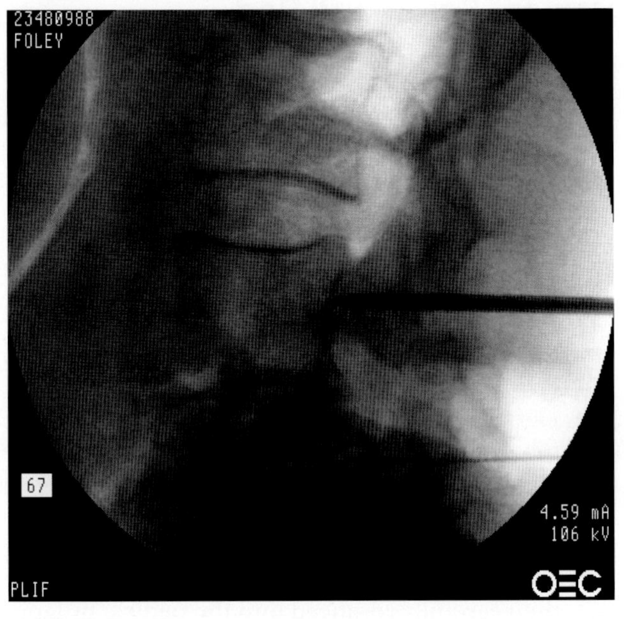

C

FIGURE 23–3 (A) Bone biopsy needle is used to gain access to the pedicle. **(B)** Pedicle entry. Anteroposterior fluoroscopy should show the tip to be located at the lateral margin of the pedicle cylinder. **(C)** As the needle reaches the pedicle–vertebral body junction, the tip should be positioned in the center of the pedicle on the anteroposterior image.

- After the K-wire has been positioned, the sequential dilators are placed, and the pedicle is tapped with the cannulated tap (Figs. 23–5, 23–6).
- Review of the preoperative CT or MRI will allow for selection of proper screw diameter; screw length can be chosen based on the calibration markings on the tap.
- Prior to placing the Sextant screws, the screw extenders must be attached. The screw extenders have inner and outer sleeves.
- A lock plug is placed in the inner sleeve by inserting the cap of the plug into the distal end of the sleeve. The cap of the lock plug is held within the sleeve, allowing the threaded end to hang freely (Fig. 23–7A).
- The inner sleeve is then placed into the outer screw extender and left at its most upward position.
- There are two positions for the inner sleeve within the outer screw extender. The first allows the threads of the lock plug to engage the saddle of the multiaxial Sextant screw but leaves an opening in the saddle for rod insertion. The second allows the lock plug to be driven into the final position, locking the rod to the Sextant screw (Fig. 23–7B).
- The saddle of a cannulated, multiaxial Sextant screw is placed in the distal end of the assembled screw extender, and the plug driver is used to engage the lock plug, thus attaching the Sextant screw to the extender.

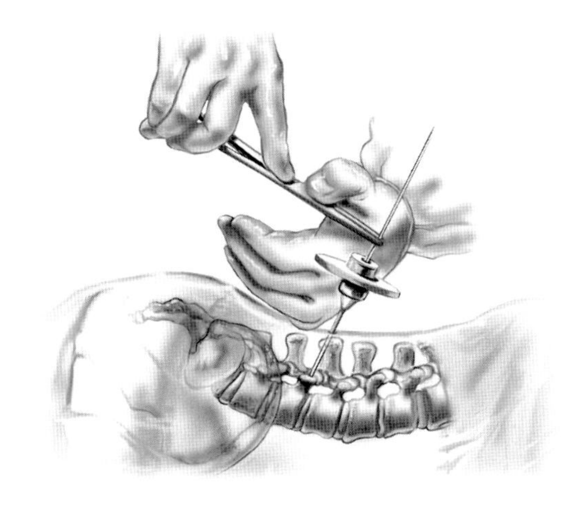

A

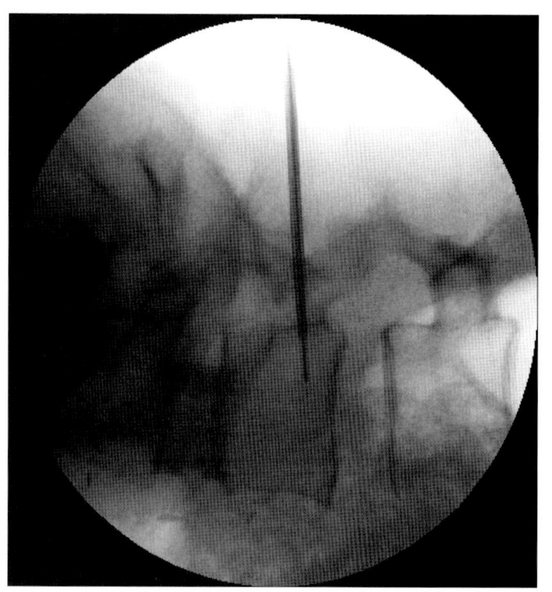

B

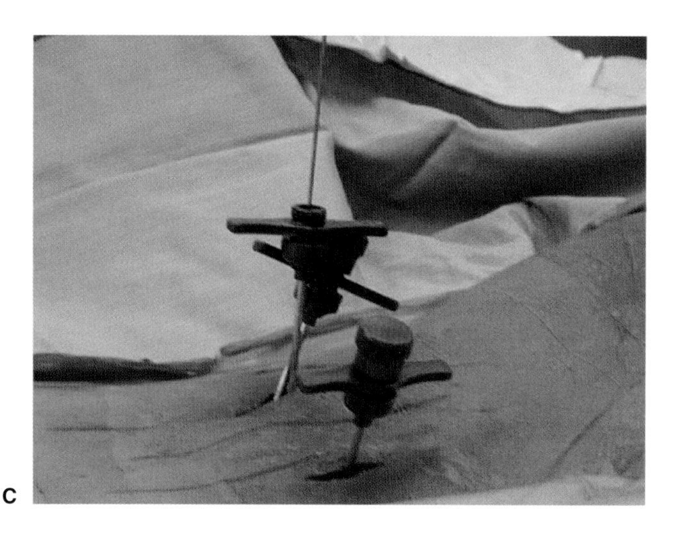

C

FIGURE 23–4 Once the needle has safely entered the vertebral body, the inner trocar is removed, and the K-wire is placed into the needle. A power driver is used to pass the wire through the pedicle under serial AP and lateral fluoroscopic guidance. **(A)** Artist depiction of a K-wire through the trocar. **(B)** Lateral x-ray. **(C)** Intraoperative picture.

- The assembly is then examined to ensure that the set screw is in the correct position, and the Sextant screw is firmly attached to the extender. A rod can also be passed immediately below the set screw into the multiaxial screw head saddle to make certain of proper assembly.
- The cannulated screwdriver is passed into the proximal screw extender; its tip passes through the set screw and engages the Sextant screw head.
- The entire screw-extender assembly is placed over the K-wire, and the screw is inserted into the pedicle under fluoroscopic guidance (Fig. 23–8).
- The K-wire is removed once the screw has traversed the pedicle to prevent inadvertent advancement.
- The exact procedure is repeated for the pedicle screw on the same side at the adjacent level.
- The proximal portion of each screw extender has a flat surface; one of these surfaces has an extrusion, and the other has a matching receptacle. The screw extenders are rotated so that their flat surfaces are flush and the extrusion from the first surface fits in the receptacle of the other (Fig. 23–9).
- The maneuver of aligning the extender surfaces external to the patient also aligns the screw saddles beneath the paraspinous muscle, readying them for rod insertion.
- Once the surfaces are flush against one another, the rod inserter is connected to the two screw-extender assemblies (Fig. 23–10).
- The rod connects to the screw-extender-inserter assembly in such a fashion that the rod is geometrically constrained to pass along an arc that intersects the openings in the screw saddles (Fig. 23–11).
- Prior to passing the rod, a trocar tip is attached to the rod inserter. A small stab wound is made where the trocar intersects the skin, and the rod inserter creates a pathway through the fascia and muscle to the first screw head under fluoroscopic guidance.

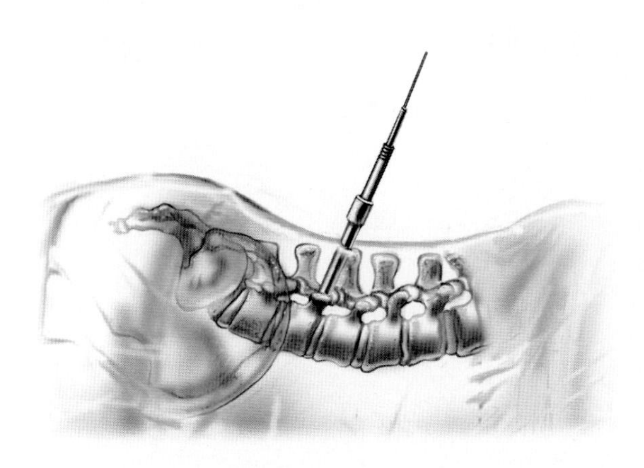

A

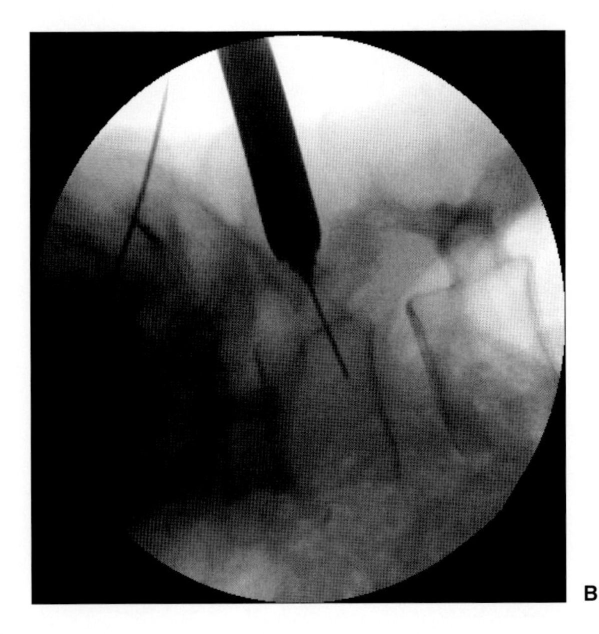

B

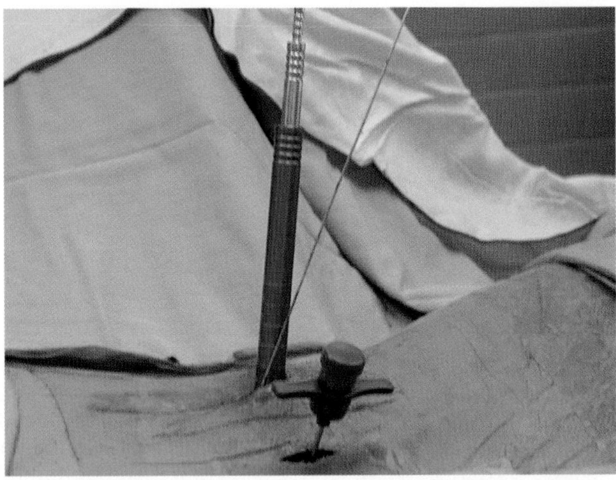

C

FIGURE 23–5 After the K-wire has been positioned, the sequential dilators are placed. **(A)** Artist depiction. **(B)** Lateral x-ray. **(C)** Intraoperative picture.

- The pathway can either be made rostral or caudal to the levels of fusion.
- One can also adjust the sagittal trajectory of the rod insertion pathway by slightly advancing one screw-extender assembly and backing out the other. If bony obstruction is encountered along the lateral aspects of the facet complexes, the screw-extender-inserter assembly can be rotated laterally (remaining connected) to allow for a more lateral rod trajectory.
- A rod template is attached to the screw extenders and determines the appropriate length rod. The trocar is then replaced by the curvilinear rod, and the rod is passed through the multiaxial screw saddles.
- Multiplanar fluoroscopic views are obtained to verify that the rod is properly positioned.
- Compressive or distractive forces can be applied to the construct prior to the final tightening.
- The inner extender sleeves are then advanced to their final position, allowing the lock plugs to be able to engage the rod. The lock plugs should tighten within 1.5 rotations.
- If the lock plugs need to be loosened for any reason, it is wise to consider removing the screw-extender assembly after first replacing a K-wire through it. The screw and extender can be properly assembled under direct vision and then simply reinserted over the K-wire. If one loosens the lock plug with the screw and extender in the patient, one risks inadvertently disassembling the extender from the screw (remember that the lock plug holds the screw to the extender).
- Final tightening is performed with the plug driver. The rod inserter serves as the countertorque device. The lock plug heads shear off and are retained

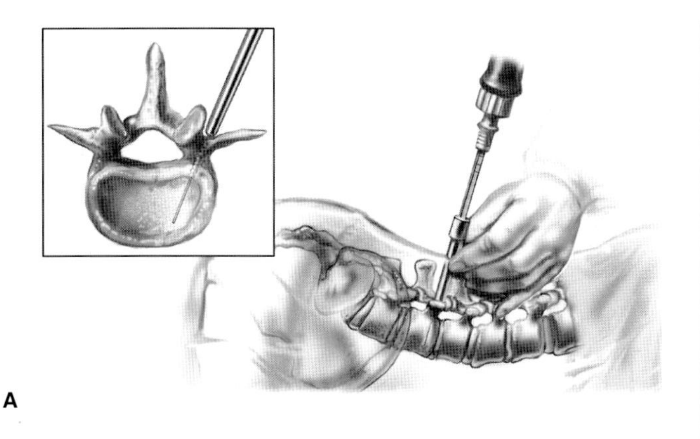

A

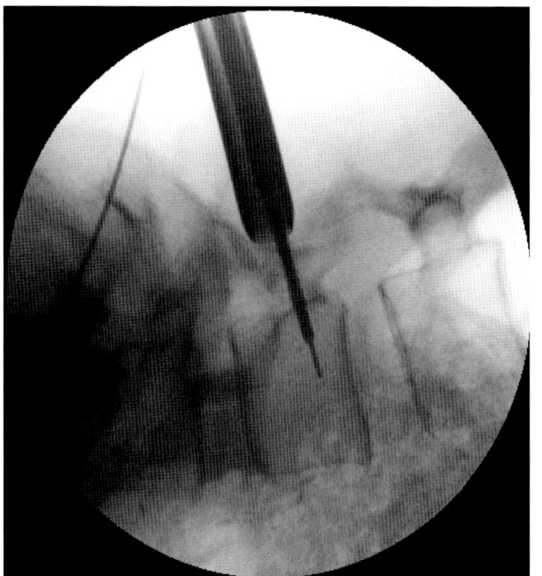

B

C

FIGURE 23–6 The pedicle is tapped with the cannulated tap. **(A)** Artist's depiction. **(B)** Lateral x-ray. **(C)** Intraoperative picture.

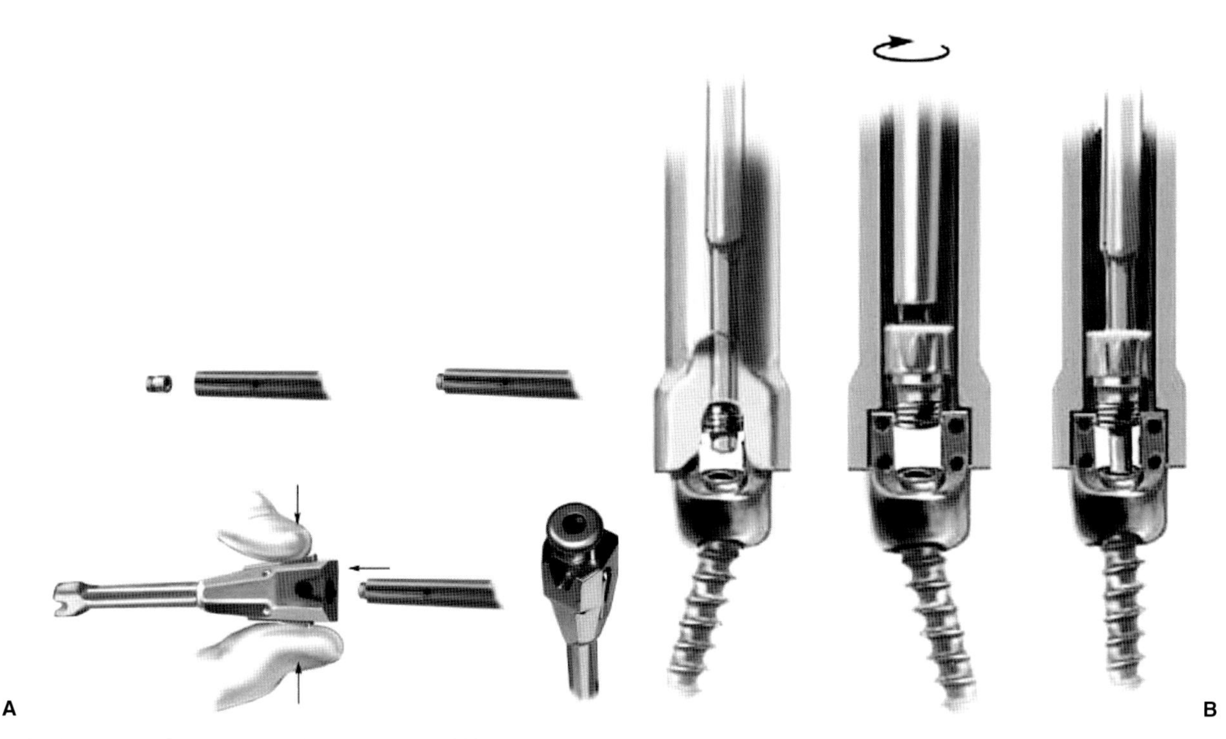

A B

FIGURE 23–7 Screw extender assembly. **(A)** Inner screw driver placed within screw extender shaft. **(B)** Engagement of the locking screw and screwdriver on the polyaxial screw head.

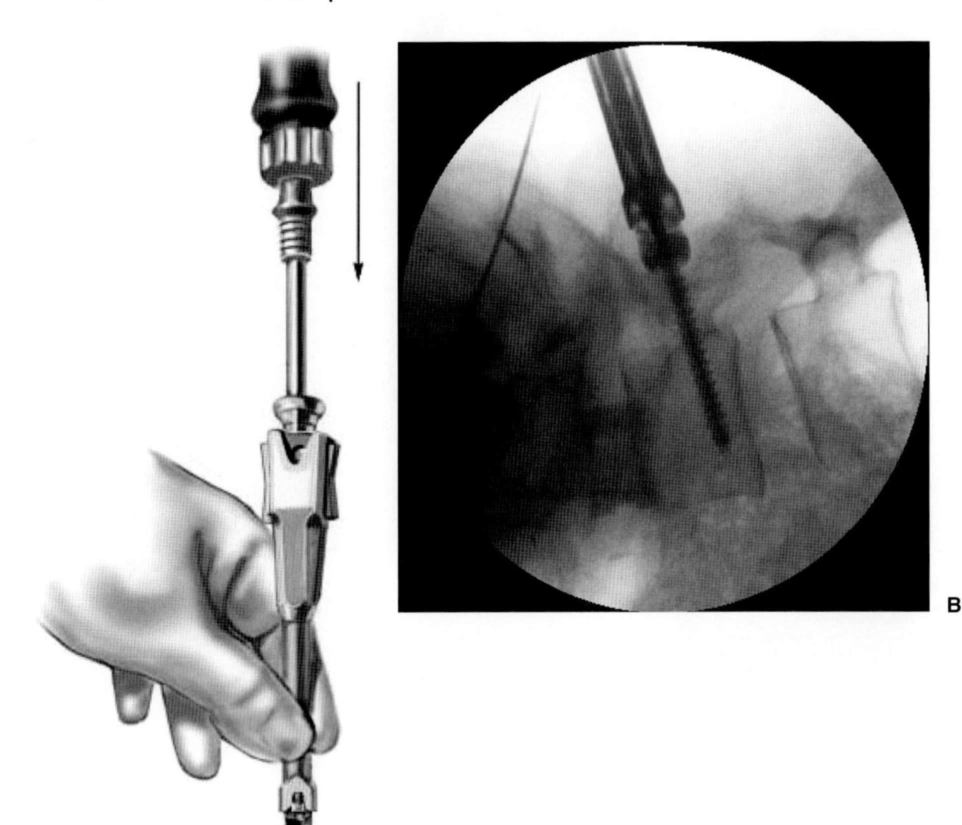

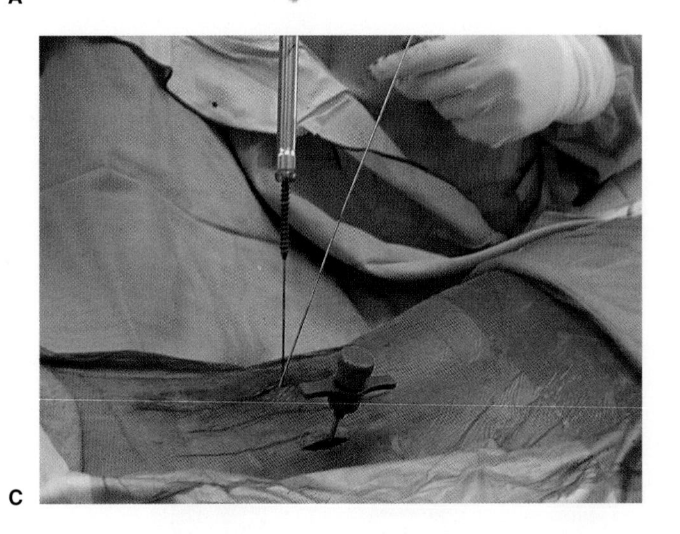

FIGURE 23–8 The entire screw-extender assembly is placed over the K-wire, and the screw is inserted into the pedicle under fluoroscopic guidance. **(A)** Artist's depiction. **(B)** Lateral x-ray. **(C)** Intraoperative picture.

within the inner sleeves, detaching the extenders from the Sextant screws.

- The rod is detached from the inserter. The extender-inserter assembly is then removed from the field. A percutaneous rod and screw construct is left in place in a traditional anatomical position (Fig. 23–12).
- The entire procedure is repeated on the opposite side, after which the wounds are irrigated and closed in layered fashion. We prefer to use an absorbable, subcuticular suture and Steri-strips for cosmetic purposes (Fig. 23–13).

Results

Sixty-three patients have undergone percutaneous pedicle screw and rod insertion with the Sextant system at our institution since March 2000. Thirty-nine of the patients have been followed for at least 12 months. Twenty-two of the patients were male, and 17 were female. Their ages ranged from 23 to 80 years, with a mean of 46 years. The diagnoses were isthmic spondylolisthesis in 17 patients (11 grade I, 5 grade II, and 1 grade III), degenerative spondylolisthesis (stenosis) in

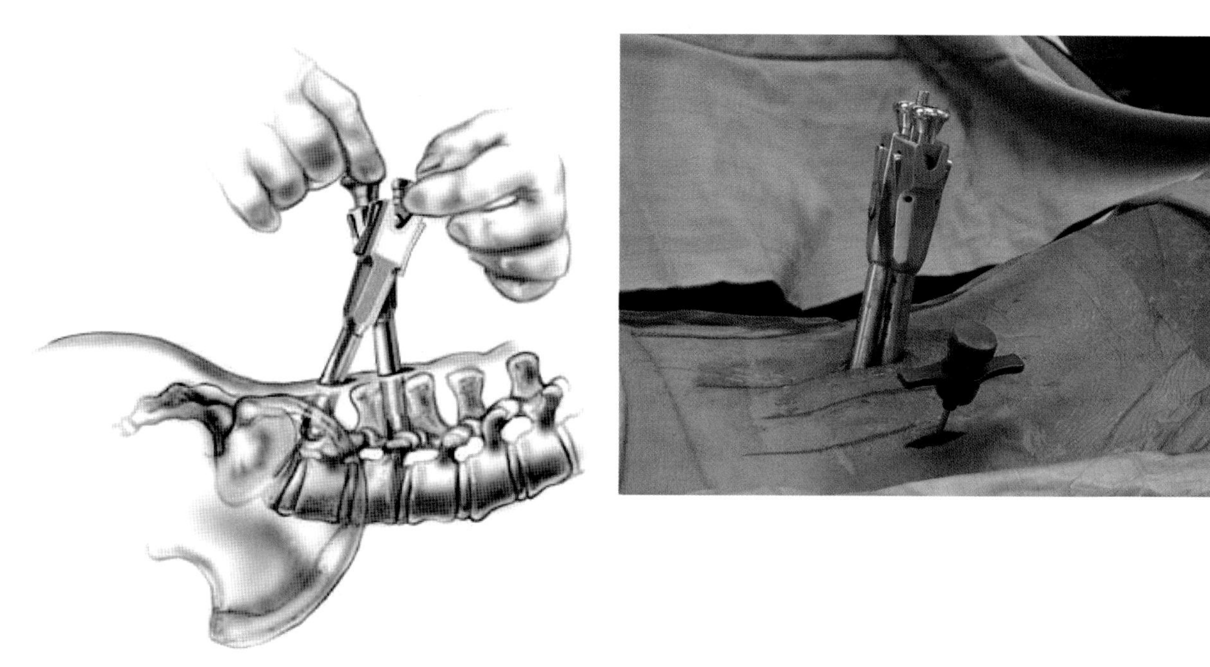

FIGURE 23–9 The maneuver of aligning the extender surfaces external to the patient also aligns the screw saddles beneath the paraspinous muscle, readying them for rod insertion. **(A)** Artist's depiction. **(B)** Intraoperative picture.

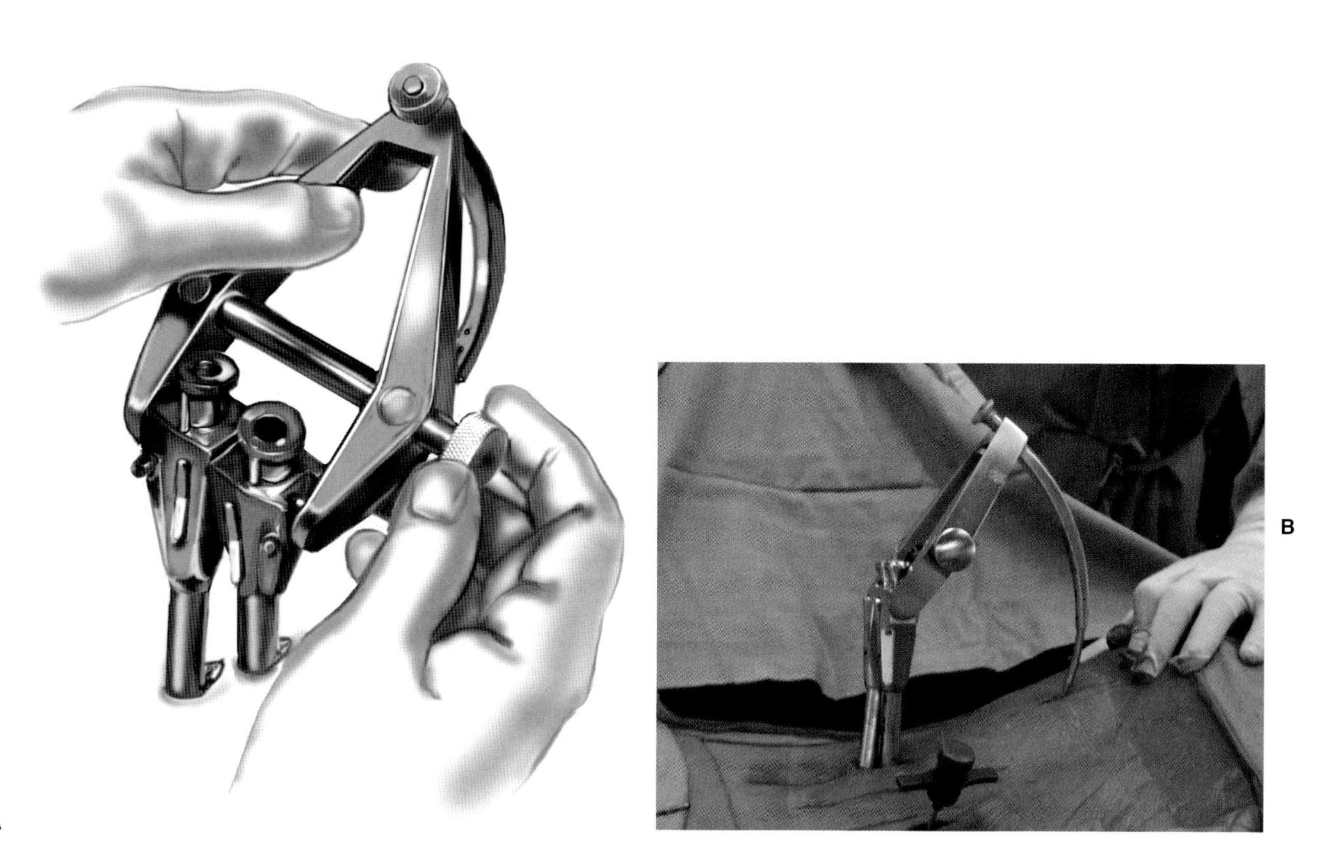

FIGURE 23–10 Once the surfaces are flush against one another, the rod inserter is connected to the two screw-extender assemblies. **(A)** Artist's depiction. **(B)** Intraoperative picture.

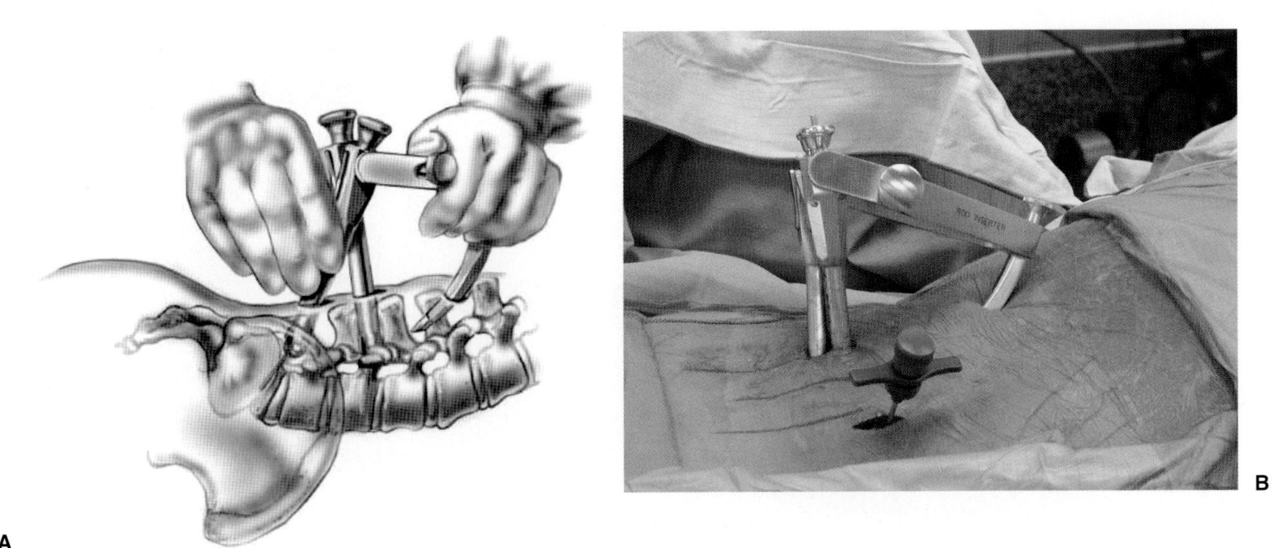

FIGURE 23–11 The rod connects to the screw-extender-inserter assembly in such a fashion that the rod is geometrically constrained to pass along an arc that intersects the openings in the screw saddles. **(A)** Artist's depiction. **(B)** Intraoperative picture.

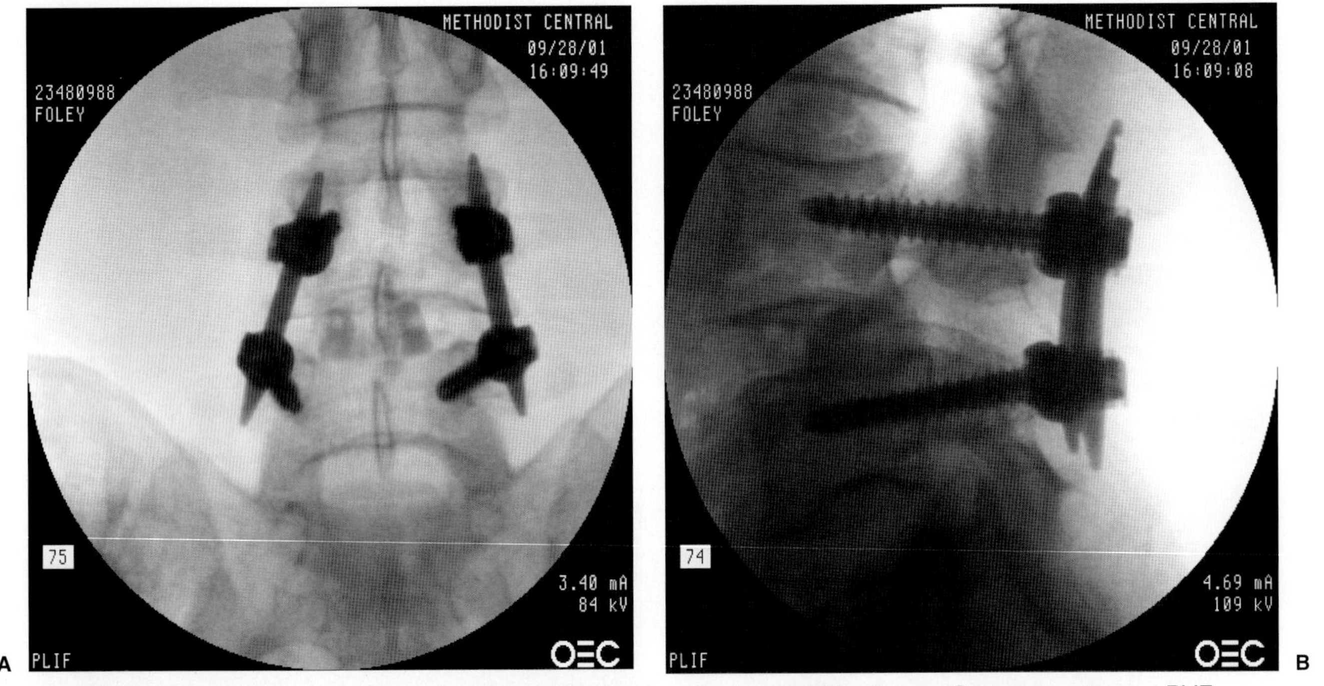

FIGURE 23–12 Postoperative anteroposterior **(A)** and lateral **(B)** x-rays after a METRx-Tangent-Sextant percutaneous PLIF.

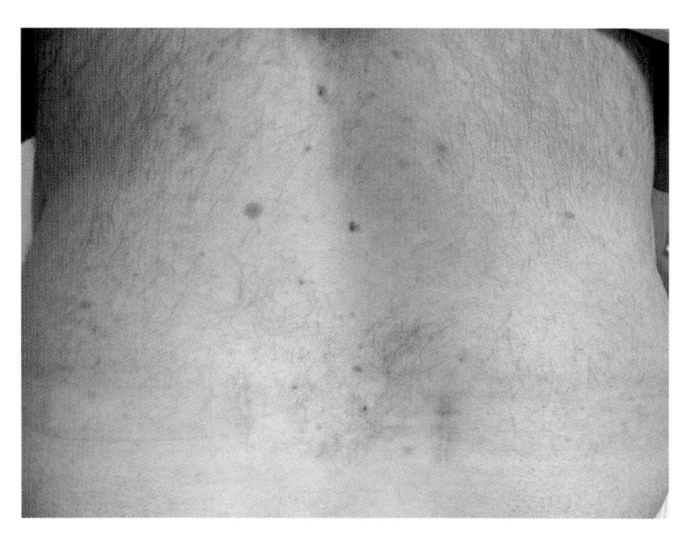

FIGURE 23–13 Postoperative scar as seen in clinic.

15 patients, degenerative disk disease in five patients, and one trauma; the remaining two patients suffered from symptomatic nonunion related to previous failed fusion. Thirty-seven patients had single-level fusions, and two had two-level fusions. Twenty-five patients underwent concomitant ALIF, 12 underwent minimally invasive PLIF or TLIF, one underwent a minimally invasive retroperitoneal approach, and one had a minimally invasive posterolateral fusion. The instrumented levels were L5–S1 in 19 patients, L4–L5 in 16 patients, L3–L4 in one patient, and L2–L3 in one patient. Two patients underwent two-level fusion and fixation (one L3–L5 and another L4–S1).

The mean length of follow-up was 22 months, with a range of 12 to 38 months. All patients but one improved clinically (26 excellent, 12 good by MacNab criteria); one patient who presented with mechanical low-back pain had persistent mechanical low-back pain despite a solid fusion. One patient required replacement of a loose lock plug 1 month postoperatively. The patient did well clinically, and the event was asymptomatic. Reoperation to replace the lock plug was performed on an outpatient basis. This event occurred early in our clinical experience and led to a redesign of the lock plug. No other device-related problems have been experienced. Solid fusions were obtained in all patients (contiguous bony bridging, no motion on flexion-extension views), and all rods and screws were placed in a satisfactory position.

Percutaneous lumbar fixation was designed, in part, to minimize the paravertebral muscle injury that occurs with conventional open procedures. Magerl[10] first reported the use of percutaneous pedicle screws combined with an external fixator in 1982. The most obvious limitation of this technique was the risk of infection, not to mention the discomfort of an external appliance. Mathews and Long[11] described the use of percutaneous pedicle screws with longitudinal connectors placed under direct vision in the suprafascial, subcutaneous space. This superficial instrumentation was uncomfortable to the patient and associated with a significant nonunion rate as well, perhaps secondary to the long lever arms of the hardware.

The Sextant system allows for placement of percutaneous screws and rods through paramedian stab incisions. The conventional anatomical position of the construct avoids the instrumentation-related discomfort that was associated with earlier versions of percutaneous fusion. The geometrically constrained arc produced by the Sextant apparatus simplifies the connection of the percutaneous rods and screws.

There are several distinct advantages of the Sextant system compared with standard open lumbar pedicle fixation. The paraspinous muscles are bluntly separated rather than stripped from their attachments and are minimally retracted using a sequential dilation technique, as described by Foley and Smith[9] for microendoscopic diskectomy. This results in significantly less intraoperative blood loss, less iatrogenic muscle injury, and less postoperative pain. Patients are therefore able to ambulate and mobilize much more quickly, resulting in a decreased rate of perioperative complications, shorter hospital stays, and decreased cost.[12] From a technical perspective, it is also easier to achieve the desired lateral to medial pedicle screw trajectory because there is not a wall of soft tissue that limits the angulation of the instruments (as can be encountered in the open surgery). This is particularly helpful in obese patients because more extensive exposure and retraction can be avoided. Operative time is also significantly lessened; it takes only 1 hour for the surgeon to place four screws and two rods.

The Sextant system is an emerging component in the rapidly developing field of minimally invasive spine surgery. It is an important advancement and serves as a complement to other newly established minimally invasive fusion techniques for ALIF, PLIF, TLIF, and posterolateral onlay fusion. As the technology continues to evolve, the indications for Sextant will certainly expand from primarily degenerative disease to include multilevel fusions for spinal disorders due to trauma and neoplastic conditions. The clinical utility of Sextant appears promising because our early experience suggests that the system is able to achieve the same clinical results as conventional open procedures while significantly reducing the exposure-related morbidity.

REFERENCES

1. Thomsen K, Christensen FB, Eiskjaer SP, et al. The effect of pedicle screw instrumentation on functional outcome and fusion rates in posterolateral lumbar spinal fusion: a prospective, randomized clinical study. *Spine*. 1997;22:2813–2822.
2. Kawaguchi Y, Matsui H, Tsuji H. Back muscle injury after posterior lumbar spine surgery: a histologic and enzymatic analysis. *Spine*. 1996;21:941–944.

3. Kawaguchi Y, Matsui H, Tsuji H. Back muscle injury after posterior lumbar spine surgery, II: Histologic and histochemical analyses in humans. *Spine.* 1994;19:2598–2602.
4. Gejo R, Matsui H, Kawaguchi Y, et al. Serial changes in trunk muscle performance after posterior lumbar surgery. *Spine.* 1999;24: 1023–1028.
5. Styf JR, Willen J. The effects of external compression by three different retractors on pressure in the erector spine muscles during and after posterior lumbar spine surgery in humans. Spine. 1998;23:354–358.
6. Mayer TG, Vanharanta H, Gatchel RJ. Comparison of CT scan muscle measurements and isokinetic trunk strength in postoperative patients. *Spine.* 1989;14:33–36.
7. Rantanen J, Hurme M, Falck B, et al. The lumbar multifidus muscle five years after surgery for a lumbar intervertebral disc herniation. *Spine.* 1993;18:568–574.
8. Sihvonen T, Herno A, Paljiarvi L, Airaksinen O, Partanen J, Tapaninaho A. Local denervation atrophy of paraspinal muscles in postoperative failed back syndrome. *Spine.* 1993;18:575–581.
9. Foley KT, Smith MM. Microendoscopic discectomy. Tech Neurosurg 1997;3:301–307.
10. Magerl F. External skeletal fixation of the lower thoracic and the lumbar spine. In Uhthoff HK, Stahl E, eds. *Current Concepts of External Fixation of Fractures.* New York: Springer-Verlag; 1982: 353–366.
11. Mathews HH, Long BH. Endoscopy assisted percutaneous anterior interbody fusion with subcutaneous suprafascial internal fixation: evolution, techniques and surgical considerations. *Orthop Int Ed.* 1995;3:496–500.
12. Foley KT, Gupta SK, Justis JR, Sherman MC. Percutaneous pedicle screw fixation of the lumbar spine. *Neurosurg Focus.* 2001;10: 1–8.

24

Minimally Invasive Transforaminal Lumbar Interbody Fusion

FAHEEM A. SANDHU AND RICHARD G. FESSLER

After 45 years of experience with lumbar spine surgery, Cloward,[1,2] the first surgeon to successfully perform a posterior lumbar interbody fusion (PLIF), declared that PLIF should replace simple diskectomy, decompressive laminectomy, and chemonucleolysis as the definitive surgical procedure for the lumbar spine. Through a single dorsal approach, 360-degree stabilization of the lumbar spine is possible. This avoids a second anterior surgery and the morbidities associated with that approach. However, the procedure is technically challenging and requires significant retraction of the thecal sac and nerve root, which can cause injury and also limits surgical treatment to the lower lumbar spine. When performed properly, good outcomes have been attained in 80 to 85% of patients.[2,3]

Harms and Rolinger[4] reported a modification of the PLIF procedure where a unilateral facetectomy was done and grafts were placed from a more lateral location.[4] This transforaminal or TLIF technique was safer because it required little or no retraction of the thecal sac or nerve root while still accomplishing a circumferential fusion. Humphreys et al[5] compared TLIF and PLIF procedures and found that PLIF was associated with significantly higher blood loss than TLIF; PLIF also resulted in multiple complications, whereas TLIF had no associated complications.[5] When compared to anterior interbody fusion with posterior instrumentation, TLIF is associated with decreased blood loss, shorter operative times, and reduced cost.[6,7]

Significant disruption of the musculoligamentous complex occurs with open PLIF and TLIF procedures. Iatrogenic injury to soft tissue support structures of the spine have been negatively correlated with long-term fusion outcomes.[8–12] In an effort to minimize damage to soft tissue but still achieve lumbar arthrodesis, a minimally invasive PLIF (MI-PLIF) technique was developed.[13] As with the open PLIF procedure, MI-PLIF has significant challenges and risks. Although the senior author's (RGF) initial experience with MI-PLIF was uncomplicated, it was felt that the procedure would be easier and safer if a transforaminal approach were used. The open TLIF procedure was modified and adapted to current minimally invasive methods. Herein we describe our technique for performing a minimally invasive TLIF (MI-TLIF).

Indications

Which fusion procedure (anterior, posterior, or both) is best to treat various lumbar spine diseases is the subject of considerable debate. PLIF has been successfully used to treat a broad range of lumbar pathologies including spondylolisthesis, segmental instability, failed back syndrome, recurrent disc herniation, massive bilateral disk herniation, disk herniation alone in a heavy laborer, and degenerative disk disease with mechanical back pain.[14–16] The indications for TLIF are identical to those for PLIF.

It is our practice to offer MI-TLIF fusion to our spondylolisthesis patients (grades I and II only) with demonstrable instability on dynamic radiographs. Patients with degenerative disk disease and mechanical back pain should have clear evidence of degenerative changes at the affected level or have reproducible symptoms on provocative testing, such as a diskogram. We generally do not recommend fusion for recurrent or massive disk herniations. Instead we recommend fragmentectomy of the disk using a microendoscopic technique. These patients may ultimately require a fusion, but by employing minimally invasive techniques, this may be postponed, perhaps indefinitely.

Surgical Equipment/OR Setup

In order to safely perform a minimally invasive TLIF procedure, several pieces of equipment are essential. C-arm fluoroscopy is a must. The use of image guidance is optional. At this time, it is not our practice to use image guidance for this procedure. An expandable tubular retractor (Ex-Tube, Medtronic Sofamor Danek, Memphis, TN) is very important for safe execution of a minimally invasive TLIF. The tube is inserted at a diameter of 26 mm and is expanded in situ to a final working diameter of 44 mm (Fig. 24-1). Use of an endoscope is optional; it is helpful for visualizing the nerve root when placing interbody grafts. We generally use loupe magnification with a headlight or the operating microscope during the procedure. The basic surgical set is essentially the same as a standard laminectomy/fusion except the instruments are slightly longer for working through the tubular retractor. It is important to have a high-speed drill (Midas Rex, Ft. Worth, TX) available as an aid for removing bone. The tools for readying the disk space for graft placement consist of distractors (7–14 mm), rotating cutters, endplate scrapers, and a chisel (Fig. 24-2A–D). Many options exist for interbody graft material. We have had good results when using either allograft bone or cages. Our current practice is to use a polyether ether ketone (PEEK) cage with bone morphogenetic protein-2 (BMP-2) (Medtronic Sofamor Danek). Marking the pedicles for placement of percutaneous screws is relatively easy and requires only an 11-gauge bone biopsy needle, a Kocher clamp, K-wires, a drill, and fluoroscopy. We use the Sextant instrumentation set (Medtronic Sofamor Danek) for placement of cannulated pedicle screws.

The operating room is arranged such that the operating table is in the center of the room, anesthesia at the head, and fluoroscopy monitor at the foot (Fig. 24–3). The C-arm base is placed on the side opposite of the TLIF as is the video monitor. Equipment tables are kept behind the surgeon on the operative side and a Mayo stand is situated over the feet to pass instruments in active use.

The patient is positioned prone on a Wilson frame, which is placed on a Jackson table (Fig. 24-3). It is helpful to use the Jackson table for ease of moving the C-arm during surgery. The arms are bent 90 degrees and placed alongside the patient's head. The knees, axilla, elbows and wrists are padded to prevent nerve palsies. The legs are elevated with pillows to reduce stretch on the sciatic nerve. The face is placed in a padded mask that has a mirrored surface (Prone View, Dupaco) so the anesthetist can view the face and endotracheal tube throughout the procedure.

Surgical Technique

Following induction and intubation, a Foley catheter is placed and leads are inserted into appropriate lower extremity muscle groups for EMG monitoring. The anesthetist is instructed to avoid the use of paralytics, muscle relaxants, and nitrous oxide, which may interfere with EMG recordings. A single dose of antibiotics, either cephazolin or vancomycin, is administered. Sequential compression devices are placed on the legs and the patient is brought to the prone position on the operating table. The C-arm is brought into position for a lateral view of the affected level. An occlusive barrier is placed at the top of the gluteal cleft, and the skin is prepped and draped in standard fashion.

Localization and Exposure

The region of pathology is localized with the aid of fluoroscopy and a Steinmann pin. Once marked, a stab incision is made 3 cm from the midline, and the Steinmann pin is inserted until it rests on bone. Ideally, the pin should be on the facet complex of the affected level. If localization is satisfactory, the skin incision is extended to a final length of 2.5 to 3.0 cm with the position of the Steinmann pin being the center of the incision. Sequential dilators are passed over one another and fluoroscopy is used to confirm adequate insertion. The appropriate-length working channel is introduced over all the dilators, brought into line with the disk space in a medial orientation, and secured to the operating table with a flexible arm clamp. The working channel is opened to its full capacity using the specially designed distractor, and when open, it should span the distance from pedicle to pedicle at the level of interest (Fig. 24-4A–D). Muscle and soft tissue are cleared from the lamina and facet with monopolar cautery (Fig. 24-5A). Next, the working channel is angled laterally, and the transverse processes are exposed. The tubular retractor is again turned medially to begin the laminotomy and facetectomy.

Laminotomy/Facetectomy

A straight curette is used to define the interlaminar space and a plane is developed between the ligamentum flavum and bone with an angled curette. Fluoroscopy is used sporadically throughout the procedure to assess position and evaluate the extent of decompression. Angled Kerrison

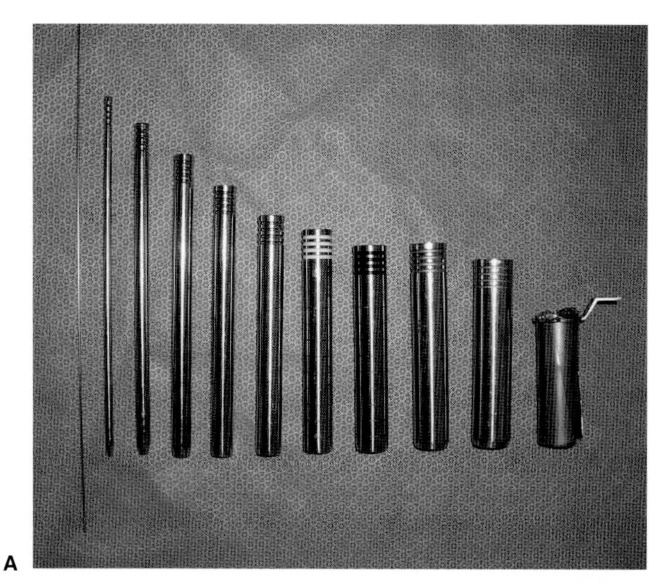
A

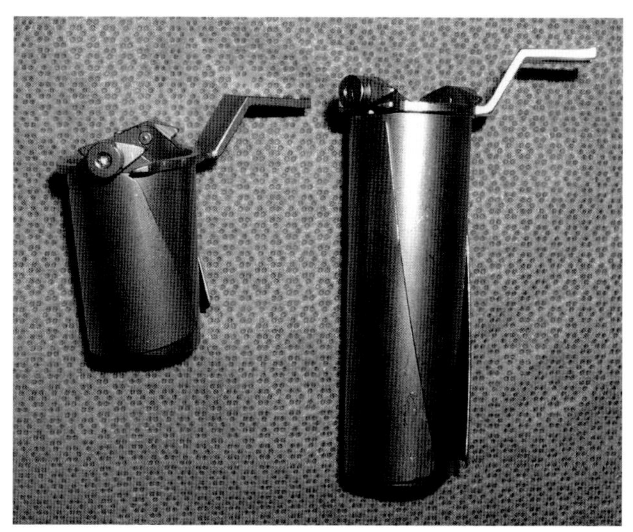
B

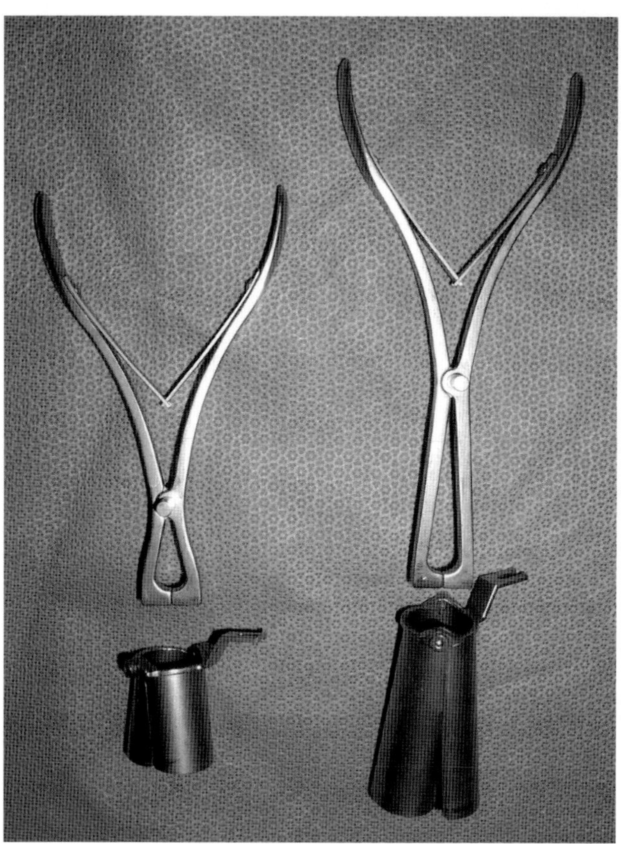
C

FIGURE 24–1 Sequential dilators **(A)** used to establish a working corridor to the spine. Ex-tubes in the closed **(B)** and open position **(C)**.

ronguers are used to begin the laminotomy and facetectomy (Fig. 24-5B). We save all the bone for later use in the transverse process fusion. The decompression should extend from pedicle to pedicle in a rostral–caudal direction. Laterally, a near-total or total facetectomy is done to provide adequate space for graft placement (Fig. 24-5C). Next, the ligamentum flavum is removed (Fig. 24-5D). Epidural veins are coagulated with bipolar cautery and divided if necessary. The lateral edge of the dura, the nerve root, and the disk space should be clearly visualized (Fig. 24-6A-F).

Interbody Fusion

A 15-blade scalpel is used cut the anulus, and disk material is removed with pituitary rongeurs (Fig. 24-7A,B).

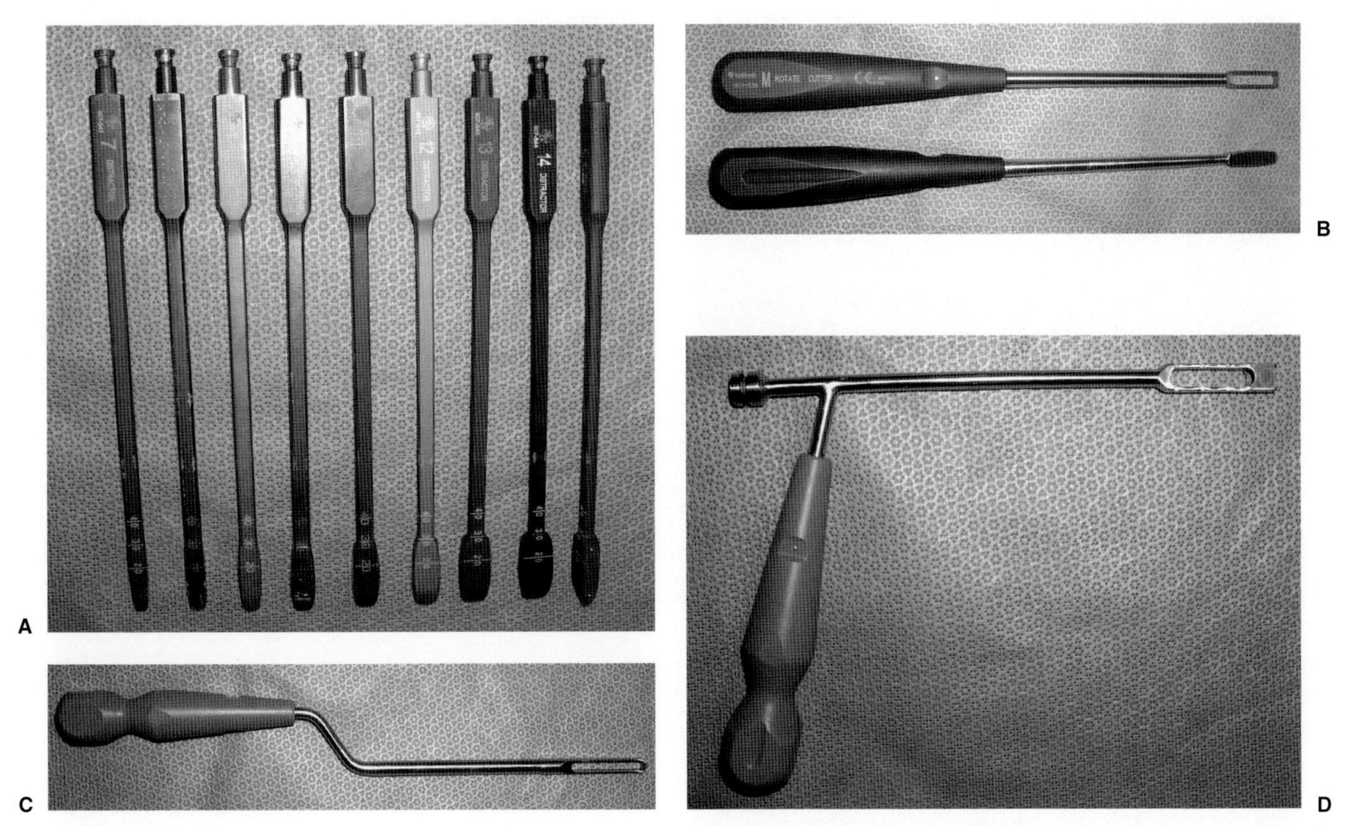

FIGURE 24–2 Instruments necessary for preparing the disk space for graft placement. **(A)** Disk space dilators (7–15 mm). **(B)** Rotating cutters. **(C)** Endplate scraper. **(D)** Chisel.

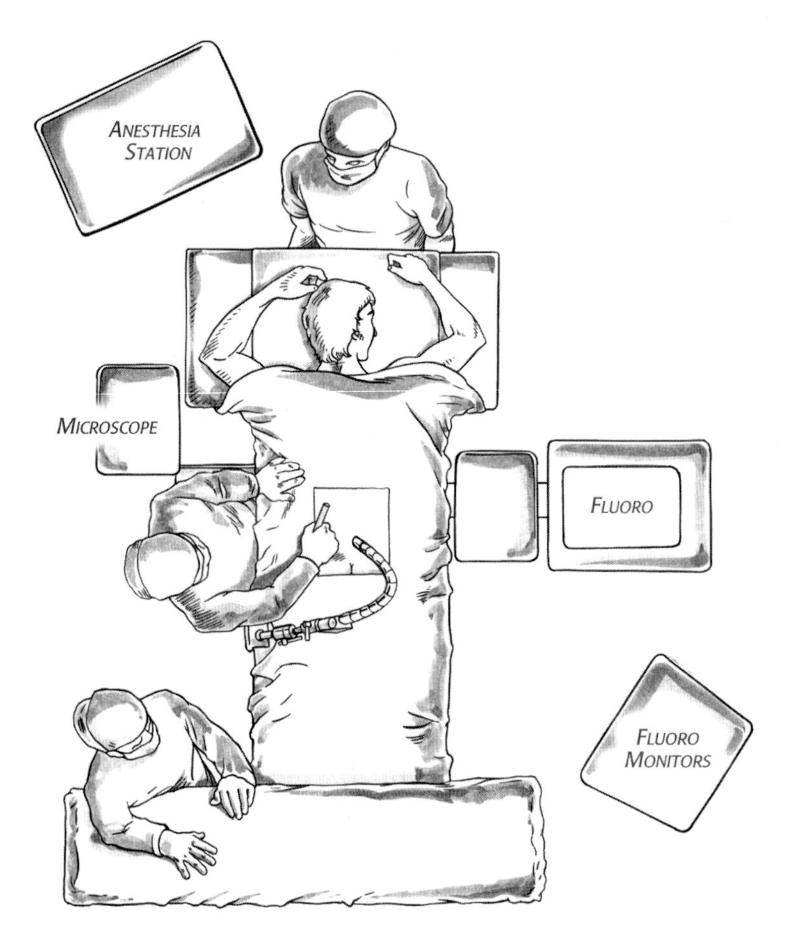

FIGURE 24–3 Operating room setup for an MI-TLIF procedure.

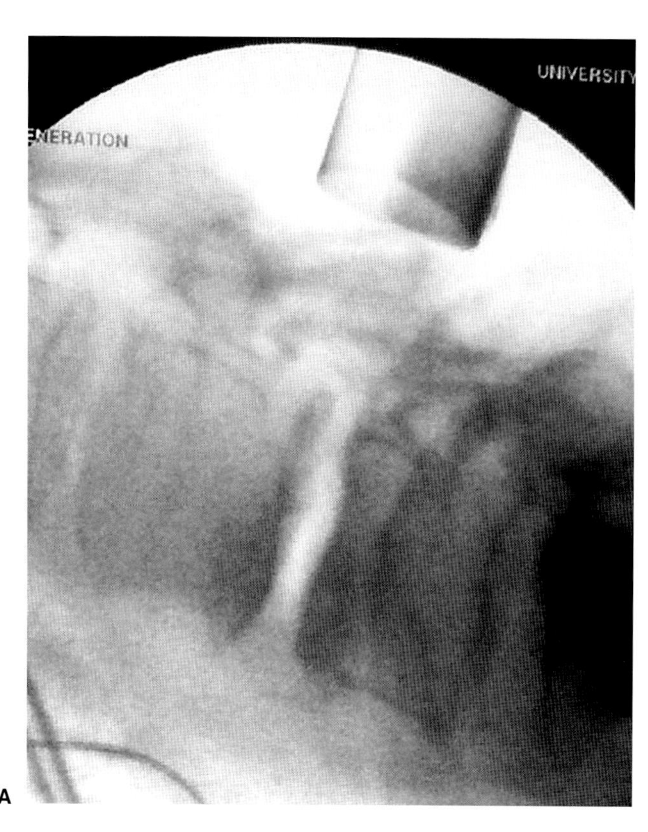

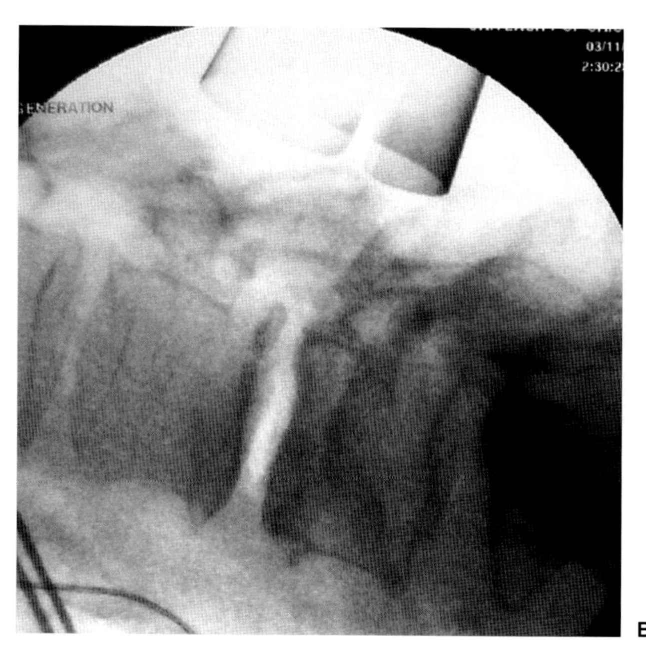

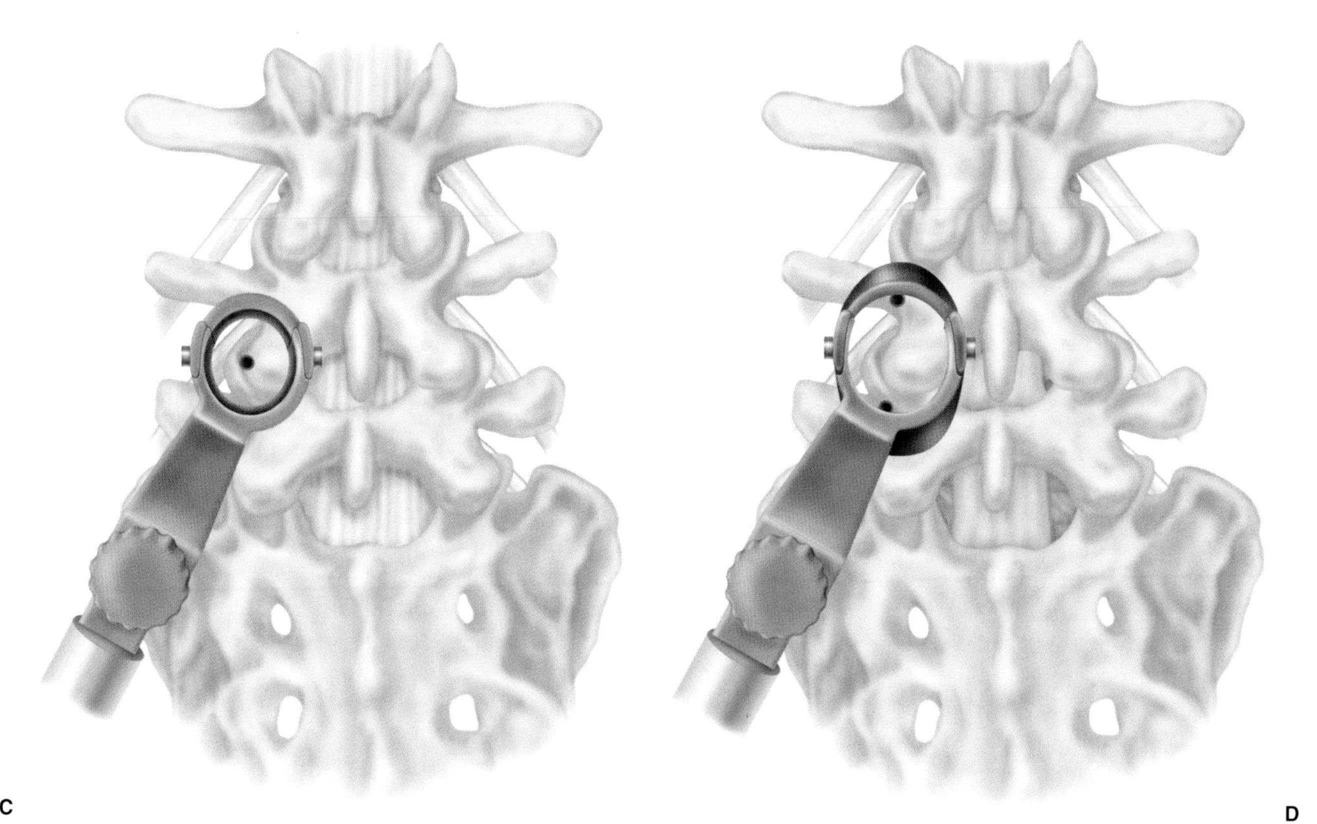

FIGURE 24–4 Intraoperative fluoroscopy **(A,B)** and illustration showing the Ex-tube in closed **(C)** and open **(D)** positions. Note that when open, the Ex-tube provides exposure from pedicle to pedicle.

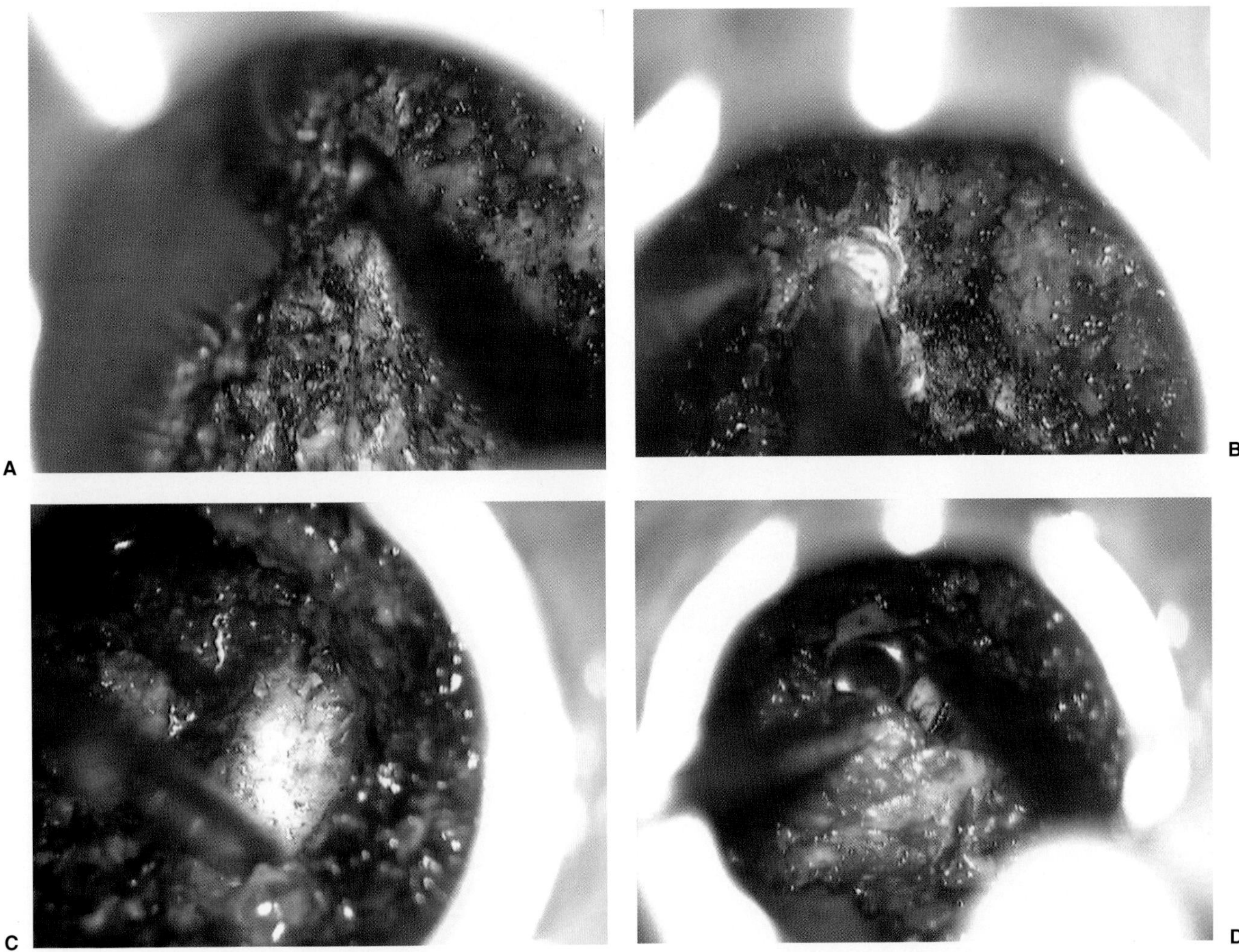

FIGURE 24–5 Intraoperative images during a typical MI-TLIF procedure. **(A)** Exposure of the lamina and facet. **(B)** Initiation of the laminotomy. **(C)** Ligamentum flavum seen after completion of the laminotomy and facetectomy. **(D)** The ligamentum flavum is removed with Kerrison rongeurs. **(E)** The thecal sac and disk space are exposed following removal of the ligamentum flavum. **(F)** The diskectomy is begun. **(G)** The end plates are prepared. **(H)** A view of the disk space prior to graft placement. **(I)** The first allograft bone graft is placed and pushed to the contralateral side. **(J)** Final appearance after placement of two allograft bone grafts.

A down-angled curette is helpful to ensure that subligamentous disk fragments and the contralateral disk are properly removed (Fig. 24-7C). Disk space dilators are then inserted to measure the interbody space for the appropriately sized graft. The disk space is sequentially dilated until disk space height is similar to adjacent levels. The maximum insertable dilator translates into the width of the interbody graft we use. Next, the rotating cutter is introduced parallel with the disk space and rotated to start preparing the vertebral body end plates (Fig. 24-8A). The end plates are scraped, and debris is removed with a pituitary rongeur (Fig. 24-8B). A chisel is used to remove osteophytes (Fig. 24-8C). Our experience has been that a chisel slightly smaller than the graft works best (e.g., a 10-mm chisel is used for a 12-mm graft). The operative site is copiously irrigated with antibiotic saline prior to graft placement. The end plates are now ready for graft placement (Fig. 24-9A–C). If allograft (Tangent, Medtronic Sofamor Danek) is used, we insert two grafts and orient them toward each other such that a circle in the center of the vertebral body is made on completion of graft placement (Fig. 24-10A–D). When placing the PEEK cage, we first lay a BMP-2 soaked sponge along the anterior annulus, place a BMP-2 pledget in the cage, and insert the cage obliquely such that it is centered in the disk space. Thrombin-soaked Gelfoam and a large cottonoid are placed over the interspace for hemostasis. Attention is next directed at the transverse processes. The tubular retractor is adjusted to visualize the transverse processes. They are decorticated with a high-speed drill and autograft bone saved from the laminectomy and facetectomy is packed between the processes. If the bone quantity seems inadequate, it is supplemented one-to-one with allograft cancellous bone chips. The working channel is collapsed and the cottonoid, Gelfoam, and working channel are removed.

Instrumentation

The next part of the procedure is insertion of the instrumentation. We use the "bull's eye" technique for marking the pedicles. The C-arm is rotated 90 degrees for a true AP view parallel with the disk space. The bone biopsy needle is localized over the pedicle and passed through the soft tissue onto the pedicle. We try to target the center of the pedicle and then orient the needle so it is directly in line with the pedicle; the needle will appear as a single spot ("bull's eye") in this orientation (Fig. 24-11A). The needle is tapped into the pedicle with a mallet and position is confirmed by fluoroscopy. Then, with the needle held firmly in the correct orientation, the stylet is removed and a K-wire is drilled ~1 cm into the pedicle. The bone needle is removed and fluoroscopy is used to confirm that the K-wire is in the center of the pedicle (Fig. 24-11B). The process is repeated for the contralateral pedicle and then for both pedicles at the adjacent affected level. The C-arm is brought to the lateral position for advancement of the K-wires.

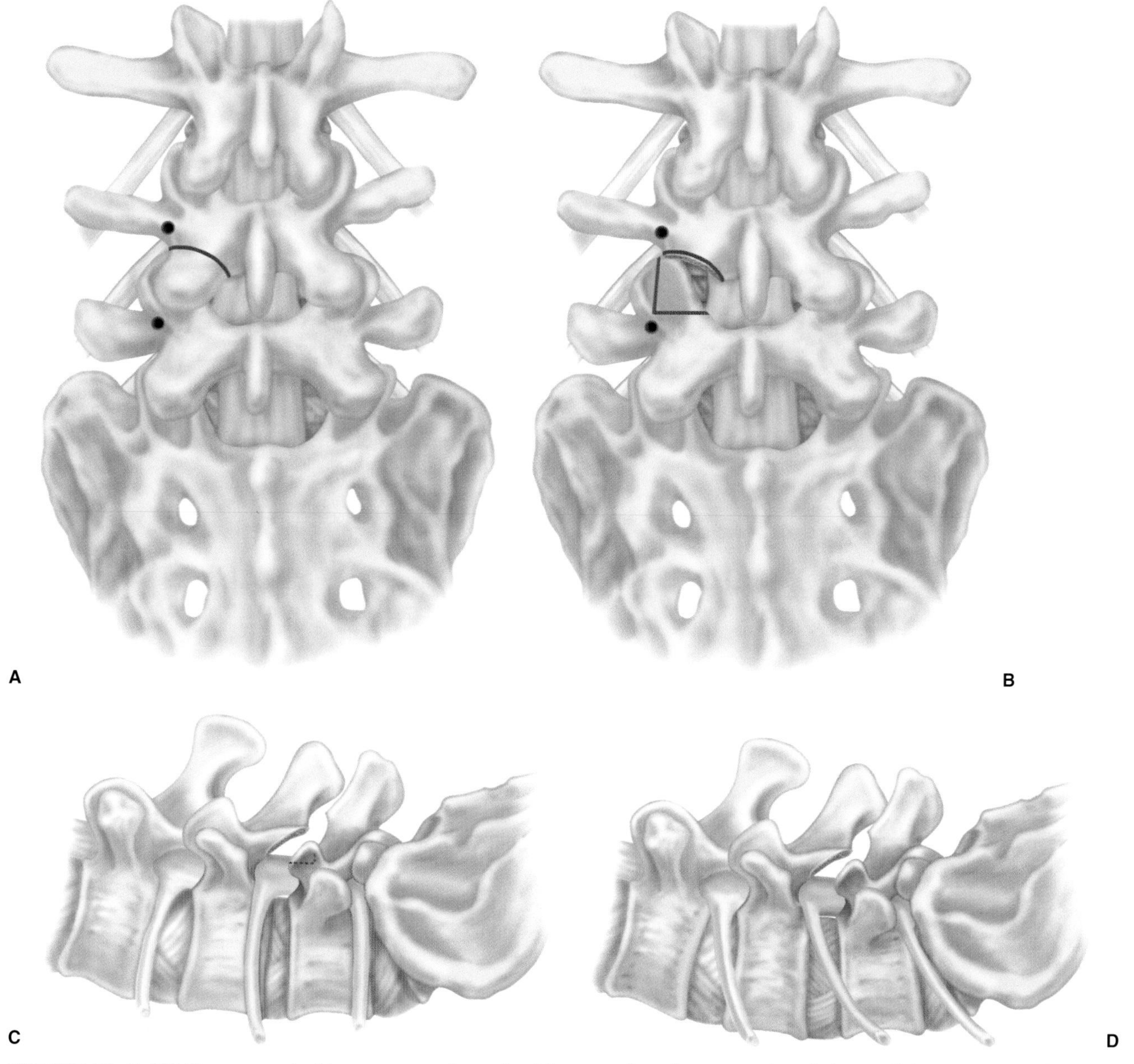

FIGURE 24–6 (A) The amount of bony removal required for a TLIF. **(B,C)** The inferior articulate surface of the facet joint is completely removed. **(D,E)** After the removal of the inferior articulate surface, the superior aspect of the superior articulate surface is removed until the pedicle is reached. **(F)** The disk space obtained after aggressive bony removal as seen through the Ex-tube.

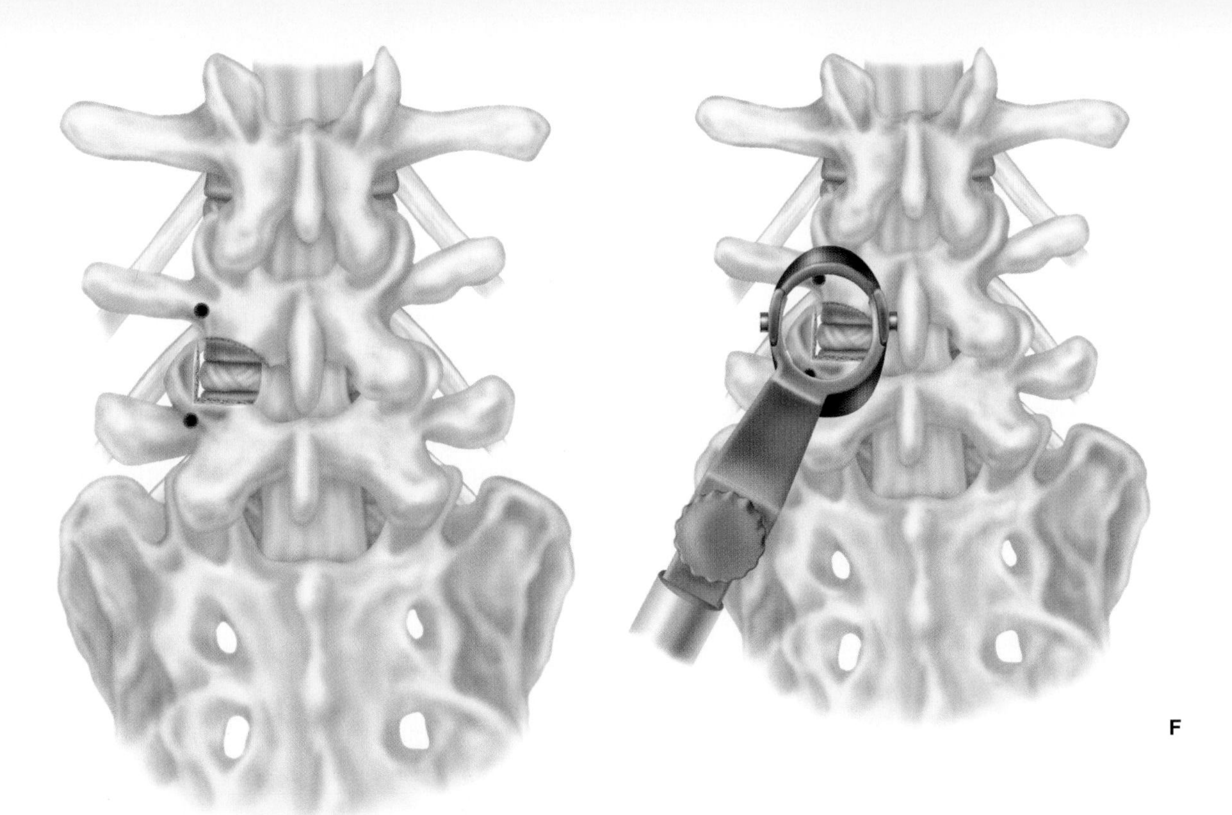

FIGURE 24–6 (*Continued*)

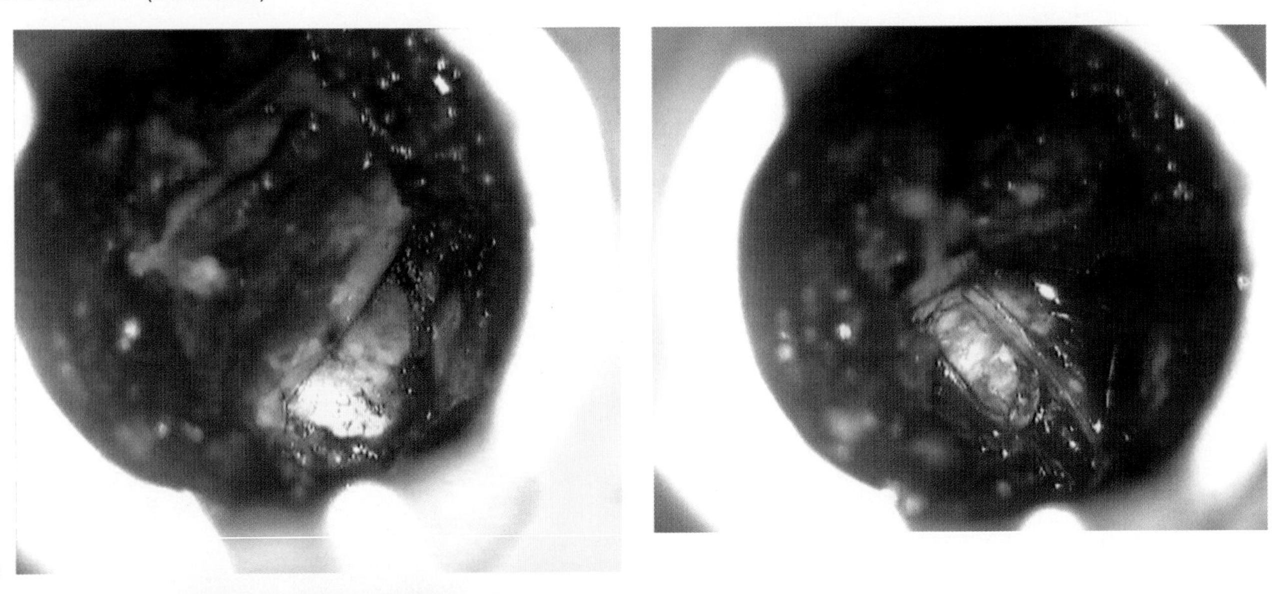

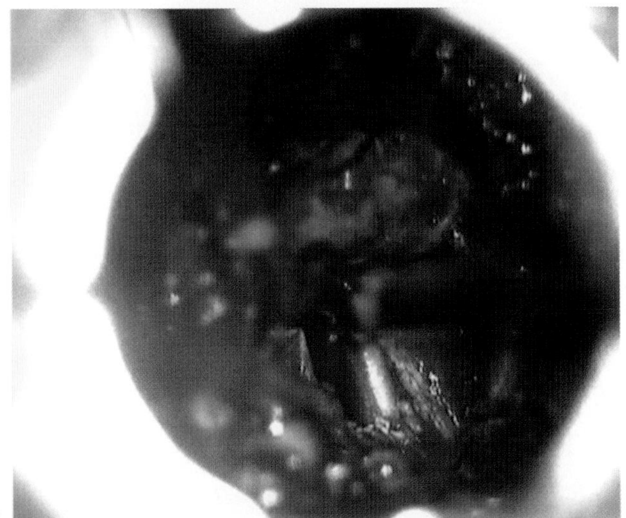

FIGURE 24–7 MI-TLIF preparation of the disk space. **(A)** The thecal sac and disk space are exposed following removal of the ligamentum flavum. **(B)** The diskectomy is begun. **(C)** The end plates are prepared.

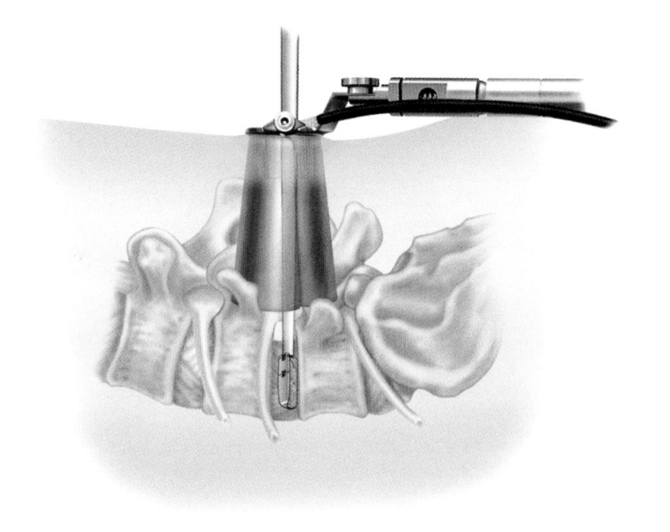

A

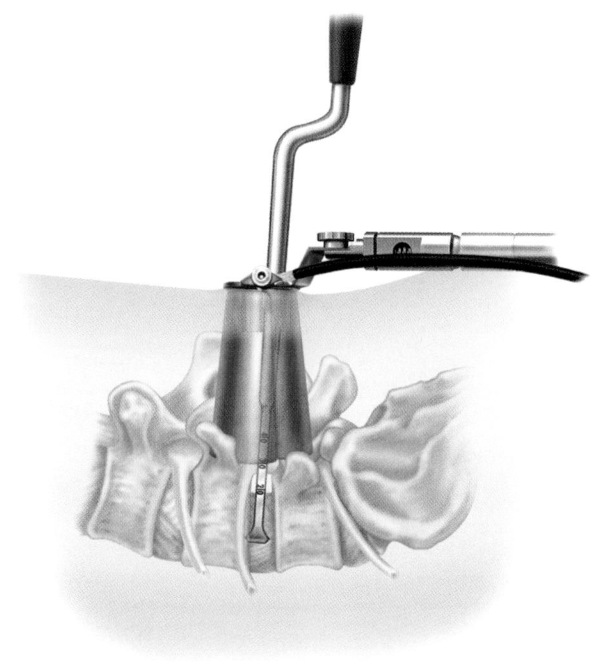

B

C

FIGURE 24–8 Endplate preparation for MI-TLIF. **(A)** Disk rotator through the X-tube for initial disk removal. **(B)** End plates are scraped in medial and lateral directions. **(C)** A chisel one size smaller than the anticipated bone graft is used in a medial direction for the first bone graft and then laterally for the second bone graft.

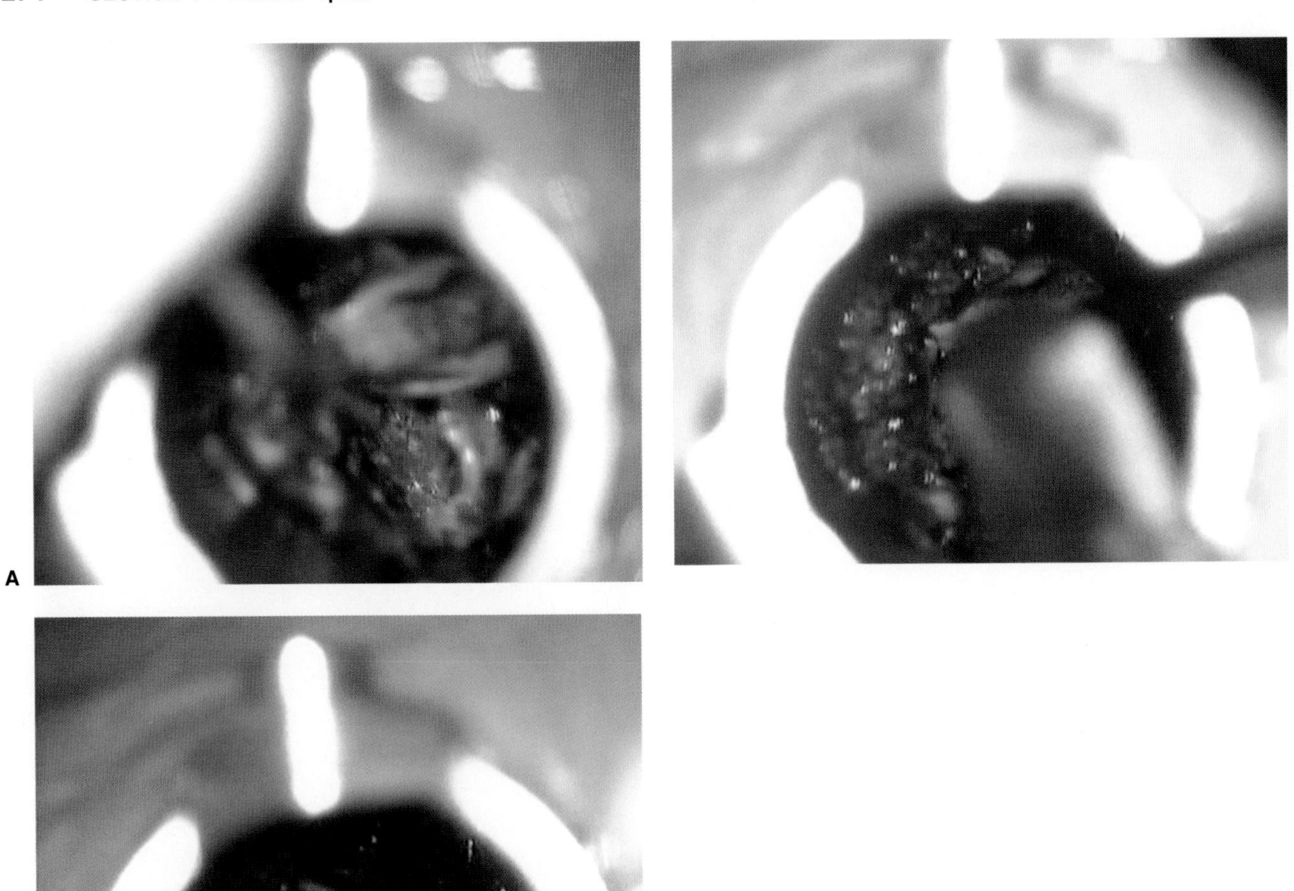

FIGURE 24–9 (A) A view of the disk space prior to graft placement. **(B)** The first allograft bone graft is placed and pushed to the contralateral side. **(C)** Final appearance after placement of two allograft bone grafts.

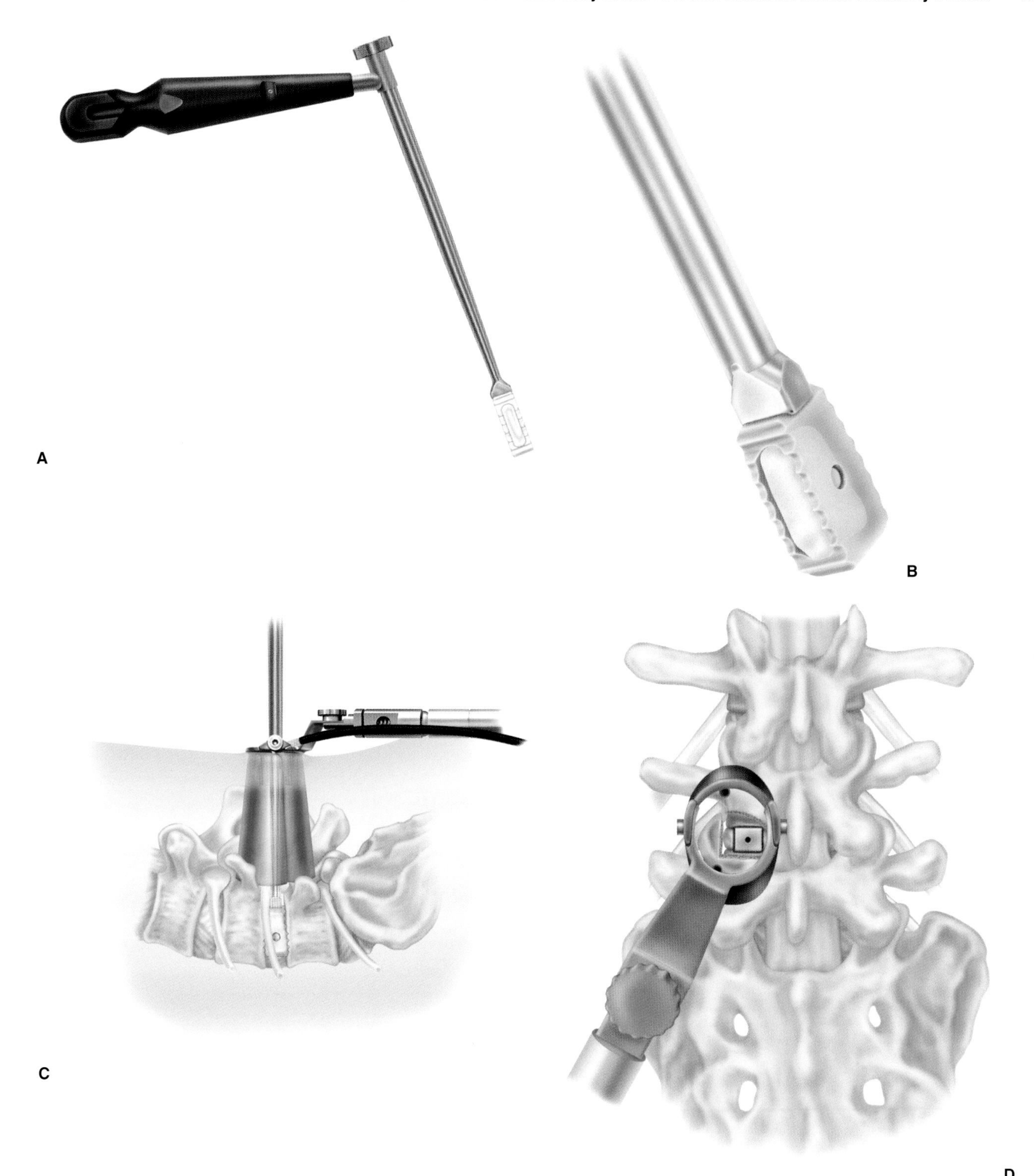

FIGURE 24–10 Bone graft placement via the Ex-tube. **(A,B)** Bone graft loaded for placement. **(C,D)** Final bone graft position as seen through the Ex-tube.

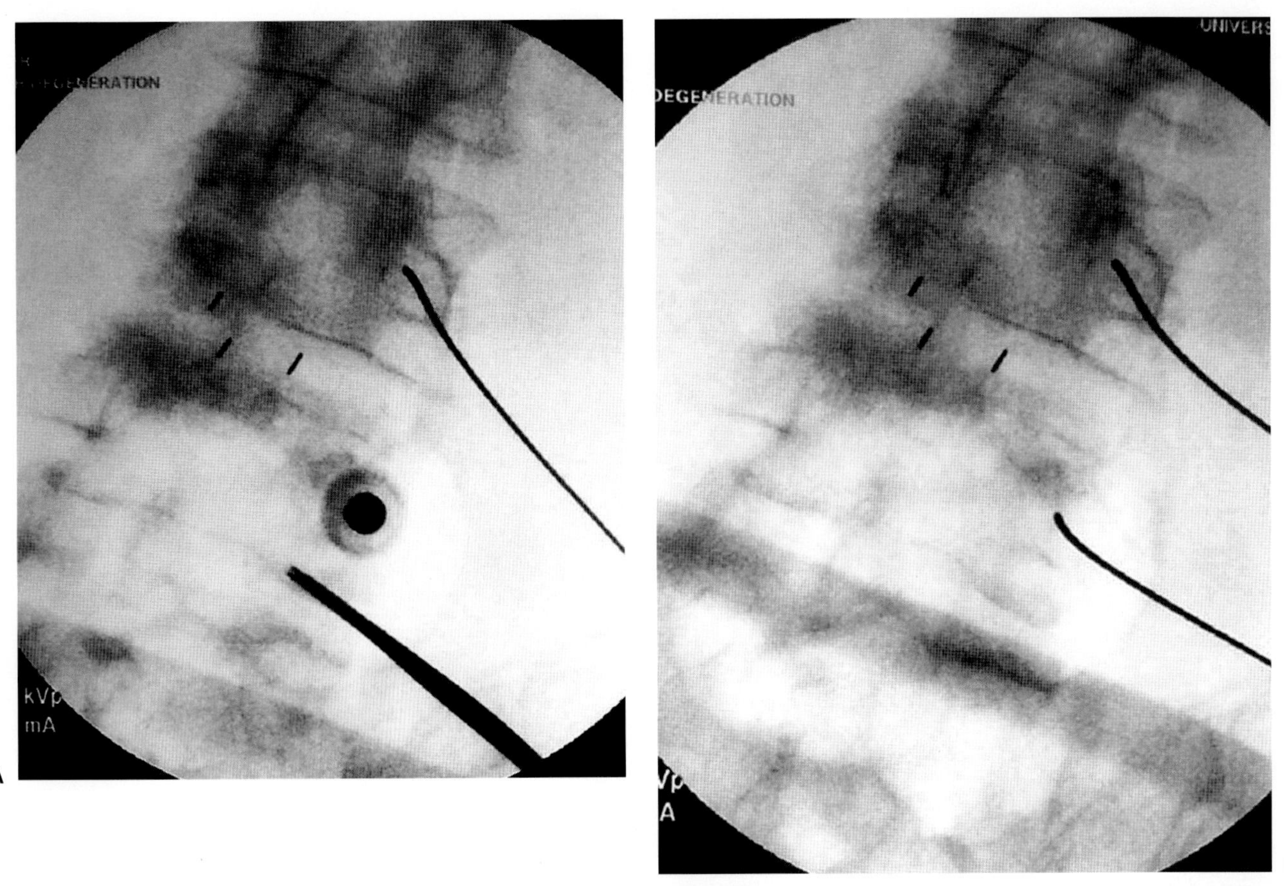

FIGURE 24–11 (A) A bone biopsy needle is placed in the "bull's eye" position over the pedicle. **(B)** K-wires are passed through the inner cannula of the biopsy needle, which centers them in the pedicles.

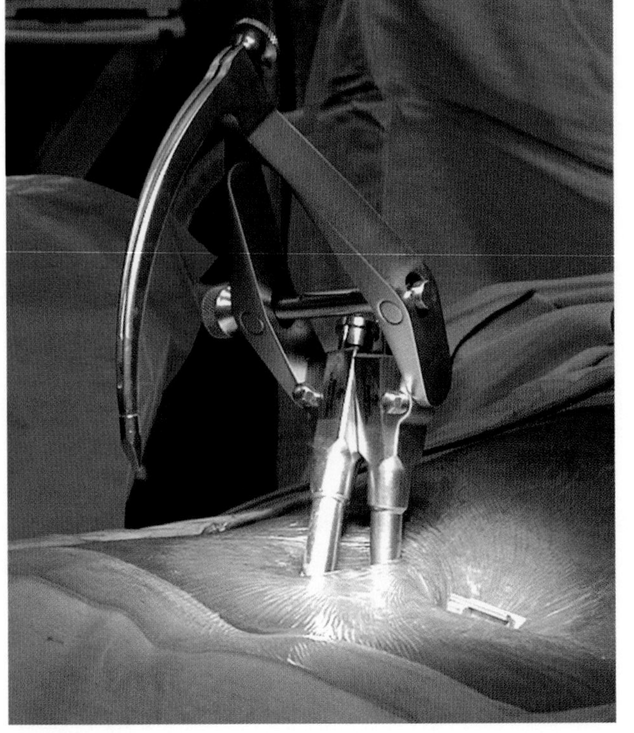

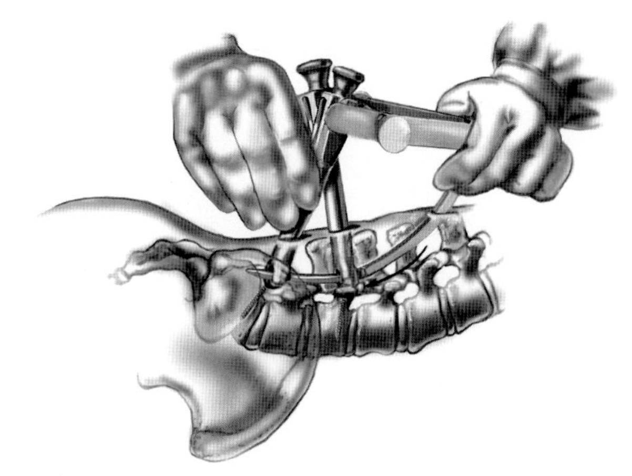

FIGURE 24–12 (A) Sextant apparatus attached to two screw extenders prior to passage of a rod. **(B)** The rod is passed subcutaneously.

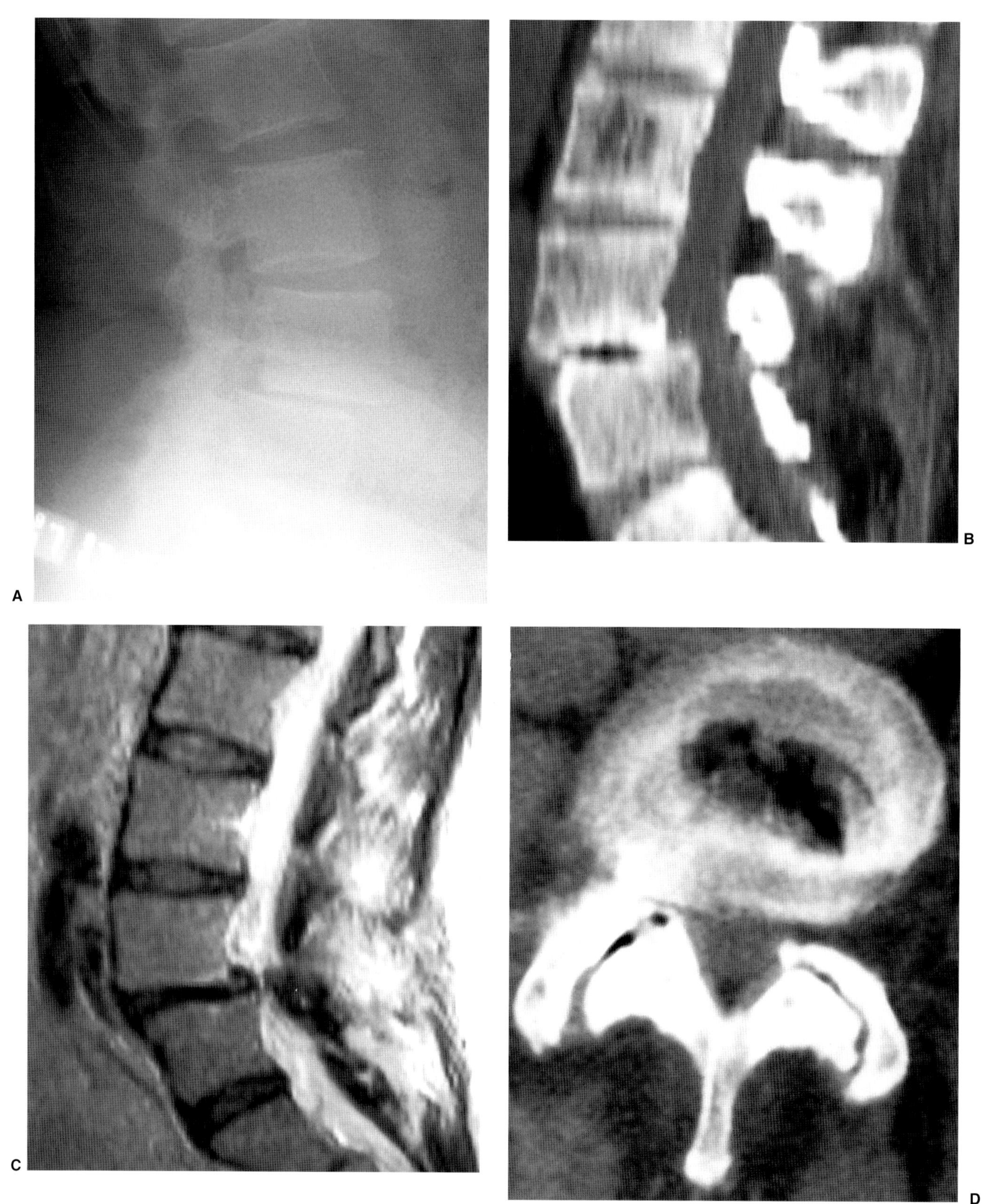

FIGURE 24–13 (A) Lateral radiograph revealing grade I spondylolisthesis at L4–5. **(B)** Sagittal CT reconstruction. **(C)** Sagittal T2-weighted MR scan. **(D)** Axial CT through the L4–5 disk space.

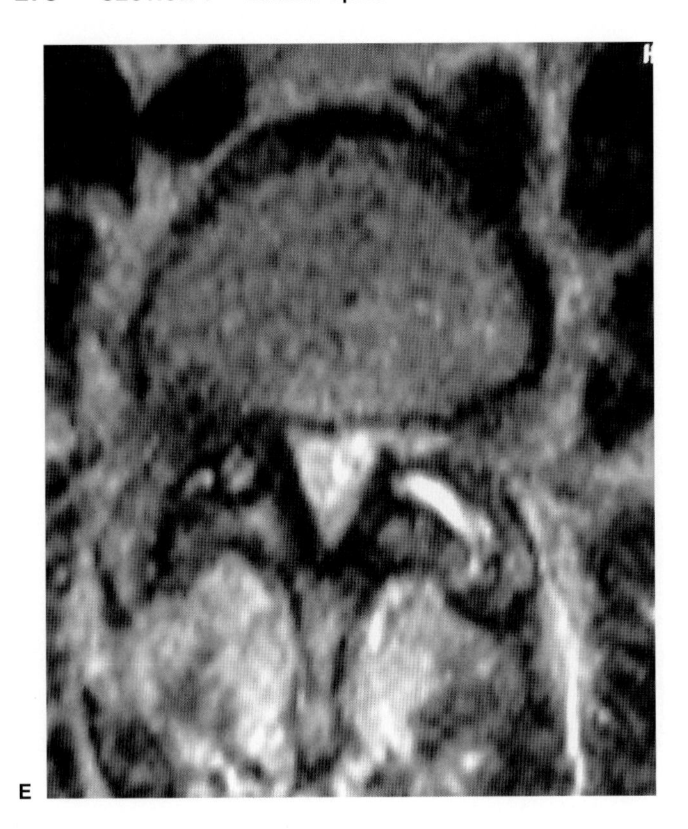

FIGURE 24–13 *(continued)* **(E)** Axial T2-weighted MR scan demonstrating stenosis at the L4–5 interspace.

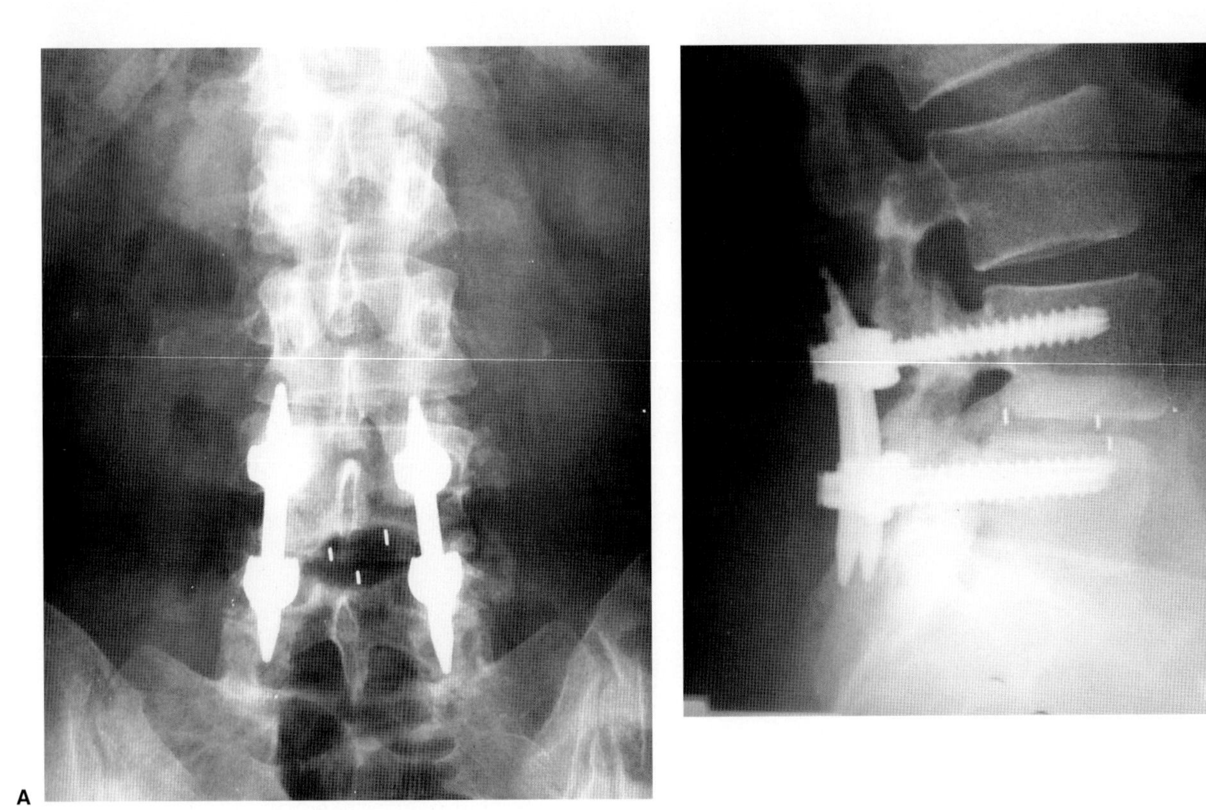

FIGURE 24–14 (A) Postoperative AP and **(B)** lateral radiographs 6 weeks after surgery showing good position of instrumentation, restoration of disk height, and reduction of the spondylolisthesis.

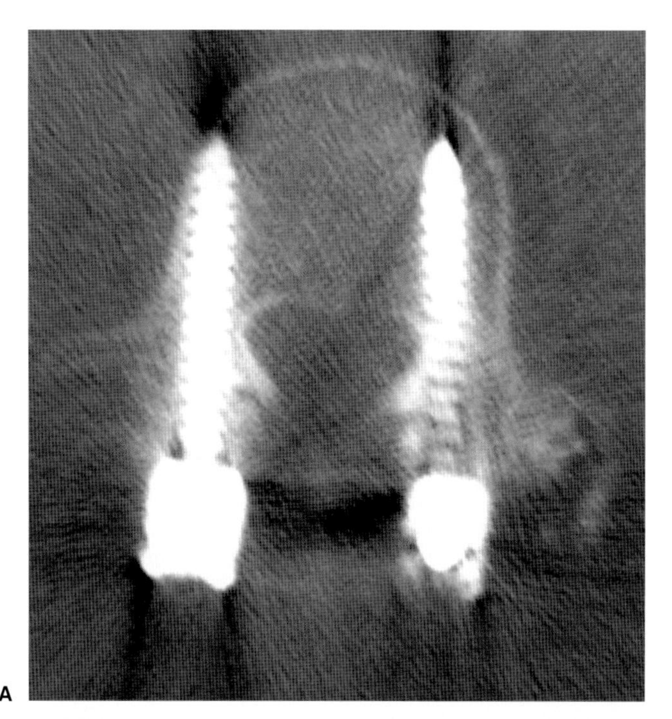

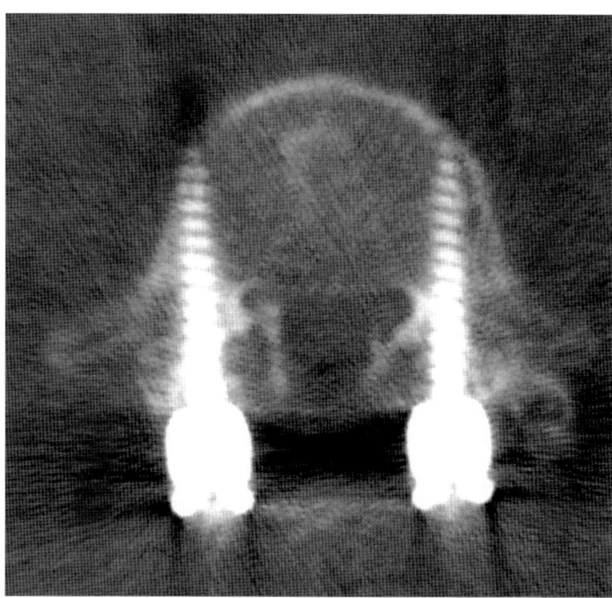

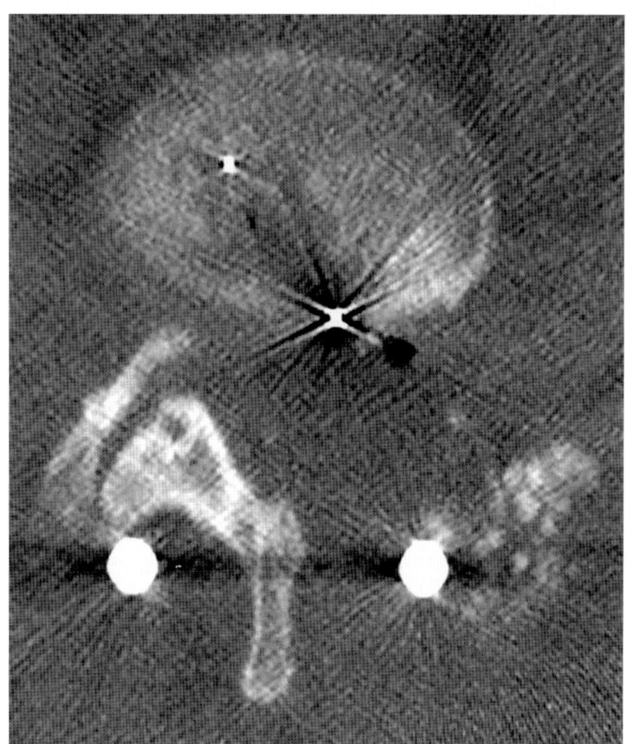

FIGURE 24–15 Axial CT images of the same case showing the position of percutaneously placed screws at **(A)** L4 and **(B)** L5 and **(C)** the position of the graft.

We insert K-wires about two thirds the length of the vertebral body parallel with the end plate. The remainder of the procedure can be completed in less than 30 minutes. Soft tissue over the K-wires is dilated, the pedicles are tapped, and cannulated screws are inserted. Care is taken not to tap too far as this can dislodge the K-wire and necessitate beginning over. The Sextant device is attached to the screw extenders and pushed through the soft tissue to create a tract for the rod (Fig. 24-12A,B). The rod size is calculated by placing templates on the Sextant at this point. The tip of the Sextant is replaced with the rod, which is pushed through the soft tissue and both screw heads. The C-arm is brought to the AP orientation to confirm that the rod has passed through both screw heads before tightening. The screws are then compressed, tightened, and broken off with a torque wrench. The Sextant is disconnected from the rod and removed. The process is repeated on the opposite side. Wounds are irrigated with antibiotic saline and closed in layers with absorbable suture. The wound is dressed with three coats of 2-octyl cyanoacrylate (Dermabond; Ethicon).

Complication Avoidance

A number of complications are possible with this technique, but with care and anticipation, most can be avoided. It is possible for the Steinmann pin or the dilators to slip into the interlaminar space and cause dural perforation or nerve injury. This can be avoided by removing the Steinman pin after passage of the first dilator and ensuring that the dilators are docked on bone with passage of successive dilators. Dural tears and nerve root injury can occur with removal of bone and ligament. Good visualization and generous use of an angled curette to define and develop a plane are the best ways to avoid these complications. Intraoperative EMG monitoring provides immediate feedback of nerve irritation throughout the procedure, especially during graft placement. Frequent use of fluoroscopy is helpful to guide decompression and for accurate screw placement.

Case Illustration

A 60-year-old woman with chronic low back pain developed muscle spasms in her left buttock of 6 months' duration. She had an episode of severe back and buttock pain that necessitated hospitalization for pain control. There was no history of prior back surgery or trauma. Physical examination revealed no abnormalities. Plain radiographs of her lumbosacral spine revealed grade I spondylolisthesis; MRI and CT scan demonstrated significant stenosis at L4-5 (Fig. 24-13A–E). She underwent a left L4-L5 MI-TLIF/Sextant with PEEK interbody graft, BMP-2, and left transverse process fusion. Good reduction of her spondylolisthesis was achieved, and the graft was in good position following surgery. Surgery was completed in 3.5 hours; blood loss was estimated at 100 cc. She was discharged from the hospital 3 days following surgery. Six weeks after surgery, she was off narcotic pain medications and had returned to work. Radiographs at this time showed good alignment of her spine and evidence of early fusion between the transverse processes (Figs. 24-14, 24-15).

Transforminal lumbar interbody fusion with instrumentation can be performed safely and effectively by minimally invasive techniques, reducing significant morbidity and pain associated with conventional open techniques. They can accomplish all the surgical goals of the open procedures and thus are likely to replace the open techniques as the standard for lumbar interbody fusion.

REFERENCES

1. Cloward RB. Posterior lumbar interbody fusion updated. *Clin Orthop.* 1985;193:16–19.
2. Cloward R. The treatment of ruptured lumbar intervertebral disks by vertebral body fusion, I: Indications, operative technique, after care. *J Neurosurg.* 1953;10:154–168.
3. Freeman BJ, Licina P, Mehdian SH. Posterior lumbar interbody fusion combined with instrumented postero-lateral fusion: 5-year results in 60 patients. *Eur Spine J.* 2000;9:42–46.
4. Harms J, Rolinger H. [A one-stager procedure in operative treatment of spondylolistheses: dorsal traction-reposition and anterior fusion (author's transl)]. *Z Orthop Ihre Grenzgeb* 1982;120:343–347.
5. Humphreys SC, Hodges SD, Patwardhan AG, et al. Comparison of posterior and transforaminal approaches to lumbar interbody fusion. *Spine.* 2001;26:567–571.
6. Whitecloud TS III, Roesch WW, Ricciardi JE. Transforaminal interbody fusion versus anterior-posterior interbody fusion of the lumbar spine: a financial analysis. *J Spinal Disord.* 2001;14:100–103.
7. Hee HT, Castro FP Jr, Majd ME, et al. Anterior/posterior lumbar fusion versus transforaminal lumbar interbody fusion: analysis of complications and predictive factors. *J Spinal Disord.* 2001;14:533–540.
8. Kawaguchi Y, Yabuki S, Styf J, et al. Back muscle injury after posterior lumbar spine surgery: topographic evaluation of intramuscular pressure and blood flow in the porcine back muscle during surgery. *Spine.* 1996;21:2683–2688.
9. Kawaguchi Y, Matsui H, Tsuji H. Back muscle injury after posterior lumbar spine surgery: a histologic and enzymatic analysis. *Spine.* 1996;21:941–944.
10. Mayer TG, Vanharanta H, Gatchel RJ, et al. Comparison of CT scan muscle measurements and isokinetic trunk strength in postoperative patients. *Spine.* 1989;14:33–36.
11. Sihvonen T, Herno A, Paljarvi L, et al. Local denervation atrophy of paraspinal muscles in postoperative failed back syndrome. *Spine.* 1993;18:575–581.
12. Wetzel FT, LaRocca H. The failed posterior lumbar interbody fusion. *Spine.* 1991;16:839–845.
13. Khoo LT, Palmer S, Laich DT, et al. Minimally invasive percutaneous posterior lumbar interbody fusion. *Neurosurgery* 2002;51 (suppl 2):S166–S281
14. Cloward RB. Spondylolisthesis: treatment by laminectomy and posterior interbody fusion. *Clin Orthop.* 1981:74–82.
15. Hutter C. Spinal stenosis and posterior lumbar interbody fusion. *Clin Orthop.* 1985;193:103–114.
16. Branch CL, Jr. The case for posterior lumbar interbody fusion. *Clin Neurosurg.* 1996;43:252–267.

25

Percutaneous Translaminar Facet Screw Fixation

JOHN S. THALGOTT AND JAMES M. GIUFFRE

Translaminar facet screws (TLFSs), invented by Magerl for posterior stabilization, were first described by Montesano et al in 1988.[1] In 1998, Rathonyi et al[2] reported their findings from a biomechanical study that comprised an intact human cadaver spine versus TLFS alone, versus Bagby and Kuslich (BAK) cages alone, versus TLFS + BAK cages at both one and two levels. They noted: "The combination of the excellent stabilizing effect of an anterior cage in axial compression, flexion, and lateral bending, with the stabilizing effect of TLFS fixation in extension and axial rotation seem optimal from a biomechanical perspective." In another biomechanical study in 1998, Deguchi et al[3] compared TLFSs with pedicle screws in a human cadaver model. They described TLFS fixation as having "similar biomechanical performance to pedicle screw fixation." Multiple investigators have reported excellent clinical results with a high rate of fusion using TLFS in a circumferential fusion model.[4–12]

TLFS fixation involves placing screws through the base of the spinous process, through the lamina, and into the facet joint in a criss-cross fashion. This is instrumental in completing the tension band, which is the goal of a circumferential instrumented environment. TLFSs are inherently less invasive than transpedicular screws, and implantation through a minimally invasive approach improves upon this concept. The importance of a minimally invasive approach to TLFS fixation cannot be overstated. The use of TLFS in lieu of transpedicular fixation is ineffective if taking down of the paraspinous muscles occurs, as with a traditional open midline approach for transpedicular fixation. If the paraspinous muscles are sacrificed with the approach, a poor biomechanical environment for healing is created, both for the fusion mass and for the return of normal function of the low back (W. Rauschning, personal communication).

The introduction of TLFS has reduced the use of pedicle screws by 70% in the senior author's (JMG) practice. In an environment of managed care and escalating surgical costs, TLFSs are, on average, 75% less expensive per level compared with pedicle screw systems currently on the market. The senior author currently uses TLFSs approved for use in the spine by the U.S. Food and Drug Administration (Discovery; DePuy AcroMed, Raynham, MA). Prior to the FDA approval of this device, 4.5 mm cancellous bone screws were used as an off-label device.

Indications

The following are indications for percutaneous translaminar facet screw fixation:

- Posterior internal fixation in place of transpedicular fixation for an instrumented circumferential lumbar fusion at one or two levels
- Stabilization following laminoplasty-type decompression of a central or far lateral spinal stenosis at one or two levels
- Degenerative spondylolisthesis less than or equal to grade II with laminoplasty-type decompression
- An adjunctive fixation at the middle levels of a transpedicular fixation construct for the treatment of fracture

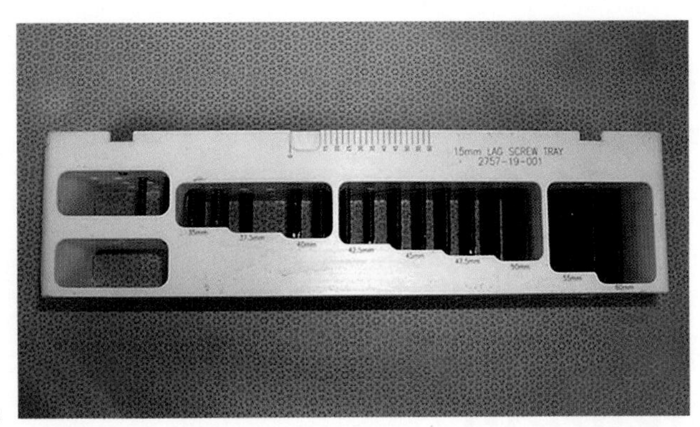

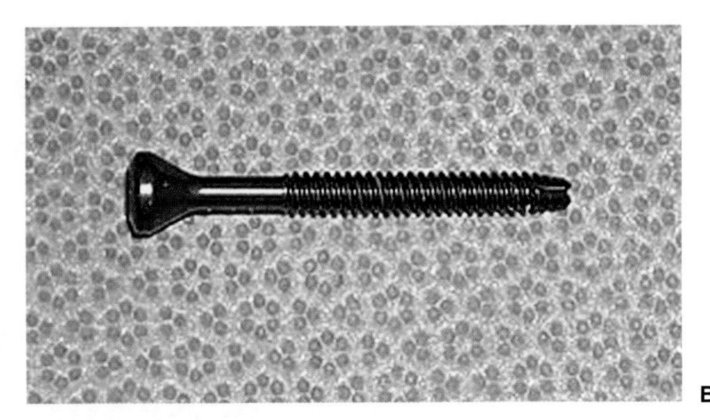

FIGURE 25–1 (A) The Discovery Translaminar Facet Screw Set (DePuy AcroMed, Raynham, MA), FDA-approved for use in the lumbar spine. **(B)** A close-up view of a titanium translaminar facet screw, which includes a hollow core.

Contraindications

Contraindications for the procedure include:

- For constructs greater than 2 lumbar levels
- A supplementary posterior fixation for a previous stand-alone anterior lumbar interbody fusion (ALIF)
- Isthmic-lytic spondylolisthesis
- Scoliosis, kyphosis, or other deformity
- A solitary fixation modality for the treatment of fracture

Surgical Procedures

Surgical Equipment

- Instruments to perform posterior lumbar surgery
- Discovery Translaminar Facet Screw Set, containing 4.5 mm diameter screws (Fig. 25–1)
- Power drill with drill bit and screwdriver bit

Operating Room Setup

A standard setup for posterior lumbar surgery is used, with the spine surgeon standing on the left or right side of the patient, depending on the pathology, and with one surgical technician and one surgical assistant.

Patient Positioning

The patient is placed in the prone position on a Jackson table. Following general anesthesia, the patient is draped and prepped in the standard fashion, and preoperative antibiotics are given. Fluoroscopy is used to find the landmarks of the appropriate lumbar level (Fig. 25–2). The skin is marked, identifying the level(s) to be addressed.

Surgical Technique

Great care is taken to limit the midline incision to 2.5 to 5.0 cm (Fig. 25–3). The incision should be made as small as possible without dissecting or denervating the

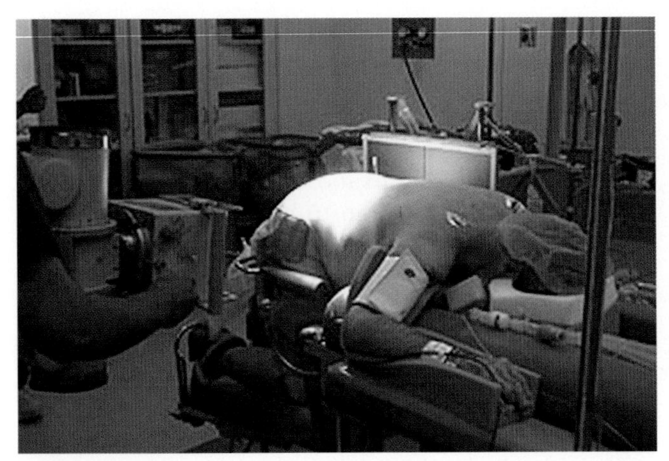

FIGURE 25–2 The patient is placed in the prone position on a Jackson table. Preoperative fluoroscopy is used to identify the appropriate level for the approach.

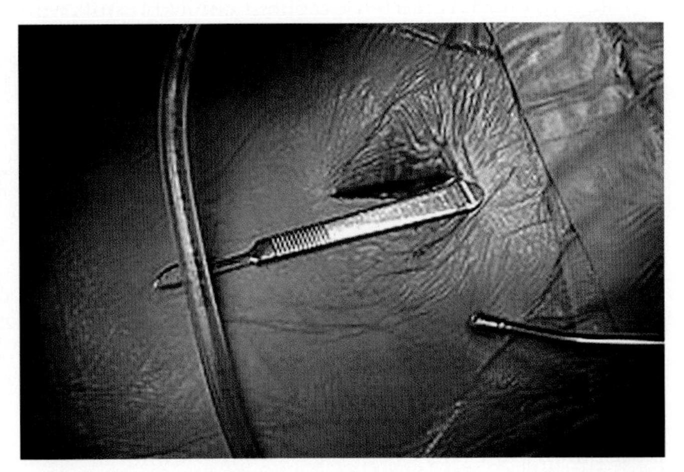

FIGURE 25–3 A 2.5 to 5.0 cm midline incision is made. The size of the incision does not change for a two-level procedure.

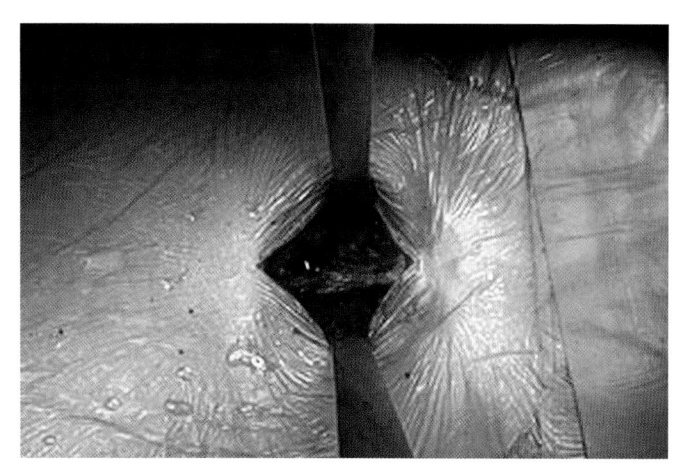

FIGURE 25–4 Posterior retractors are placed bilaterally at the lateral edges of the incision.

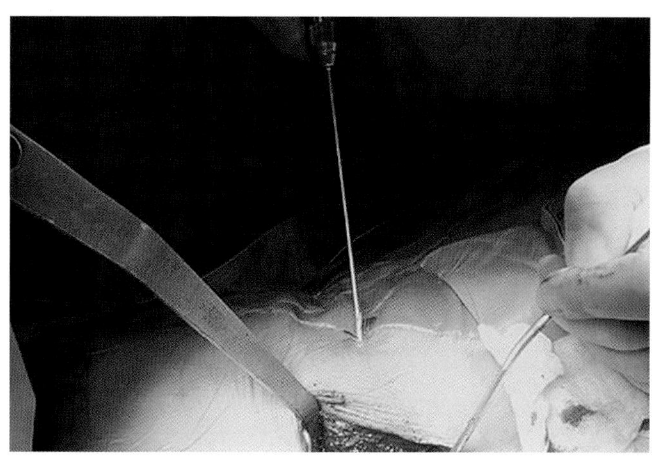

FIGURE 25–6 Small percutaneous incisions are placed above and lateral to the primary incision. The drill is placed through this incision.

paraspinous muscles. Posterior retractors are then placed at the edge of the incision laterally on each side (Fig. 25–4). A laminoplasty-type decompression must be performed. The laminar arch and at least 50% of the facet joints must also be left intact (Fig. 25–5). Following decompression, percutaneous incisions are made to the left and right, lateral and cranial to the midline incision. The surgeon stands on the left side of the patient. A 3.2 mm drill is placed through the incision (Fig. 25–6) to the base of the spinous process. A hole is drilled through the base of the spinous process, across the lamina, and to the contralateral facet joint, from left to right (Fig. 25–7). This is then repeated from right to left, with the surgeon standing on the right side of the patient. Once this is completed, the drill bit is changed to a screwdriver bit, and the appropriate-length screws are selected. The screws can be placed either through the lateral percutaneous incisions or through the midline incision, with power, depending on the anatomy and surgeon's preference (Fig. 25–8). Following screw placement (Fig. 25–9), bone graft is placed in the midline (Fig. 25–10),

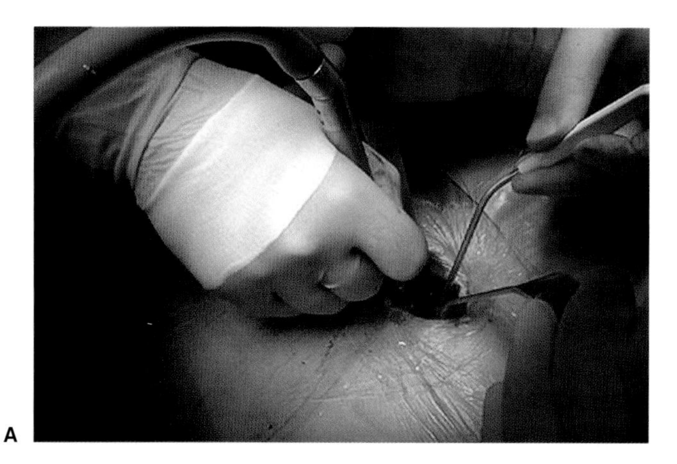

A

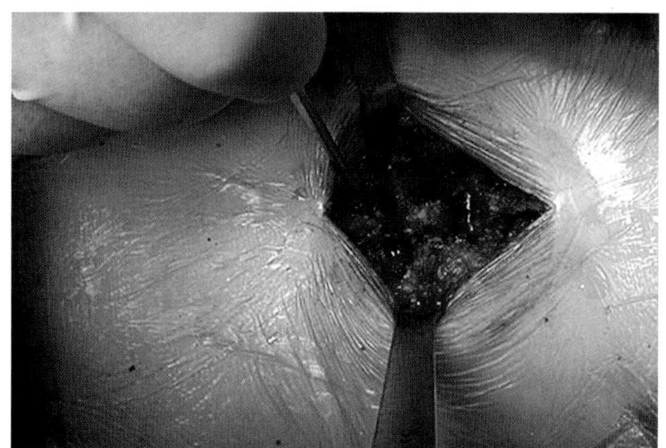

B

FIGURE 25–5 (A) Standard instruments (e.g., a Midas Rex drill) can be used through this minimally invasive incision. A laminoplasty-type decompression technique is necessary for this approach. **(B)** The laminar arch must be kept intact, and there cannot be more than 50% removal of the facet joints.

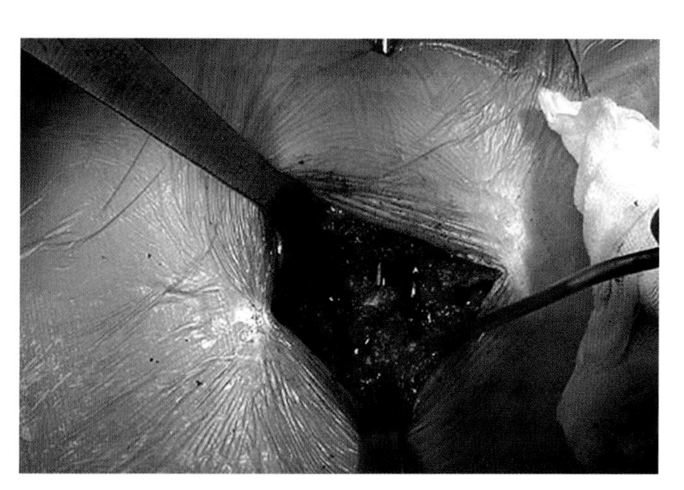

FIGURE 25–7 The drill is shown penetrating the base of the spinous process and across the lamina.

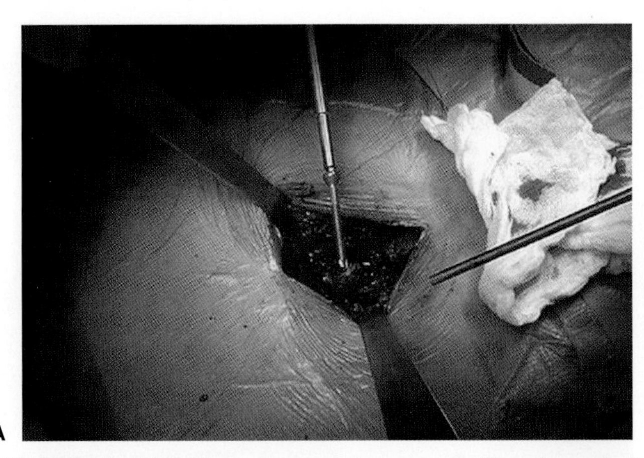

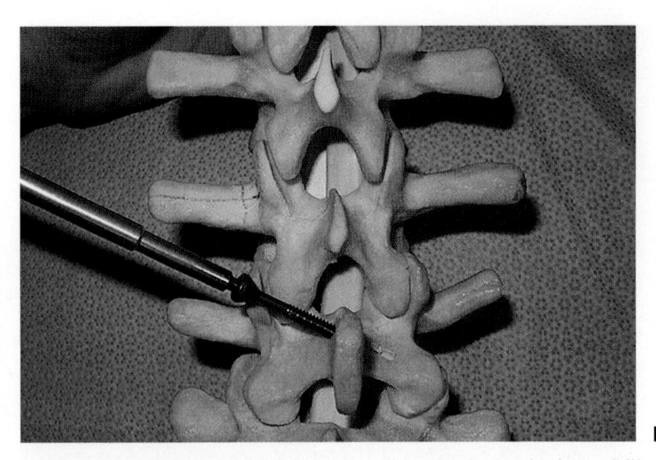

FIGURE 25–8 (A) The screw can be placed either through the percutaneous lateral incisions or directly through the midline incision. **(B)** Sawbones model view of implantation of the screw from left to right.

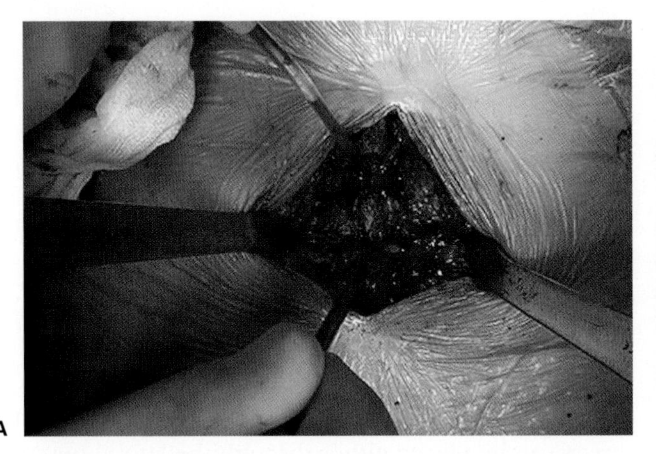

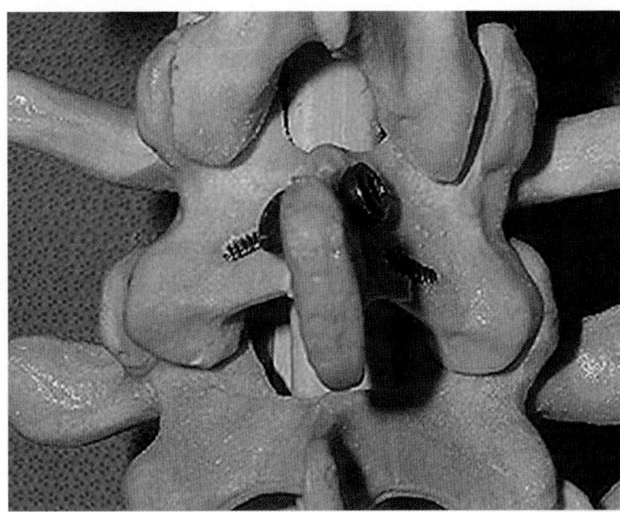

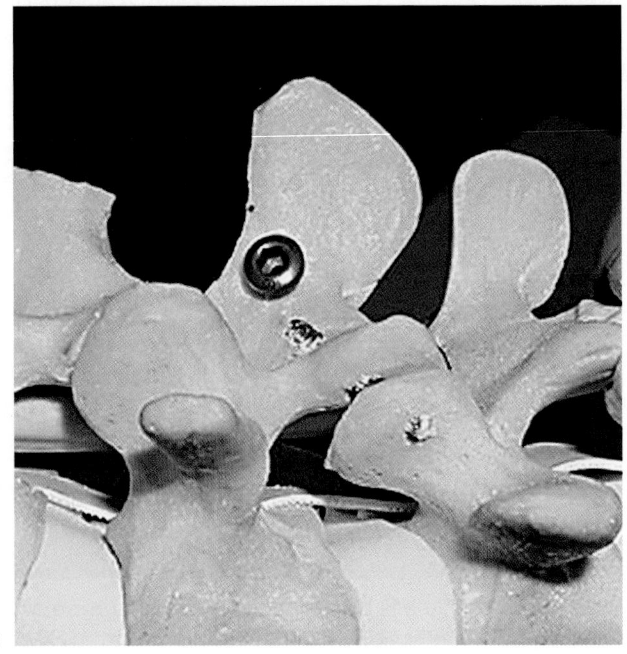

FIGURE 25–9 (A) Perioperative anteroposterior view of a completed one-level construct. **(B)** Sawbones model anteroposterior view of a completed one-level construct. **(C)** Sawbones model lateral view of a completed one-level construct.

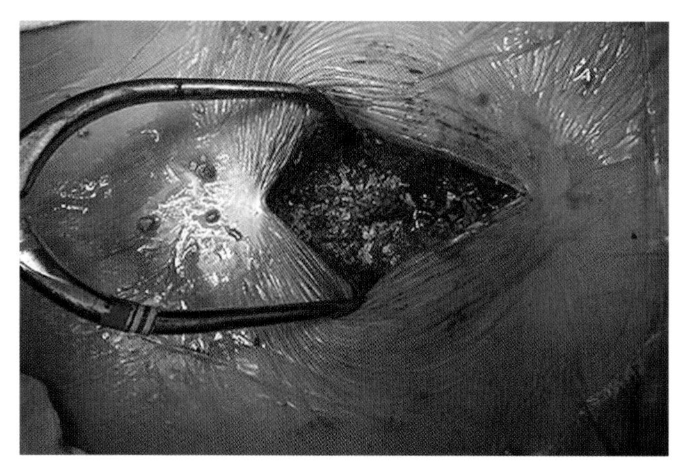

FIGURE 25–10 Bone graft (here, local bone mixed with coralline hydroxyapatite) is placed in the midline for a midline posterior fusion. This patient had an ALIF procedure previously.

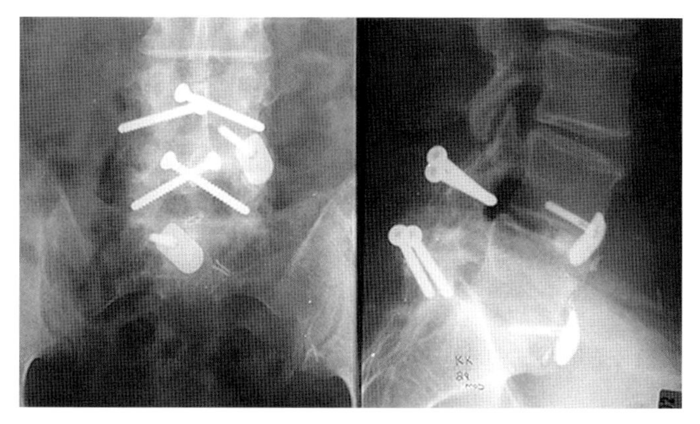

FIGURE 25–12 Anteroposterior **(A)** and lateral **(B)** radiographs of a 50-year-old male patient at 29 months postop with notable fusion. The patient presented with internal disk disruption and degenerative disk disease at L4–L5 and L5–S1. Femoral rings were implanted anteriorly via a gasless endoscopic approach. The patient had a 70% reduction in pain and returned to work at 5 months following surgery.

not in the lateral gutters, which are not exposed with this approach.

Postoperative Care

Patients who undergo either circumferential minimally invasive instrumented fusion or only minimally invasive translaminar fixation are discharged from the hospital 1 to 3 days postoperatively. The posterior incision heals completely in 6 weeks (Fig. 25–11). Patients are placed in a Neoprene lumbar corset for at least 4 weeks postop. They begin aquatic physical therapy at 10 to 14 days postop and advance to weight training, treadmill, and range-of-motion therapy as tolerated. Return to work depends largely on the patient's motivation and occupational circumstances (Fig. 25–12).

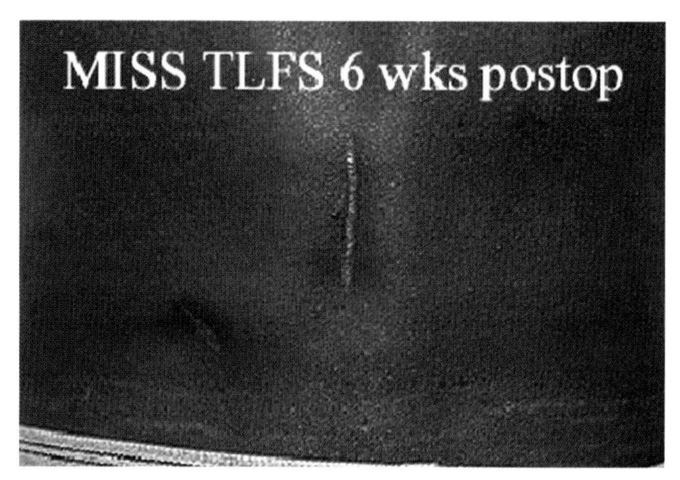

FIGURE 25–11 Healed incisions at 6 weeks following surgery. The smaller incision in the lower left quadrant is from the minimally invasive bone graft harvest of the posterior iliac crest.

Complications and Avoidance

Nerve Root Irritation Caused by the Screw

Care must be taken to place the screws subforaminally to avoid irritation of the nerve root. If a patient develops a radiculopathy postoperatively, a CT scan should be obtained to discern the presence or absence of nerve root impingement. If nerve root impingement or irritation is evident, percutaneous removal of the screw is advised. Immediate postoperative CT scans are helpful in assessing any nerve root irritation issues if the patient awakens in the recovery room with burning radiculopathy.

Inadequate Decompression

The laminoplasty-type decompression may be difficult to accomplish in some patients. If the decompression cannot be performed in this manner, a standard laminectomy or laminotomy should be performed with transpedicular fixation. These cases are rare.

Malposition of the Screw

Perioperative imaging should be used to verify alignment and placement of the screws. If the placement of a screw is suboptimal, the screw should be removed and reimplanted in the proper position.

Translaminar facet screw fixation using a minimally invasive approach can be done in place of transpedicular fixation for an instrumented circumferential lumbar fusion at one or two levels. TLFSs are inherently less invasive than transpedicular screws, and they are less expensive per level compared with pedicle screw systems. Other indications for use of TLFS include stabilization following laminoplasty-type decompression at one or two levels and as adjunctive fixation at the middle levels of a transpedicular fixation construct for the treatment of fracture.

REFERENCES

1. Montesano PX, Magerl F, Jacobs RR, Jackson RP, Rauschning W. Translaminar facet joint screws. *Orthopedics*. 1988;11:1393– 1397.
2. Rathonyi GC, Oxland TR, Gerich U, Grassmann S, Nolte LP. The role of supplemental translaminar screws in anterior lumbar interbody fixation: a biomechanical study. *Eur Spine J*. 1998;7:400–407.
3. Deguchi M, Cheng BC, Sato K, Matsuyama Y, Zdeblick TA. Biomechanical evaluation of translaminar facet joint fixation: a comparative study of poly-L-lactide pins, screws, and pedicle fixation. *Spine*. 1998;23:1307–1313.
4. Thalgott JS, Chin AK, Ameriks JA, et al. Minimally invasive 360 degree instrumented lumbar fusion. *Eur Spine J*. 2000;9(suppl 1): S51–S56.
5. Kumar N, Wild A, Webb JK, Aebi M. Hybrid computer-guided and minimally open surgery: anterior lumbar interbody fusion and translaminar screw fixation. *Eur Spine J*. 2000;9(suppl 1):S71–S77.
6. Grob D, Humke T. Translaminar screw fixation in the lumbar spine: technique, indications, results. *Eur Spine J*. 1998;7:178–186.
7. Liljenqvist U, O'Brien JP, Renton P. Simultaneous combined anterior and posterior lumbar fusion with femoral cortical allograft. *Eur Spine J*. 1998;7:125–131.
8. Humke T, Grob D, Dvorak J, Messikommer A. Translaminar screw fixation of the lumbar and lumbosacral spine: a 5-year follow-up. *Spine*. 1998;23:1180–1184.
9. Reich SM, Kuflik P, Neuwirth M. Translaminar facet screw fixation in lumbar spine fusion. *Spine*. 1993;18:444–449.
10. Grob D, Rubeli M, Scheier HJ, Dvorak J. Translaminar screw fixation of the lumbar spine. *Int Orthop*. 1992;16:223–226.
11. Heggeness MH, Esses SI. Translaminar facet joint screw fixation for lumbar and lumbosacral fusion: a clinical and biomechanical study. *Spine*. 1991;16(suppl):S266–S269.
12. Jacobs RR, Montesano PX, Jackson RP. Enhancement of lumbar spine fusion by use of translaminar facet joint screws. *Spine*. 1989; 14:12–15.

26

Laparoscopic Fusion of the Lumbosacral Spine

STEPHEN E. HEIM, ANTHONY ALTIMARI, AND JOHN L. ANDRESHAK

The evolution of threaded interbody fusion cages has presented a significant new form of segmental fixation (interbody fixation devices) for application to the lumbar and lumbosacral spine. These devices serve as carriers for such fusion material as autogenous cancellous bone or, more recently, bone morphogenetic protein, while restoring segmental stability to the involved motion segment.

The biomechanics of these devices greatly surpass those of the interbody spacers commonly used (i.e., femoral ring composite grafts, tricortical wedges, and various impacted "containment devices" for cancellous bone), which have not offered significant stability in flexion/extension or torsion. In fact, several biomechanical studies have shown this recent class of construct to compare quite favorably with the segmental pedicular fixation/posterior lumbar interbody fusion (PLIF) constructs.[1]

Interbody spacers have traditionally been utilized as a component of an overall construct employing segmental posterior instrumentation. In contrast, when applied effectively, the threaded interbody cages are able to confer a degree of stability to the symptomatic motion segment so as to function as stand-alone constructs. The biomechanics of the interbody cage constructs are generally based on significant preoperative disk space narrowing. The act of reconstituting the anterior column height restores the annular tension, which is a key factor in the proper construct mechanics (Fig. 26–1). It is in such an application that the favorable comparison to pedicular fixation/PLIF constructs can be obtained.

Inappropriate size and/or placement of the threaded interbody devices may ineffectively create tension in the anulus fibrosus, resulting in a biomechanically compromised stand-alone construct. In these instances, the lack of annular tension results in the cage system functioning as an interbody spacer rather than as an interbody fixation device; supplemental stabilization techniques may be required. This failure to obtain adequate distraction of the anulus fibrosus has been among the most common reasons for failure of the procedure. With regard to the degree of disk space narrowing, the authors generally consider patients with 50% or more disk space narrowing to be appropriate candidates for a stand-alone interbody construct. In addition, radiographic findings of significant end-plate sclerosis and significant traction spurs correlate well with the ability to tension the anulus fibrosis intraoperatively. Increasing the tension of the anulus fibrosus in the interbody construct was found to be associated with higher biomechanical strength in biomechanical studies.

Laparoscopic Application of Threaded Interbody Fusion Devices

The laparoscopic application of interbody cage devices is simply a variance in the surgical approach to the spine. It is of paramount importance that the surgeon remains cognizant of the biomechanics of stand-alone interbody constructs regardless of the surgical approach selected for their placement. With adherence to these concepts, the authors have found laparoscopic techniques to offer

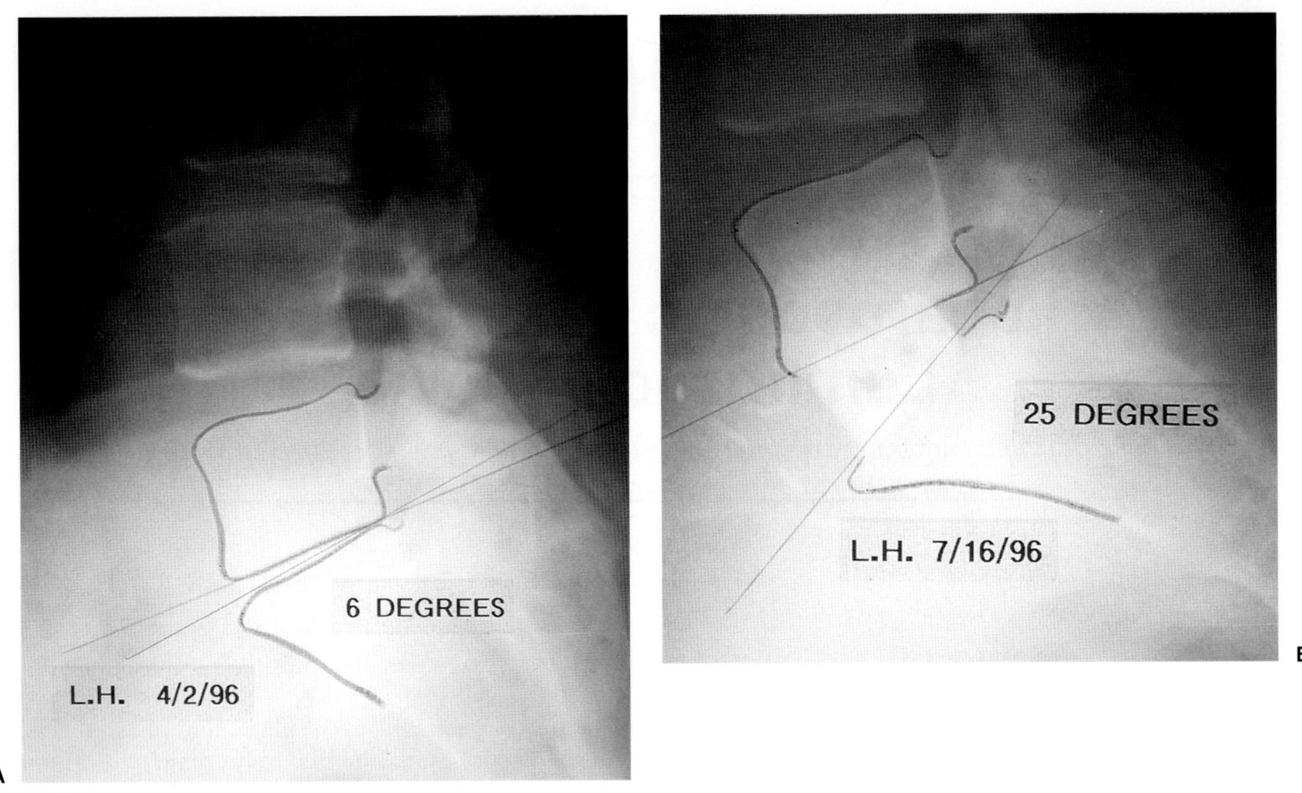

FIGURE 26–1 (A) Plain radiograph showing markedly narrowed preoperative disk space at the L5–S1 disk space. **(B)** Postoperative radiograph showing restoration of anterior column height and annular tension by interbody fixation device.

a significant reduction in the operative morbidity associated with the anterior approach.

Initial Clinical Results of Laparoscopic Interbody Fusion

The authors have had the opportunity to participate at one of the initial clinical centers for the development of the laparoscopic application of the BAK, threaded femoral cortical bone dowel, and tapered LT Interbody Cage systems (Medtronic-Sofamor Danek, Memphis, TN) since early 1994. The first cases of the laparoscopic technique of interbody cage placement utilized the BAK cage.[2] This initial experience demonstrated an important pattern of learning curves associated with this procedure: operative time, length of hospitalization, and complications. In comparing the open and laparoscopic insertion techniques of the BAK cage during the initial learning curve phase of the procedure, the authors were able to demonstrate a significant decrease in operative morbidity by the reduction in the length of hospitalization.

With further experience following this initial clinical trial, we were able to further decrease the length of hospitalization to an average of 23 hours for each of these cage systems, as well as the cylindrical Interfix cage. The open application of interbody cages has produced an average 3-day hospitalization over the same time period.

More recently, the authors participated at one of the initial pilot trial centers studying the use of recombinant bone morphogenic protein (rhBMP-2; InFuse, Medtronic-Sofamor Danek) with the LT Interbody Cage system (Medtronic-Sofamor Danek). We utilized the laparoscopic application technique for cage/BMP placement while the additional study sites employed a retroperitoneal open approach. The laparoscopic technique provided a remarkable 12-hour average hospitalization compared with the 3-day hospitalization for patients who underwent the open retroperitoneal technique.

On the one hand, the further reduction in the length of hospitalization (vs. 23 hours) realized with the use of rhBMP-2 (InFuse) is believed to represent the procedural morbidity of the iliac bone graft harvesting in the earlier clinical trials. On the other hand, the consistent 3-day hospitalization of the retroperitoneal open procedure with either rhBMP-2 (InFuse) or iliac crest bone graft represents the morbidity of the open exposure technique itself. With the possibility of a true same-day discharge, the approach to patient education must address this. Furthermore, the nursing unit staff will need to be educated on both this possibility as well as on the

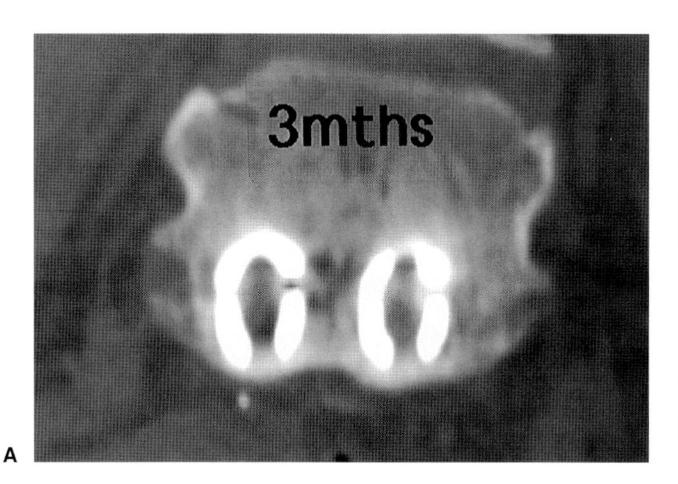

A

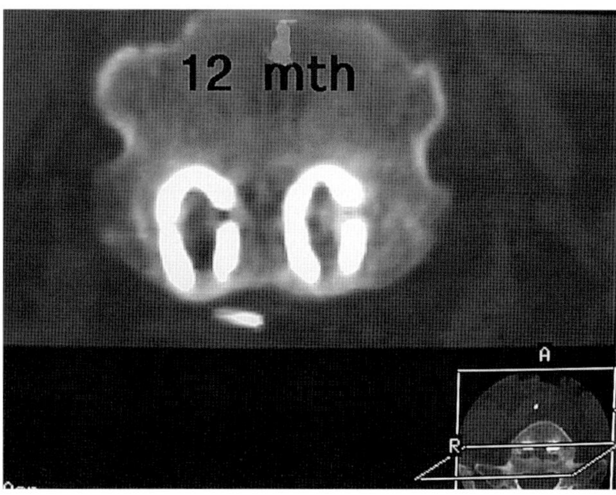

B

FIGURE 26–2 Postoperative CT of the LS–S1 interspace of the fusion using the LT Interbody cage system and rhBMP-2 (InFuse). **(A)** 3 months. **(B)** 12 months.

generally much more rapid mobilization of these patients compared with those who undergo an open anterior approach, or certainly the more common posterior instrumented spinal fusion procedures.

The radiographic appearance of the pattern of fusion in laparoscopic patients is of even greater experience. Whereas the open patient group underwent complete diskectomies, laparoscopic patients underwent "channel diskectomies"; that is, only the disk material specifically was removed. In all of these patients (i.e., open or laparoscopic) no bone graft material was used. Figure 26–2 demonstrates the postoperative CT images of a patient who underwent an L5–S1 laparoscopic anterior interbody fusion with rhBMP-2 (InFuse) and the LT Interbody Cage system. Ossification within the confines of the disk space is clearly visible, as are the areas where the intervertebral disk had not been excised. This is felt to represent a biological induction of the remaining nucleus pulposus to ossify.

Indications

The current indications for the use of threaded interbody cages, either metallic or allograft, include:

- One- or two-level degenerative disk disease at L2–S1 (particularly disk resorption)
- Discogenic pain/painful annular tear
- Revision of failed posterior fusions
- Grade I spondylolisthesis
- Segmental instability

As has been previously mentioned, the "stand-alone" use of the threaded interbody cages requires a significant preoperative narrowing of the symptomatic motion segment (Fig. 26–1). If the application is to a wide disk space, the use of supplementary posterior segmental instrumentation is appropriate.

In cases of spondylolytic spondylolisthesis, the lack of integrity of the pars intra-articularis seems to be associated with a greater laxity in the anulus fibrosus—this laxity, in fact, is one of the primary sources of the actual translatory deformity present. This fatigue, or laxity, of the anulus fibrosus can lead to a less definitive end point in disk space distraction with possible implications for fixation. This has led the authors to treat spondylolytic spondylolisthesis with an interbody cage device (as a stand-alone construct) only when there is marked disk space narrowing. The radiographic findings of end plate sclerosis and significant traction spur formation correlate clinically with the reasonable expectation of being able to place tension the anulus fibrosus and thereby produce a stable standalone construct. If distraction does not seem to produce an appropriate annular tension, however, the surgeon must recognize this and consider supplementary posterior fixation.

Last, in the instance of L5–S1 spondylolisthesis, the surgeon must ensure that the angle of the disk space does not pass into or below the pubic symphysis on the lateral radiograph. The anterior application of interbody cage devices requires a colinear approach to the disk space. Such an angulation would therefore prohibit appropriate cage placement.

Contraindications

Commensurate with the importance of significant preoperative narrowing of the involved disk space, a symptomatic motion segment with a well-preserved disk space would be contraindicated for a stand-alone interbody construct. The general contraindications include:

- A well-preserved disk height leading to difficulty in fitting a large enough implant within the width of the disk space
- Lack of annular tensioning producing the biomechanics of an interbody spacer rather than an interbody fixation device
- A previously attempted interbody fusion
- Grade II or higher spondylolisthesis
- Significant intra-abdominal/retroperitoneal scarring from previous surgeries, radiation therapy, or infection

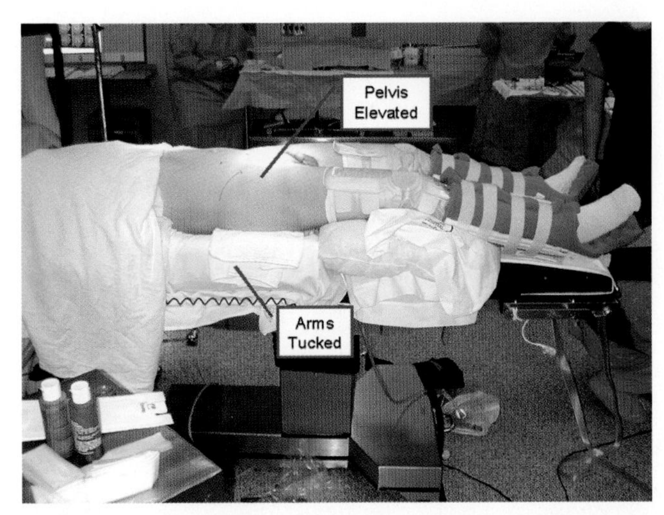

FIGURE 26–3 Patient positioning. Bucks traction boots help keep the patient from sliding up while in Trendelenburg's position.

Surgical Technique

The surgical team is composed of:

- Laparoscopic general surgeon
- Spine surgeon
- Anesthesiologist
- Camera operator (generally an OR nurse or technician)
- Scrub nurse/OR technician (familiar with both the spine and laparoscopic aspects of the procedure)
- Circulating nurse
- Radiology technician

It is imperative that the general/access surgeon and the spine surgeon truly view themselves as a team. The access surgeon will need to realize the magnitude of exposure required for the spinal portion of the procedure, particularly the degree to which the great vessels will need to be mobilized. It is especially important that the spine surgeon/access surgeon team first experience the procedure together in a series of open interbody cage fusions prior to progressing to the laparoscopic approach.

Preprocedural preparation is of primary importance in ensuring a neutral orientation of the spine and in avoiding difficulties in obtaining intraoperative fluoroscopic images. These are each key factors in the determination of cage placement within the disk space. Whether performed via an open or a laparoscopic approach, this is truly a "procedure of millimeters."

The patient is positioned supine on a radiolucent operating table. The authors prefer to elevate the patient's pelvis and lumbar spine from the surface of the operating table with folded surgical blankets. This then permits the arms to be positioned along the patient's side (tucked and padded) without obscuring the lateral fluoroscopic visualization of the symptomatic motion segment (Fig. 26–3). The spine should not be placed into a position of lordosis by way of bolsters or other positioning influences.

The ability to maneuver the C-arm into position and to visualize the pathologic motion segment clearly must also be assessed—the table upright will determine how high on the table the patient must be placed. Double-check the fluoroscopy with the requisite Trendelenburg positioning to be used during the procedure. In addition to visualizing the motion segment on the lateral image, the anteroposterior/Ferguson view must show a neutral motion segment rotation prior to proceeding.

The bladder is decompressed with a Foley catheter and the stomach with an orogastric tube, with both removed at the completion of the procedure. All routine positioning checks (i.e., padding of neurovascular structures/bony prominences) are also rechecked. It must be recalled that the laparoscopic procedure requires up to 30 degrees of Trendelenburg position throughout its duration, as opposed to the open anterior application of the interbody cages.

General Laparoscopic Technique

Exposure

For L4–L5 and L5–S1, the standard portal placement includes a periumbilical laparoscopic portal, 5 mm right and left of the lower abdominal quadrant dissection/retraction portals, and a suprapubic spinal working portal (Fig. 26–4A). The initial portals placed include the camera and right/left lower quadrant sites. Using these portals, the dissection is performed, and the symptomatic motion segment is exposed. The suprapubic spinal working portal is created only after the involved disk space is verified. This portal must present a colinear approach to the disk space, the line

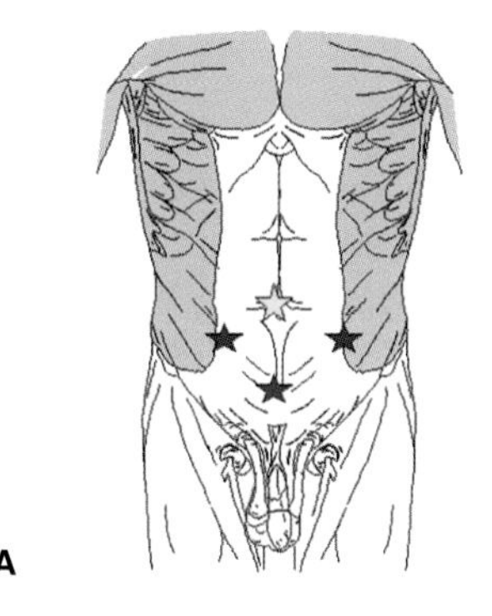

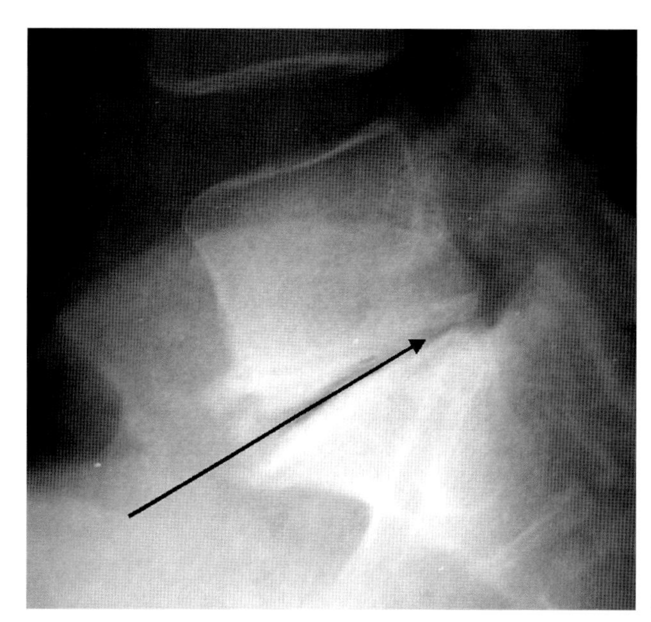

FIGURE 26–4 (A) Laparoscopic portal placement. **(B)** Determining the placement of the suprapubic spinal working portal. The authors place a percutaneous long spinal needle and fluoroscopically verify the optimal spinal working portal location.

of approach, which will represent the orientation of the interbody cage within the disk space. In other words, if a nonlinear approach from the spinal working portal to the disk space exists, then this is the same orientation the implanted cage will take with the motion segment (Fig. 26–4B).

In the course of dissection, it is important to avoid the use of monopolar cautery upon opening the posterior peritoneum. This minimizes the risk of retrograde ejaculation. It also avoids extraneous marks on the anterior anulus fibrosus. The midline of the motion segment is determined with fluoroscopy, again ensuring the neutral rotation of the spine as well. The accurate placement of the interbody cages is very much dependent upon this landmark—again, this is truly an "operation of millimeters," whether performed open or laparoscopically.

Cage Insertion

Depending on the specific cage system being used, the sequence of cage placement may vary; however, there are several points that are generally not system dependent:

- At each step, verify the midline, right, and left diskal entry sites. This will help ensure that the cage is being placed in the desired right or left diskal entry site (not inadvertently in the midline).
- Clear the diskal entry site of any debris following each step with pituitary rongeurs. Fluoroscopy will assist in demonstrating that the depth of rongeur insertion is appropriate to reach the desired depth of the disk space truly without risking dural/neural injury.
- Save the final reaming/tapping images on the fluoroscopy monitor to serve as a reference during cage insertion to minimize the risk of stripping the cage.
- Monitor the medial edge of the spinal working cannula. This medial edge should generally approximate the midline disk mark. If a gap exists, the cannula has worked itself laterally. If the midline mark is covered by the cannula, the cages may impinge on one another.
- Carefully verify appropriate end-plate preparation and engagement fluoroscopically; avoid placing undersized cages.
- If concern exists on the orientation/placement of the cage, obtain additional fluoroscopic images without hesitation.
- Utilize good-quality autogenous iliac crest bone graft material, or bone morphogenetic protein.
- Proceed with each step only after verifying that the laparoscopic access surgeon is satisfied with the exposure and retraction.
- If suboptimal motion segment stability is realized intraoperatively, strongly consider supplementary segmental posterior instrumentation.

Technique for Laparoscopic Placement of LT Interbody Cages

- Do careful preoperative templating on the adjacent normal-height disk using standard anteroposterior, lateral, and Ferguson spinal radiographs.

- Template axial CT or MRI scans to assess the fit of LT cages within the motion segment end plates.
- Use the lateral radiograph to determine the depth-stop setting for the end-plate reamers.
• Induce general anesthesia with the patient on the transportation gurney.
- Place orogastric tube and Foley catheters.
- Apply the TED hose.
• Transfer patient to the prepared bed.
- Fold surgical blankets to the width of the patient's pelvis to allow the arms to be padded and tucked at the sides (Fig. 26–3).
- Apply Bucks boots to prevent cranial migration of the patient while in the Trendelenburg position.
- Ensure that all monitoring lines and IVs are out of the lateral fluoroscopic image view.
- Do not extend the spine with bolsters or other padding.
• Laparoscopic exposure:
- The autonomic plexus rests in the retroperitoneal fat layer. Open the posterior retroperitoneum with laparoscopic scissors rather than with cautery.
- Incise the posterior peritoneum to the right of the midline.
- Ligate and divide middle sacral vessels for both L4–L5 and L5–S1 procedures.
- Ligate and divide the iliolumbar vessel for L4–L5 procedures.
- Expose the entire width of the disk space (Fig. 26–5).
• Harvest the iliac cancellous bone graft if rhBMP-2 (InFuse) is not utilized.
• Mark the midline of the disk space using anteroposterior fluoroscopy.
- Check the skin midline before making the spinal working portal.

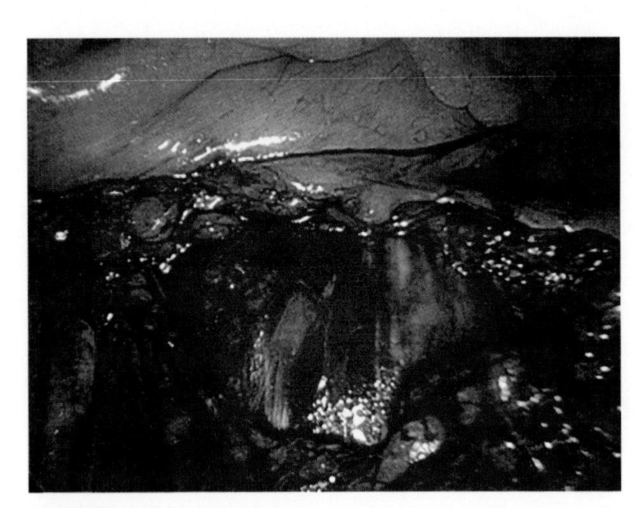

FIGURE 26–5 Operative photograph showing the complete exposure of the L5–S1 disk.

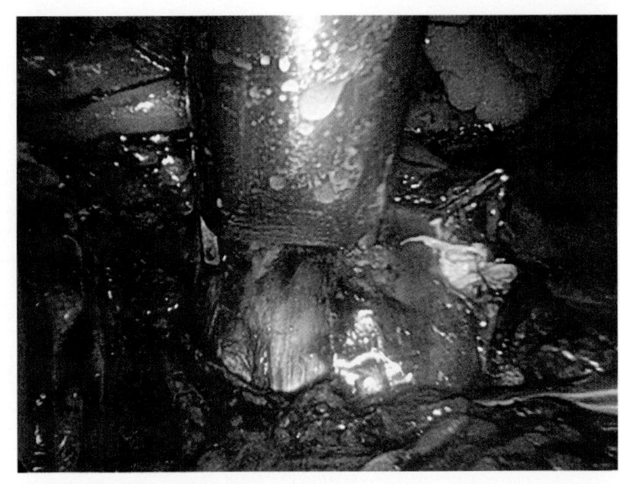

FIGURE 26–6 Operative photograph showing starting guide being positioned to open the left L5–S1 discal entry site.

- Keep the midline mark in view throughout the procedure.
- The medial edge of the spinal working cannula should approximate this midline mark throughout the procedure.
• Open the right and left diskal entry sites.
- Use the starting guide appropriate for the templated implant size (Fig. 26–6).
- Use the largest trephine that will fit in the disk space.
• Clear the diskal entry sites using the pituitary rongeurs.
- Perform this debridement with each step.
- Utilize fluoroscopy to ensure the rongeur reaches the depth of the disk space.
• Distract the disk space, beginning on the right diskal entry site.
- Use the distractor size appropriate for the templated cage size.
- Assess and confirm that this has resulted in firm annular tensioning. If not, determine if a larger implant should be used.
• Seat the spinal working cannula over the distraction plug, and remove the distractor.
• Ream the adjacent end plates at the right diskal entry site (parallel reaming of end plates).
• Move to the left diskal entry site.
- Repeat the sequence of disk space distraction and end-plate reaming on the left.
- Save the lateral fluoroscopic image of the final reaming depth.
- Debride the left diskal entry site with pituitary rongeurs.
• Prepare the implant.
- The implant holder secures the cage.

- Pack cancellous bone firmly within the cage (if used).
- If Infuse (rhBMP-2) is used, do not use suction over the implants from this point on.
- Place the left implant.
- Monitor the saved image of reaming depth to avoid stripping the implant.
- Slightly recess the cage from the anterior vertebral margin, but maintain contact with the ring apophysis.
- Orient the implant to the vertebral end plates.
- Do not suction over the InFuse sponges.
- Switch back to the 18 mm Ethicon laparoscopic cannula.
- Center the spinal working cannula over the prepared right diskal entry site.
- The end plates were previously reamed in a parallel manner.
- Seat the spinal working cannula again.
- Debride the disk space once again (debris can be pushed into the void of the right discal entry site with the process of preparing/placing the left cage).
- Place the right implant.
- Seat the right implant to an equal depth as the left.
- Orient the implant to the end plates.
- Do not suction over the InFuse sponges
- Use the Adjuster instrument to fine-tune cage rotation.
- Obtain final anteroposterior and lateral fluoroscopic images.
- Close the posterior peritoneum (this helps avoid the risk of adhesions to the surgical site).
- Surgeon's preference as to the use of laparoscopic staples
- Close 10 mm or larger fascial openings.
- Skin closure and dressings
- Remove the orogastric tube and Foley catheter.
- Mobilization on the nursing unit:
- Educate the floor nurses on early mobilization as opposed to the typical open fusion patient.
- Oral postoperative analgesics are typically sufficient.
- Discharge when ambulatory, voiding, and tolerating oral intake (thorough preoperative patient and family education is key).
- Schedule of postoperative visits:
- Plane anteroposterior, lateral, and Ferguson radiographs at each visit
- Flexion/extension radiographs at each visit except the initial 2-week visit
- CT scan (1.25 mm sections with sagittal and coronal reconstructions) at 3 months
- Postoperative bracing at the surgeon's discretion
- Rehabilitation:
- Encourage early ambulation.
- Physical therapy beginning at 6 weeks for InFuse patients (12 weeks if autologous iliac bone graft is used)

Complications

As stated earlier, the initial laparoscopic BAK series revealed a significant learning curve with regard to complications. It appears that the most significant and highest frequency of complications occur in the first 10 to 15 cases in a surgeon's experience. The importance of the laparoscopic access surgeon and the spine surgeon working as a team on several open interbody cage procedures prior to evolving to the laparoscopic technique cannot be overemphasized.

The complications in the original 118 laparoscopic BAK cases among the five clinical trial sites are shown in Table 26–1. Recall that these complications occurred as each of the study sites were indeed passing through their "learning curve" phase. Also, the initial clinical sites involved in this first laparoscopic clinical series were truly the first to perform the procedure. For that reason, the technique was evolving while the surgical teams progressed through their learning curve. It is for these reasons that the authors feel these may represent a worst-case scenario. With the availability of hands-on surgical technique courses and the opportunity to visit surgical teams well established in the procedure, it is reasonably expected that the current learning curve should be safer.

In terms of fusion, each of the cage series utilizing iliac crest bone graft resulted in a 5 to 10% pseudarthrosis rate. No pseudarthroses occurred in the InFuse (rhBMP-2) patients.

Case Illustrations

A 62-year-old female underwent an L5–S1 laparoscopic interbody fusion with the LT interbody cage and InFuse (rhBMP-2). The preoperative diagnosis was a grade I L5–S1 spondylolytic spondylolisthesis and functionally limiting mechanical low back pain. Preoperative provocative diskography had confirmed the pain origin and also shown L4–L5 to be asymptomatic (Fig. 26–7).

The laparoscopic interbody fusion was performed uneventfully, and the patient was discharged to home that afternoon, independent in ambulation and requiring

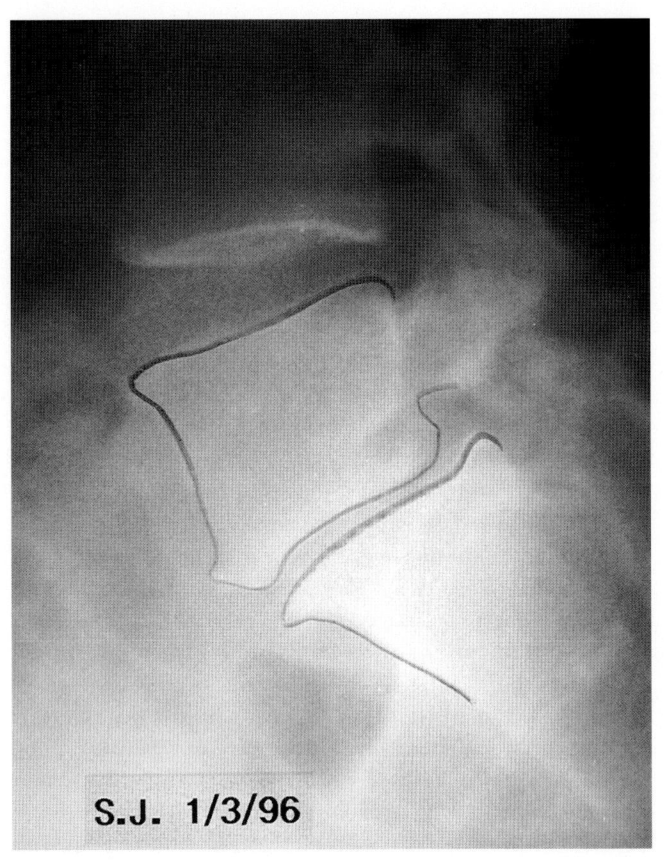

FIGURE 26–7 Preoperative lateral radiograph showing narrowing of the L5–S1 disk space.

only limited oral analgesics. The preoperative mechanical low-back pain was relieved immediately, and her incisional discomfort resolved over the ensuing 2 weeks as expected. At 3 months a CT scan to assess fusion was performed (Fig. 26–8) and revealed a well-developed interbody fusion mass.

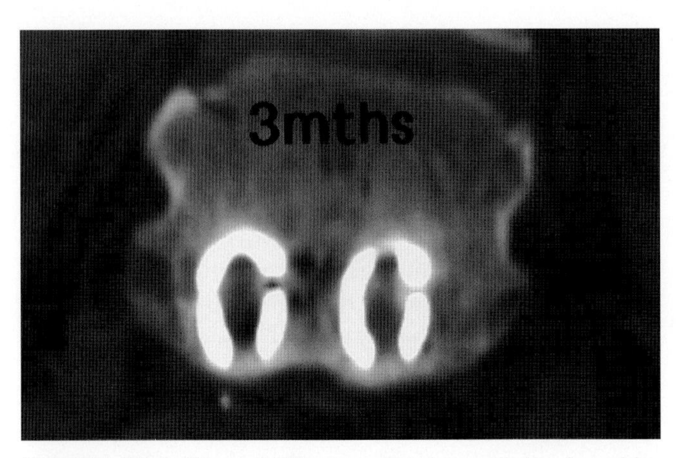

FIGURE 26–8 Coronal CT scan showing well-developed interbody fusion mass at 3 months following surgery.

The formation of bone throughout the anatomical confines of the interspace was of particular interest, despite the fact that the disk space was debrided only where the interbody cages were placed. Furthermore, there was no evidence of heterotopic ossification. Repeat CT scans performed at 1 year revealed the further maturation of the interbody fusion without heterotopic extension (Fig. 26–9).

The patient recovered and rehabilitated very well clinically. She voiced complete resolution of the preoperative mechanical low-back pain and indicated she was functionally unlimited. In the authors' experience, the same-day discharge is typical for patients treated with the laparoscopic approach to the spine and InFuse/LT interbody devices.

The particular advantages of interbody cages include the beneficial effects on bone healing associated with the anterior column location, the stabilization potential in appropriate motion segments, the ability to restore anterior column height and foraminal volume, the correction of segmental lordosis with the LT interbody device, and the avoidance of the fusion disease phenomenon. These advantages are not dependent on whether the approach of insertion is open or laparoscopic. The specific and demonstrated chief benefit of the laparoscopic approach to interbody cage insertion is the reduction in surgical morbidity. This is especially evident when the laparoscopic technique is combined with the use of bone morphogenic protein (rh-BMP2/InFuse). It is our belief that this significant reduction in patient morbidity will drive the further acceptance of the laparoscopic approach in a manner similar to the evolution of arthroscopic orthopedic surgery and laparoscopic general surgery.

The main disadvantage of the laparoscopic approach is the initial learning curve of the surgical team with the technique. In addition, the anterior approach to cage placement (open or laparoscopic) is limited, at this time, with regard to the inability to decompress the spinal canal directly.

It is recommended that interbody cages be considered as only one option in the stabilization of symptomatic motion segments. With care in patient selection, their ability to function in a stand-alone configuration has been successfully demonstrated. To evolve to the laparoscopic placement technique of interbody cages, the access surgeon and spine surgeon should begin as a team with the open approach, placing the particular instrumentation system they plan to use laparoscopically. Together, the access surgeon and spine surgeon should attend a hands-on laparoscopic course for the specific instrumentation system. In terms of initial case selection, they should begin with nondeformity L5–S1 cases and, most importantly, allow for time for the cases.

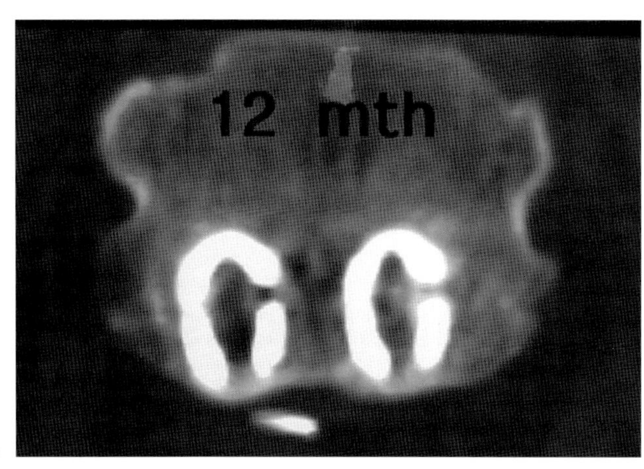

A

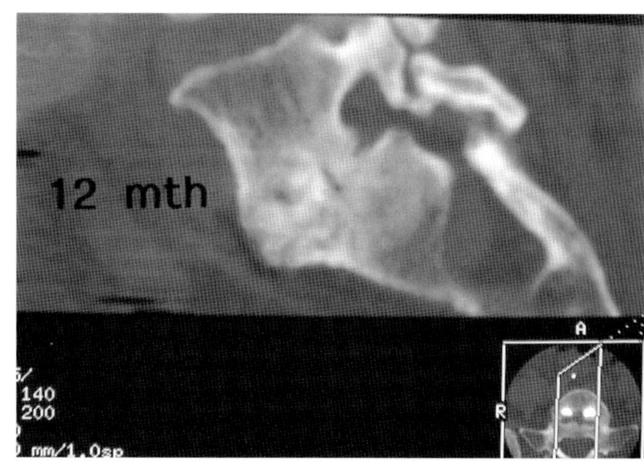

B

FIGURE 26–9 Coronal **(A)** and lateral **(B)** CT reconstruction images showing interbody fusion at 12 months. Note the absence of heterotopic ossification and the essentially complete ossification of the disk space.

REFERENCES

1. Zdeblick TA, Warden KE, Zou D, McAfee PC, Abitbol JJ. Anterior spine fixators: a biomechanical in vitro study. *Spine*. 1993;18:513–517.
2. Zucherman JF, Zdeblick TA, Bailey SA, Mahvi D, Hsu KY, Kohrs D. Instrumented laparoscopic spinal fusion: preliminary results. *Spine*. 1995;20:2029–2034.

27

Endoscopic Lateral Transpsoas Lumbar Spine Fusion

JOHN J. REGAN AND DARREN BERGEY

Anterior approaches for lumbar interbody fusion have been increasingly used in an attempt to lower the incidence of pseudoarthroses and to re-create the patient's normal sagittal alignment.[1–9] The majority of complications associated with anterior lumbar interbody fusion (ALIF) are associated with the surgical exposure. Most of these techniques usually require the presence of an experienced general or vascular surgeon due to the risk of serious complications.[10,11] Although low, the incidence of injury to the great vessels or sympathetic plexus is not negligible, and the consequences of such potential injuries can be debilitating for the patient.[6]

Retroperitoneal lumbar fusion and stabilization offers several advantages over conventional anterior approaches. Retroperitoneal approaches eliminate intra-abdominal adhesions that cause bowel obstruction. The lateral retroperitoneal approach eliminates dissection of the great vessels and the sympathetic plexus, minimizing the complications of bleeding or retrograde ejaculation. This approach also minimizes nerve injury because dissection, drilling, and reaming are directed laterally rather than posteriorly toward the spinal canal.

It was not until 1992, with the introduction of threaded spinal fusion cages, that laparoscopic spine fusion began to evolve. In 1998, McAfee, Regan, and colleagues[5] described a minimally invasive, endoscopic anterior retroperitoneal approach to the lumbar spine with an emphasis on the lateral BAK cage. This technique did not require CO_2 insufflation, Trendelenburg positioning of the patient, entrance into the peritoneum, or anterior dissection near the great vessels. Following entry into the retroperitoneal space from a direct lateral approach, the trajectory of this approach is anterior to the psoas muscle, requiring a considerable amount of retraction of the psoas posteriorly. This causes significant muscular swelling and weakness postoperatively. A transpsoas muscle-splitting approach through its anterior third provides a more direct approach to the lumbar interbody space and is the approach preferred at this time.

Indications

The indications for lateral endoscopic transpsoas lumbar fusion are single- or two-level symptomatic degenerative disk disease, segmental spinal instability, progressive lumbar scoliosis, and pseudarthrosis. This approach may be used for lumbar levels 1 through 4. Low-grade spondylolisthesis, two-level degenerative disk disease, and lumbar scoliosis may be corrected with this approach by surgeons with experience (Figs. 27–1, 27–2, 27–3, 27–4, 27–5).

Patients with discogenic pain should be selected for surgery based on a history of mechanical symptoms and failed conservative therapy. Patients with a strong mechanical back pain history who have conformed to a physical therapy program for 4 months without relief are good candidates for the procedure. Radiographic findings of disk space narrowing, end-plate sclerosis, and osteophyte formation indicate degenerative disk changes. MRI should provide confirmation of degenerative disk disease with evident Modic changes. Diskography is performed in all patients with more than single-level degenerative disk disease.

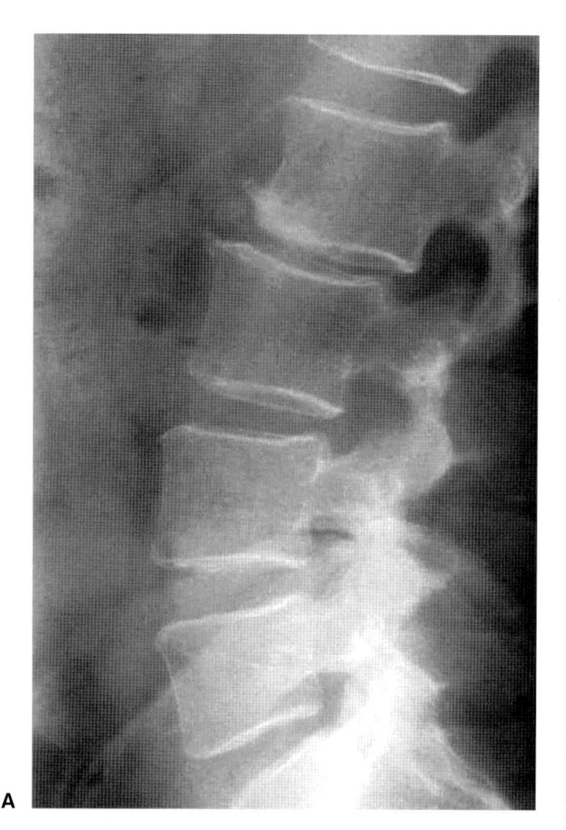

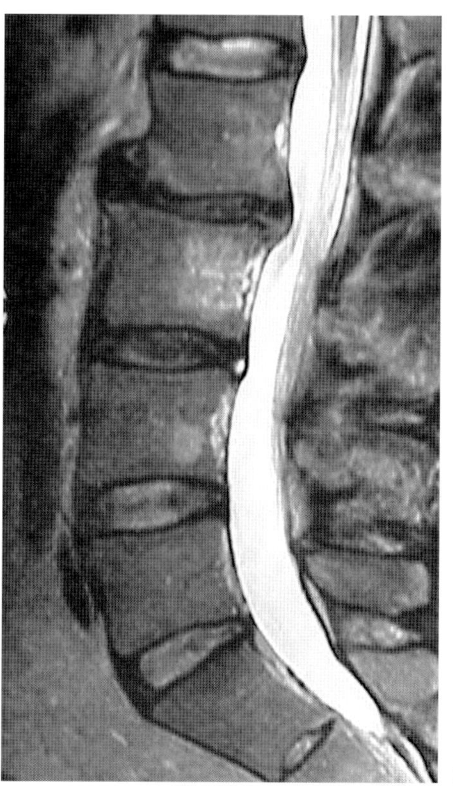

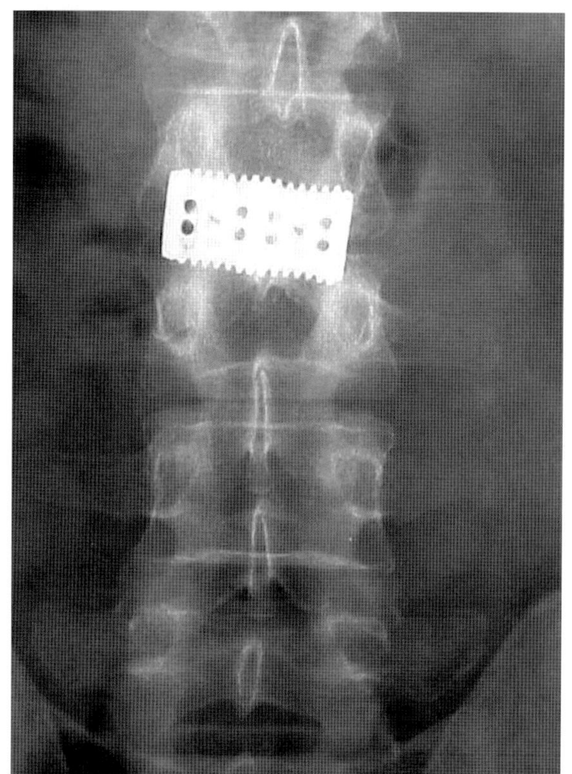

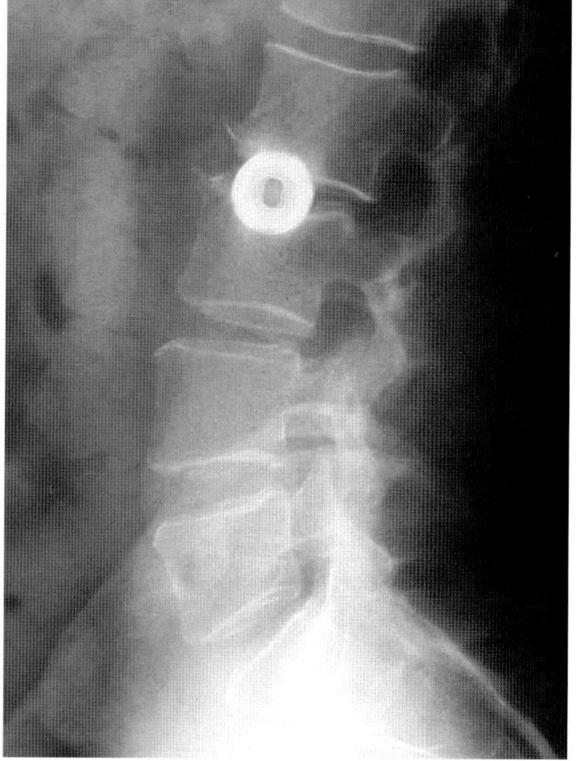

FIGURE 27–1 This 43-year-old patient presented with intractable mechanical back pain radiating into the anterior thigh. Lateral x-ray **(A)** and MRI **(B)** show degenerative changes and retrolisthesis, with no evidence for nerve root impingement. Postoperative x-rays **(C,D)** show lateral BAK. This patient was treated in a brace for 12 weeks and went on to solid fusion.

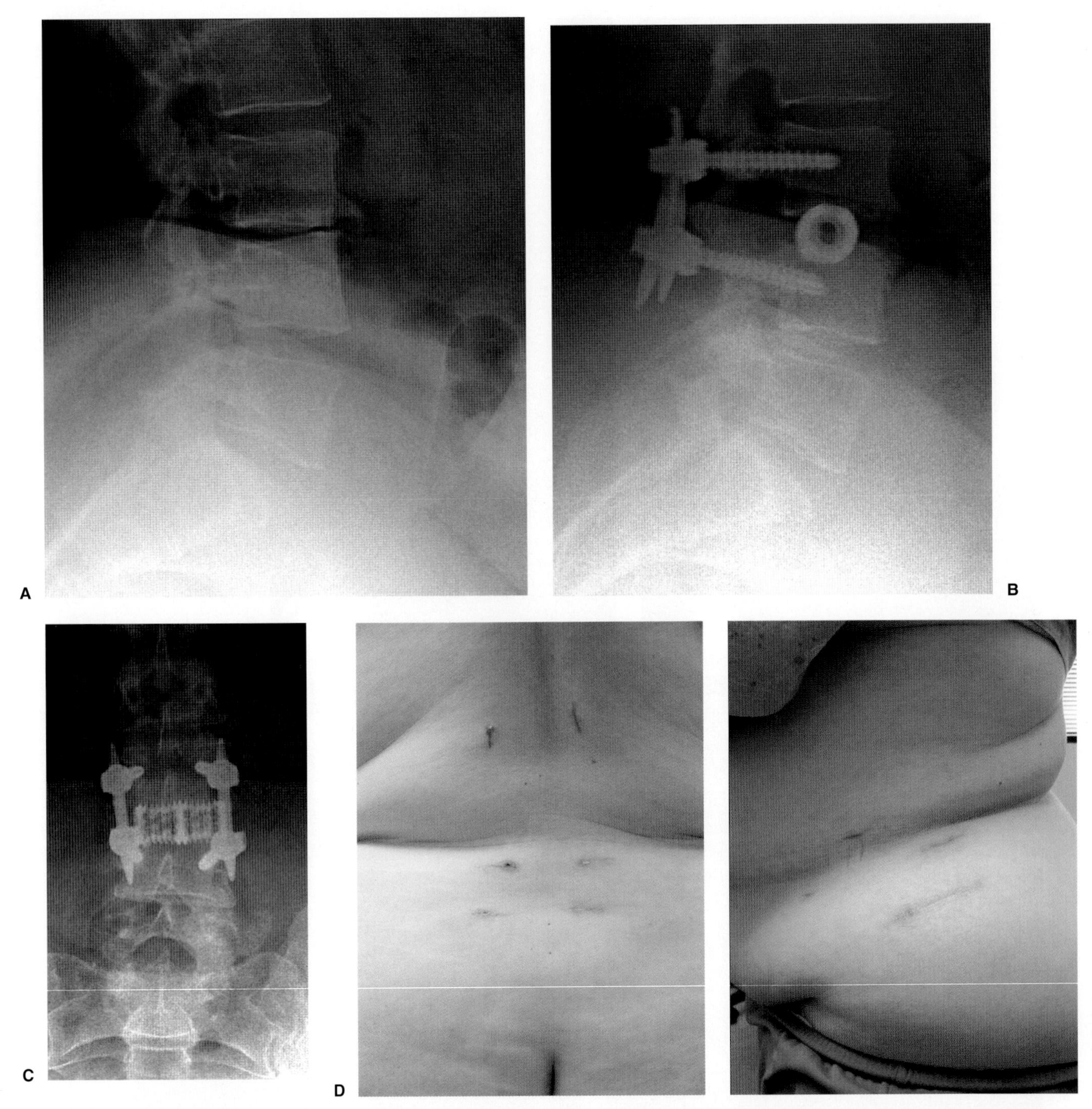

FIGURE 27–2 This 46-year-old patient with mechanical back pain and demonstrated single-level degenerative disk disease **(A)** was treated with lateral endoscopic fusion followed by percutaneous Sextant pedicle fixation (**B,C**). Posterior and lateral skin views **(D,E)** show healed incisions. Bone graft was taken from the lateral iliac crest, as shown by the larger incision on the lateral view.

Contraindications

Patients with extensive peritoneal adhesions from previous surgery or inflammatory or infectious disease affecting the peritoneum should be excluded from the lateral endoscopic approach. Patients who have overlying psychological conditions or positive Waddell's signs or who are habitual narcotics users are not candidates for fusion surgery.

Surgical Technique

Following the induction of general endotracheal anesthesia, the patient is turned in a right lateral decubitus position (left side up) (Fig. 27–6A,B) on a beanbag on a radiolucent table, with the kidney rest elevated. Anteroposterior and lateral intraoperative fluoroscopy is then used to verify the approximate level of the desired

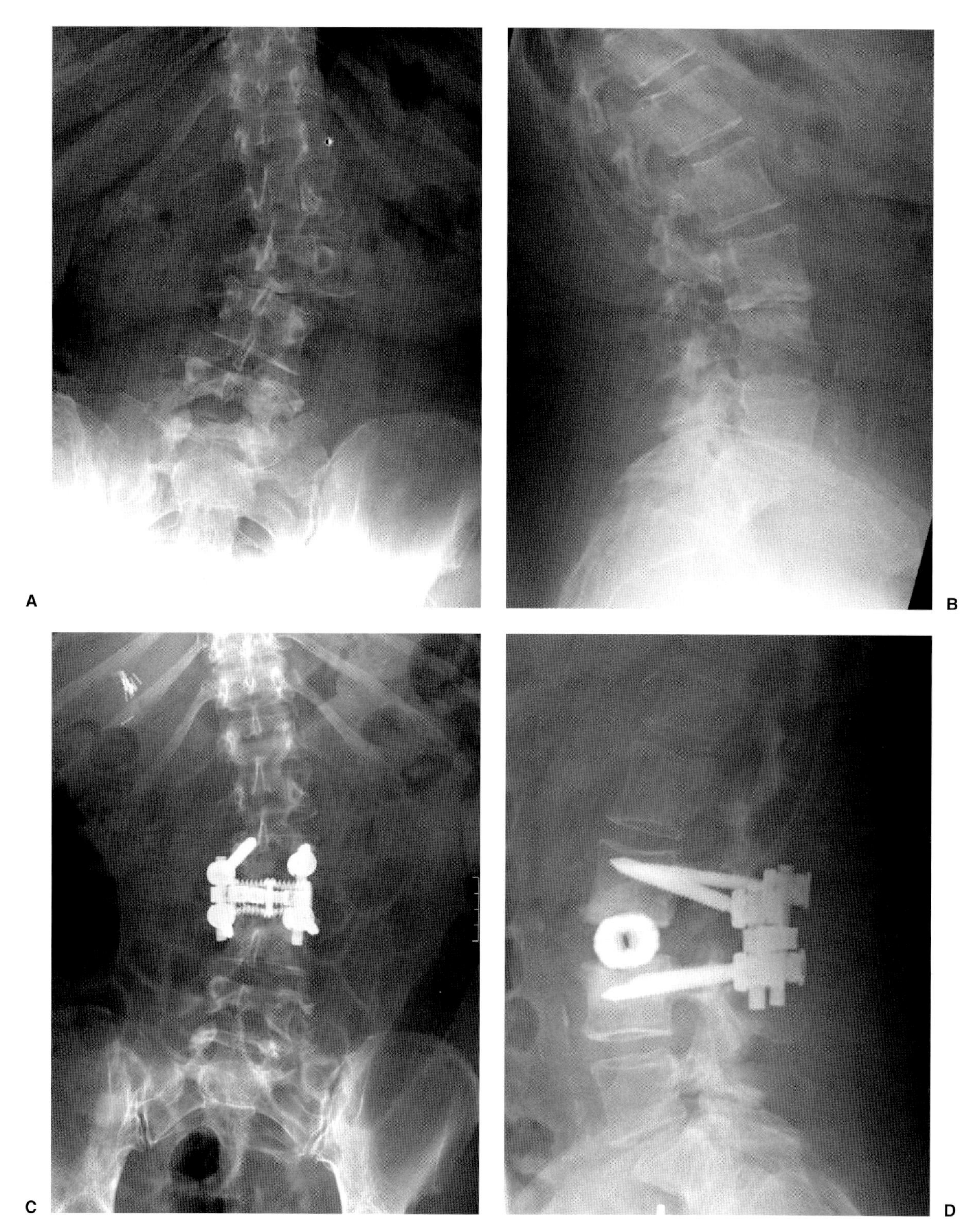

FIGURE 27–3 This 49-year-old patient developed progressive scoliosis during a 5-year period with severe back and anterior thigh pain. Preoperative x-rays **(A,B)** show lateral listhesis at L2–L3 with resulting severe scoliosis. Lateral endoscopic diskectomy and insertion of BAK cage followed by posterior laminectomy for stenosis and internal fixation with pedicle system **(C,D)** resulted in significant correction of scoliosis and resolution of back and leg complaints.

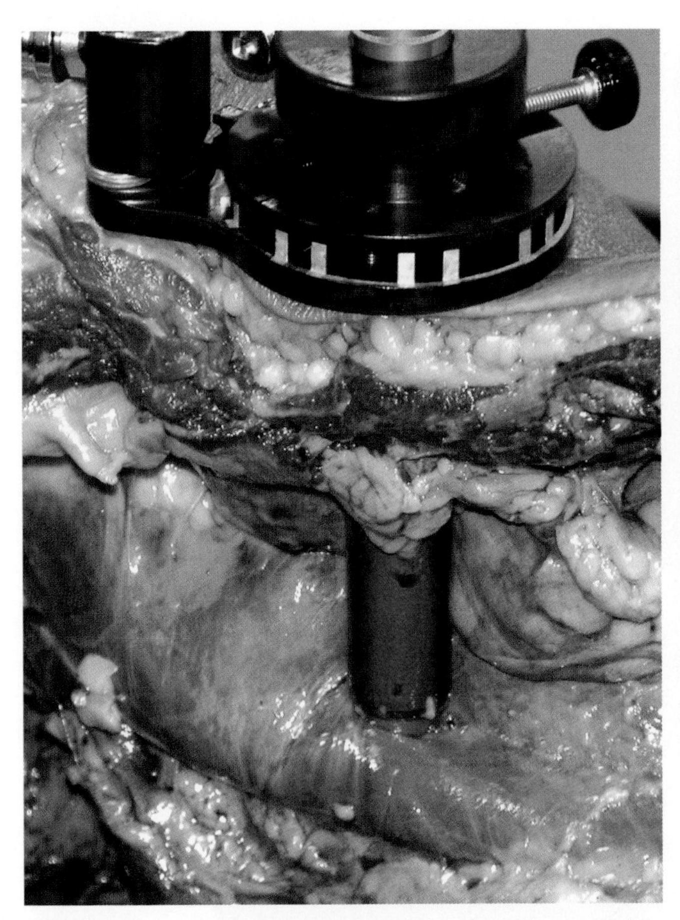

FIGURE 27–4 Cadaver dissection depicts lateral approach to the lumbar spine, with the endoscopic tube penetrating the anterior third of the psoas muscle at the disk space.

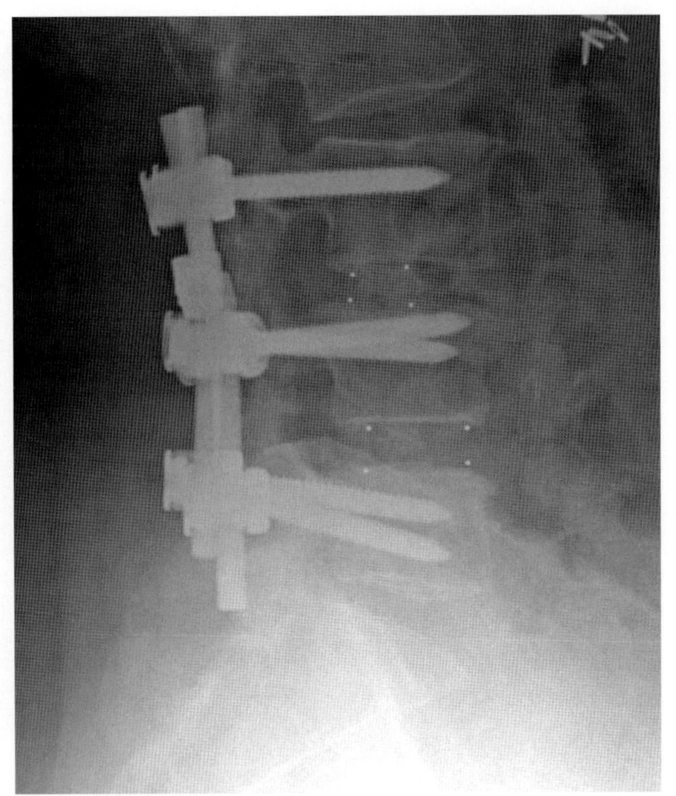

FIGURE 27–5 This 62-year-old patient presented with degenerative scoliosis at L2–L3 and L3–L4. She was treated with anterior carbon fiber cages through the lateral endoscopic approach, followed by posterior internal fixation using an open pedicle screw system.

disk space, with a metal marker on the skin in the midaxillary line. This method optimizes the placement of the working portal directly over the desired disk space. The patient is prepped and draped in the standard fashion. A 1 cm skin incision is made at the level of the disk space, and an optical trocar is inserted. The 10 mm laparoscope is then inserted into the optical dissecting trocar and focused on the subcutaneous tissue to allow visualization of the tissue planes. The trocar has two "winged keel" cutting surfaces that will not penetrate a fascial layer such as the peritoneum unless the trocar is twisted. The three abdominal muscular layers that overlie the peritoneum are penetrated in sequence under direct visualization until the preperitoneal fat is encountered. One or a combination of three different techniques may be used at this point to create a potential space that is superficial to the peritoneum (the retroperitoneal space). The trocar is most frequently used as a dissecting device under direct visualization until the laterally oriented fibers of the psoas major muscle are viewed. Blunt finger dissection can then be used to increase this space. A dissection balloon (Origin, Menlo Park, CA) can be filled with 1 L of air to dissect the retroperitoneal space, more correctly referred to as the retrotransversalis fascia. CO_2 insufflation can be used as an alternative in the retroperitoneal cavity up to a pressure of 20 mmHg to create a working space. The longitudinal fibers of the psoas major muscle are then identified. The genitofemoral nerve is usually visualized on the surface of the psoas muscle.

Following enlargement of the retroperitoneal space, two additional 1 cm incisions are made. The original portal, which is directly orthogonal with the disk space, is used as the working portal for use of the high-speed drill, curettes, and Kerrison and pituitary rongeurs. The second portal is necessary for the 10 mm laparoscope. A third portal is used for retraction of the psoas muscle fibers, and a fourth 10 mm portal is required for suctioning (Fig. 27–6C,D). The dissection is carried in a longitudinal fashion in line with the muscle fibers and through the anterior two thirds of the psoas muscle. When the psoas major muscle is separated during retroperitoneal endoscopy, there is a potential risk of injury to the lumbar plexus or nerve roots. Understanding the relationship between the greater psoas muscle and the lumbar plexus is essential to avoid nerve injury. The

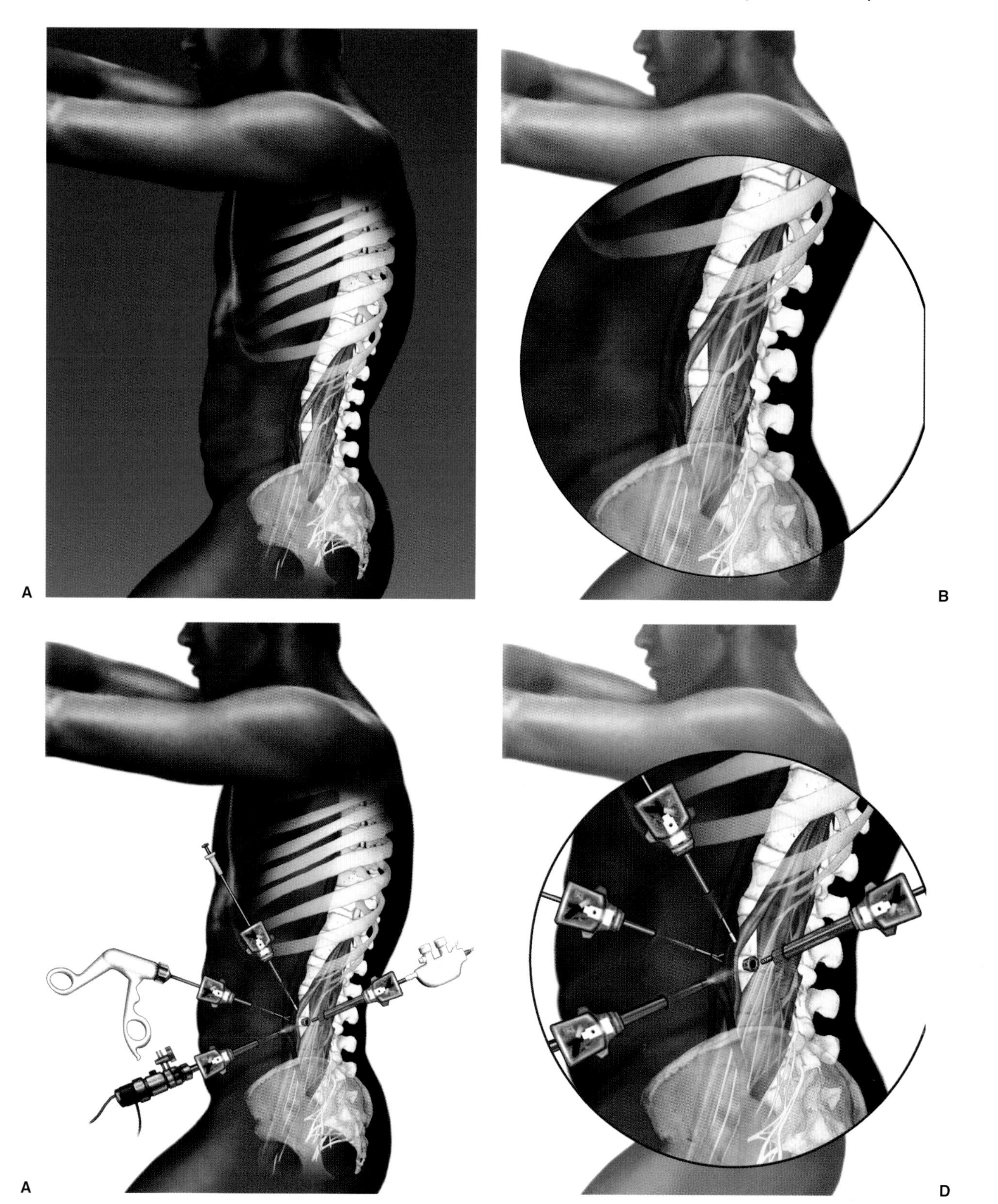

FIGURE 27–6 This series of illustrations depicts the lateral approach to L3–L4. **(A,B)** The patient is in a straight lateral position, where the skin will be marked directly over the disk after fluoroscopy is obtained. **(C,D)**

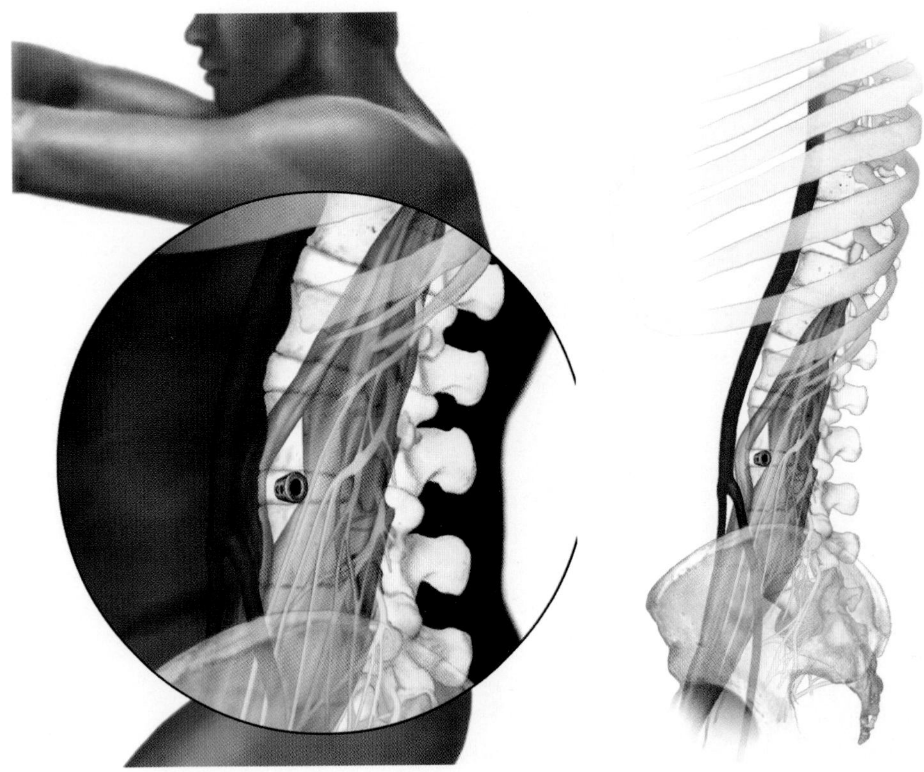

FIGURE 27–6 (*Continued*)The initial trocar is placed from the lateral position directly over the disk. Once insufflation is complete, three additional anterior trocars are placed. This is done after using the 10 mm endoscope to dissect the peritoneum toward the midline. **(E,F)** The final position of a cage with respect to the psoas muscle. It is critical to dissect only the anterior third of the muscle to avoid the femoral plexus.

genitofemoral nerve branches from the L1 and L2 nerve roots pierces the psoas muscle toward the anterior side of the muscle, and subsequently descends in accordance with the abdominal surface of the psoas major. The level that the genitofemoral nerve passes through the psoas muscle varies from the cranial third of the L3 vertebral body to the caudal third of the L4 vertebral body. In the case of spreading the psoas muscle, it is thought that the more caudal the muscle is spread, the more likely transitory genitofemoral nerve paralysis will occur. For protecting the lumbar plexus or roots and the genitofemoral nerve, the safe zone is in the anterior third of the psoas muscle. The muscle should be split more anteriorly with respect to the vertebral body from the cranial part of L3 and above. Based on anatomical studies, the plexus lies in the posterior half of the vertebral body at L4 and above. The safety zone with respect to the lumbar plexus is at the abdominal edge of the vertebra. The surgical approach should therefore be directed at or above L4 in the anterior half of the vertebral body with respect to a lateral view of the spine. At the L4–L5 disk and below, the plexus can pass anterior to the midaxis of the vertebra as seen on a lateral view. Retraction of the psoas muscle posteriorly should also be avoided because this can trap the exiting root against the base of the pedicle and transverse process. The relatively avascular intervertebral disk space can often be palpated through the anterior portion of the psoas muscle and is exposed first. The midportions of the adjacent vertebral bodies are then exposed. If necessary, the lumbar segmental vessels are ligated and divided. In most cases this is not necessary.

Once the vertebral level is confirmed fluoroscopically, the transversalis fascia, perinephric fascia, and retroperitoneal contents are retracted anteriorly. A Harmonic scalpel (Ethicon Endosurgery, Cincinnati, OH) is used to mark the intervertebral disk space. At this point, it is important for the surgeon to have access to various methods of hemostasis. We most frequently utilize the harmonic scalpel, but we also have bipolar endoscopic electrocautery, Endo-Avitene Microfibrillar Collagen (Humacao, Peurto Rico), and Gelfoam soaked in thrombin available to us. If necessary, the segmental vessels are dissected from the underlying bone and elevated with a right-angled clamp. It is important to use two vascular clips or an endoloop ligature on the high-pressure side of the vessels. The vessels are divided with endoscopic scissors. The 5 mm Harmonic scalpel is also used to ligate segmental vessels. The segmental vessels are ligated and divided in the anterior half of the vertebral body to allow maximal possible collateral circulation to the neural foramen and spinal cord. The disk space is incised using the Harmonic scalpel. Graduated endoscopic curettes and pituitary rongeurs are used to perform a complete diskectomy. The disk space height is restored by using a distraction plug placed from the side. A drill tube is placed over the distraction plug. The position of the distraction plug is monitored with anteroposterior and lateral fluoroscopy. The center of the distraction plug will correspond to the center of the BAK interbody fusion cage.[2] It is important to countersink the cage and pack additional bone graft superficial to the cage. The presence of a solid trabecular bone bridge in this location (lateral "Sentinel sign") allows for confirmation of the arthrodesis after ~3 to 6 months following surgery. The BAK or carbon fiber cages are packed with autogenous iliac graft obtained through a separate incision over the ipsilateral anterior iliac crest (Fig. 27–6E,F).

Using the technique described here at L4–L5, it is sometimes necessary to remove part of the iliac crest or place a docking portal through the iliac wing to be orthogonal to the disk space.[6,12] A carbon cage can alternatively be inserted at L4–L5 using a portal orthogonal to the L4–L5 space and slightly anterior to the iliac crest, angling obliquely in a slight anterior-to-posterior direction.

Patients are repositioned prone for pedicle screw instrumentation when posterior fixation is indicated. Traditional posterior fusion methods are used for scoliosis cases; however, single- or two-level anterior interbody fusions performed through this endoscopic lateral approach may be combined with percutaneous posterior pedicle screw fixation. This combination allows for a minimally invasive approach to 360 degree fusion. The Sextant (Medtronic, Memphis, TN) and Atavi (Endius, Plainville, MA) systems have been used successfully for one- and two-level fusions (Fig. 27–7).

Results and Complications

In the McAfee et al[5] series, 18 patients underwent a lateral endoscopic retroperitoneal approach for lumbar spinal fusion. There was a short postoperative stay of 2.9 days. All patients obtained a solid arthrodesis, and there were no cases of great vessel injury, retrograde ejaculation, or implant migration.

Regan has subsequently compiled a series of 27 consecutive lateral endoscopic transpsoas lumbar spinal fusions. The average operative time was 145 minutes (range: 120 to 170 minutes) for the anterior approach. Average blood loss was 150 ml (range: 50 to 650 ml). Twenty-two of 27 patients (85%) had a good to excellent outcome and

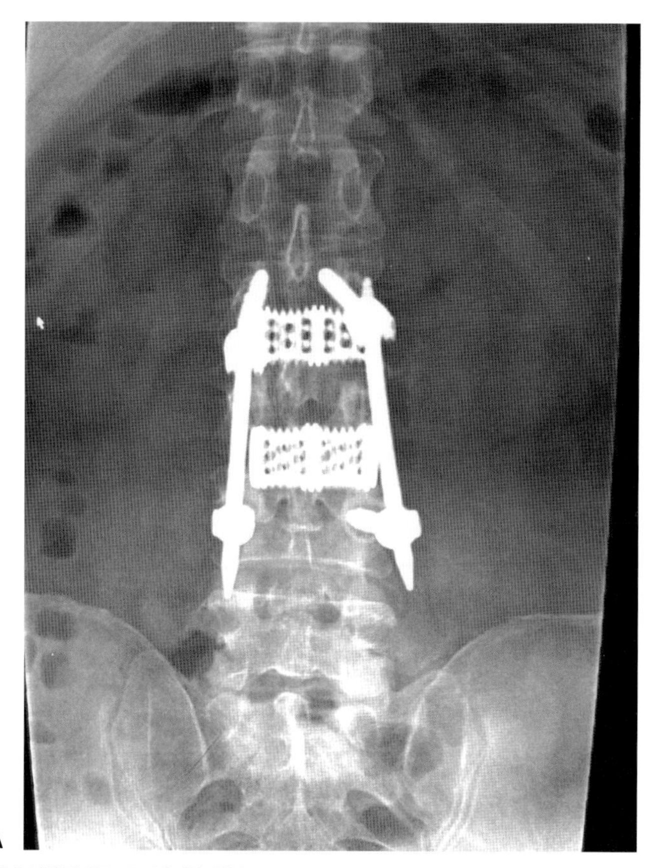

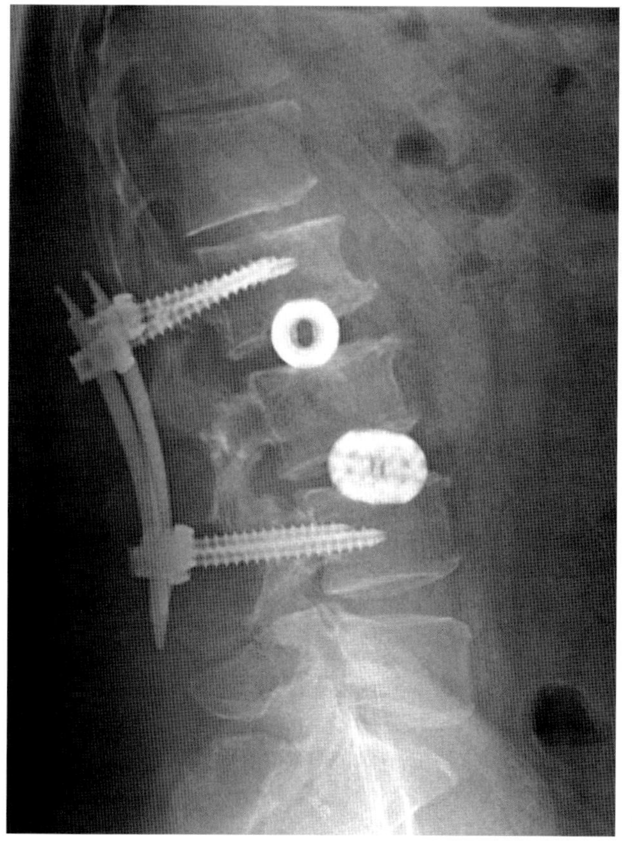

FIGURE 27–7 (A,B) This patient underwent endoscopic lateral fusion through the anterior endoscopic approach, followed by posterior two-level Sextant percutaneous fixation.

would undergo the surgery again. Visual analogue scale (VAS) improved postoperatively by 5.9 for all patients. There were no mortalities, infections, pseudarthroses, implant migrations, or subsidence in this series.

There was an incidence of postoperative groin and anterior thigh paresthesias or pain in 8 of 27 patients (30%). These symptoms were self-limiting and resolved within 8 weeks postoperatively. This complication is due to the dissection of the psoas muscle and subsequent postoperative edema/hematoma causing irritation of the genitofemoral nerve. The genitofemoral nerve arises from the L1 and L2 roots. It passes obliquely through the substance of the psoas and emerges from its inner border at a level corresponding to the L3–L4 interspace. It then descends on the surface of the psoas muscle, normally under the cover of the peritoneum, and divides into the genital and femoral branches. The genital branch passes outward on the psoas major and pierces the fascia transversalis, or passes through the internal abdominal ring. It then descends along the back part of the spermatic cord to the scrotum and supplies, in the male, the cremaster muscle. In the female, it accompanies and ends in the round ligament. The femoral branch of the genitofemoral nerve descends on the external iliac artery, sending a few branches to it, and after passing beneath Poupart's ligament to the thigh, supplies the skin of the anterior aspect of the thigh down about midway between the pelvis and the knee.

Two patients underwent conversion from an endoscopic to a mini-open approach. One patient was converted due to adhesions from prior surgery and one patient due to bleeding from a segmental vessel.

Vraney et al[10] reported that access to the L4–L5 disk space via an endoscopic transperitoneal approach would be readily accessible in only ~33% of patients and in others would require significant dissection. This was based on a review of computer-generated series of abdominal arterial studies and not actual surgical cases or directly observed anatomy. Regan et al[7,9] reviewed the results of 58 consecutive patients who underwent laparoscopic ALIF at the L4–L5 level using BAK cages in an attempt to describe variations in the approach used to address anatomical variations in the location of the great vessel bifurcation when approaching this region. The L4–L5 disk space was accessed above the great vessel bifurcation in 30 patients (50%), below the bifurcation in 18 patients (30%), and between the vessels in the remaining 10 patients.

Tiusanen et al[13] reported a 5.9% incidence of retrograde ejaculation following anterior transabdominal lumbar interbody fusion. There were 12 cases (5%) of retrograde ejaculation that occurred as a complication of laparoscopic BAK interbody fusion and stabilization in the first series of 240 patients submitted to the U.S. Food and Drug Administration.[9] The retroperitoneal exposure has not been associated with this postoperative complication.[3]

The lateral endoscopic retroperitoneal approach for lumbar fusion avoids dissection of the great vessels regardless of the level of bifurcation. Because the autonomic plexus is not dissected, there is a reduced risk of retrograde ejaculation compared with anterior approaches.[6] In addition, the lateral decubitus position facilitates exposure of the lumbar spine, as gravity helps in pulling the abdominal contents anteriorly. It is also easier to position a trocar orthogonal to the disk space with a laterally directed interbody fusion device, as opposed to the supine Trendelenburg position required for transperitoneal laparoscopy. Unlike standard anterior approaches, the anterior longitudinal ligament and posterior longitudinal ligament are not violated with the lateral retroperitoneal approach. This confers a significant biomechanical advantage. Moreover, with the transperitoneal approach, if the surgeon reams, taps, or drills too deeply, the spinal canal contents are at risk. With the lateral retroperitoneal approach, these activities are directed toward the contralateral psoas muscle instead of the spinal canal contents.[6] In the FDA laparoscopic BAK study,[9] the incidence of iatrogenic intraoperative disk herniation in patients undergoing surgery at one level was 2.8% (3 of 25 patients). Overall, for BAK implants inserted via a straight anterior-to-posterior direction, the incidence of reoperation for iatrogenic penetration or for pushing intervertebral disk material into the spinal canal was 2.3%.

Posterior instrumentation was used in all patients. Stand-alone anterior lumbar interbody fusion remains controversial, and we feel that providing a posterior tension band reduces the pseudarthrosis rate significantly. We utilize percutaneous pedicle screw fixation on all single- and two-level cases. Scoliosis cases require a traditional posterior approach. This combination provides a minimally invasive approach and allows for 360-degree fusion.

There has been a surge in the use of laparoscopic approaches to the lumbar spine for interbody fusion using threaded cages. These techniques are attractive in that they offer the potential for less perioperative pain and morbidity, shorter hospital stays, quicker recovery times, and a faster return to work and the patient's normal lifestyle. The lateral endoscopic approach to the lumbar spine offers several advantages over traditional techniques. Mobilization of the great vessels is not required, and dissection of the sympathetic plexus is eliminated.

REFERENCES

1. Obenchain TG. Laparoscopic lumbar discectomy: case report. *J Laparoendosc Surg.* 1991;1:145–149.
2. Bagby G. Arthrodesis by the distraction-compression methods using a stainless steel implant. *Orthopedics.* 1988;11:931–934.
3. Mayer MH. Mini ALIF: a new microsurgical technique for minimally invasive anterior lumbar interbody fusion. *Spine.* 1997;6: 691–700.

4. McAfee PC. Complications of anterior approaches to the thoracolumbar spine: emphasis on Kaneda instrumentation. *Clin Orthop.* 1994;306:110–119.
5. McAfee PC, Regan JJ, Geis WP, Fedder IL. Minimally invasive anterior retroperitoneal approach to the lumbar spine: emphasis on the lateral BAK. *Spine.* 1998;23:1476–1484.
6. McAfee PC, Regan JJ, Zdeblick T, et al. The incidence of complications in endoscopic anterior thoracolumbar spinal reconstructive surgery: a prospective multicenter study compromising the first 100 consecutive cases. *Spine.* 1995;20:1624–1632.
7. Regan JJ, Aronoff RJ, Ohnmeiss DD. Laparoscopic approach to L4–5 for interbody fusion using BAK cages: experience in the first 58 cases. *Spine.* 1999;24:2171–2174.
8. Regan JJ, McAfee PC, Guyer RD, Aronoff RJ. Laparoscopic fusion of the lumbar spine in a multicenter series of the first 34 consecutive patients. *Surg Laparosc Endosc.* 1996;6:459–468.
9. Regan JJ, Yuan H, McAfee PC. Laparoscopic fusion of the lumbar spine, minimally invasive spine surgery: a prospective multicenter study evaluating open and laparoscopic lumbar fusion. *Spine.* 1999;24:402–411.
10. Vraney RT, Philips FM, Wetzel FT, Brustein M. Peridiscal vascular anatomy of the lower lumbar spine: an endoscopic perspective. *Spine.* 1999;24:2183–2187.
11. Vollmar B, Olinger A, Hildebrandt U, Menger RD. Cardiopulmonary dysfunction during minimally invasive thoraco-lumboendoscopic spine surgery. *Anesth Analg.* 1999;88:1244–1251.
12. Osman SG, Marsolais EB. Endoscopic transiliac approach to L5–S1 disc and foramen: a cadaver study. *Spine.* 1997;22:1259–1263.
13. Tiusanen H, Seitsalo S, Osterman K, Soini J. Retrograde ejaculation after anterior interbody lumbar fusion. *Eur Spine J.* 1995;4:339–342.

28

Gasless Endoscopic ALIF: The BERG Approach

JOHN S. THALGOTT AND JAMES M. GIUFFRE

The evolution of endoscopic anterior lumbar interbody fusion (ALIF) began with the first laparoscopic diskectomy performed by Obenchain.[1] From that, a combination of vascular surgeons and anterior lumbar spine surgeons developed the gas-mediated laparoscopic approach for ALIF.[2–7] For a brief window in time, this approach was the gold standard for minimally invasive access to the anterior lumbar column. This would not have occurred had it not been for the introduction of small cylindrical fusion cages because cylindrical cages were the only interbody fusion implant that could fit through the ports at that point in time.

Despite the fact that the gas-mediated approach was well publicized, it is not without its drawbacks. Access above L5–S1 is severely limited. Access to L4–L5 is possible in some cases, but mobilization of the vessels at L4–L5, as well as bowel retraction, is extremely difficult. The approach requires the use of long, thin instruments due to the small size of the valved ports. These endoscopic instruments have fulcrums that are too far from the surgical field, which creates an unnatural operative technique, compared with open anterior lumbar surgery. There are also issues concerning the maintenance of the pneumoperitoneum because suction often eliminates gas from the abdominal cavity faster than the insufflator can supply it. This causes an undesirable loss of exposure.

Because of these limiting problems with the gas-mediated approach, a gasless approach, balloon-assisted endoscopic retroperitoneal gasless (BERG), was developed as the next step in minimally invasive anterior lumbar surgery.[8–9] The BERG approach utilizes a balloon to perform the initial dissection followed by a combination of a mechanical lifting arm and fan retractor to distend the abdomen without the use of gas insufflation. This is a true retroperitoneal approach to the anterior lumbar column, which allows for access up to L2 and in some cases up to L1. Because there are no pressurized ports with this approach, the surgeon can use standard anterior instruments for lumbar fusion surgery. There is no pneumoperitoneum to maintain, so loss of exposure due to suction is not a problem. Vascular and bowel retraction is similar to an open anterior retroperitoneal approach.

Indications

By definition, BERG is a retroperitoneal approach to the anterior lumbar spine. Indications for the BERG approach are exactly the same as they are for the open retroperitoneal approach:

- ALIF at one, two, or three levels from L2 to the sacrum
- For stand-alone ALIF or as part of a circumferential fusion
- In patients indicated for ALIF with a diagnosis of degenerative disk disease, internal disk disruption, spinal stenosis, spondylolisthesis, failed laminectomy syndrome, severe disk herniation, or prior posterior pseudarthrosis

Non-ALIF Indications

Indications for the non-ALIF approach are

- Tumor resection
- Irrigation and debridement of a deep wound infection
- Anterior reconstruction of lumbar vertebral fracture
- Anterior release for deformity correction

Contraindications

The BERG approach has no absolute contraindications, although there are some relative contraindications. It is the role of the vascular surgeon to examine the physical health and surgical history of the patient closely prior to surgery. The vascular surgeon should have strong input as to whether or not to attempt a BERG approach with a contraindicated patient.

Contraindications include

- Excessive obesity
- Multiple prior abdominal surgeries, particularly on the left side
- In most cases, ALIF above L2 and definitely above L1

Surgical Equipment

The following instruments and equipment are necessary to perform the BERG approach to ALIF properly:

- Clear-ended endoscopic dissecting port
- Two flexible, nonvalved ports with 3 cm diameter
- Dissecting balloon and inflator

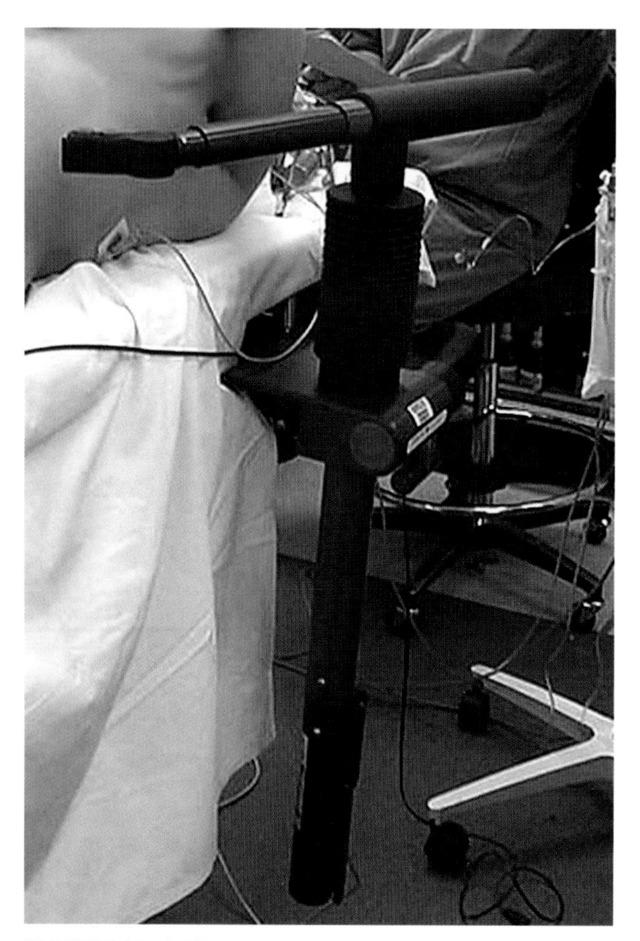

FIGURE 28–1 The mechanical lifting arm is used to lift the fan retractor and distend the abdominal wall.

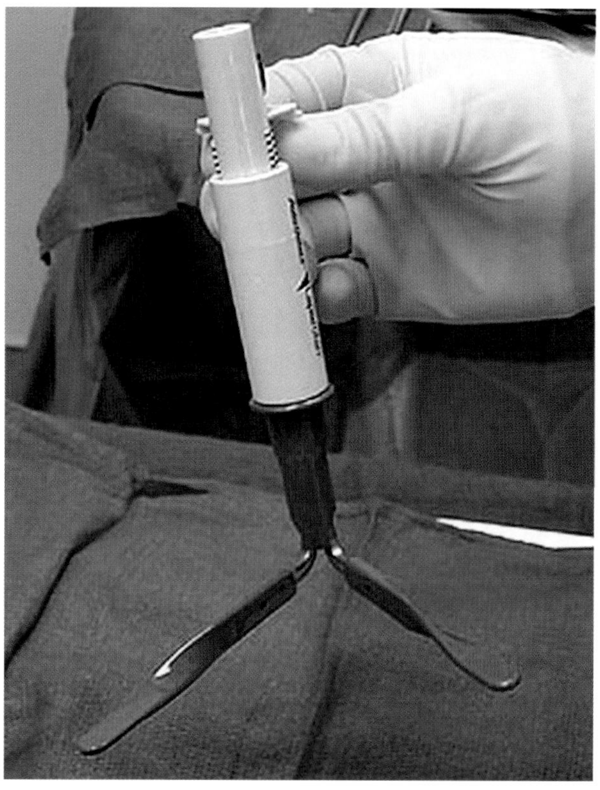

FIGURE 28–2 The fan retractor is used to distend the abdominal wall.

- Scalpel
- Laprolift mechanical arm (Fig. 28–1)
- Laprofan fan retractor (Fig. 28–2)
- Balloon retractor for retracting peritoneal contents (Fig. 28–3)
- 0-degree endoscope
- Two video monitors
- Standard set of instruments for anterior lumbar surgery, including a disk knife, end-plate dissectors,

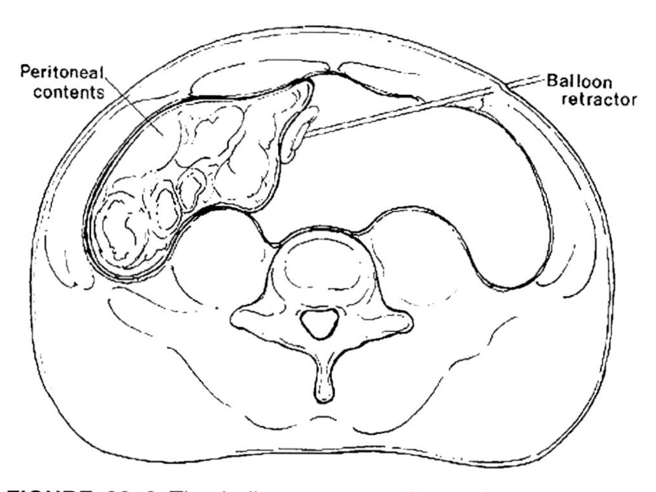

FIGURE 28–3 The balloon retractor is used to retract the peritoneal contents to the right.

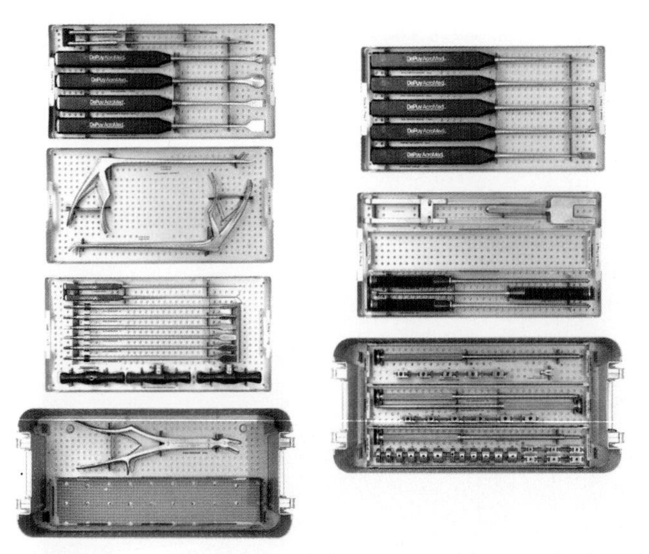

FIGURE 28–4 A standard set of instruments for anterior lumbar surgery.

rongeurs, curettes, and vascular retractors (Fig. 28–4)

- Fusion device and instrumentation of implantation: cage or femoral ring

Operating Room Setup

The spinal surgeon stands on the left side of the patient; the vascular surgeon stands on the right. Video monitors are aligned and angled next to each surgeon, providing cross-table visualization. An endocopically trained technician stands to the right of the spinal surgeon and operates the endoscope following exposure (Fig. 28–5).

Patient Positioning

The patient is placed in the supine position. Following general anesthesia, the patient is draped and prepped in standard fashion, and preoperative antibiotics are given. Fluoroscopy is used to find the landmarks of the appropriate lumbar level. The skin is marked, identifying the level and angle of the pathologic disk interspace(s). These are drawn on the lateral aspect of the left abdomen, marking the angles of the disk spaces to be addressed (Fig. 28–6).

Surgical Technique

A transverse, 20 mm left flank incision is made ~1 cm above the left iliac crest in the midaxillary line (Fig. 28–7). The dissection is taken down through the external oblique, internal oblique, and transversus muscles under direct vision to the preperitoneal fat layer using a clear-ended, endoscopic dissecting port. As the preperitoneal fat layer is penetrated by the clear-ended dissecting port,

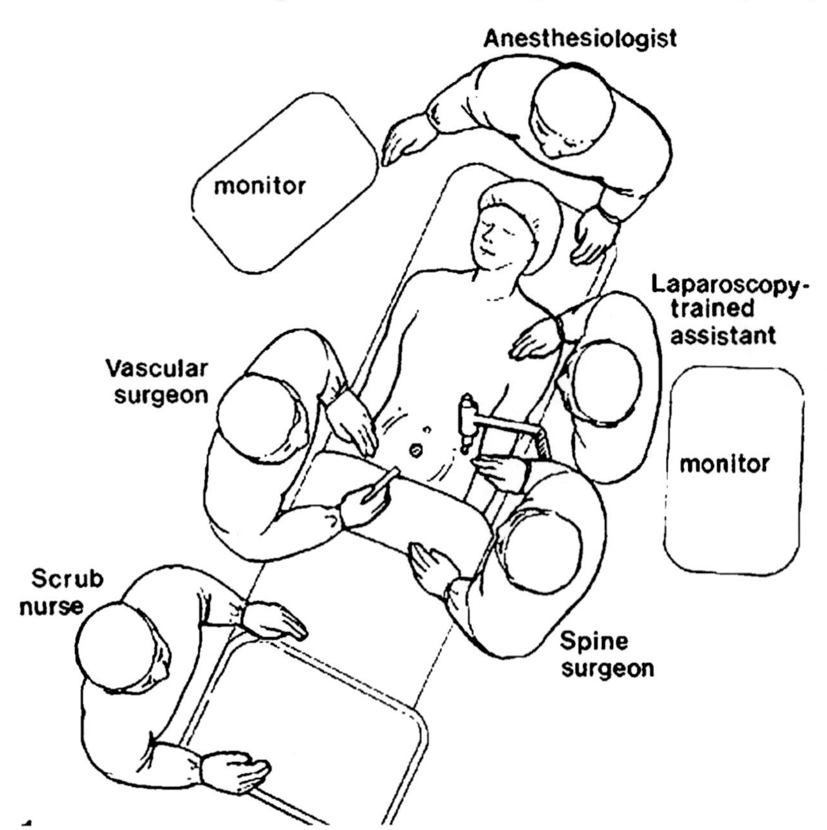

FIGURE 28–5 The operating room setup for the BERG approach.

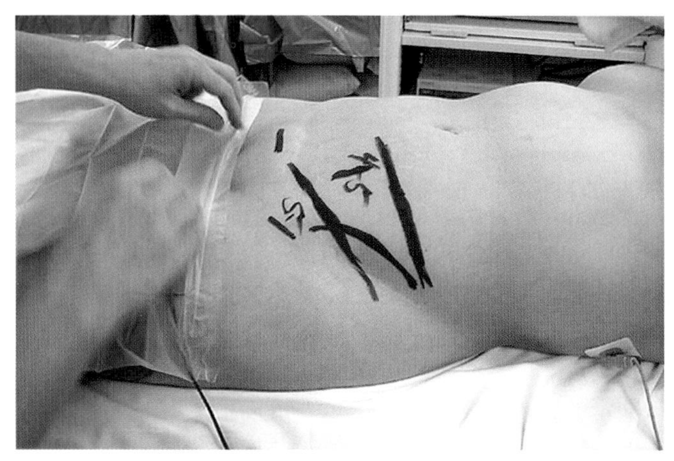

FIGURE 28–6 Preoperative markings on the abdomen demonstrating the angle and location of the interdiscal segments.

there is a color change to yellow, which lets the surgical team know that layer has been reached and that they should proceed with caution.

The retroperitoneal space is then gently insufflated with a bulb syringe and digitally dissected into the iliac fossa to allow for balloon insertion. An undeployed elliptical-shaped preperitoneal balloon is advanced through the incision until the entire balloon is within the retroperitoneal space.

A 0-degree angled endoscope is placed through the lumen of the dissection cannula, and the balloon is expanded to an approximate volume of 1 L. The endoscope is directed toward the anterior abdominal wall. This allows the identification of the peritoneal reflection on the anterior abdominal wall, at the rectus sheath, above and below the line of Douglas (Fig. 28–8). The peritoneal reflection is used as a landmark for the anterior working port. The anterior working port is located lateral to the peritoneal reflection on the rectus sheath. This port is formed at a level determined by the preoperative markings on the abdomen, which correspond to the interspace angulation. A 2 to 3 cm paramedian incision is made through the anterior abdominal wall and carried down through the fascia. This is done lateral to the peritoneal reflection and with great care to avoid the peritoneal sac. This creates the anterior working/retraction port. The balloon is removed after a 1 cm malleable retractor is placed between the two ports under direct endoscopic vision. Once the retroperitoneal space has been mobilized, the next goal is the retraction of the abdominal wall.

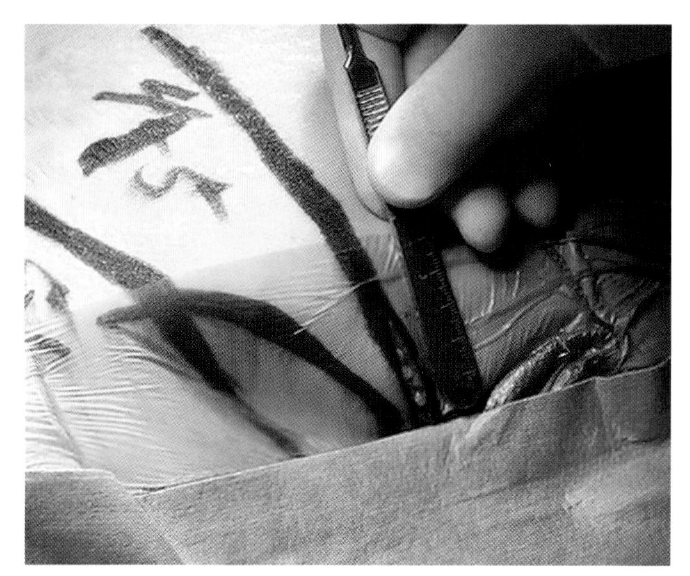

FIGURE 28–7 The initial left flank incision. This will become the area of abdominal distention as well as the port for the endoscope and the balloon retractor used to retract the peritoneal contents.

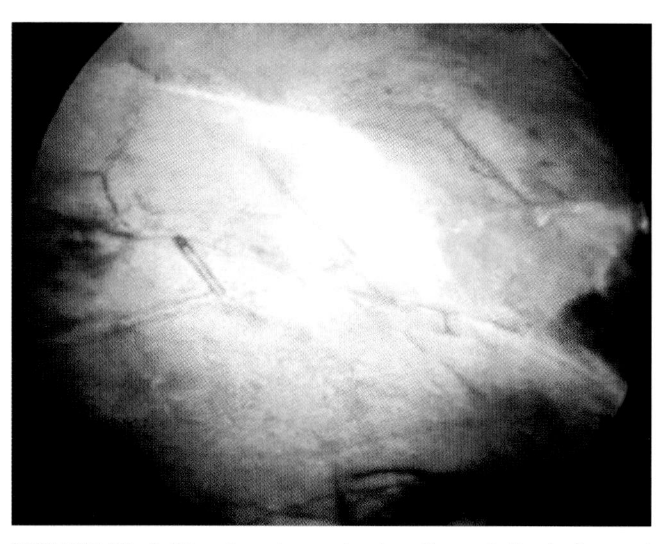

FIGURE 28–8 Direct endoscopic view through the balloon at the peritoneal reflection, used as a landmark to create the anterior working port.

There are three levels of retraction necessary to access the anterior lumbar spine. The first of these is distraction of the anterior abdominal wall. This is accomplished by the insertion of a fan retractor into the initial flank port. The fan retractor is expanded under direct endoscopic vision. Once expanded, the fan retractor is attached to a mechanical lifting arm. The abdominal wall is elevated by this combination, creating the retroperitoneal space and replacing the need for gas. A flexible nonvalved port, utilized for lateral visualization and retraction, is placed directly below the legs of the fan retractor to provide a clear path for the endoscope.

The second level of retraction is necessary to displace the peritoneal contents past the midline to provide access to the lumbar spine and vascular anatomy. A long retractor with an inflatable end is inserted through the newly created lateral working port in the initial left flank incision to push the peritoneal sac and intra-abdominal

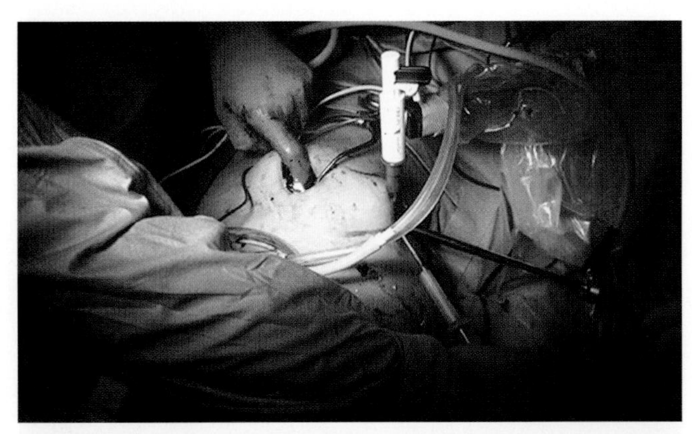

FIGURE 28–9 The entire setup for the approach with fan retractor and lifting arm to the right, endoscope and balloon retractor in place within the left flank incision, and anterior working port to the left.

contents aside, creating the working space (Fig. 28–9). Once the retractor is in place, the technician stands with his or her abdomen against the retractor handle, leaving two hands free for endoscope operation, cleaning, and so on.

The third level of retraction is vascular. Following establishment of the operative cavity, the psoas muscle and vascular anatomy are used as reference landmarks. The psoas muscle is bluntly dissected to expose the pathologic disk space(s). The L5–S1 vascular retraction begins by identifying the right iliac vein and utilizing a vascular retractor to retract the fascia and presacral veins, thereby exposing the anterior aspect of the L5–S1 interspace. Through the visualization/retraction port, a standard vein retractor is passed and is used to retract the iliac vein laterally. Once this is done, the presacral veins are ligated or cauterized with bipolar cautery if necessary. Great care must be used in dissecting the anterior soft tissues to maintain the integrity of the presacral plexus.

The L4–L5 exposure is more complex. It begins by using an anterior vessel retractor and displacing the vena cava or left iliac vein. This is placed on tension, and the iliolumbar vein is identified. If necessary, the iliolumbar vein is ligated using corporeal knot tying. This is generally reinforced with two specific ligatures. Once the iliolumbar vein is ligated, gentle dissection is used to retract the left iliac vein, exposing the L4–L5 interspace past the midline. The vascular retraction for L3–L4 is performed in a similar way, but it does not require ligation of the iliolumbar vein.

Following psoas dissection and vessel retraction, a spinal needle is placed into the pathologic disk(s), and fluoroscopy is used to confirm the operative level. The anterior working port allows for both vascular retraction and the introduction of such standard spinal instruments as dissectors, rongeurs, curettes, and end-plate elevators.

Our experience with the BERG approach has been primarily with ALIF. The technique for ALIF is essentially the same as it is with an open anterior retroperitoneal approach. Diskectomy begins by incising the anterior anulus with a long-handled scalpel, both cranially and caudally, as well as left and right. End-plate elevators, rongeurs, and curettes are introduced and utilized through the anterior working port. Once the disk is removed, the surgical team has several options for fusion (e.g., anatomical cages, screw-in cages, allograft, and autograft). After the allograft, disk prosthesis, or cage is placed, the option of buttress plate fixation is possible. Following this, the implant position is confirmed through fluoroscopy.

Upon satisfactory imaging, the retroperitoneum is inspected, and the three levels of retraction are removed. The incision is closed in layers in standard fashion.

Postoperative Care

Patients undergoing stand-alone ALIF or circumferential minimally invasive instrumented fusion are discharged from the hospital at 1 to 3 days postoperatively. Patients are placed in a neoprene lumbar corset for at least 4 weeks postoperatively. They begin aquatic physical therapy at 10 to 14 days postoperatively and advance to weight training, treadmill, and range-of-motion therapy as tolerated. Return to work depends largely on the patient's motivation and occupational circumstances (Fig. 28–10).

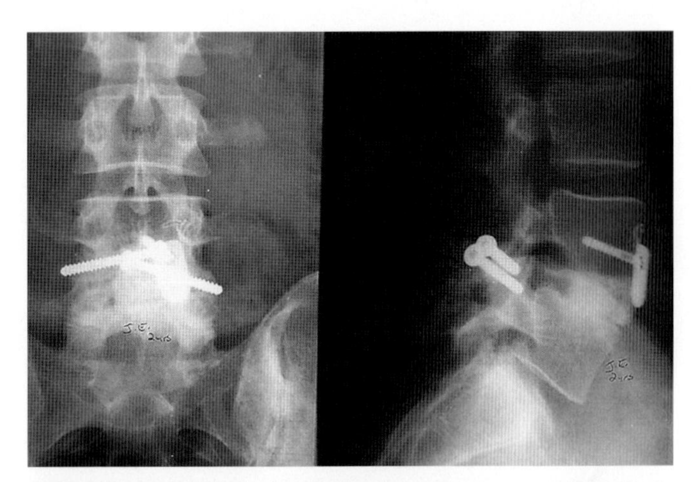

FIGURE 28–10 Lateral radiograph at 2 years postoperatively of a 30-year-old male presenting with failed laminectomy syndrome and mild degenerative disk disease at L4–L5. He had an ALIF with femoral ring allograft via BERG and minimally invasive posterolateral instrumented fusion. The patient was discharged within the following day and returned to work at 2 months postoperatively. He has a solid fusion radiographically. **(A)** AP x-ray. **(B)** Lateral x-ray.

Complications and Avoidance

All of these postoperative complications are known to occur with anterior lumbar surgery, and the BERG approach is no exception.

- *Inadvertent vessel laceration:* The complication of largest concern is the inadvertent vessel laceration. In a minimally invasive, two-dimensional environment where visualization is limited, a vessel laceration, especially a laceration of one of the great vessels, can cause serious problems for the surgical team. In our initial experience with this approach, a vessel laceration became an automatic conversion to an open approach. As the surgical team became more proficient in repairing these vessels endoscopically, however, the complication no longer caused an automatic conversion. The key to handling a vessel laceration is to have a vascular surgeon on the surgical team. Although it is possible to perform the BERG approach without a vascular surgeon, it is not recommended. Utilizing the same vascular surgeon or same two vascular surgeons on a rotating basis for all BERG approaches is the optimal arrangement.
- *Peritoneal tear:* This is another very good reason for a vascular (or general) surgeon to be part of the surgical team. The thickness of a patient's peritoneum cannot be assessed preoperatively. Much greater care must be used to avoid tearing a thin peritoneum if it is identified perioperatively. It is possible to repair a torn peritoneum; however, if it cannot be repaired, or if the approach cannot be reworked around the tear, the approach will have to be converted to open.
- *Ileus:* A bowel prep should be given with patients having nothing but liquids for 12 hours prior to surgery.
- *Retrograde ejaculation:* As with an open approach, great care should be taken not to disrupt the sympathetic chain.
- *Bladder incontinence:* The ureter is usually visible following balloon dissection. As with an open approach, care should be taken not to injure the ureter.
- *Deep vein thrombosis:* Pneumatic stockings may be used in patients with circulatory comorbidities . If a vessel laceration occurs, a postoperative venogram may be indicated.
- *Incisional herniation:* Proper suturing of the abdominal wall in layers should suffice to avoid an incisional heriation.
- *Infection:* Perioperative antibiotics should be administered by the anesthesiologist.

Balloon-assisted endoscopic retroperitoneal gasless is a true retroperitoneal approach to the anterior lumbar column. Indications for the BERG approach are exactly the same as they are for an open retroperitoneal approach. Because there are no pressurized ports with this approach and no pneumoperitoneum to maintain, the surgeon can use standard anterior instruments for lumbar fusion surgery. To minimize complications, the BERG approach should be performed in conjunction with a vascular surgeon.

REFERENCES

1. Obenchain TG. Laparoscopic discectomy and fusion: a case report. *J Laparoendosc Surg.* 1991;1:145–149.
2. Olsen D, McCord D, Law M. Laparoscopic discectomy and anterior interbody fusion of L5–S1. *Surg Endosc.* 1996;10:1158–1163.
3. McAfee PC, Regan JJ, Geis WP, Fedder IL. Minimally invasive anterior retroperitoneal approach to the lumbar spine: emphasis on the lateral BAK. *Spine.* 1998;23:1476–1484.
4. Regan JJ, Yuan H, McAfee PC. Laparoscopic fusion of the lumbar spine, minimally invasive spine surgery: a prospective multicenter study evaluation open and laparoscopic lumbar fusion. *Spine.* 1999;24:402–411.
5. Regan JJ, McAfee PC, Guyer RD, Aronoff RJ. Laparoscopic fusion of the lumbar spine in a multicenter series of the first 34 consecutive patients. *Surg Laparosc Endosc.* 1996;6:459–468.
6. Sachs BL, Schwaitzberg SD. Lumbosacral (L5–S1) discectomy and interbody fusion technique. In: Regan JJ, McAfee PC, Mack MJ, eds. *Atlas of Endoscopic Spine Surgery.* St. Louis, MO: Quality Medical Publishing; 1994:275–291.
7. Zucherman J, Zdeblick TA, Bailey SA, Mahvi D, Hsu KY, Kohrs D. Instrumented laparoscopic spinal fusion: preliminary results. *Spine.* 1995;20:2029–2035.
8. Thalgott JS, Chin AK, Ameriks JA, et al. Gasless endoscopic anterior lumbar Interbody Fusion Utilizing the BERG Approach. *Surg Endosc* 2000;14:546–552
9. Thalgott JS, Chin AK, Ameriks JA, Jordan FT, Giuffre JM, Fritts K, Timlin M. Minimally invasive 360° instrumented lumbar fusion. *Eur Spine J.* 2000;9(suppl 1):S51–S56.

■ SECTION FIVE ■

Percutaneous Procedures

29

Percutaneous Vertebroplasty for Painful Vertebral Body Compression Fractures

HUY M. DO AND BRIAN S. KIM

Approximately 700,000 vertebral fractures associated with osteoporosis occur each year.[1] As a result of osteoporosis, the lifetime risk of symptomatic vertebral fracture is 16% for women and 5% for men.[2] *Vertebral compression fractures* are defined as the reduction in vertebral body height by 15% or greater and can be classified by the degree and type of deformity, which include wedge, biconcavity, and compression fractures.[2–4] The most commonly compressed vertebral levels are T8, T12, L1, and L4, and most occur spontaneously from normal or trivial stress. Traditional conservative management of vertebral body compression fractures includes analgesics, immobilization, muscle relaxants, physical therapy, and external bracing when indicated.

Percutaneous vertebroplasty is a minimally invasive, radiologically guided, therapeutic procedure for the treatment of pain caused by a vertebral body compression fracture. This procedure was initially described in the treatment of symptomatic vertebral hemangiomas, multiple myeloma, and metastases.[5–8] Percutaneous vertebroplasty has gained popularity as a viable and potential standard of care for the management of pain and disabilities associated with vertebral body compression fractures. There are multiple case series in the medical literature reporting high clinical success rates with percutaneous vertebroplasty in the treatment of vertebral compression fractures related to various etiologies.[2,7–15]

Percutaneous vertebroplasty is performed by placing a needle percutaneously into the compressed vertebral body under fluoroscopic monitoring and guidance. Once the needle is in position, polymethyl methacrylate (PMMA) mixed with sterile barium sulfate powder for added radiopacity is injected into the vertebral body fracture (Fig. 29–1). PMMA, a medical-grade cement, is believed to work by strengthening the weakened fractured vertebra, immobilizing microfractures, and relieving stress on the remaining bone by increasing tensile strength. These properties lead to pain relief in the patient and strengthen the treated fractured vertebra against initial failure and subsequent collapse.

Indications

Treatment criteria for percutaneous vertebroplasty include:

- Pain unrelieved by narcotics
- Radiographic evidence of compression fracture with pain localized to the fracture level(s)
- Pain in a focal bandlike radiation that is worse with weight bearing and is relieved with rest or when in a recumbent position

Percutaneous vertebroplasty is indicated in the following situations:

- Compression fractures of the vertebrae due to osteoporosis, aggressive hemangiomas, metastatic disease, osteogenesis imperfecta, trauma, or vertebral osteonecrosis

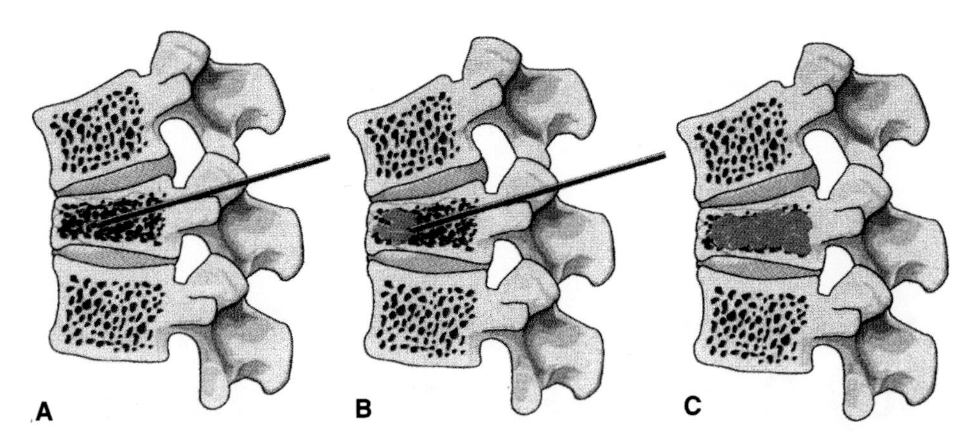

FIGURE 29–1 Schematic showing needle placement **(A)**, injection of PMMA **(B)**, and completed filling of the vertebral body fracture with PMMA **(C)**.

- Chronic traumatic fracture with nonunion of the fracture fragments
- Presurgical stabilization of a partially compressed vertebral body or internal stabilization of unstable traumatic fractures
- Patients with multiple compression fractures for whom further vertebral body collapse would result in pulmonary compromise

Contraindications

Percutaneous vertebroplasty is absolutely contraindicated in the following situations:

- Patients with asymptomatic vertebral compression fracture
- Patients with a fracture that is clearly responding to medical therapy
- Osteomyelitis of target vertebra
- Prophylactic treatment with no evidence of fracture
- Acute traumatic fracture of nonosteoporotic vertebra
- Uncorrected coagulation disorders
- Allergy to any required component

Percutaneous vertebroplasty has a relative contraindication in the following situations:

- Patients with a retropulsed fragment that is causing spinal canal compromise of greater than 20%
- Patients unable to lie prone for the entire procedure
- Patients with pain due to herniated disks, facet arthropathy, spinal stenosis, or degenerative changes
- Pathologic fracture with tumor extension into the epidural space
- Severe vertebral body collapse (vertebra plana)

Instruments and Preparations

Vertebroplasty Equipment

A standard spinal intervention patient preparation tray should include betadine and alcohol solutions for sterilization, sterile patient drape cover, 25- or 22-gauge spinal needles for local anesthesia, sterile towels and sponges, #11 scalpel for dermatotomy, 11- or 13-gauge bone biopsy–type needles at least 6 inches long and with various inner stylet tips (Fig. 29–2A), PMMA cement, sterile barium sulfate powder (opacifying agent), and screw-down injector reservoir syringes or 1 ml Luer-lock syringes (Fig. 29–2B).

High-quality single or biplane fluoroscopy should be used for adequate visualization of the spinal bony anatomy and opacified PMMA. One should avoid poor-quality C-arm fluoroscopic units.

Anesthesia

Conscious sedation with intravenous fentanyl and midazolam is generally adequate for this procedure. General anesthesia may be indicated in select situations (e.g., patients with multiple compression fractures requiring extended operating time and in patients in whom movement is a problem with the targeting and introduction of the needle). In addition, patients who experience difficulties with ventilation or who are unable to tolerate the prone position during the procedure may require general anesthesia or deep sedation. Local anesthesia with 1% lidocaine or 0.25% bupivacaine should be applied to the skin and deep structures, including the periosteum of the bone at the intended site.

Positioning

The patient is positioned prone on the fluoroscopy table with padding under the body. The hips are slightly bent, and the arms are positioned over the shoulder (Fig. 29–3).

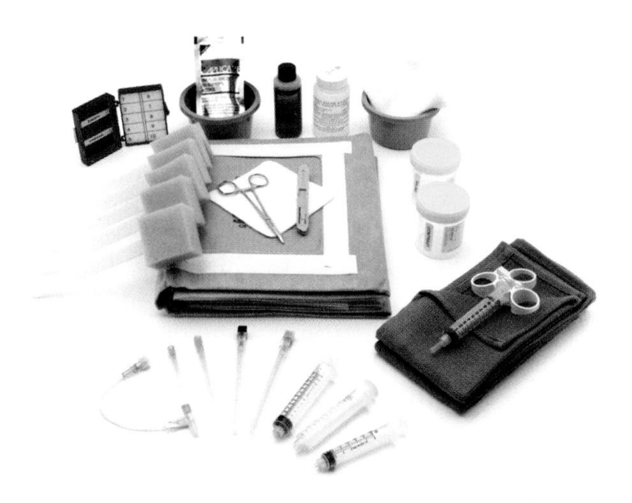

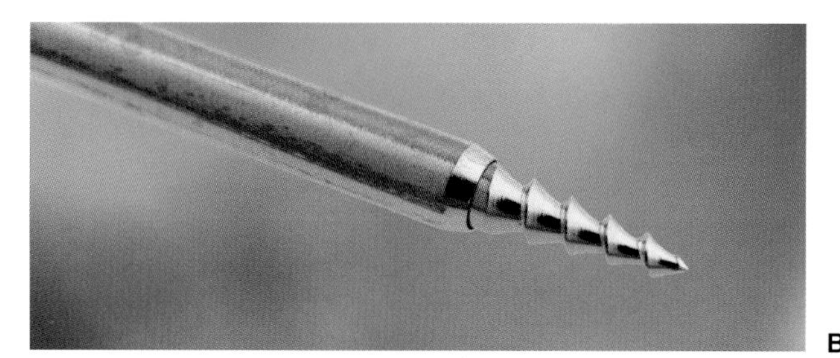

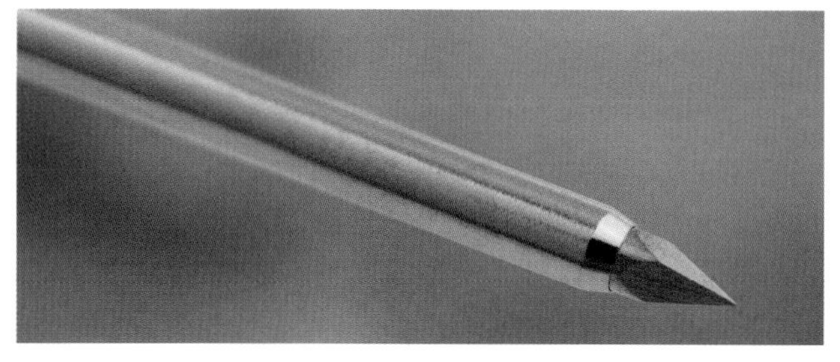

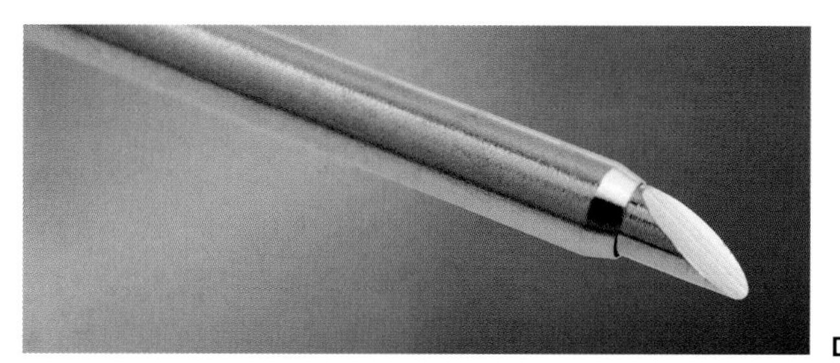

FIGURE 29–2 (A) Standard spinal intervention patient prep tray. Images of different inner stylets that can fit through the vertebroplasty needle, including screw tip **(B)**, diamond point tip **(C)**, and beveled tip **(D)**.

Techniques with Relevant Radiographic Anatomy

The procedure time can vary from 30 to 120 minutes. In experienced hands, a single-level vertebroplasty should usually take no more than 45 minutes. Potential risks discussed during the informed consent process include potential extravasation of PMMA beyond the confines of the vertebral body with possible worsening pain, paralysis, loss of bowel or bladder function, and pulmonary embolism, infection, bleeding, allergies to iodinated contrast or other drugs, rib or pedicle fracture,

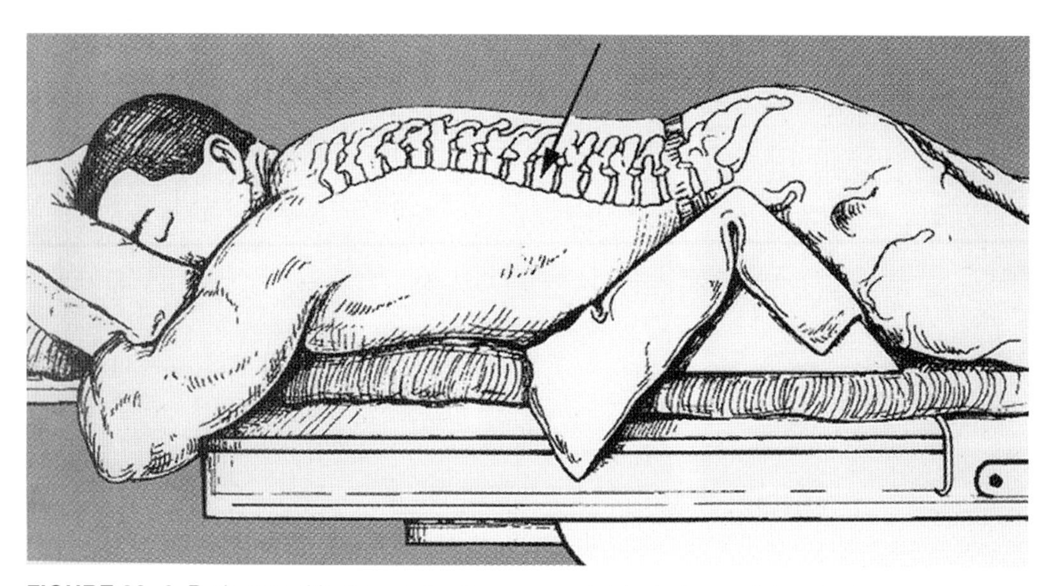

FIGURE 29–3 Patient positioning on the fluoroscopy table during vertebroplasty procedure.

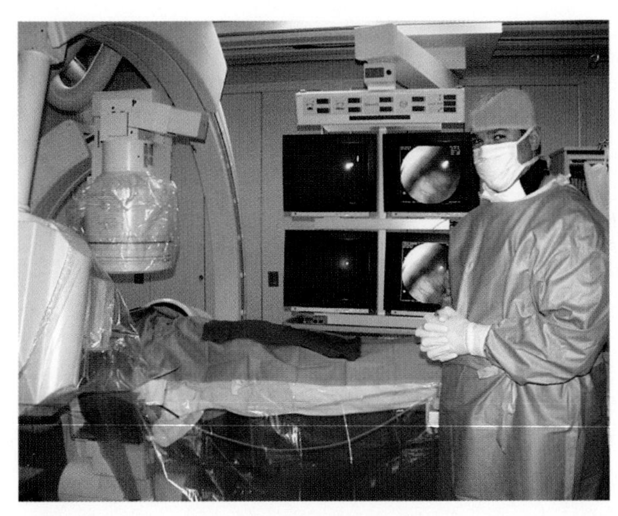

FIGURE 29–4 All involved personnel, including physicians, nurses, and technologists, are required to be sterilely dressed. The AP image intensifier and the lateral x-ray tube are also sterilely draped.

pneumothorax, dural tear with cerebrospinal fluid leak, and death.

Preoperative prophylactic antibiotics of 1.0 g of cephazolin or 500 mg of vancomycin should be given intravenously 30 minutes prior to the procedure.[16] If antibiotics are administered with the cement, 1.2 g of tobramycin powder should be added to the mixture.[10]

Pedicle Targeting

The vertebral body to be treated is isolated on both true anteroposterior (AP) and lateral planes. A single series should be obtained for reference. The pedicle to be punctured, most often the left, is isolated on the lateral plane for positioning in the inferior to superior plane and under AP oblique fluoroscopy for the lateral to medial approach. The overlying skin is marked. Strictly sterile technique is used throughout the procedure to minimize the risk of deep-seated infection. All room personnel, including physicians, nurses, and technologists, are required to don surgical masks and hats prior to patient prepping and opening of sterile trays and equipment. AP image intensifier and lateral tube should be sterilely draped (Fig. 29–4). A simple "bull's-eye" approach to the pedicle can be used for both straight AP and AP oblique approaches. In the straight AP approach, the needle tip is positioned in the midportion of the ipsilateral pedicle and advanced gradually until the needle tip ends in the anterior one third of the vertebral body. With this approach, the PMMA delivered will usually stay on the ipsilateral hemivertebra and will not adequately cross midline into the contralateral hemivertebra, and a contralateral transpediculate needle placement and PMMA injection will be required (Fig. 29–5A,B). If the pedicle is visualized in the more AP oblique, "Scottie-dog" view, then the needle track will start more lateral to the superior articular facet and pass through the pedicle in a steeper lateral-to-medial course.[3] The final positioning of the tip of the needle will therefore be more anterior and near the midline and will likely allow for a single transpediculate injection that will fill most of the vertebral body, obviating the need for a contralateral needle puncture (Fig. 29–6A,B). The 25-gauge spinal needle used for induction of local anesthesia can also

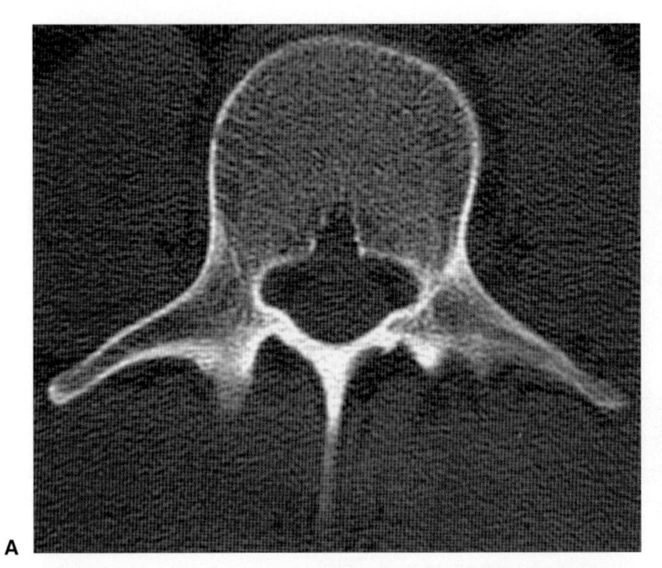

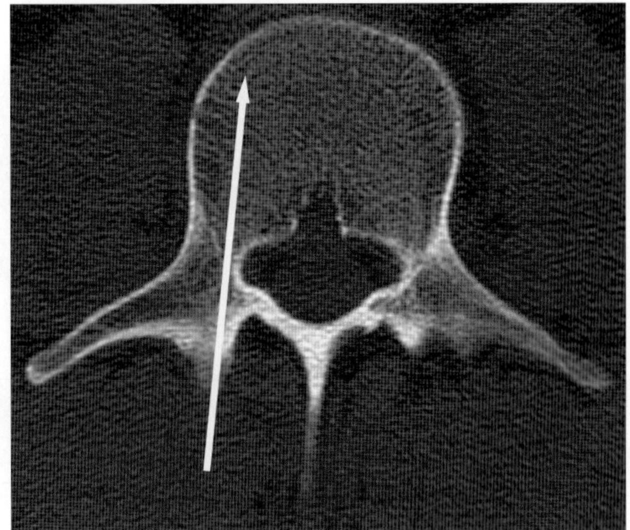

FIGURE 29–5 Axial radiographs of a spine model. **(A)** Using AP projection, the outline of the pediculate cortex is distinct, and the "bull's-eye" lucent needle track can be seen. **(B)** Needle advancement in AP projection results in the needle tip in the anterior one third and midportion of the right hemivertebra and adequate filling of the contralateral left hemivertebra is not likely.

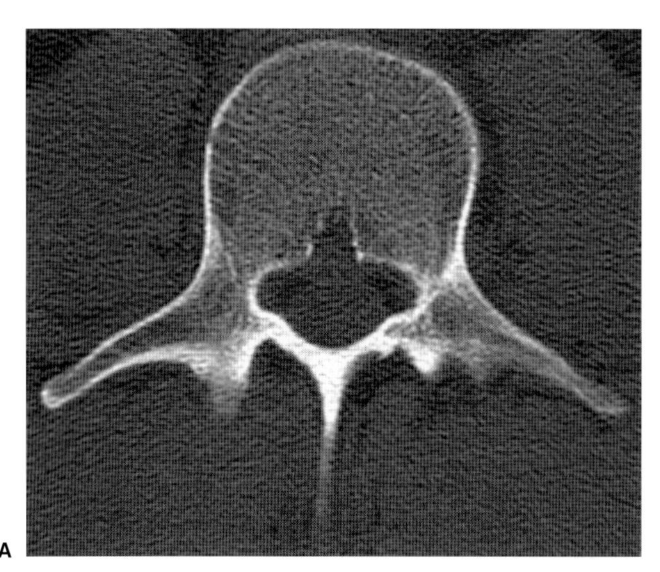

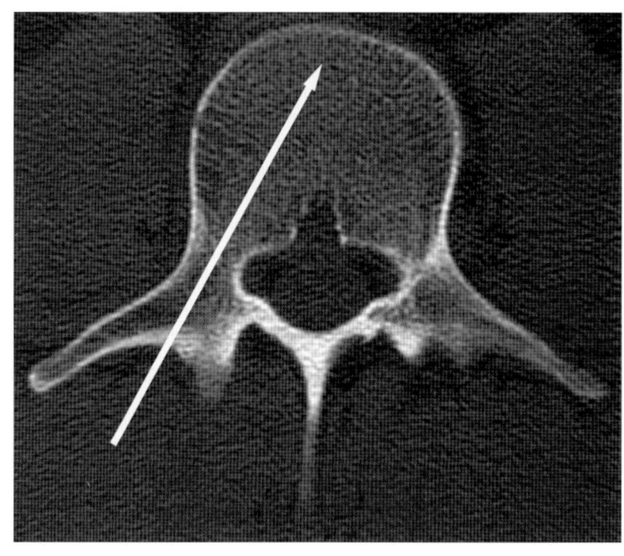

FIGURE 29–6 Axial radiographs of a spine model. **(A)** From the AP oblique position, the pediculate cortex is less distinct but adequate. **(B)** Needle advancement guided by this projection is better for bihemispheric filling. Note midline and more anterior location of the needle tip.

aid in correct tube positioning prior to introduction of the vertebroplasty needle (Fig. 29–7). A small skin dermatotomy is made with a scalpel, and the needle is advanced through the pedicle under biplane fluoroscopic guidance.

Intraosseous Venography (Vertebrography)

After needle placement, a short extension tube is attached to the needle hub, and 2 to 5 ml of diluted contrast medium (Omnipaque 300; Nycomed, Princeton, NJ) is mixed with saline at a ratio of 1:1. Biplane digital subtraction angiography is performed at a rate of two frames per second during the contrast injection. Rapid flow of contrast into the vena cava or paravertebral veins without visibility of the vertebral bone marrow indicates communication of the needle tip with a major venous outlet and requires needle advancement.[10]

Differences of opinion and controversy exist regarding the utility of antecedent venography in improving clinical outcome or decreasing complications during vertebroplasty (Fig. 29–8). It is thought that intraosseous venography can decrease potential complications associated with incorrect or suboptimal needle placement within the basivertebral venous plexus or in direct connection with a paravertebral vein.[10] Venography can also delineate the potentially dangerous route of possible escape of PMMA cement outside the confines of the vertebral body through cortical defects and within venous structures.[17] Some studies, however, have shown no difference in efficacy, safety, or clinical outcome in patients treated with percutaneous vertebroplasty with or without venography when performed by experienced interventional neuroradiologists.[9,16,18–20]

Although venography may not augment the safety of vertebroplasty in experienced operators, it may very well guide novice or inexperienced operators to perform

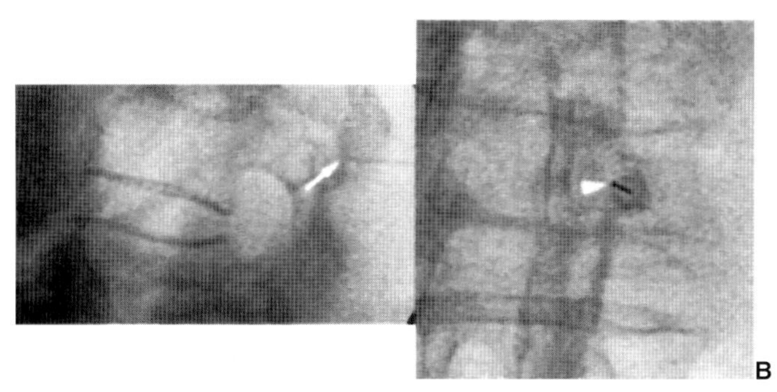

FIGURE 29–7 Lateral **(A)** and AP oblique **(B)** views showing the 25-gauge needle used for local anesthesia and the needle tip (*arrow* in A, *arrowhead* in B) in relation to the target pedicle.

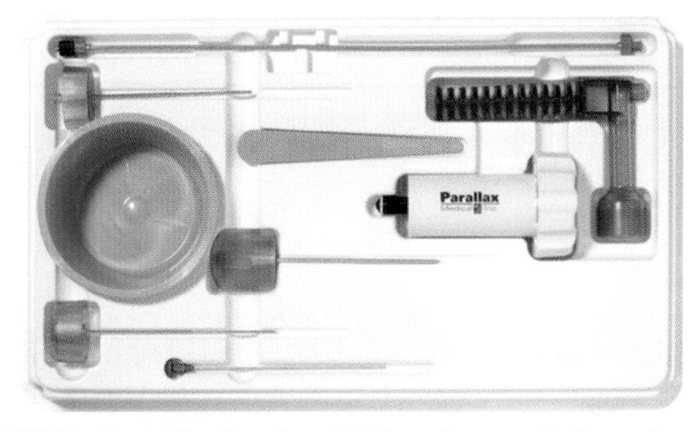

FIGURE 29–8 The Parallax EZ Flow Cement Delivery System (Parallax Inc, Mountain View, CA), which comes with needle, reservoir, twist-type plunger for injection, and high-pressure tubing.

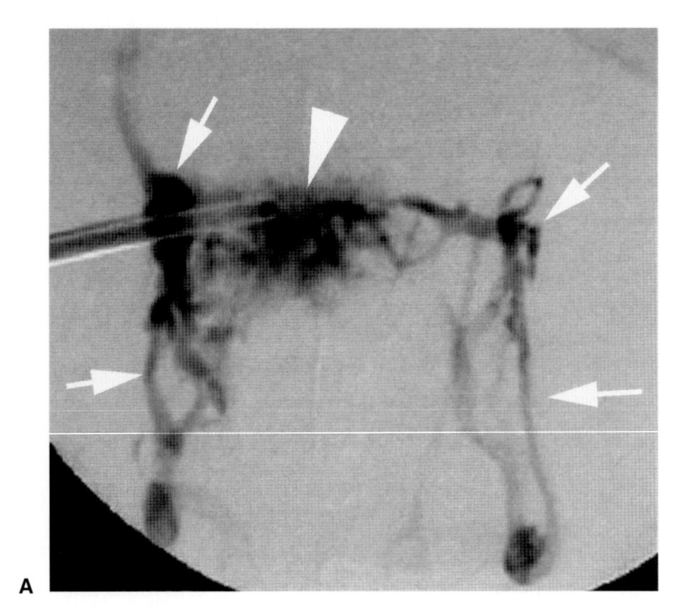

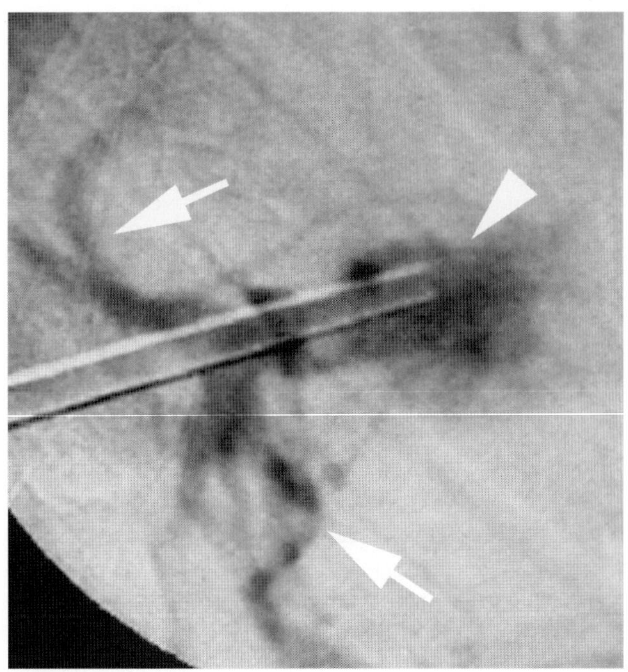

FIGURE 29–9 Intraosseous venography. Anteroposterior **(A)** and lateral **(B)** lumbar venograms demonstrate mottled spongiform trabecular opacification (*arrowhead*) prior to opacification of paravertebral veins (*arrows*).

vertebroplasty more safely. Furthermore, even though venography may not be absolutely correlated with actual extravasation of cement, the additional information provided by delineation of the venous anatomy around the vertebral body may be of benefit, especially to less-experienced physicians.[19]

Cement Opacification

Powdered PMMA polymer (CMW Laboratories, Blackpool, England) is added to 6 g of sterile barium sulfate powder (Tracers from Parallax Medical, Scotts Valley, CA) to fill the receiving cylinder to the 18 ml mark. The bottle should then be capped and shaken to disperse the barium throughout the PMMA powder. Eight milliliters of liquid PMMA monomer is then added to the PMMA polymer/barium mixture, and the cylinder is securely capped. The cylinder is shaken vigorously for 30 seconds, then placed on its side for 3 minutes to allow for adequate mixing. The PMMA mixture should be in a thin, "cake frosting" consistency prior to injection. PMMA can be injected under fluoroscopic control using 1 ml Luer-lock syringes or into a commercially available cement reservoir delivery system (E-Z Flow Cement Delivery System, Parallax Medical, Mountain View, CA; Fig. 29–9A). With this delivery system, instead of using multiple syringes, the PMMA is loaded into the barrel of the injection device, and the screw-type plunger is applied (Fig. 29–9B). The system is attached to the needle through high-pressure tubing, and each turn of the plunger delivers ~0.25 ml of PMMA material. Injection should be stopped as a rule when the cement reaches the posterior one fourth of the vertebral body on the lateral projection (Fig. 29–10), complete cement filling of an osteonecrotic cavity in Kümmell's disease (Fig. 29–11), if significant amounts of cement leak across an end-plate fracture, or with persistent filling of the epidural or paravertebral veins despite needle repositioning. The needle is removed, and the puncture site is cleaned and sterile dressed with antibiotic ointment and a large bandage.

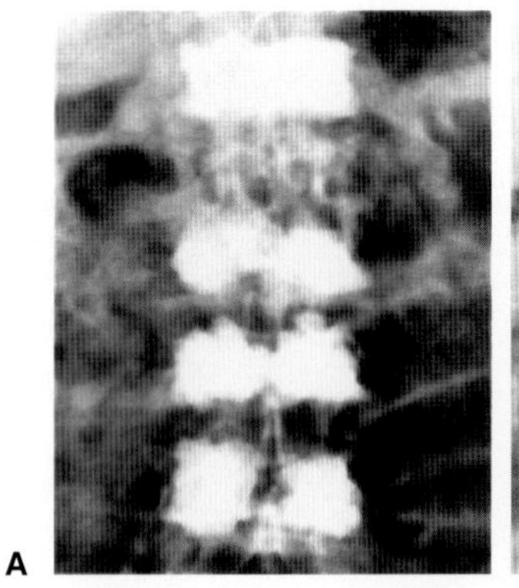

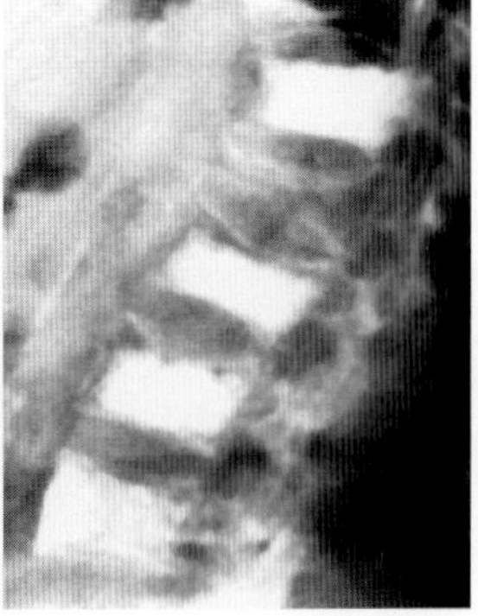

FIGURE 29–10 AP **(A)** and lateral **(B)** radiographs of the lumbar spine in a patient who developed painful compressions fractures of L1, L3, L4, and L5, which were treated on three separate sessions. The chronic compression of L2 was not tender and therefore was not treated.

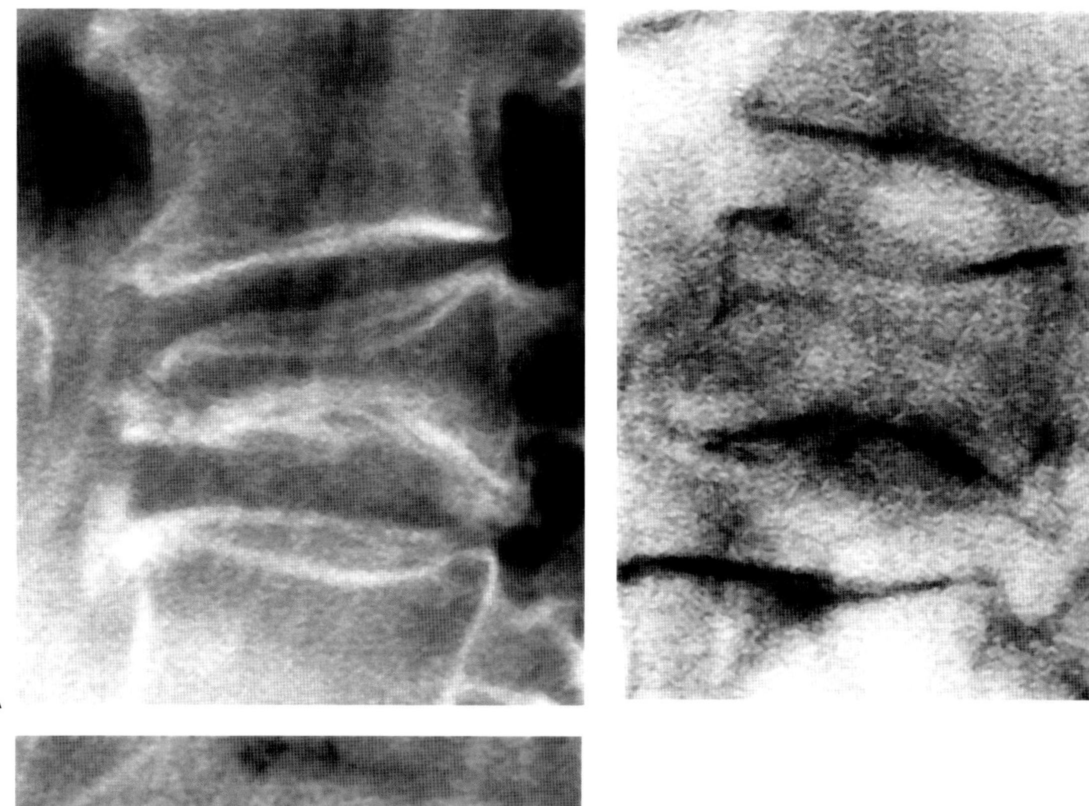

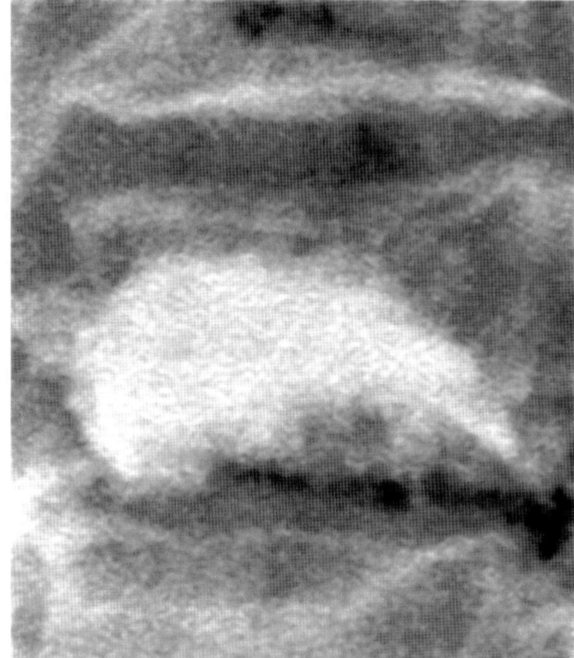

FIGURE 29–11 Lateral radiographs of painful compression fracture due to vertebral osteonecrosis with instability. Upright pretreatment film **(A)** demonstrates severe anterior wedge deformity. The compression reexpands with recumbent positioning **(B)**. Upright postvertebroplasty film **(C)** several weeks after treatment shows stabilization of fracture deformity.

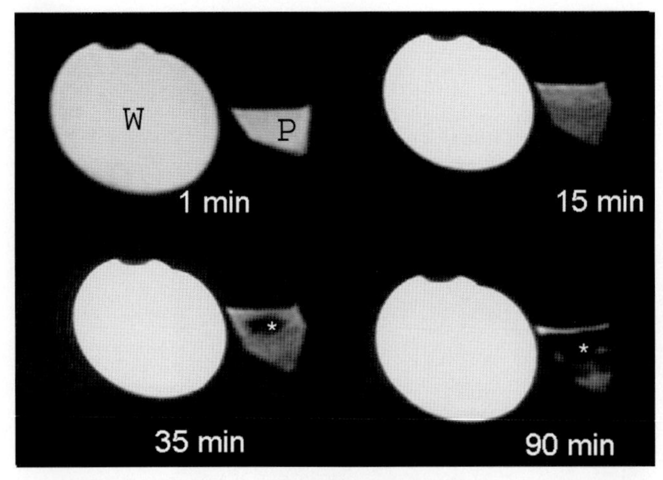

FIGURE 29–12 MRI of PMMA polymerizations. Sequential T2-weighted MRIs at 1 minute, 15 minutes, 35 minutes, and 90 minutes after preparation of PMMA mixture for injection. PMMA is hypointense to reference water signal. Note the progressive loss of signal in a centrifugal pattern at 35 and 90 minutes. PMMA = P; water = W.

Postoperative Care

After the procedure, the patient is required to remain supine for 2 hours to allow complete curing or polymerization of PMMA and for the anesthesia to wear off. In vitro MRI demonstrates that PMMA mixed for vertebroplasty begins to polymerize at 25 to 35 minutes (Fig. 29–12). Outpatients can be discharged to home under the care of a responsible adult. Inpatients should return to the ward for further observation and can be discharged home once mobile. The patient can then gradually increase activity as tolerated, with optional physical therapy and short-term use of bracing. Finally, the patient should be instructed to contact the treating physician if there is worsening pain, fever, difficulty breathing, or neurologic change.

Results

A prospective randomized trial comparing percutaneous vertebroplasty to medical therapy for acute (less than 6 weeks) osteoporotic vertebral body compression fractures is currently under way at Stanford University. The early results have been very impressive. Of the 40 patients enrolled, 21 were randomized to percutaneous vertebroplasty, and 19 were randomized to continued medical therapy. The crossover point is defined as 6 weeks from the onset of the symptomatic fracture(s). Outcome variables measured at 6 weeks are an 11-point visual analogue scale (VAS, 0–10), and 6-point activity and analgesic intake scales (0–5) (Table 29–1). All patients offered vertebroplasty had significant improvement in measured outcomes regardless of whether they were offered vertebroplasty first or after a trial of medical therapy. For the group that was offered vertebroplasty first, the mean pre- and postoutcome scores are 9.5 and 3.7 (VAS), 3.7 and 1.8 (activity), 3.8 and 1.8 (analgesic), respectively ($p < .001$). There was no significant improvement in outcomes of patients offered medical therapy. Only three out of 19 (16%) patients had mild to moderate improvement in their pain score; therefore, these patients were not offered vertebroplasty. Sixteen out of 19 (85%) patients who were randomized to medical therapy had either no improvement or worsening in their pain scores and were offered vertebroplasty. When this group was offered vertebroplasty, their outcome scores improved significantly pre- and postaugmentation: 8.7 and 2.1 (VAS), 3.3 and 1.5 (activity), 3 and 1.1 (analgesic), respectively ($p < .001$).

TABLE 29–1 Analgesic Use and Activity Level Scoring System

Score	Medication Use	Activity Level
0	No medication	Unrestricted activity
1	Aspirin, over-the-counter NSAIDs	Ambulatory with assistance
2	Physician prescribed nonnarcotic	Restricted to wheelchair use
3	Oral narcotic, as needed	Upright in bed or chair, nonmobile
4	Oral narcotic, scheduled	Flat in bed
5	Parenteral narcotic	

NSAIDs = nonsteroidal anti-inflammatory drugs.

Potential Technical Difficulties

During Pedicle Targeting

Care and caution must be used in performing the oblique, "Scottie-dog" AP view because the pediculate cortex is not as well seen as it is on the AP view. If the needle position is placed too far laterally, the transverse process may be fractured. If the target pedicle is not well seen under fluoroscopy in the AP oblique projection (due either to overlying calcific or ossific structures or to extreme osteoporosis), then the straight AP approach should be used to decrease potential misplacement of the needle.

During PMMA Injection

Cement compaction should be identified by the lack of movement of the opacified PMMA down the needle during injection and crowding of the suspended barium particles at the distal tip of the needle lumen. If injection is immediately difficult, the syringe or delivery

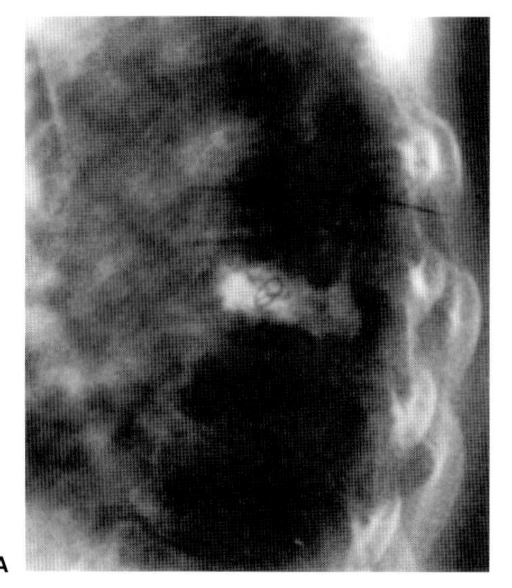

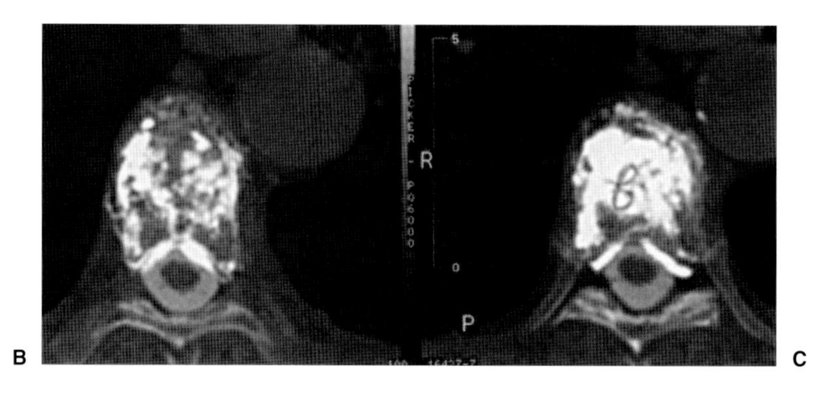

FIGURE 29–13 Untoward delivery of PMMA in a patient who developed worsening back pain several hours after vertebroplasty treatment of a thoracic compression fracture. Lateral radiograph **(A)** shows PMMA delivery posterior to the vertebral body. Posttreatment axial CT images **(B,C)** show the presence of radiopaque PMMA not only in the vertebra but also within the spinal canal, likely to be within the epidural venous plexus. There is no evidence of spinal cord compression.

system should be disconnected and evaluated for plug formation at the tip of the syringe or injection tubing. Clearing of the needle will require a plunger or stylet to push some of the cement into the vertebra. This maneuver should be done under constant fluoroscopic control. If there is continued difficulty of delivery of cement, the needle may need to be pulled back slightly and the injection tried again. Sometimes careful evaluation of cement flow pattern with comparison to intraosseous venography will aid in the detection of early venous extravasation. If adequate cement crosses the midline to the contralateral hemivertebra, a contralateral transpediculate approach is not performed.

Potential Complications

Potential complications of percutaneous vertebroplasty that have been documented include infection, bleeding, back pain, rib fracture, pneumothorax from punctured lung, fever, optic neuritis, and various other neurologic complications.[8,10,19,21–24] If any neurologic symptoms develop, a CT scan of the treated vertebra and adjacent regions should be ordered to assess for possible pedicle fracture, PMMA distribution within the vertebral body, and potential extravasation of PMMA.

Although cement extravasation will occur, it is the volume and amount of extravasation that will cause potential clinical complications. PMMA cement can escape posteriorly into the spinal canal, causing spinal canal stenosis or cord compression and potential paralysis (Fig. 29–13). PMMA extravasation to the intervertebral foramina can potentially cause nerve root compression, or to the vena cava and pulmonary arteries can potentially cause pulmonary embolism.[25] In the setting of a right-to-left cardiac shunt (e.g., patent foramen ovale or ductus arteriosus) an ischemic cerebral infarction could theoretically occur, although this has never been reported. Other reports have found transient arterial hypotension induced by PMMA injection during percutaneous vertebroplasty.[26] When reviewing all major vertebroplasty series in well-trained experienced hands, the complication rate ranges from 1 to 10%, with osteoporotic patients having ~1 to 3% complication rate, hemangioma patients having a 5% complication rate, and patients with metastases to the vertebra having a 10% complication rate.[8]

Operator injury from PMMA vapor exposure may be of concern to treating physicians and members of the treating staff, but exposures of less than 5 ppm to physicians performing vertebroplasty in a standard ventilation neuroangiography suite are considered safe.[27] The U.S. Occupational Safety and Health Administration limits for personnel are set at 100 ppm per 8-hour shift. Finally, toxicities of PMMA in nonvertebroplasty procedures and from experimental animal models have shown PMMA to cause decreased pulmonary function, decrease in systemic arterial blood pressure, and acute bronchospasm.[28–30] PMMA use in hip arthroplasty has been associated with cardiovascular derangement, but no generalized association has been found between

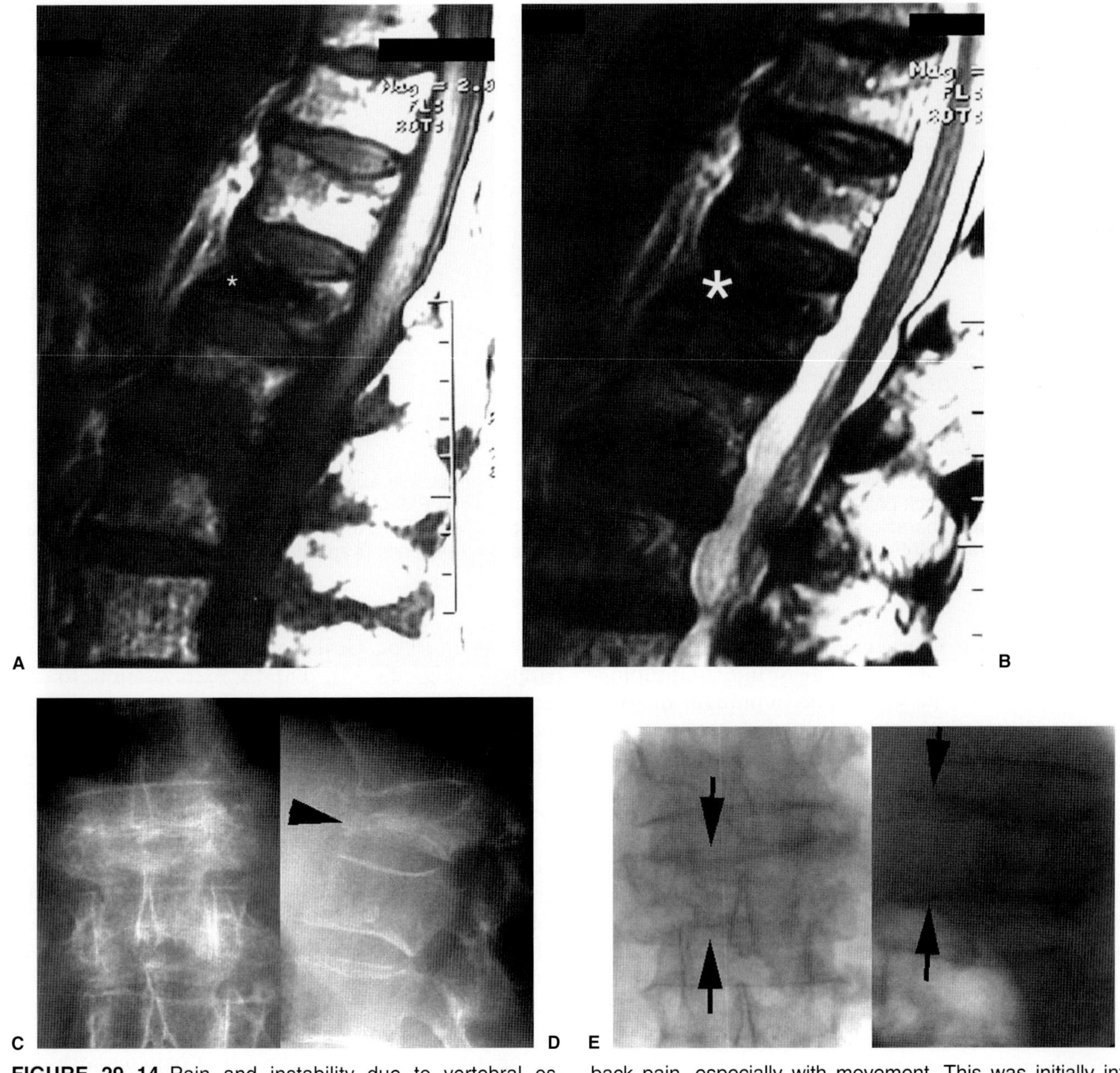

FIGURE 29–14 Pain and instability due to vertebral osteonecrosis (Kummel's disease). Sagittal T1-weighted **(A)** and T2-weighted **(B)** MRIs from an outside study show marked hypointense signal (asterisk) within a seemingly partially compressed L1 vertebra in this patient with severe back pain, especially with movement. This was initially interpreted as chronic compression fracture with sclerosis; however, subsequent plain films in upright weight-bearing **(C,D)** and recumbent non-weight-bearing positions **(E,F)** reveal that the MRI hypointense signal actually represents gas.

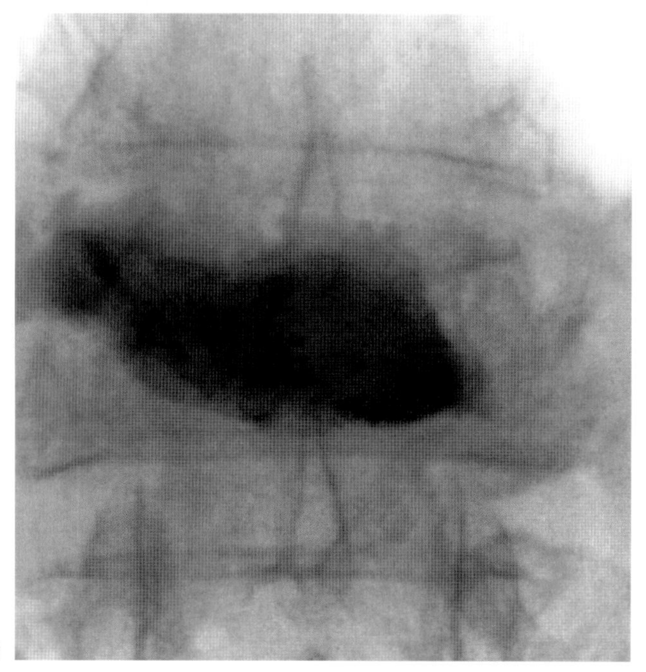

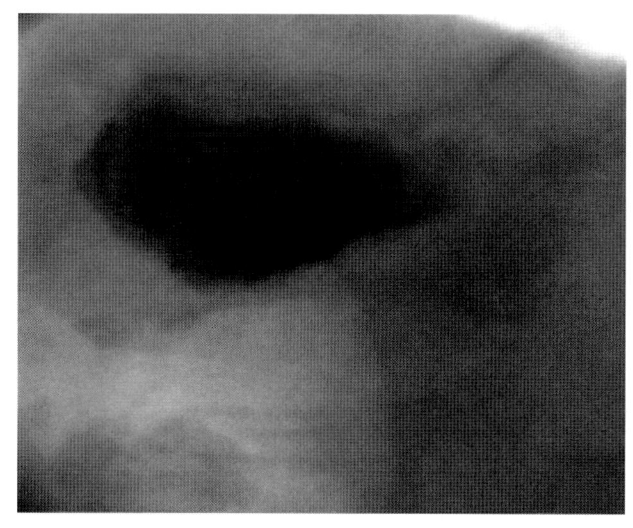

FIGURE 29–14 (*Continued*) Note the severe compressive change of the vertebra on upright films (*arrowhead* in D), which expands to near normal on prone films (*arrows* in E and F). Postvertebroplasty images in the upright weight-bearing position show stabilization of fracture **(G,H)**.

PMMA use in percutaneous vertebroplasty and cardiovascular derangement.[31]

Avoidance

Events to be wary of include patients on warfarin, which should be discontinued prior to the procedure and then switched to heparin. Patients with elevated white blood cell counts that indicate a possible infection should wait until the cause is diagnosed and treated. The patient's primary care physician should be consulted regarding corticosteroid use to discuss decreasing or ceasing its use. In patients with atypical back pain, one should consider other potential rare causes (e.g., a perforated ulcer).

Complications are most commonly associated with:

- Inappropriate patient selection and poor patient cooperation
- Poor visualization because of inadequate fluoroscopic equipment
- Unsatisfactory cement opacification
- Operator error resulting from lack of knowledge of radiographic spinal anatomy, particularly the bony and venous anatomy
- Poor fluoroscopic triangulation skills and embolization technique
- Unfamiliarity with the equipment, devices, and PMMA
- Lack of patient monitoring
- Improper nonsterile technique

Case Illustrations

Case 1 is a patient with painful compression fracture due to osteoporosis complicated by vertebral osteonecrosis (Fig. 29–14). The necrotic gas-filled intraosseous cavity was interpreted on an outside MRI as consistent with chronic compression fracture due to very low intensity signal on both T1- and T2-weighted images. This unstable fracture was only diagnosed by comparing the change in vertebral body heights on weight-bearing and recumbent views. Vertebroplasty treatment of this fracture resulted in complete pain relief and resumption of normal daily activities 2 days postprocedure.

Case 2 is a patient with known breast carcinoma metastasis to L4 vertebral body 8 years ago. At that time, the focal tumor deposit was treated with surgical partial corpectomy, followed by PMMA packing of the resultant surgical cavity. The patient was pain free until she presented with new onset of pain in the same level and with MRI evidence of recurrent tumor. This level was successfully treated with percutaneous PMMA injection and resulted in complete pain relief (Fig. 29–15).

Percutaneous transpediculate vertebroplasty is an innovative and beneficial treatment option for painful osteoporotic and pathologic compression fractures

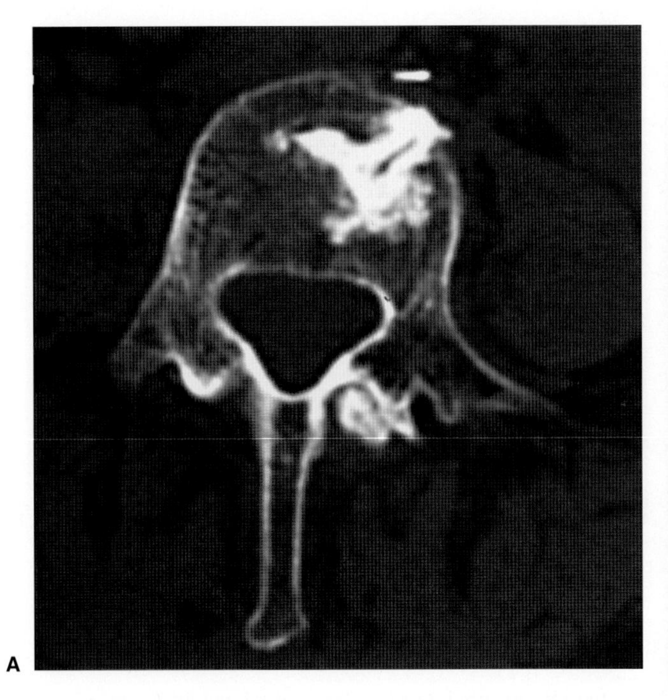

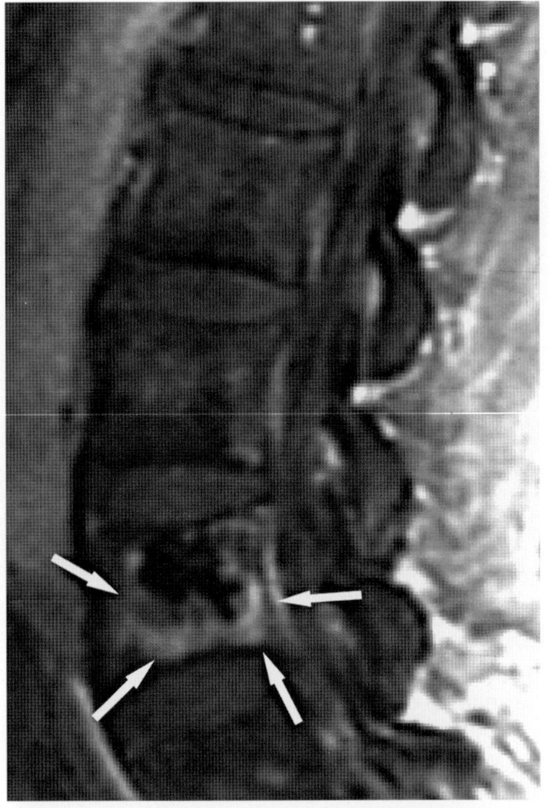

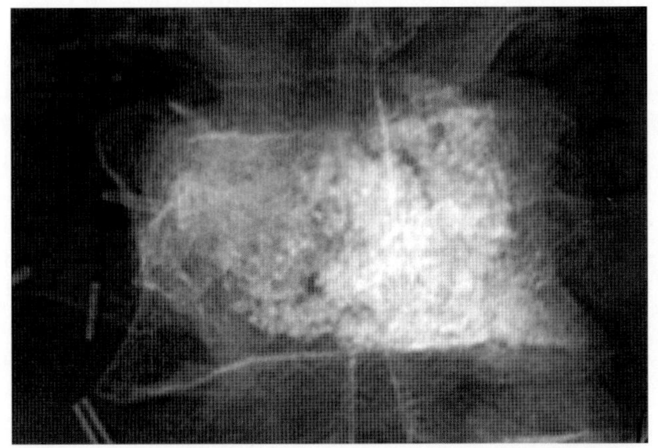

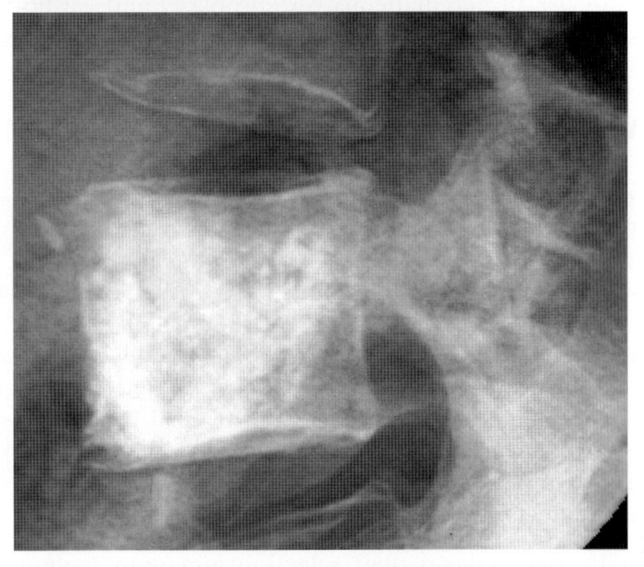

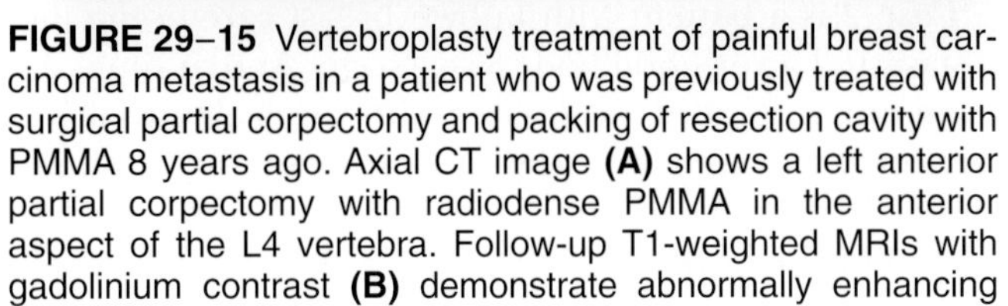

FIGURE 29–15 Vertebroplasty treatment of painful breast carcinoma metastasis in a patient who was previously treated with surgical partial corpectomy and packing of resection cavity with PMMA 8 years ago. Axial CT image **(A)** shows a left anterior partial corpectomy with radiodense PMMA in the anterior aspect of the L4 vertebra. Follow-up T1-weighted MRIs with gadolinium contrast **(B)** demonstrate abnormally enhancing tumor surrounding the surgically placed PMMA, which appears marked hypointense (dark) on all MRI sequences. Postvertebroplasty AP **(C)** and lateral **(D)** radiographs of the L4 vertebra show good filling of the vertebra with PMMA. The patient was symptom free several hours posttreatment, and she underwent additional radiotherapy to this region without complications.

that are refractory to medical therapy. Large clinical series have shown that vertebroplasty can provide significant pain relief with a very low complication rate. With the accumulation of scientific data, technological advances, and acceptance by the general community, vertebroplasty may become the standard of care for treatment of painful vertebral body compression fractures.

REFERENCES

1. Riggs BL, Melton LJ III. The worldwide problem of osteoporosis: insights afforded by epidemiology. *Bone.* 1995;17:505S–511S.
2. Melton LJ III. Epidemiology of spinal osteoporosis. *Spine.* 1997; 22:2S–11S.
3. Jensen ME, Dion JE. Percutaneous vertebroplasty in the treatment of osteoporotic compression fractures. *Neuroimaging Clin N Am.* 2000; 10:547–568.
4. Ross PD. Clinical consequences of vertebral fractures. *Am J Med.* 1997;103:30S–42S.
5. Eastell R, Cedel SL, Wahner HW, et al. Classification of vertebral fractures. *J Bone Miner Res.* 1991;6:207–215.
6. Galibert P, Deramond H, Rosat P, et al. Preliminary note on the treatment of vertebral angioma by percutaneous acrylic vertebroplasty. *Neurochirurgie.* 1987;33:166–168.
7. Cotten A, Dewatre F, Cortet B, et al. Percutaneous vertebroplasty for osteolytic metastases and myeloma: effects of the percentage of lesion filling and the leakage of methyl methacrylate at clinical follow-up. *Radiology.* 1996;200:525–530.
8. Deramond H, Depriester C, Galibert P, et al. Percutaneous vertebroplasty with polymethylmethacrylate. *Radiol Clin North Am.* 1998; 36:533–546.
9. Weill A, Chiras J, Simon J, et al. Spinal metastases: indications for and results of percutaneous injection of acrylic surgical cement. *Radiology.* 1996;199:241–247.
10. Jensen ME, Evans AJ, Mathis JM, et al. Percutaneous polymethylmethacrylate vertebroplasty in the treatment of osteoporotic vertebral body compression fractures: technical aspects. *Am J Neuroradiol.* 1997;18:1897–1904.
11. Cyteval C, Baron Sarrabere MP, Rouz JO, et al. Acute osteoporotic vertebral collapse: open study on percutaneous injection of acrylic surgical cement in 20 patients. *Am J Roentgenol.* 1999;173:1685–1690.
12. Debussche-Depriester C, Deramond H, Fardellone P, et al. Percutaneous vertebroplasty with acrylic cement in the treatment of osteoporotic vertebral crush fracture syndrome. *Neuroradiology.* 1991; 33:149–152.
13. Depriester C, Deramond H, Toussaint P, et al. Percutaneous vertebroplasty: indications, technique, and complications. In: Connors JJ III, Wojak JC, eds. *Interventional Neuroradiology: Strategies and Practical Techniques.* Philadelphia: WB Saunders; 1999; 347–357.
14. Gangi A, Dietemann JL, Guth S, et al. Computed tomography (CT) and fluoroscopy-guided vertebroplasty: results and complications in 187 patients. *Semin Intervent Radiol.* 1999;16:137–142.
15. Rami PM, McGraw JK, Heatwole EV, et al. Percutaneous vertebroplasty in the treatment of vertebral body compression fracture secondary to osteogenesis imperfecta. *Skeletal Radiol.* 2002;31:162–165.
16. Mathis JM, Barr JD, Belkoff SM, et al. Percutaneous vertebroplasty: a developing standard of care for vertebral compression fractures. *Am J Neuroradiol.* 2001;22:373–381.
17. McGraw JK, Heatwole EV, Strand BT, et al. Predictive value of intraosseous venography before percutaneous vertebroplasty. *J Vasc Interv Radiol.* 2002;13:149–153.
18. Gangi A, Kastler B, Dietemann JL. Percutaneous vertebroplasty guided by a combination of CT and fluoroscopy. *Am J Neuroradiol.* 1994;15:83–86.
19. Gaughen JR, Jensen ME, Schweickert PA, Kaufmann TJ, Marx WF, Kallmes DF. Relevance of antecedent venography in percutaneous vertebroplasty for treatment of osteoporotic compression fractures. *Am J Neuroradiol.* 2002;23(4):594–600.
20. Vasconcelos C, Gailloud P, Beuchamp NJ, et al. Is percutaneous vertebroplasty without pretreatment venography safe? Evaluation of 205 consecutive procedures. *Am J Neuroradiol.* 2002;23:913–917.
21. Barr JD, Barr MS, Lemley TJ, Mc Cann RM. Percutaneous vertebroplasty for pain relief and spinal stabilization. *Spine.* 2000;25: 923–928.
22. Padovani B, Kasriel O, Brunner P, et al. Pulmonary embolism caused by acrylic cement: a rare complication of percutaneous vertebroplasty. *Am J Neuroradiol.* 1999;20:375–377.
23. Harrington KD. Major neurological complications following percutaneous vertebroplasty with polymethylmethacrylate: a case report. *J Bone Joint Surg Am.* 2001;83:1070–1073.
24. Lee BJ, Lee SR, Yoo TY. Paraplegia as a complication of percutaneous vertebroplasty with polymethylmethacrylate: a case report. *Spine.* 2002;27:E419–E422.
25. Jang JS, Lee SH, Jung SK. Pulmonary embolism of polymethylmethacrylate after percutaneous vertebroplasty: a report of three cases. *Spine.* 2002;27:E416–E418.
26. Vasconcelos C, Gailloud P, Martin JB, et al. Transient arterial hypotension induced by polymethylmethacrylate injection during percutaneous vertebroplasty. *J Vasc Interv Radiol.* 2001;12:1001–1002.
27. Cloft HJ, Easton DN, Jensen ME, et al. Exposure of medical personnel to methylmethacrylate vapor during percutaneous vertebroplasty. *Am J Neuroradiol.* 1999;20:352–353.
28. Phillips H, Cole PV, Letton AW. Cardiovascular effects of implanted acrylic bone cement. *BMJ.* 1971;3:460–461.
29. Wong HY, Vidovich MI. Acute bronchospasm associated with polymethylmethacrylate cement. *Anesthesiology.* 1997;87:696–698.
30. Convery FR, Gunn DR, Hughes JD, Martin WE. The relative safety of polymethylmethacrylate: a controlled clinical study of randomly selected patients treated with Charnley and ring total hip replacements. *J Bone Joint Surg Am.* 1975;57:57–64.
31. Kaufmann T, Jensen M, Ford G, et al. Cardiovascular effects of polymethylmethacrylate use in percutaneous vertebroplasty. *Am J Neuroradiol.* 2002;23:601–604.

30

Kyphoplasty

CHRISTOPHER M. BONO AND STEVEN R. GARFIN

Methods of reduction and internal stabilization of spine fractures typically require extensive open procedures. With a growing demand for minimally invasive methods, an interest in percutaneous techniques of fracture reduction and fixation has arisen. Kyphoplasty has been developed for the treatment of painful osteoporotic compression fractures of the thoracic and lumbar spine. Using an inflatable balloon tamp inserted into the vertebral body, anterior height loss in a compressed segment can be restored and maintained with the insertion of methacrylate cement.[1,2] This technique offers a unique option to patients who would otherwise be managed with prolonged nonoperative care or by extensive open anteroposterior surgery.[3–5]

Fractures at multiple levels can result in progressive anterior column shortening and thoracolumbar kyphosis. This can potentiate disability, lung dysfunction, and eating disorders by decreasing thoracic and abdominal volumes, especially in the elderly.[6–9] Because of this, interest in a minimally invasive method of kyphosis correction has gained attention. Preliminary clinical data indicate consistent restoration of vertebral height in addition to durable pain relief in 90% of cases with low complication rates.[1,10]

Kyphoplasty is not limited to the treatment of osteoporotic vertebral compression fractures (VCFs). It has been used to stabilize pathologic fractures secondary to multiple myeloma, and it may be indicated for metastatic tumors as well.[11–13] With continuing advances in bioresorbable materials, the procedure will likely have a place in the future treatment of traumatic vertebral fractures in normal bone.

Indications

The clinical indications of kyphoplasty are (1) treatment of painful osteoporotic VCFs, (2) restoration of height loss and correction of kyphosis secondary to VCFs, and (3) pain relief from neoplastic lytic bone lesions that do not require excision.

Osteoporotic Pain Relief

The primary indication for kyphoplasty is the relief of pain related to osteoporotic VCFs. Although deformity correction (i.e., vertebral height restoration) is achievable in more acute fractures, it should be considered a secondary benefit. A patient with a nonpainful, static deformity associated with osteoporotic VCFs should not be considered an operative candidate unless kyphosis is rapidly progressive. In most cases, however, this is associated with intractable pain. Vertebral augmentation, either kyphoplasty or vertebroplasty, can relieve pain in more than 90% of patients treated.[1,14–16] The most likely mechanism of pain relief is fracture stabilization, although some experts believe the exothermic effects of methacrylate curing can "denervate" the vertebral body.

Optimal results with kyphoplasty rely on a careful physical examination and correlative imaging studies to identify the most symptomatic level(s). Systematic percussion of the spinous processes can localize pain to a particular level, which can then be marked with a radiopaque marker before plain radiographs are made. This information should be considered along with results of MRI of the spine, which can display increased T2 signal in acutely fractured vertebrae.[17] STIR images are helpful in differentiating fracture from tumor, which may be difficult based on plain films and clinical history alone. If MRI is not possible, a CT and bone scan can be used as an alternative to determine the most acute level.[18]

Osteoporotic Kyphosis

Kyphoplasty is a deformity-correcting procedure; however, the presence of a compressed vertebral body is not an automatic indication for kyphoplasty. Spinal balance must be considered, as with other deformity operations. Because the osteoporotic spine is usually rigid, bending films are of limited utility. Long plate anteroposterior and lateral views are essential in evaluating the location of the weight-bearing line. In older fractures, kyphoplasty may have minimal effects on correcting balance, whereas acute fractures are more amenable to restoration. Further investigation is required to demonstrate a positive balance between the potential benefits of kyphosis correction versus procedural risks more clearly.

Kyphosis is quantitated using the Cobb method. Extrapolating from recommendations for Scheuermann's disease, correction might be warranted for curves of 75 to 80 degrees or those that do not correct to less than 50 degrees. Considering the percutaneous nature of kyphoplasty with minimal morbidity, smaller curves might be considered if spinal balance is compromised. Fracture risk increases after an intitial VCF.[19–21] The surgeon must consider the projected amount of kyphosis that the patient is likely to exhibit in his or her lifetime. Furthermore, rigid deformities from multiple healed fractures might be better addressed by other procedures. Restoring spinal balance may help reduce fracture risk, although this remains to be demonstrated in a prospective clinical investigation.

VCFs and kyphosis can negatively affect pulmonary function, especially in the elderly patient.[9,22] Schlaich et al[9] demonstrated a strong correlation between the severity of kyphosis and compromise of measured lung capacity. In addition, mortality rates associated with pulmonary complications are significantly higher in patients with kyphotic VCFs than they are in those without deformity.[22] Such procedures as kyphoplasty that can either arrest or correct kyphosis secondary to osteoporotic VCFs would therefore be useful. Further study to determine if deformity correction can reverse these negative effects is required.

Lytic Bone Tumors

Kyphoplasty is indicated in the management of pain associated with lytic lesions of the vertebral body secondary to neoplastic processes. Experience treating multiple myeloma lesions in the spine has been encouraging.[13] The procedure may also be involved in the treatment of metastatic tumors. The best results can be expected when one or two symptomatic lesions can be localized in patients without neurologic compromise. Preoperative imaging should confirm that the posterior vertebral body is not disrupted to avoid cement extrusion or balloon tamp blowout into the spinal canal.

Contraindications

Kyphoplasty should not be performed in stable, healed, painless fractures. Bleeding abnormalities, either intrinsic or pharmacologic, must be corrected preoperatively to avoid epidural hematoma formation, particularly if the pedicle cortex or posterior vertebral body has been penetrated. Although we do not routinely perform kyphoplasty on osteoporotic burst fractures because of concern of posterior cement extrusion, it may have a role in select cases with minimal to no canal compromise in a neurologically intact patient. Other fracture patterns, (e.g., vertebra plana) make it difficult or impossible to cannulate the vertebral body.

Operating Room Setup

Both general and local anesthesia can be used. It is the authors' preference to use general anesthesia for patients undergoing multilevel procedures. Local with sedation is suitable for one-segment procedures with the advantage of the ability to monitor neurologic status intraoperatively. The disadvantage of local anesthesia is discomfort sometimes experienced during cannulation of the pedicle and the need for the awake patient, who is often elderly, to remain absolutely still throughout the procedure.

With either anesthesia type, the patient is positioned prone on a radiolucent table, carefully protecting all pressure points. Transverse rolls under the chest and thighs help extend the spine and fracture reduction. A radiolucent Jackson table or a Kambin frame can be used as an alternative. For work at the L1 level and above, the arms should be tucked at the sides to allow access for the image intensifier (C-arm). Before starting the procedure, it is imperative that an adequate lateral can be obtained because the arms can sometimes obscure the view of the spine.

One or two C-arms can be used. If two machines are used, they must be adjusted so that the PA and lateral views can be taken at the same time (Fig. 30–1). The PA machine must be raised up enough to allow the surgeon ample room to place the instruments. A single C-arm can be used successfully, but it requires frequent moves to see both the posteroanterior (PA) and the lateral images.

The PA view should be adjusted so that the pedicle "halo" is clearly seen. Although this is more easily afforded on a PA view in the thoracic spine, medial pedicle angulation in the lumbar spine may be better seen with the "en face" view. This is achieved by angling the beam 10 degrees toward the midline. During each step of pedicle cannulation, the instruments should be perfectly centered within the pedicle on the en face view.

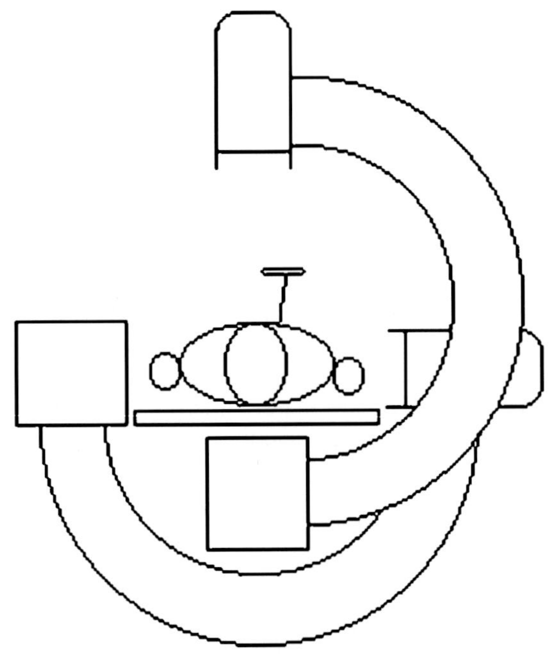

FIGURE 30–1 Two C-arms are optimally used. This allows simultaneous PA and lateral fluoroscopic views.

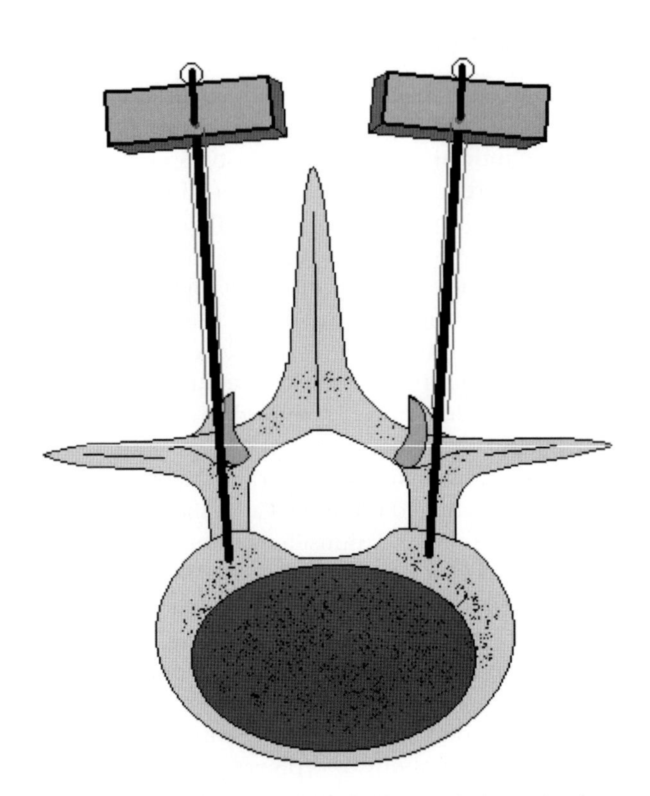

FIGURE 30–2 The transpedicular technique is the most commonly used approach.

Once adequate radiographic visualization is confirmed, the patient is prepped and draped in the usual sterile fashion.

Surgical Technique

Transpedicular Approach

The most often used approach for kyphoplasty, the transpedicular approach, can be used from T8 to L5 and requires a pedicle diameter of at least 4 to 5 mm (Fig. 30–2). In the upper thoracic spine, the pedicles usually are too thin to safely accept the instruments, making other approaches (extrapedicular, see later) a better choice. This determination should be made preoperatively based on CT or MRI axial image measurement. Structures endangered using the transpedicular technique are the spinal cord or cauda equina medially, the nerve root superiorly and inferiorly, and in the thoracic spine the pulmonary cavity laterally. If the anterior vertebral body is violated, which may occur in any of the three approaches, the great vessels may be injured.

The midline is marked by palpation, and the correct vertebral level is identified using the C-arm. Using the PA view, a Jamshidi needle or guide pin is introduced through the skin just lateral to the lateral pedicle border. The instrument is advanced to the bone at approximately a 10-degree angle toward the midline. Once the bone can be felt with the needle, orthogonal images confirm proper orientation. On the lateral it should be aligned with the midline of the pedicle. On the PA view, it should appear to be just medial to the lateral border of the pedicle halo, remembering that the halo represents the pedicle waist, which is anterior and medial to the point of needle entry. The needle tip should be within the confines of the pedicle at all times.

The appropriate starting point is crucial. With this confirmed, the instrument is advanced through the pedicle and into the vertebral body. In severely osteoporotic patients, this can be difficult to discern because of poor bone quality, making frequent C-arm images necessary. The Jamshidi is advanced to just beyond the junction of the vertebral body and pedicle. In this position, the needle may appear medial to the pedicle on the PA view. Although this appearance is acceptable, the tip should not cross the midline on this view at any point during insertion. If it does, the surgeon must try to determine if the medial pedicle cortex has been breached. If doubt exists, the instrument should be repositioned until safe placement is confirmed.

Because the instruments' diameters are generally smaller than the pedicle dimensions, they may be slightly cranially or caudally directed to target a particular region of the fractured vertebra. For instance, the device is directed toward the inferior vertebral body in a

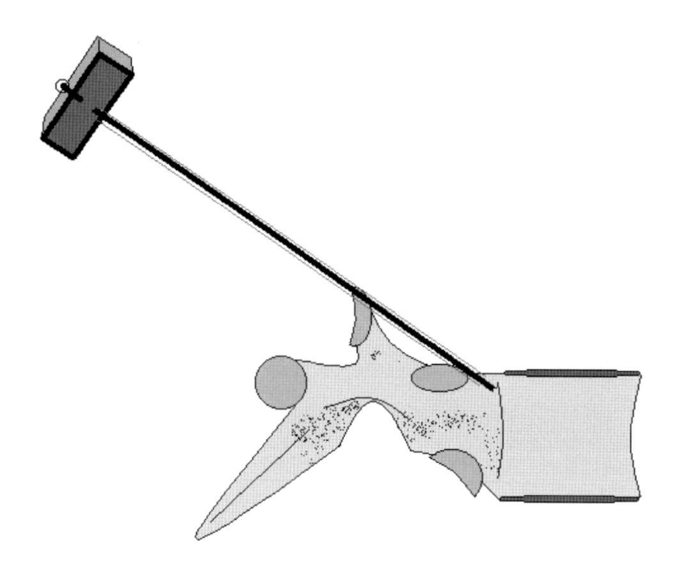

FIGURE 30–3 The extrapedicular approach utilizes the interval between the rib and the pedicle. Optimal placement is obtained by starting at the posterosuperior aspect of the vertebral body, aiming for the anteroinferior aspect.

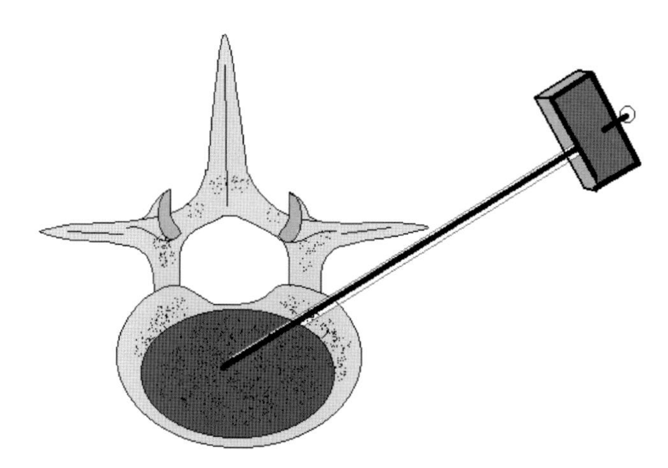

FIGURE 30–4 The PA technique utilizes a "diskogram" type of approach aimed toward the midportion of the vertebral body. It risks injury to the segmental vessel and the exiting nerve roots.

superior end-plate fracture. This places more cancellous bone between the inflatable tamp and the injured end plate. With uniform vertebral body compression, the tools are directed toward the midaspect.

Extrapedicular Approach

The extrapedicular approach should be used in thoracic vertebrae with pedicles too small to accept the kyphoplasty tools. Because it employs the interval between the pedicle and the rib, it is not an option in the lumbar spine. Under C-arm guidance, the Jamshidi needle is inserted just lateral and superior to the pedicle on the PA view (Fig. 30–3). On the lateral view, it should be centered within the pedicle, although anatomically it will be lateral to it. On the PA view, the needle should appear to enter the bone at the superolateral aspect of the vertebral body, aiming inferomedially (~20 degrees) toward the spinous process. On the lateral view, it is directed toward the anteroinferior aspect of the vertebral body. The spinal cord is at less risk with a more lateral starting position than the transpedicular approach, although it may still be injured with medial misplacement. Lateral deviation risks pneumothorax, which may not be detected until high-quality postoperative plain radiographs are taken. Lateral vertebral body violation can injure the segmental artery, great vessels, or lungs.

Posterolateral Approach

The posterolateral approach for kyphoplasty can be used in the L2 to L4 vertebrae. The bone is entered through the posterolateral cortex, anterior to the transverse process. Although the transpedicular and lateral extrapedicular approaches can be used bilaterally, the posterolateral technique is a unilateral approach. The needle trajectory is similar to that for a diskogram, except that it is aligned with the vertebral body instead of the disk (Fig. 30–4). Skin entry is 8 to 10 cm lateral to the midline, with the needle directed ~45 degrees toward the midline. The PA view should confirm that the needle is confined to the borders of the vertebral body, optimally positioned within the center of the bone. The lateral view ensures that the needle tip does not pass anterior or posterior to the vertebral body, which can have disastrous sequelae. With proper placement, the instruments pass anterior to the transverse process and the neural foramen, avoiding injury to the exiting nerve root. Dangers encountered with this approach include injury to the nerve root if the needle is not anterior to the transverse process. Anterior or posterior migration can injure the great vessels or cauda equina, respectively. Passage of the instruments through the psoas muscle can injure components of the lumbar plexus. It is best if the patient is awake during this technique to help avoid transecting the nerve roots because the patient can vocalize leg pain during the procedure.

Bone Tamp Insertion

The center stylet of the Jamshidi needle is removed, and a flexible guidewire is inserted. Holding the guidewire in place, the Jamshidi is removed from the body. C-arm images should confirm maintenance of wire orientation. An initial dilator is passed over the guidewire and advanced to the junction of the vertebral body and pedicle. This must be performed with frequent lateral images

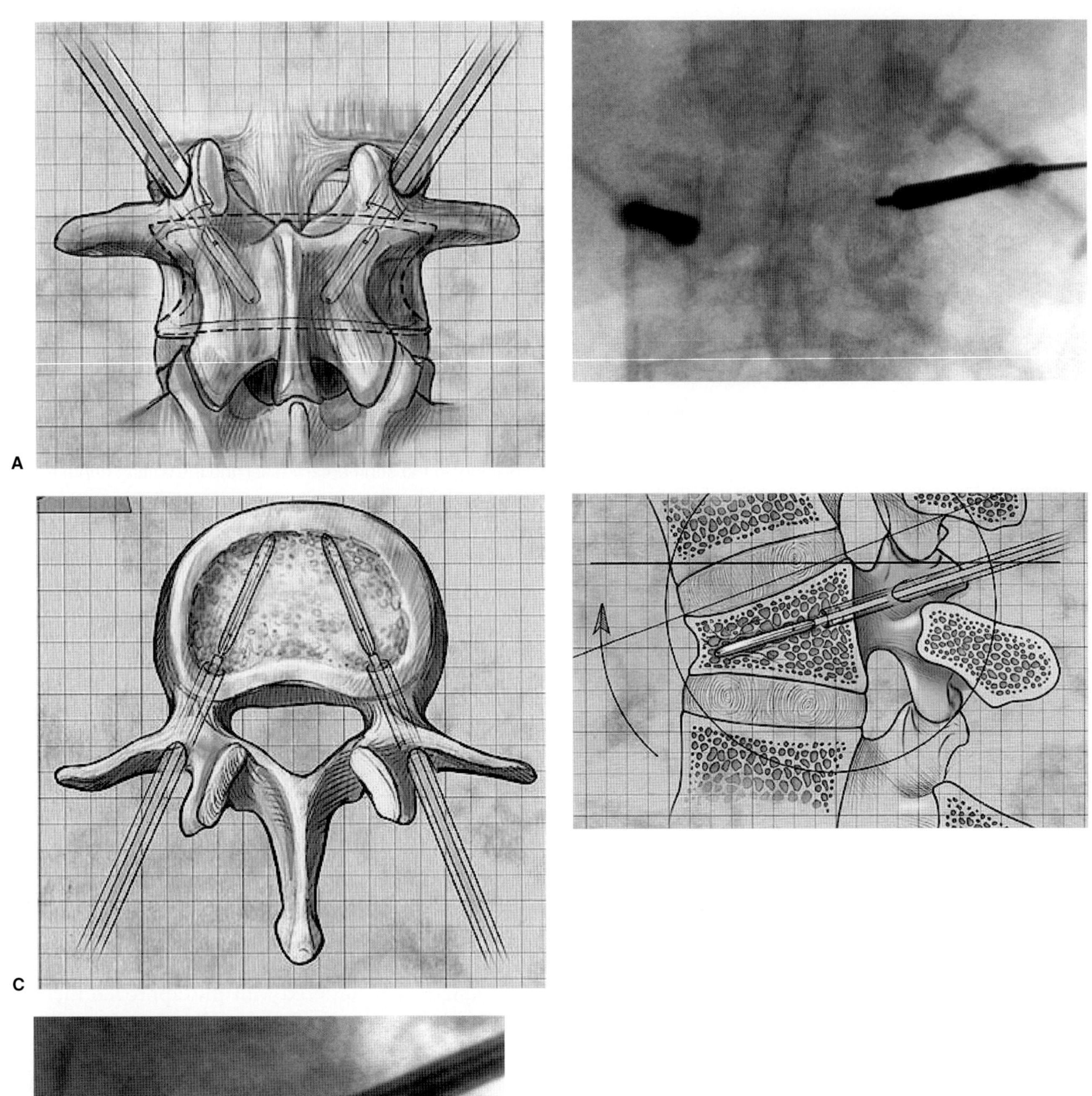

FIGURE 30–5 Illustrative and radiographic views of the optimal positioning of the instruments and the balloon tamp. **(A)** The PA view confirms that the instruments are within the "halo" of the pedicle. **(B)** Note that the tamp is aimed toward the midline **(C)** and the anterointerior edge of the vertebral body **(D,E)**.

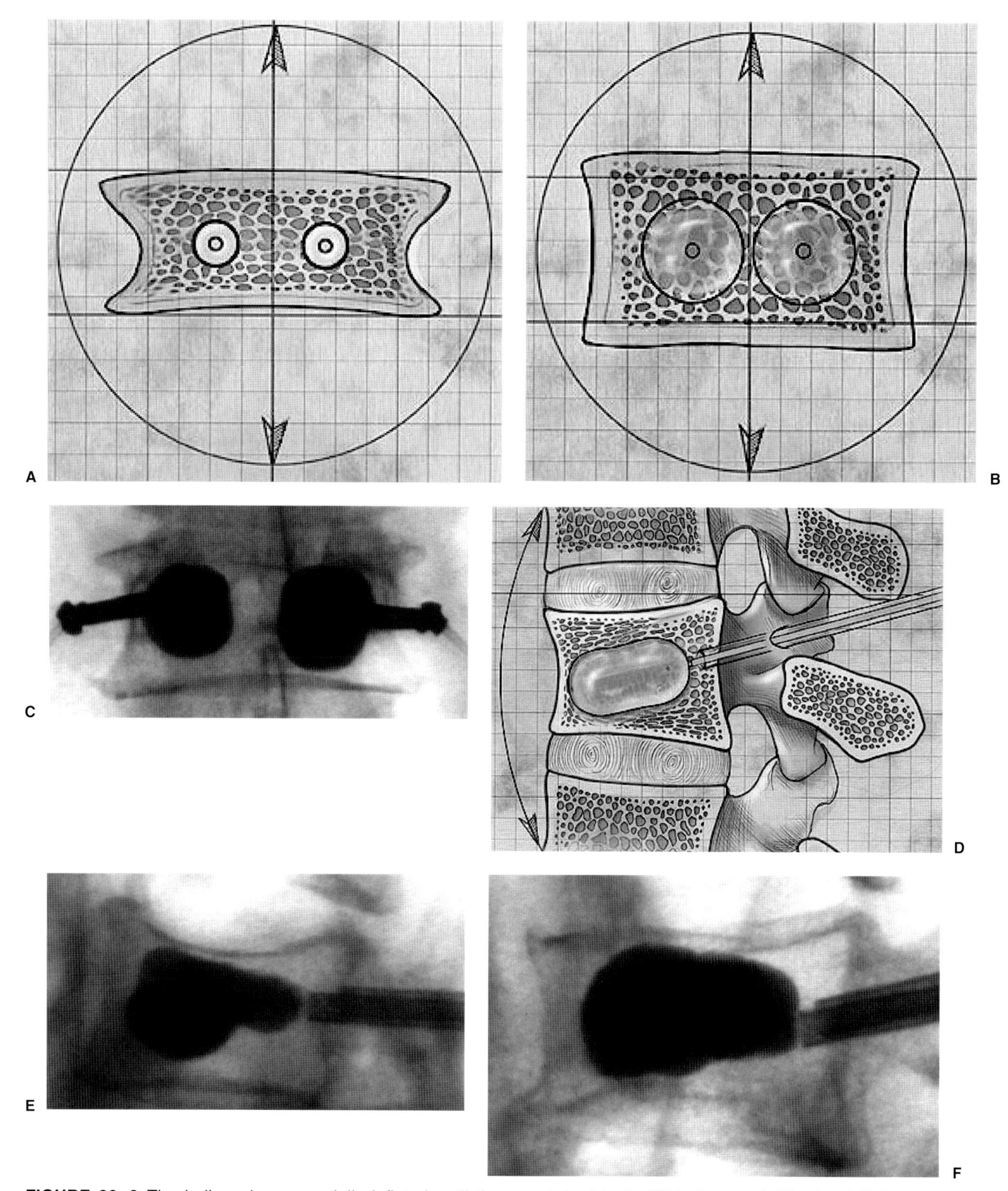

FIGURE 30–6 The balloon is sequentially inflated until the fracture is reduced. Inflation is stopped if pressures become too high (greater than 350 psi) or breakout beyond the vertebral body cortex appears imminent. Artist's depiction of the vertebral body **(A)** before and **(B)** after inflation of the balloons. **(C)** AP fluoroscopy of balloon inflation. **(D)** Lateral depiction of balloon inflation. **(E, F)** Lateral fluoroscopy during inflation.

because the guidewire can be inadvertently advanced through the anterior cortex. Next, a working cannula is inserted over the dilator. The dilator and guidewire can then be removed. A finger twist drill is inserted through the cannula and advanced incrementally to the anterior vertebral body cortex. We must warn that, as the bone is soft, this must be performed under radiographic guidance to avoid penetration of the cortex.

The twist drill is removed. Small pieces of bone within the flutes of the drill can be sent for microscopic analysis, if warranted. Next, the inflatable balloon tamp (Kyphon, Inc., Santa Clara, CA) is inserted through the cannula (Fig. 30–5). The surgeon must choose between a small (15 mm) or large (20 mm) balloon. This can be determined preoperatively using CT or MRI measurements. Upper and middle thoracic vertebrae can often accommodate only a small balloon tamp, whereas lower thoracic and lumbar vertebrae may accept the larger one.

Instead of being a concentric sphere, the tamp is slightly narrowed in its midpoint, creating "anterior and posterior" tamps. Though not a flat surface, this facilitates better "en masse" reduction of the fractured end plate. The anterior and posterior limits of the tamp are delineated with small radiopaque markers. Because the tamp itself is radiolucent, this facilitates proper positioning within the vertebral body before inflation. The balloon is then inflated under controlled pressure, using a digital manometer, with a radiopaque contrast liquid. Fracture reduction and tamp location are judged on both the PA and lateral C-arm views (Fig. 30–6). In addition to height restoration, the surgeon

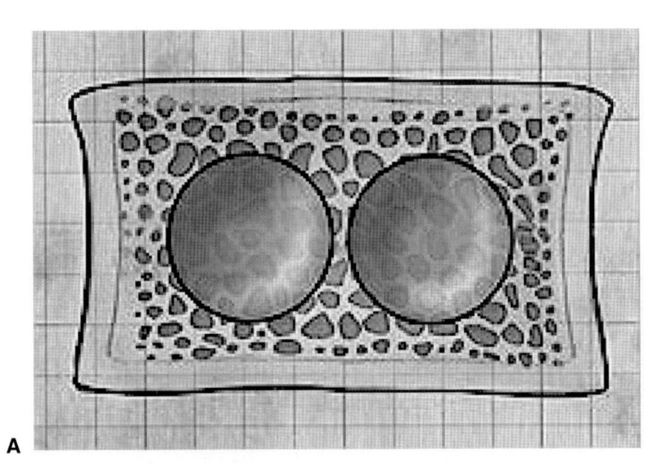

A

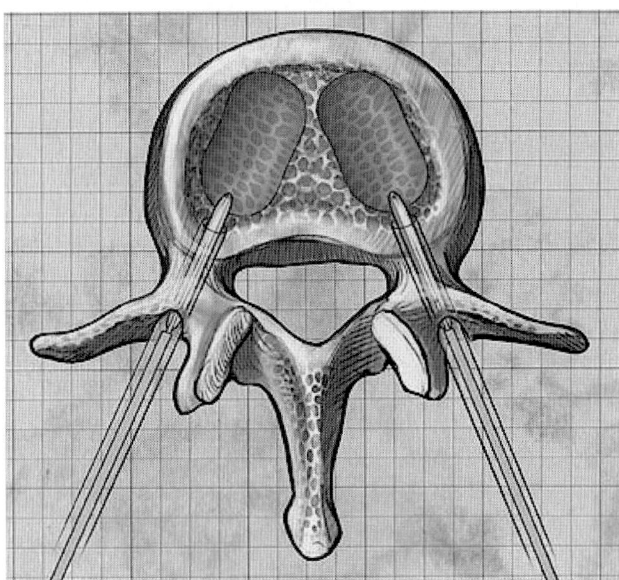

B

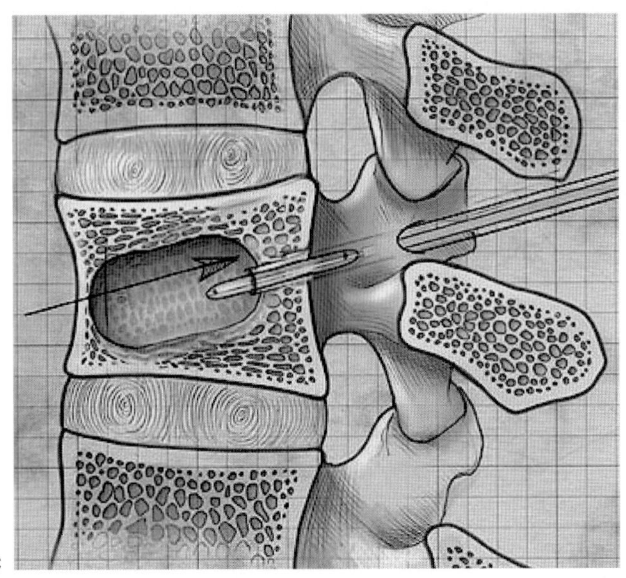

C

FIGURE 30–7 The balloon tamp creates a void within the soft cancellous bone of the osteoporotic vertebral body. This facilitates low-pressure injection of cement. **(A)** Anteroposterior, **(B)** axial, and **(C)** sagittal images.

must ensure that the balloon is maintained within the limits of the bone. Small "blebs" of the balloon can puncture through the superior or inferior end plates that may allow cement leakage. The lateral wall may also be "blown out" if care is not taken. Overinflation can risk spinal canal violation. In acute fractures treated within 2 to 3 months, up to 99% of predicted height can be restored. The correction is not as reliable with older fractures.

Cement Composition

The use of polymethyl methacrylate (PMMA) in the spine is considered "off label" use. Regardless, it is currently

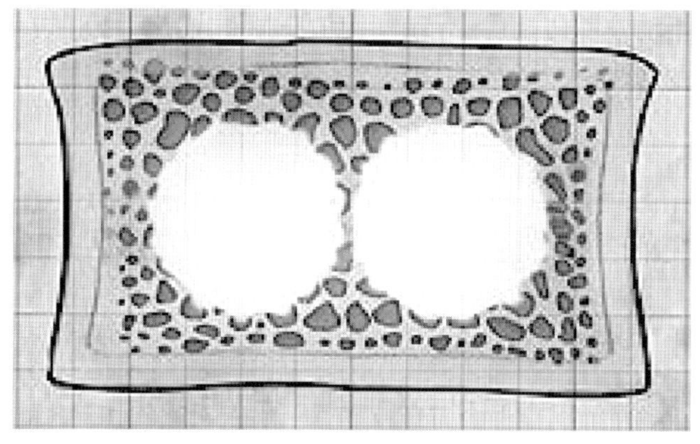

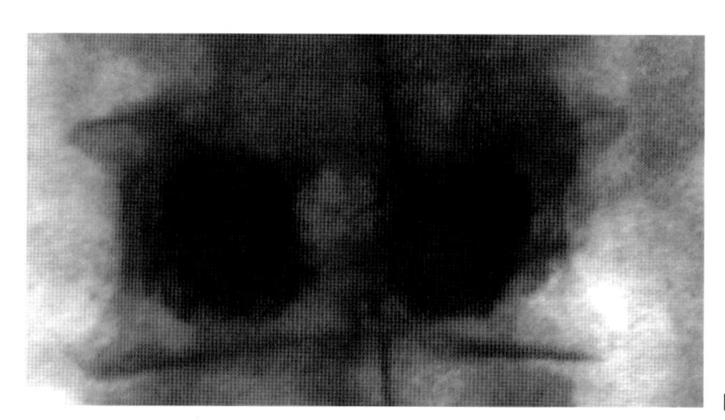

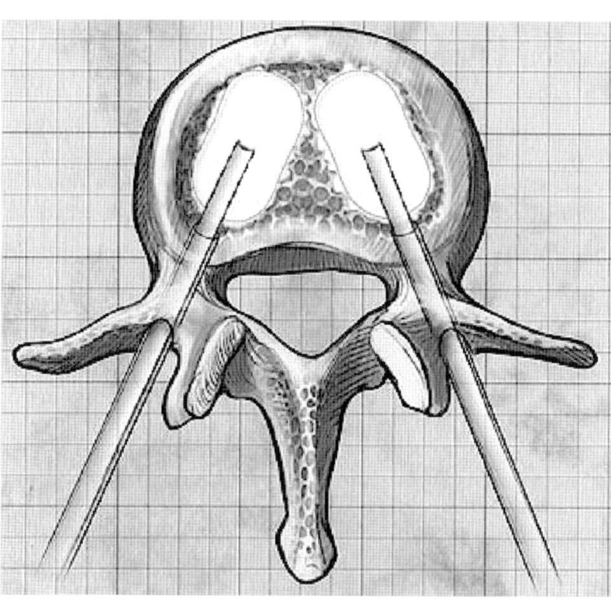

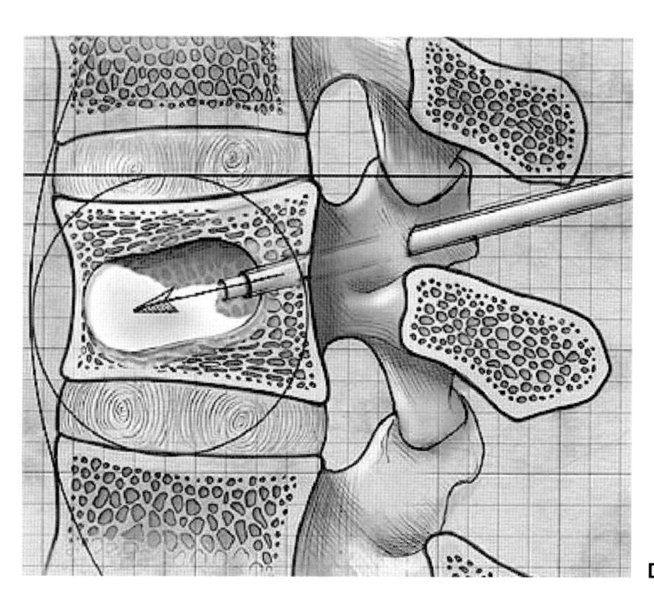

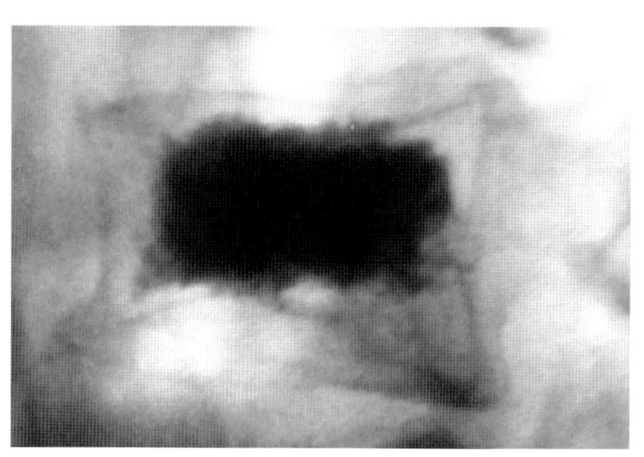

FIGURE 30–8 Cement is inserted in 1.5 ml increments using bone filler devices. This is monitored with frequent fluoroscopic images to ensure that the cement remains within the vertebral body. Cement injection is stopped once material has reached the posterior aspect of the vertebral body/anterior aspect of the pedicle or if cement appears to be leaking. In most cases, cement extravasation is clinically insignificant. **(A)** AP artist's depiction and **(B)** fluoroscopy. **(C)** Axial and **(D)** sagittal depiction with **(E)** lateral fluoroscopy after PMMA injection.

the only accepted material for vertebral body augmentation in humans. To increase its radiopacity, 6.0 g of barium sulfate are added to each 40 ml bag of cement, as well as 1.0 g of a heat-stable antibiotic powder (i.e., cefazolin, vancomycin, or tobramycin). The dry substances are mixed thoroughly before adding 10 ml of the liquid monomer. The combination is then blended until homogeneous. Although still liquid, the cement is injected into long tubular bone-filler devices. These fit snugly into the working cannula. The cement is allowed to cure to a much more viscous state than required for vertebroplasty. The cement is ready for injection when a long bead of cement can be suspended from the tip of a syringe.

Cement Delivery

The balloons are deflated (Fig. 30–7). Bone-filler devices are inserted into both cannulas. A central pusher is used to deliver the cement into the bone, which is carefully monitored using the C-arm. In unstable fractures, the contralateral tamp can be kept inflated to maintain reduction while cement is injected through the ipsilateral side. Cement injection is continued until cement (1) has filled the anterior two thirds of the vertebral body, (2) begins leaking through the vertebral body, or (3) starts to fill the posterior aspect of the body (Fig. 30–8). If the cement is too liquid, it may leak through small cracks in the vertebra walls or end plates. In this case, injection can be temporarily stopped, allowing the peripheral cement to begin to cure and seal any potential leaks. Depending on the volumes achieved during tamp inflation, 2 to 6 ml of cement can be injected on each side.

The cement is allowed to cure for 5 to 10 minutes. After hardening, the instruments are twisted and carefully removed. Final images are taken to confirm cement placement, fracture reduction, and restoration of alignment.

Complications

Few complications have been reported with kyphoplasty. In an ongoing multicenter study,[1] clinical complications occurred in 1.2% of patients and 0.7% of fractures. The most common technical complication is cement leakage, which may be as high as 8.6%, although this is rarely associated with clinically detectable sequelae. Neurologic injury has unfortunately been reported secondary to cement extrusion into the canal or neural foramina.[1,23,24] These complications do not appear to be related to the use of the balloon tamp per se, but were more likely secondary to original, improper Jamshidi needle placement. The most common clinical complication of vertebral augmentation is transient pyrexia, probably from a mild systemic reaction to the PMMA, and appears to be more frequent after vertebroplasty than kyphoplasty. Intraoperative hypotension has been reported during cement injection with vertebroplasty, although this has not been reported during kyphoplasty. Other potential complications are epidural hematomas, which are more likely with anticoagulant administration, and pneumothorax, if instruments are inserted too lateral in the thoracic spine. For safety, anticoagulants should be stopped 1 week before surgery and reinitiated no earlier than 4 days postoperatively. If anticoagulation cannot be stopped for risk of a massive thromboembolic pulmonary event, placement of an inferior vena cava filter before kyphoplasty should be considered.

REFERENCES

1. Garfin SR, Yuan H, Lieberman IH. Early outcomes in the minimally-invasive reductions and fixation of compression fractures. *Proc N Am Spine Soc.* 2000;184–185.
2. Belkoff SM, Mathis JM, Fenton DC, Scribner RM, Reiley ME, Talmadge K. An ex vivo biomechanical evaluation of an inflatable bone tamp used in the treatment of compression fracture. *Spine.* 2001;26:151–156.
3. Hirano T, Hasegawa K, Washio T, Hara T, Takahashi H. Fracture risk during pedicle screw insertion in osteoporotic spine. *J Spinal Disord.* 1998;11:493–497.
4. Kostuik JP. Anterior Kostuik-Harrington distraction systems for the treatment of kyphotic deformities. *Spine.* 1990;15:169–180.
5. Hu SS. Internal fixation in the osteoporotic spine. *Spine.* 1997;22:43S–48S.
6. Leech JA, Dulberg C, Kellie S, Pattee L, Gay J. Relationship of lung function to severity of osteoporosis in women. *Am Rev Respir Dis.* 1990;141:68–71.
7. Lyles KW, Gold DT, Shipp KM, Pieper CF, Martinez S, Mulhausen PL. Association of osteoporotic vertebral compression fractures with impaired functional status. *Am J Med.* 1993;94:595–601.
8. Leidig-Bruckner G, Minne HW, Schlaich C, et al. Clinical grading of spinal osteoporosis: quality of life components and spinal deformity in women with chronic low back pain and women with vertebral osteoporosis. *J Bone Miner Res.* 1997;12:663–675.
9. Schlaich C, Minne HW, Bruckner T, et al. Reduced pulmonary function in patients with spinal osteoporotic fractures. *Osteoporos Int.* 1998;8:261–267.
10. Lieberman IH, Dudeney S, Reinhardt MK, Bell G. Initial outcome and efficacy of "kyphoplasty" in the treatment of painful osteoporotic vertebral compression fractures. *Spine.* 2001;26: 1631–1638.
11. Heary RF, Bono CM. Metastatic spine tumors. *Neurosurg Focus.* 2001;11:1–9.
12. Cotten A, Dewatre F, Cortet B, et al. Percutaneous vertebroplasty for osteolytic metastases and myeloma: effects of the percentage of lesion filling and the leakage of methyl methacrylate at clinical follow-up. *Radiology.* 1996;200:525–530.
13. Dudeney S. Hussein, Lieberman IH. Kyphoplasty in the treatment of vertebral fractures secondary to multiple myeloma. Paper presented at: Annual Meeting of the North American Spine Society; 2001; Seattle.
14. Deramond H, Depriester C, Galibert P, Le Gars D. Percutaneous vertebroplasty with polymethylmethacrylate: technique, indications, and results. *Radiol Clin North Am.* 1998;36:533–546.

15. Jensen ME, Dion JE. Percutaneous vertebroplasty in the treatment of osteoporotic compression fractures. *Neuroimaging Clin N Am.* 2000;10:547–568.
16. Jensen ME, Dion JE. Vertebroplasty relieves osteoporosis pain. *Diagn Imaging.* 1997;19:68,71–72.
17. Do HM. Magnetic resonance imaging in the evaluation of patients for percutaneous vertebroplasty. *Top Magn Reson Imaging.* 2000;11: 235–244.
18. Maynard AS, Jensen ME, Schweickert PA, Marx WF, Short JG, Kallmes DF. Value of bone scan imaging in predicting pain relief from percutaneous vertebroplasty in osteoporotic vertebral fractures. *Am J Neuroradiol.* 2000;21:1807–1812.
19. Wasnich RD. Epidemiology of osteoporosis. In: Favus M, ed. *Primer on the Metabolic Bone Diseases and Disorders of Mineral Metabolism.* Philadelphia: Lippincott/Williams & Wilkins; 1999:257–259.
20. Ross PD, Davis JW, Epstein R, Wasnich RD. Pre-existing fractures and bone mass predict vertebral fracture incidence in women. *Ann Intern Med.* 1991;114:919–923.
21. Wasnich RD, Davis JW, Ross PD. Spine fracture risk is predicted by non-spine fractures. *Osteoporos Int.* 1994;4:1–5.
22. Kado DM, Browner WS, Palermo L, Nevitt MC, Genant HK, Cummings SR. Vertebral fractures and mortality in older women: a prospective study: study of Osteoporotic Fractures Research Group. *Arch Intern Med.* 1999;159:1215–1220.
23. Harrington KD. Major neurological complications following percutaneous vertebroplasty with polymethylmethacrylate: a case report. *J Bone Joint Surg Am.* 2001;83:1070–1073.
24. Wenger M, Markwalder TM. Surgically controlled, transpedicular methyl methacrylate vertebroplasty with fluoroscopic guidance. *Acta Neurochir (Wien).* 1999;141:625–631.

31

Intradiskal Electrothermal Therapy

CURTIS W. SLIPMAN, SARJOO M. BHAGIA, AND RUSSELL V. GILCHRIST

Until recently, treatment for predominant axial back pain caused by discogenic disease has consisted of a variety of noninvasive measures. These interventions encompass oral analgesics, oral anti-inflammatory agents, physical therapy, and epidural space steroid instillation. With these interventions, some patients experience relief, but many do not. A portion of those with intractable back pain are candidates for more aggressive measures and, in particular, a lumbar fusion. Prior to the advent of intradiskal electrothermal annuloplasty, there was no intervening therapeutic tool between rehabilitation and fusion. This new procedure involves placing a navigable electrothermal catheter within a symptomatic lumbar disk. Thermal energy is then conducted into the posterior annular wall during a timed protocol. The heating of the annular wall is theorized to cause coagulation and collagen denaturation that may result in a stabilizing effect to the disk.[1,2] Ablation of nociceptors within the disk by thermal treatment has also been postulated.[3] The U.S. Food and Drug Administration approved its use in 1998, and over 30,000 procedures have been performed in the United States to date.

Since its inception, several outcome studies have been performed with varying results. Karasek and Bogduk[4] reported on the 1-year outcome of 35 patients treated with intradiskal electrothermal therapy (IDET) and compared them with a control group of 17 patients similarly diagnosed but denied insurance authorization for IDET. Although both groups received similar rehabilitation measures, suggesting no treatment bias, the same conclusion is not applicable when considering the inclusion criteria. It must be emphasized that there was an inherent bias in the control group because they were denied this new and potentially conclusive procedure. Sixty percent of the treatment group experienced satisfactory results, which were defined as at least 50% reduction of their preprocedure visual analogue scale (VAS) rating, return to work, and a final VAS score of less than 4. Of the entire group receiving this intervention, 23% of the patients had complete relief of pain. Correcting for the relatively small sample size, this complete pain-free success rate of 23% carries a 95% confidence interval of ± 14%. Thus, were this study to be repeated, complete relief could be observed in as much as 37% or as little as 9% of patients. The 95% confidence interval for the satisfactory group resulted in a range of 44 to 76%. Only one patient in the control group improved, whereas the remainder continued to have their preprocedure pain intensity. Bogduk and Karasek[5] reported on this same population with 2-year follow-up documenting stable and enduring outcomes. Satisfactory success rates at 2 years marginally decreased to 54%, and complete relief of pain was observed in 20% of patients.

Derby et al[6] reported that 62.5% of IDET-treated patients had a favorable outcome, defined as improvement in three of the following four outcome tools: the Roland-Morris Low Back Pain and Disability Questionnaire (RM), VAS, the North American Spine Society Low Back Pain Outcome Assessment Instrument Patient Satisfaction Index (PSI), and a general activities of daily living questionnaire (ADL) modified from the same instrument. Twenty-five percent of patients showed no change at 12 months, whereas 12.5% patients had an unfavorable outcome, defined as worsening of three of the four outcome scales. Although a 62.5% favorable outcome is significant, the mean improvement in individual scores is unimpressive and may not be clinically significant. The mean decrease in the VAS was 1.84 (*SD* = 2.38) and in the RM was 4.03 (*SD* = 4.82). With respect to specific activities, 41% were improved in sitting, 50% in standing, 45% in walking, and 41% in sleeping, although the magnitude of improvement was not quantified. An interesting aspect of this study is the conclusions that can be drawn concerning technique. Seventy-three percent of the IDET-treated patients experienced a favorable outcome if the active catheter tip incorporated 75 to 100% of the posterior annular wall. In contrast, 16.7% of the treated patients had a favorable outcome when less than 50% of the posterior annular wall was treated.

Saal and Saal reported on the outcome of patients treated with IDET at a minimum of 6 months,[7] 12 months,[8] and 2 years[9] follow-up. In the latter study,[9] consisting of 58 patients, a statistically and clinically significant improvement in VAS and bodily pain scores on the Medical Outcomes Study Short-Form General Health Survey (SF-36) was observed. The study group demonstrated a clinically significant improvement in physical function as supported by statistically significant improvement in sitting tolerance and physical function SF-36 scores. The conclusion that these results were clinically significant stem from two studies that have validated the SF-36 as a reliable instrument. Patrick et al[10] had reported that a change in score of 17.7 on the physical function scale or 21.5 on the bodily pain scale is clinically significant. Subsequently, Deyo et al[11] demonstrated that a 7-point change on any of the subscales is clinically significant. Consequently, the outcome study by Saal and Saal, in which a change in score of 31.33 on physical function and of 21.86 on bodily pain were reported, is indeed clinically significant.

In a prospective nonrandomized clinical trial involving 27 consecutive patients with a follow-up of 1 year, Gerszten et al[12] noted that 75% of them improved based on the Oswestry low back pain disability questionnaire. Only 48% of patients were found to improve according to the SF-36 survey. There was no relationship identified between outcome and duration of symptoms ($p = .32$), number of levels treated ($p = .20$), or workers' compensation ($p = .38$).

In a prospective case series consisting of 33 patients with a mean follow-up of 15 months, Lutz et al[13] demonstrated a mean change in the VAS score of 3.9 ($p < .001$), a mean change in the lower extremity VAS score of 3.7 ($p < .001$), and a mean change in the RM of 7.3 ($p < .001$). Seventy-five percent of patients reported that they would undergo the same procedure for the same outcome. Complete pain relief was achieved in 24% of the patients and partial pain relief in 46% of the patients.

The exact mechanism by which IDET produces its reported clinical effects remains unknown. Kleinstuck et al[14] attempted to study intradiskal temperature dispersion from the SpineCATH. They were able to measure temperatures of greater than 42°C (temperature sufficient to thermocoagulate unmyelinated nerve fibers) at distances greater than 10 mm from the probe. It has been suggested that their use of previously frozen cadaveric disks and the placement of the heating elements in the nuclear cavity rather than in the anulus, as is done in clinical practice, may have limited the peak temperatures.[9] There is a dearth of peer-reviewed published literature assessing in vivo temperature dispersion from the SpineCath and the hypothesized resultant protein denaturation. In a recent report, Shah et al[1] found microscopic evidence of acute collagen modulation in cadaveric disks heated with a SpineCATH. In an earlier cadaveric biomechanical study, Lee et al[2] did not note any change in stability of the lumbar spine before and after treatment with IDET. Long-term follow-up studies need to be performed to delineate the biomechanical consequences of denaturation of intradiskal collagen.

Based on the above studies, and in particular the 2-year report by Bogduk and Karasek,[5] IDET represents a minimally invasive option for a select group of patients with chronic discogenic pain, proven by nonsedated provocative diskography, who have failed to improve with a comprehensive, exercise-based rehabilitation care program and who desire functional improvement but are reticent to undergo a lumbar fusion.

Indications

The IDET procedure is indicated in patients with low back pain caused by internal disk disruption syndrome. The inclusion criteria consist of function-limiting low back pain of at least 6 months' continuous duration and failure to improve from an appropriate nonsurgical, conservative rehabilitation program of at least 4 months' duration. In our view, an appropriate regimen comprises progressive intensive exercise, at least two fluoroscopically guided epidural space corticosteroid injections, a trial of manual therapy (provided it is early in the course), oral anti-inflammatory medication, nonnarcotic analgesics, and activity modification. An MRI study should demonstrate a degenerative disk without a focal protrusion or any evidence of neural compression at the proposed IDET disk level. A concordant pain response must be obtained with provocative diskography at low pressurization at one or more disk levels with adjacent control levels not demonstrating pain reproduction.[5,7,8]

Contraindications

Contraindications to the IDET procedure include systemic infection, osteomyelitis, diskitis, cellulitis, complete collapse of the disk space, the presence of sequestered or extruded disk herniations, cauda equina syndrome, gross instability, and uncorrectable bleeding diathesis. The presence of hardware previously used for a lumbar fusion or a spinal cord stimulator theoretically precludes the performance of IDET. Performing IDET under these latter circumstances could result in inadvertent heating of nondiskal structures, so extreme caution is suggested. Moderately degenerated disks represent a relative contraindication. Such disks create a technical challenge, and even when the procedure is performed properly, the outcome may be disappointing.

Instruments and Preparations

Instruments

The following instruments are essential: ORA-50 S Electrothermal Spine generator, single-use SpineCATH intradiskal electrothermal catheter, 17-gauge introducer needle, connector cable from the spine generator to the electrothermal catheter, fluoroscopy machine, standard sterile prep kit, sterile towels, sponge clamp, four 3 cc syringes, one 6-inch, 25-gauge needle, sterile gloves, and blood pressure and pulse oximeter. The SpineCath catheter is a flexible device with a curved tip (Fig. 31–1).

Anesthesia

Intravenous access is obtained prior to the procedure, and light conscious sedation is given. We have found the combination of Versed and fentanyl to work extremely well in our patients. For most patients, a starting dose of fentanyl of 75 μg is typically sufficient, provided the introducer needle and catheter are placed expeditiously. When difficulty is encountered, another 25 to 50 μg may be required. One milligram of Versed is appropriate for most patients. Of course, the doses must be modified according to patient size, debility, narcotic use history, and degree of anxiety. Heavy sedation should be avoided secondary to its potential cardiac and pulmonary complications. In addition, the patient needs to be responsive during the procedure to communicate any sudden onset of pain, dysesthesias, or paresthesias during advancement of the introducer needle and during the heating protocol. If the patient is not alert enough to recognize or inform the physician of such symptoms, then permanent neural injury may transpire.

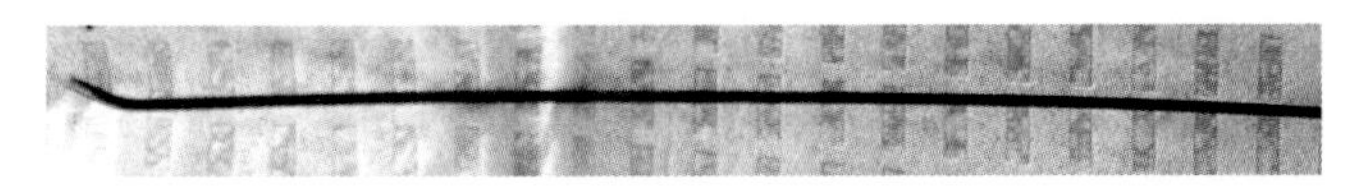

FIGURE 31–1 IDET catheter revealing curved tip.

Positioning

The positioning is physician-dependent and relates to the surgeon's usual diskography technique. The patient is placed in the prone or prone oblique position on the fluoroscopy table. An extraforaminal approach is used, because IDET should never be performed via transdural placement.

Surgical Technique

A standard diskography technique is used to gain access to the disk. This involves securing an oblique view of the lumbar spine in which the superior articular process (SAP) of the vertebral body crosses the intervertebral disk and divides it into half posterior to the SAP and half anterior to the SAP for the L4–L5 and L5–S1 disk. Lumbar disks cephalad to the L4–L5 level should have the SAP bisect the disk in a 60:40, rather than 50:50, proportion. In the oblique view, the superior and inferior vertebral end plates should be aligned in parallel to allow the introducer needle to be placed in the midportion of the disk. Such placement enhances the operator's ability to slink the catheter within the disk and not abut the end plates. The low back area is then prepped and draped in the usual sterile manner. Using a sponge clamp for a marker, the subcutaneous skin and tissues are anesthetized with 1% lidocaine. The 17-gauge introducer needle is then advanced to the posterolateral border of the disk. To avoid injuring the exiting nerve root, the introducer needle should remain just ventral to the SAP. Again, the introducer needle should enter the disk midway between the end plates to avoid injury to these sensitive structures.

Once proper positioning is achieved, the needle is advanced through the posterolateral anulus. The needle tip is placed near the central nucleus, as confirmed in two planes by fluoroscopy. At this juncture, the needle should be aimed in a trajectory that would result in the catheter reaching the ventral and contralateral corner of the disk (approximately 10 o'clock if the middorsal disk represents 6 o'clock). Such placement is essential because the catheter will need to deflect off this "corner" and curve back toward the dorsal aspect of the disk. Intradiskal catheter function is then verified prior to placing it into the introducer needle. This is accomplished by attaching the connector cable to the generator and catheter. At this point, the generator should have been set in AutoTemp mode. Once connected, the actual temperature gauge should display room temperature. The impedance gauge should read within normal limits (85–230 ohms). If the impedence exceeds this amount, the catheter must be replaced because it is defective. Following the impedance check, the cable is detached from

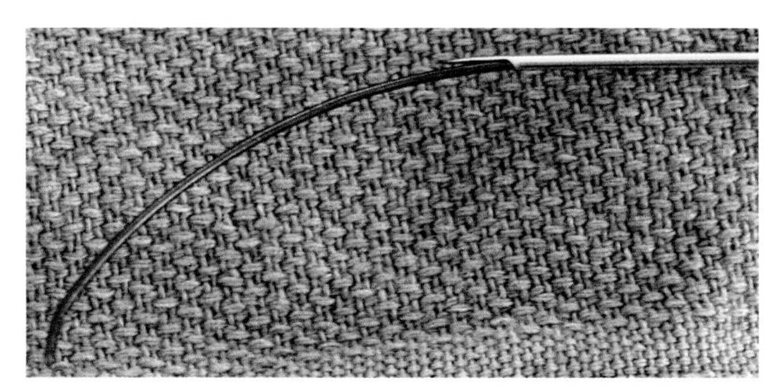

FIGURE 31–2 IDET catheter advanced through introducer needle, demonstrating development of a curve in the direction of the curved catheter tip and away from the sharp edge of the introducer needle.

the catheter. The intradiskal catheter is inserted and advanced through the introducer needle until a change of resistance is appreciated, at which point the catheter has just exited the introducer needle and is now within the substance of the nucleus. It is then navigated intradiskally while viewing in the lateral plane. Gentle advancement and real-time fluoroscopic imaging of the catheter are strongly advised because it is easily bent and can crack. If a crack develops, the catheter will no longer be able to perform its heating task. In some instances, the catheter will circumnavigate the disk without difficulty. In other cases, the catheter may move superiorly or inferiorly and bounce off the end plate. When that occurs, the catheter must be withdrawn and advanced again using a different orientation. Reorientation of the catheter must always be accomplished in synchrony with the introducer needle to avoid damaging the catheter (Fig. 31–2). Remember that the introducer needle has a sharp beveled edge. Attempting to move the catheter in a manner that deposits the catheter against this edge with any degree of force can result in shearing of the catheter. There are times when the catheter is advanced, and the tip just sinks into the eroded anteroinferior margin of the disk. Again, the catheter must be reoriented before another attempt is made. Immediate reorientation is emphasized because there are only a limited number of passes that can be attempted before the catheter becomes unusable. Repeated unsuccessful attempts in which the catheter cannot be advanced without substantial force will result in fatigue and then fracture. If the catheter advances beyond an imaginary line connecting the most dorsal aspect of the vertebral bodies above and below the disk being treated, then the catheter must be withdrawn. At no point should the catheter rest in a position that could result in inadvertent heating of the neural elements in the epidural space. Similarly, the catheter should not enter or rest within the neural foramen.

As the catheter is advanced in the lateral plane and curves around the anulus, it can pierce its outer border

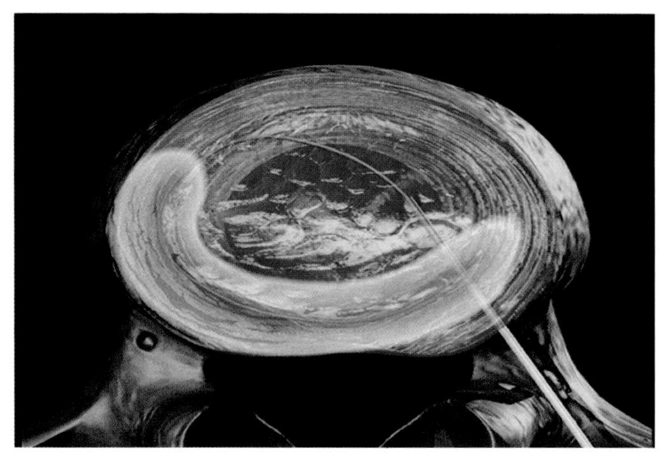

FIGURE 31–3 Schematic diagram showing placement of the catheter from 3 to 9 o'clock position, covering almost 100% of posterior anulus.

and enter the foramen. During advancement of the catheter the objective is to lodge the active portion adjacent to the inner anulus and across the entire posterior anulus. In other words, ideal placement involves covering the anulus from 3 to 9 o'clock (Fig. 31–3). This recommendation stems from our experience and two peer-reviewed papers. Derby et al[6] demonstrated superior outcomes when a greater portion of the posterior anulus is covered. Slipman et al[15] demonstrated that the annular tear in and of itself is not the painful structure, but an associated factor. Therefore, the goal is not "to cover the tear," as some have insisted. Confirmation of proper positioning is aided by the presence of radiopaque markers on the catheter, which define the borders of the heating elements.

Once the catheter is appropriately placed, attention is then directed to the radiofrequency generator (Fig. 31–4). The set power gauge should display P90, which sets the peak temperature of the catheter tip. Standard protocol peak temperature is 90°C. The generator is then turned on by pressing the RF button once. As the heating process unfolds, the generator will

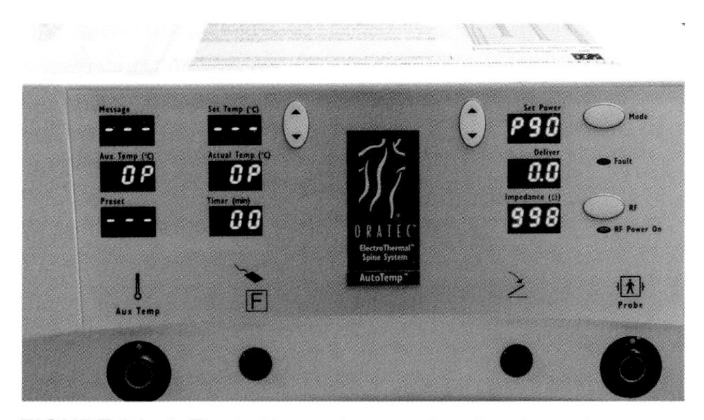

FIGURE 31–4 Electrothermal generator showing set power.

automatically incrementally raise the set temperature by 1° every 30 seconds until the peak temperature is reached. At peak temperature, heating ensues for 4 minutes until the generator automatically discontinues energy delivery. Heating will transpire over a 16.5-minute duration provided the patient does not experience any clinically significant symptoms. If the patient describes leg pain, intolerable back pain, lower extremity paresthesias or dysesthesias, or involuntary leg contractions, then an alteration in the heating scheme must be initiated. Energy delivery can be manually discontinued by pressing and releasing either the foot pedal or the RF button at any time. If severe back pain is experienced, the heating protocol can be delayed, enabling the delivery of additional fentanyl or other analgesic. It is common for patients to experience some pain, frequently their usual discomfort, but it should be tolerable. Lower extremity symptoms other than mild diffuse discomfort automatically raise the concern of accidental neural injury. Heating must be discontinued and the placement of the catheter rechecked. Once heating is completed, the cable is disconnected from the catheter. The catheter is subsequently removed from the introducer needle while viewing under fluoroscopy. Hasty withdrawal could result in shearing of this very malleable catheter. Some advocate the administration of an intradiskal dose of antibiotic prior to removal of the introducer needle. Our preference is to avoid intradiskal placement of antibiotics. Instead, we routinely administer a dose of antibiotic through the IV 1 hour prior to the procedure. The introducer needle is then removed, and a 4 × 4 pressure dressing is placed over the insertion site.

Postoperative Care

The patient is observed for 1 hour after the procedure for any complications and to allow the conscious sedation time to resolve. The IV is then removed, and the patient dons a soft lumbar orthosis and is discharged to home with an appointment to follow-up in the office in 2 weeks. The patient is instructed to wear the orthosis continuously over the initial 6-week postoperative interval, removing it only to shower or change clothes. The orthosis primarily serves as a reminder for the patient to limit his or her activities. We usually advise the patient to avoid all activities and rest for the first 3 days postop. After 3 days, the patient may begin walking short distances. Sitting is limited to 1-hour intervals with at least a 20-minute break between episodes for the first 2 weeks, then patients may increase their sitting time to tolerance. If they have a sedentary job, they may return to work as early as day 14. If their job entails heavy lifting, return to work is not recommended until 3 to 4 months postprocedure. Driving and light housework duties are allowed after 3 weeks. We typically restrict lifting to 0 to 10 lbs for the first 2 weeks, 10 to 25 lbs for 4 weeks, 25 to 50 lbs for 8 weeks, and then advance as tolerated. No bending or twisting activities are allowed through the first 6 weeks, at which time a graded flexibility and strengthening rehabilitation program is instituted. Progression to more advanced rehabilitation measures depends on the ultimate goal of each patient and is therefore individualized.

Complications

Intraoperative/Perioperative

The spectrum and incidence of potential intraoperative complications of the IDET procedure are relatively small. While advancing the introducer needle past the SAP, one could pierce the traversing nerve root. Dural puncture, annular injury, and vertebral end plate injury are also complications that may occur while advancing the introducer needle into the disk. If the heating catheter migrates into the spinal canal, there exists the potential for cauda equina syndrome secondary to thermal injury. To date, there has been one reported case of cauda equina due to IDET.[16] Uncontrolled bleeding and infection are potential complications. There has been one literature report of vertebral osteonecrosis associated with IDET, although the mechanism by which this complication occurred is unknown.[17] Adverse reactions to anesthetic, conscious sedation medications, and antibiotic prophylaxis are also potential complications. Poor intravenous fluid management can result in peripheral edema and heart failure in patients at risk.

Postoperative

Diskitis, osteomyelitis, and epidural abscess are the primary infection-related complications. Nuclear herniation through the introducer needle diskal insertion site is a theoretical complication; however, there have been no such reported cases. Most patients experience an increase in their low back pain for approximately the first week following the procedure.

Case Illustration

A 32-year-old patient described back pain without leg pain that escalated over a 9-month interval. Although he had prior episodes of back pain during the past 6 years, each episode was limited to no more than 6 weeks' duration. Between recurrences he experienced baseline low back pain that he rated 30 to 40 on a 100 mm VAS. During this recurrence, he could not perform his usual

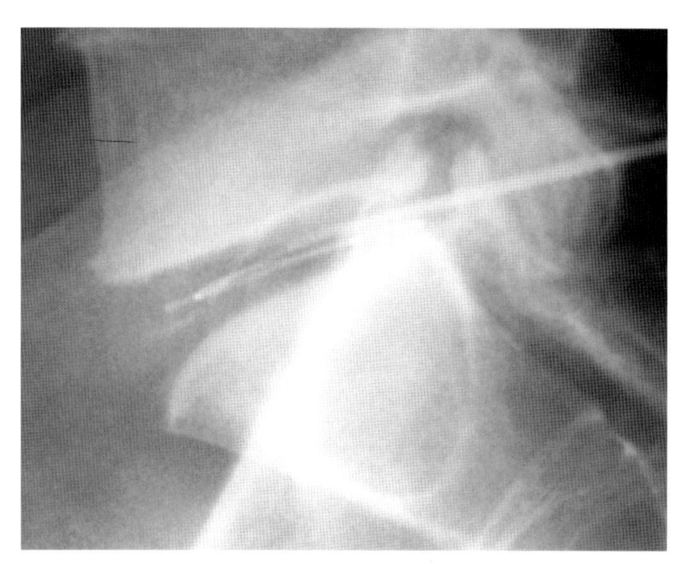

FIGURE 31–5 Lateral view of the introducer needle and catheter within the L5–S1 disk space.

sedentary activities because of impaired concentration resulting from continued pain and because of a limited sitting tolerance. He participated in active therapy with experienced physical therapists, used oral anti-inflammatory agents, and underwent three epidural space steroid instillations. Despite these efforts, his symptoms were not ameliorated. At that juncture, he was prepared to undergo IDET or a fusion procedure provided it was indicated. A nonsedated provocative diskogram demonstrated the level of involvement to be L5–S1. IDET was then performed (Figs. 31–5, 31–6). At 1 month postop there was 90% symptom reduction, which progressed to 98% at 2 months. Thereafter the symptoms remained at this level, less than 5 on a 100 mm scale, for the ensuing 2 years.

Intradiskal electrothermal therapy IDET is a minimally invasive procedure for treatment of patients with a diagnosis of lumbar internal disk disruption syndrome. Peer-reviewed publications have demonstrated that it is

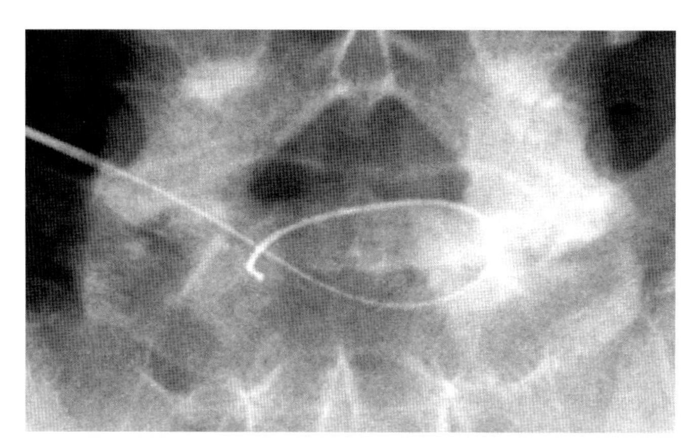

FIGURE 31–6 Posteroanterior view of the introducer and needle within the L5–S1 disk.

a safe procedure with minimal adverse events. Its advantages in the treatment of discogenic pain as compared with open surgery reside in its ability to minimize tissue destruction, decrease hospital expenses, reduce potential complications, and allow for quicker recovery time. Although the outcome studies that have been published suggest this is a worthwhile intervention for patients with internal disk disruption, the results are not overwhelming. Perhaps further inquiry will identify the inclusion and exclusion criteria that will afford higher success rates in a constant and predictable manner.

REFERENCES

1. Shah RV, Lutz GE, Lee J, et al. Intradiskal electrothermal therapy: a preliminary histologic study. *Arch Phys Med Rehabil.* 2001;82:1230–1237.
2. Lee J, Lutz GE, Campbell D, et al. Stability of the lumbar spine after intradiskal electrothermal therapy. *Arch Phys Med Rehabil.* 2001;82:120–122.
3. Smith HP, McWhorter JM, Challa VR. Radiofrequency neurolysis in a clinical model: neuropathological correlation. *J Neurosurg.* 1981;55:246–253.
4. Karasek M, Bogduk N. Twelve-month follow-up of a controlled trial of intradiskal thermal annuloplasty for back pain due to internal disc disruption. *Spine.* 2000;25:2601–2607.
5. Bogduk N, Karasek M. Two-year follow-up of a controlled trial of intradiskal electrothermal annuloplasty for chronic low back pain resulting from internal disc disruption. *Spine J.* 2002;2:343–350.
6. Derby R, Eck B, Chen Y, et al. Intradiskal electrothermal annuloplasty (IDET): a novel approach for treating chronic discogenic back pain. *Neuromodulation.* 2000;3:69–75.
7. Saal JS, Saal JA. Management of chronic discogenic low back pain with a thermal intradiskal catheter: a preliminary report. *Spine.* 2000;25:382–388.
8. Saal JA, Saal JS. Intradiskal electrothermal treatment for chronic discogenic low back pain: a prospective outcome study with minimum 1-year follow-up. *Spine.* 2000;25:2622–2627.
9. Saal JA, Saal JS. Intradiskal electrothermal treatment for chronic discogenic low back pain: prospective outcome study with a minimum 2-year follow-up. *Spine.* 2002;27:966–974.
10. Patrick DL, Deyo RA, Atlas SJ, et al. Assessing health related quality of life in patients with sciatica. *Spine.* 1995;20:1899–1909.
11. Deyo RA, Battie M, Beurskens AJH, et al. Outcome measures for low back pain research: a proposal for standardized use. *Spine.* 1998;23:2003–2013.
12. Gerszten PC, Welch WC, McGrath PM, et al. A prospective outcomes study of patients undergoing intradiskal electrothermy (IDET) for chronic low back pain. *Pain Physician.* 2002;5:360–364.
13. Lutz C, Lutz GE, Cooke PM. Treatment of chronic lumbar discogenic pain with intradiskal electrothermal therapy: a prospective outcome study. *Arch Phys Med Rehabil.* 2003;84:23–28.
14. Kleinstuck F, Diederich C, Nau W, et al. Acute biomechanical and histological effects of intradiskal electrothermal therapy on human lumbar discs. *Spine.* 2001;26:2198–2207.
15. Slipman CW, Patel RK, Zhang L, et al. Side of symptomatic annular tear and site of low back pain: is there a correlation? *Spine.* 2001;26:E165–E169.
16. Hsui A, Isaac K, Katz J. Cauda equina syndrome from intradiskal electrothermal therapy. *Neurology.* 2000;55:320.
17. Djurasovic M, Glassman SD, Dimar JR, et al. Vertebral osteonecrosis associated with the use of intradiskal electrothermal therapy: a case report. *Spine.* 2002;27:E325–E328.

32

Nucleoplasty

CURTIS W. SLIPMAN AND ZACHARIA ISAAC

In 1934, Mixter and Barr[1] publicized the potential and probable link between a herniated nucleus pulposus and radicular pain. Their study provided evidence that laminectomy and disk excision could successfully relieve pain associated with radiculopathy. Modern treatment of radicular pain employs a spectrum of treatment options, including the use of nonsteroidal anti-inflammatory medications, physical therapy, selective nerve root injections,[2–5] percutaneous disk decompression techniques, and open diskectomy.

The earliest percutaneous disk decompression technique utilized chymopapain, a proteolytic enzyme derived from papaya latex with a selective affinity for chondromucoprotein. Chemonucleolysis developed subsequent to the report of Smith and Brown,[6] in which they infused chymopapain into the intervertebral disk. Instantaneous hydrolysis of the chondromucoprotein portion of the nucleus was observed, while surrounding tissues were seemingly spared. The underlying theory behind its potential efficacy was that the removal of disk material would lead to a clinically significant reduction of external pressure on the involved nerve root. Although several outcome studies reported 70 to 90% success rates,[6,7] a controlled study initiated by the U.S. Food and Drug Administration found chymopapain no more effective than placebo.[8] Closer analyses of this investigation revealed numerous methodological flaws. Nevertheless, its impact, in part, contributed to chymopapain's severely diminished role in the treatment of radicular pain. It was ultimately no longer FDA approved or available for clinical use in the United States. Well-designed follow-up trials demonstrated the efficacy of chemonucleolysis. A prospective, placebo-controlled, double-blind, multicenter, crossover trial of 88 patients demonstrated a 73% success rate in the chemonucleolysis group and a 42% success rate in the placebo group.[9] The failures in the placebo group later underwent chemonucleolysis and had a 90% success rate. The primary end point for considering a patient a failure was if the patient had pain severe enough to consider another intervention for treatment. Another prospective, double-blind, randomized, controlled trial of 60 patients reported a 77% success rate for chemonucleolysis and a 47% success rate for placebo.[10] Success was defined as the patient stating he or she had moderate or complete relief of pain. Another study reported the 10-year outcome of a double-blind, randomized, placebo-controlled trial of 60 patients with an 80% success rate for chemonucleolysis and 34% for placebo.[11]

Reports of such side effects as transverse myelitis and anaphylaxis raised clinical concerns regarding the safety of chymopapain. Purified collagenase was demonstrated in animals to have a very low allergenicity and subsequently led to its investigation as a chemonucleolytic alternative to chymopapain. A prospective, double-blind, randomized, controlled study, however, reported 5-year good to excellent outcomes in 72% of the chymopapain group and 52% of the collagenase group.[12] They concluded that chymopapain was more effective than collagenase for the treatment of sciatica. Today, although chymopapain is no longer available in the United States, it is widely preferred in other countries in properly selected patients because of its proven success rate and minimal allergenic side effects.

Newer percutaneous disk decompression techniques have used mechanical and energy-mediated rather than biochemical processes. A rudimentary form of manual percutaneous diskectomy was initially reported by Hijikata in 1975. He used a specially designed cannula and rongeurs to remove disk material percutaneously through a posterolateral approach. In 1978, Hijikata reported that good to excellent results had been achieved in 68% of 80 patients.[13] Kambin[14] improved upon this technique because he employed a biportal posterolateral approach with direct visualization of the nuclear mass (arthroscopic microdiskectomy). In 1985, Onik and colleagues[15] developed the nucleotome, an automated suction shaver that allows for the performance of an automated percutaneous lumbar diskectomy (APLD). The shaver functioned by drawing the nucleus pulposus into a small cutting port and eliminated a portion of the nucleus via a reciprocating "guillotine-like" blade. APLD utilized a 20.3 cm needle inserted through a 2.8 mm diameter cannula. Onik et al reported an 85% success rate independent of the amount of disk material removed.

Despite these unique advances and promising preliminary reported results, prospective controlled double-blind trials demonstrated APLD to have lower success rates than chemonucleolysis and open microdiskectomy. A prospective randomized, controlled trial comparing APLD to chemonucleolysis for the treatment of sciatic pain reported a 1-year outcome of 66% success in the chemonucleolysis group and 37% in the APLD group.[15] Another prospective randomized, controlled trial comparing APLD with microdiskectomy in 71 patients reported 29% satisfactory outcomes for APLD and 80% satisfactory outcomes for open microdiskectomy. Of the patients with APLD failures who subsequently underwent microdiskectomy, a 65% success rate was reported.[16] This raised the immensely important clinical concern that outcomes of open diskectomy could be adversely affected by undergoing APLD. In an effort to improve on APLD, Mayer and Brock[17] described percutaneous endoscopic lumbar diskectomy (PELD). This technique uses a medium-sized rigid endoscope that is inserted into the posterolateral border of the disk, which opens the disk space with an annular trephine. Under intermittent endoscopic guidance, the nuclear material is removed with forceps and an automatic shaver system. In 1993, Mayer and Brock[17] detailed the results of a 6- to 17-month follow up of the PELD procedure, indicating that the majority of their first 30 patients reported 70 to 100% relief of symptoms.

Laser disk decompression was initiated by Choy and Altman in 1986.[18] They put forth the theory that a small change in disk volume could result in a large change in intradiscal pressure. Disadvantages of this technique included moderate to severe intraoperative pain secondary to the thermal effect of the laser, postoperative low back pain and spasm, and inability to visualize the tip of the laser beam under fluoroscopy. As with the earlier percutaneous decompression techniques, these success rates were not reproduced by independent outcome studies.

Various deficiencies of each of the aforementioned percutaneous disk decompression techniques has created an ongoing demand for an improved and/or novel technique that can achieve the theoretical advantages of percutaneous disk decompression without the previously experienced shortcomings; marginal success rates, disk space collapse, allergic reaction, end plate fracture, and, perhaps most importantly, limitation of the potential impact of microdiskectomy. It is with this intent and optimism that nucleoplasty has been developed. Nucleoplasty, using coblation technology, involves a 1 mm diameter bipolar instrument that achieves disk decompression using energy and potentially heat (Fig. 32–1). A 17-gauge introducer cannula is inserted into the posterolateral aspect of the disk (Fig. 32–2). Following proper placement, a bipolar catheter is threaded though the introducer needle

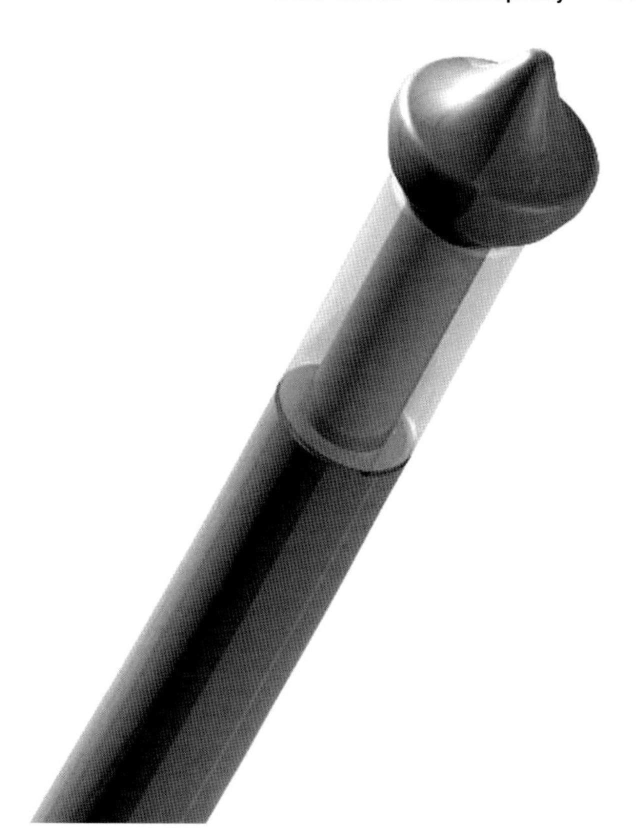

FIGURE 32–1 Coblation catheter tip.

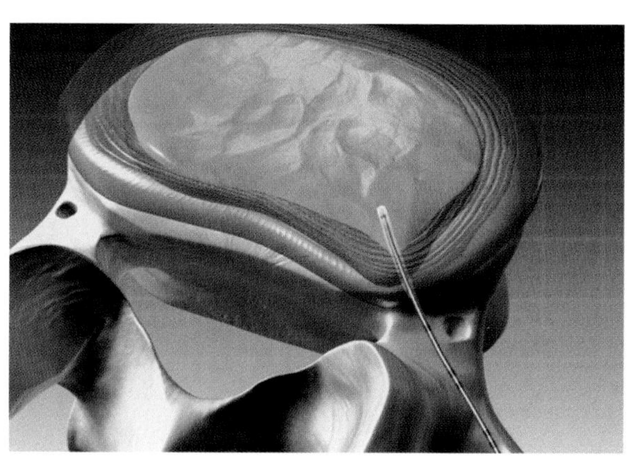

FIGURE 32–2 Coblation catheter entering the posterolateral aspect of the disk.

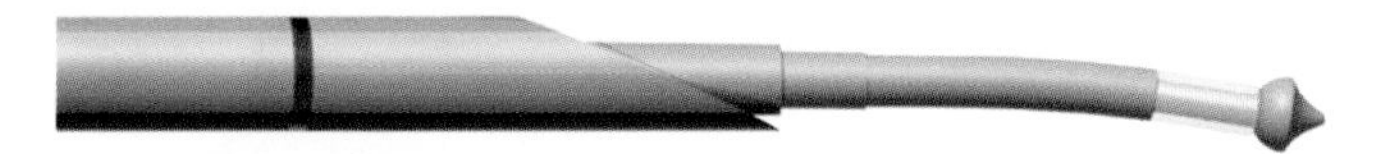

FIGURE 32–3 Catheter inserted through the introducer needle.

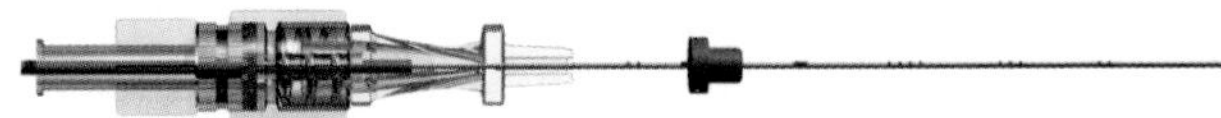

FIGURE 32–5 Cervical coblation catheter inserted through the introducer needle. The catheter terminates as a loop.

and inserted into the disk (Fig. 32–3). The catheter tip is capable of two modes, ablation and coagulation. Ablation generates ~120 V of energy at the leading edge of the catheter. Temperatures of 50 to 70°C are achieved, but they are limited to the initial 2 mm extending from the distal end of the catheter. A plasma field, which is a millimicron-thick field of highly energized particles, is generated at the tip of the catheter. It is within this plasma field that molecular dissociation of disk material occurs.[18] Serial passes of the catheter create a sequence of closely approximated channels extending from the posterolateral anulus to the anteromedial anulus (Fig. 32–4). The coagulation mode can be used during withdrawal. The coagulation mode is 60 V of energy and a tip temperature of 70°C. It is postulated that the thermal effect results in denaturization of the type II collagen, with resultant shrinkage of the surrounding collagen and widening of the channel. Temperatures 1 mm from the catheter tip range from ~40°C for ablation to 50°C for coagulation. This relatively low temperature coblation process minimizes the potential for thermal injury to the disk, anulus, or end plate.

Two peer-reviewed studies assessed the outcomes of percutaneous nucleoplasty. Sharps and Isaac[19] reported on a prospective consecutive series of 48 patients with complaints of axial or radicular pain and an associated contained focal protrusion. Follow-up ranged from 3 to 12 months postprocedurally. Sharps and Isaac reported statistically significant improvements in pain on a 10-point visual analogue scale, with a mean VAS reduction of 4.28, 4.66, 4.75, and 3.6 at 1-, 3-, 6-, and 12-month intervals, respectively. Success was defined as meeting all of the following criteria: greater than two-point VAS reduction, cessation of narcotic use, return to work, and patient satisfaction. Seventy-nine percent of patients met these success criteria. Sharps and Isaac's study had a relatively small number of patients with 1-year follow up and no control group. Singh and Slipman[20] reported on 67 consecutive patients with axial and/or radicular pain treated with nucleoplasty. Success was defined as at least 50% pain relief. Follow-up data were collected for 100% of the patients at 3 months postprocedure, 91% of the patients at 6 months, and 48% of the patients at 1 year. The percentage of patients with greater than 50% VAS reduction was 81% at 1 month, 78% at 3 months, 59% at 6 months, and 50% at 1 year. Singh and Slipman's study lacked a control group and had a very high dropout rate due to patients being lost to follow-up. These two studies independently concluded that nucleoplasty may be an effective treatment for low back pain or radicular pain associated with a contained herniation. Although these studies raise optimism for using coblation technology as a percutaneous decompression technique, prospective, controlled, randomized trials with subgroup analysis are required to determine the efficacy of this procedure.

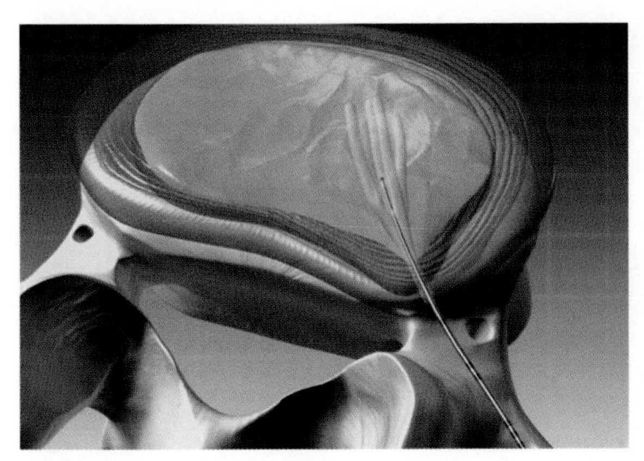

FIGURE 32–4 Catheter being withdrawn; channels have been created exclusively within the nucleus.

Coblation technology has evolved such that it is now applicable to the cervical and upper thoracic spine (Fig. 32–5). There is unfortunately a paucity of literature that would enable us to compare this technique with others when attempting to decompress the more cephalad regions of the spine.

Indications

Nucleoplasty is indicated for the treatment of radicular pain secondary to a contained herniation and is not a potential intervention when there is an extruded or sequestered disk. Many clinicians believe it should be considered as a treatment option when less aggressive measures have failed. According to that perspective, patients with acute radicular pain should engage in a minimum 6-week trial of active physical therapy, Cox-2 selective nonsteroidal anti-inflammatory drugs, and selective nerve root blocks for the treatment of acute radicular pain. Nucleoplasty can be instituted when these measures fail. It must be mentioned that there are some spine clinicians who believe that this intervention should be considered a reasonable and viable alternative to the aforementioned initial management program. Although nucleoplasty has been proposed as a treatment for acute radicular pain resulting from contained disk herniations, there is some evidence suggesting it is a legitimate therapeutic intervention for axial low-back pain. Of course, the contained herniation must be demonstrated to be painful with provocative diskography. A preliminary study evaluating patients with axial low-back pain demonstrated that patients with a contained central focal protrusion proven symptomatic by provocative diskography have a 65% success rate compared with 35% for patients with disk degeneration without a central focal protrusion following coblation. In this study, success was defined as greater than 75% VAS reduction and absence of narcotic usage.

The fact that clinical success rates reported for all percutaneous procedures do not rival the 90% success rate of open microdiskectomy is of note; however, it is critical to be aware that the highest success rate of microdiskectomy is experienced by patients with sequestered fragments. Patients with sequestered fragments are not percutaneous nucleoplasty candidates because there is no biomechanical mechanism by which that fragment would be resorbed. In a study by Chatterjee et al[21] comparing APLD with microdiskectomy for contained herniations, the microdiskectomy group had an 80% success rate. In a study by Carragee and Kim[22] examining outcomes of open diskectomy, it had been shown that herniations larger than 6 mm generally did well with diskectomy, whereas smaller herniations were associated with a poor outcome (26% success). These studies suggest that patients with smaller herniations are ideal candidates for percutaneous nucleoplasty.

The indications are straightforward for the cervical spine. Radicular symptoms must be due to a corroborative focal protrusion without advanced degenerative changes. It is unreasonable to assume that percutaneous decompression of radicular pain due to uncovertebral exostosis would be effective even in the presence of some foraminal disk material. Whether patients with severe myotomal deficits will display a good or excellent result remains to be determined, so such examination findings need to be carefully considered. Our orientation is to perform nucleoplasty and, if it fails, to move ahead with an open microdiskectomy with or without a fusion. Although the emphasis on the indications for coblation pertains to patient selection, this is not the entire issue for thoracic and especially cervical percutaneous decompression. Only physicians who have demonstrated skill in the performance of diskography in these regions should entertain the notion of using coblation. Extraordinary skill is required to avoid any of the potentially severe consequences of a less than perfect technique.

Absolute contraindications include systemic infection, cellulitis, diskitis, osteomyelitis, collapse of disk space, sequestered or extruded herniations, cauda equina syndrome, uncorrectable bleeding diathesis, and gross instability. Relative contraindications include spinal stenosis and prior surgery. Spinal stenosis is a relative contraindication because narrowing of the canal is a multifactorial process representing a combination of disk protrusion, ligamentum flavum buckling, and zygapophyseal joint hypertrophy. In cases where the disk appears to be the predominant contributor to the stenosis, it may be an effective intervention, whereas it is less likely to be successful in cases of bony or ligamentous causes of stenosis. Those instances typically occur when a patient with developmental stenosis develops an acute small protrusion initiating radicular pain that presents with a stenosis picture; standing and walking are provocative. Prior surgery is another relative contraindication. In a study comparing outcomes of patients with axial versus radicular symptoms, Sharps and Isaac[19] included a subgroup analysis of patients with prior fusion surgery at another level and prior percutaneous intradiskal procedures at the same level. Four patients with prior fusion surgery revealed only one with a successful outcome. Of four patients with prior intradiskal therapies, three had percutaneous diskectomy, and one had prior intradiskal electrothermal therapy (IDET). In this small subgroup, all four had successful outcomes. A subgroup that needs further analysis in large trials is patients with prior surgeries.

Surgical Equipment and Positioning

Nucleoplasty is an outpatient procedure performed using local anesthesia. Intravenous access and monitoring of blood pressure and pulse oximetry are suggested. Light conscious sedation can be used based on physician and patient preference. We suggest that sedation be used for patients who may be technically more difficult to obviate the muscle spasm that occurs with multiple attempts to accurately place the introducer needle. Those instances typically present with L5–S1 disk involvement and concurrent retrolisthesis, excessive collapse of the dorsal aspect of the disk and minimal height alteration of the middle and anterior portions, and/or a high iliac crest. As would be expected, light sedation should be used for obese and/or anxious patients. Heavy sedation or general anesthesia should never be considered with the percutaneous approach because of the real risk of injury to the traversing nerve root during placement of the introducer needle and/or while performing coblation with the catheter. Perioperative antibiotic prophylaxis to cover skin flora is recommended. Intravenous administration of cefazolin 1 hour preoperatively and oral cephalexin for 48 hours postoperatively is acceptable. Patients with severe penicillin allergy should alternatively use vancomycin. Although implied, it must be stated that this technique must be performed using fluoroscopic guidance. Upon signing consent forms for intravenous sedation, intravenous analgesia, and coblation/percutaneous diskectomy, the patient is positioned prone on the fluoroscopy table. Usual sterile technique is then used.

Surgical Technique

The fluoroscopy unit is positioned such that an oblique view of the spine is obtained, similar to that employed for diskography using the posterolateral approach.[23] Transdural entry into the disk is not recommended for patients undergoing nucleoplasty. The gantry angle should be orientated such that the superior articular process (SAP) of the inferior vertebral body crosses the intervertebral disk and divides it into one third medial to the SAP and two thirds lateral to the SAP for the L4–L5 and L5–S1 disks. A ratio of half and half is used for the more cephalad lumbar disks. The fluoroscopic view of the most superior and inferior aspect of each end plate should be superimposed such that the introducer needle can be positioned perpendicular to the disk or parallel with the gantry angle. When this view cannot be attained, the patient must be repositioned, the C-arm must change its cephalocaudal tilt, or the physician must alter the entry point of the needle to make up for the malalignment. After the skin is prepped and draped in sterile fashion with Betadine, the skin and subcutaneous tissues are anesthetized with 1% Xylocaine. A 3.5- to 6-inch 25-gauge needle can be used to effect the deeper anesthetization. Thereafter, a 17-gauge introducer needle is advanced toward and then into the posterolateral border of the disk, approximating the posterior annular/nuclear interface. It is important that the introducer needle is positioned in such a manner that it ensures the catheter will course parallel to the vertebral end plates. This will avoid injury by the catheter tip of the end plate during coblation (Fig. 32–6). It is also important that the introducer needle does not course too lateral (ventral) to the SAP to avoid injury to the traversing nerve root. Once accurate placement is confirmed following viewing in a minimum of two planes, posteroanterior and lateral, the catheter is advanced into and through the introducer needle. Within the disk, blunt dissection occurs by slowly advancing the catheter until it reaches the anterior annular/nuclear interface. The catheter is then withdrawn 2 mm and slowly rotated 360 degrees. The former maneuver obviates ablation of the most dorsal aspect of the anterior (ventral) annular-nuclear interface. During performance of the latter technique, there should not be any excessive resistance appreciated to guarantee the end plates are not inadvertently ablated. Coblation is then performed using a power level setting of 2 with a minimum of 6 passes oriented at the 2, 4, 6, 8, 10, and 12 o'clock

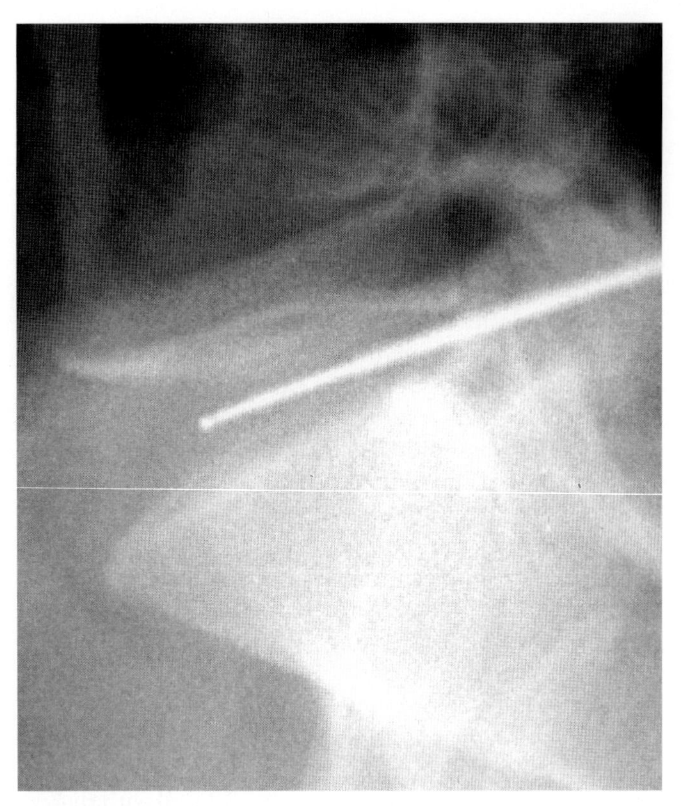

FIGURE 32–6 Introducer needle and coblation catheter are parallel with the end plates, precluding inadvertent damage to these vital structures.

positions. Each 8- to 15-second pass is comprised of an ablation component during the advancement of the catheter and a coagulation component while withdrawing the catheter. Continuous communication with the patient is essential during this part of the procedure. The patient must be reminded on multiple occasions that if any pain is experienced, the operating physician should immediately be informed. This level of interaction prevents injury and makes the patient that much more comfortable. In cases where more decompression is desired, the physician may choose to perform the technique bilaterally or put a little bend in the catheter or introducer needle to ablate additional tissue. Additional passes can also affect further volume reduction. The procedure is completed when there is no resistance to advancement and retraction of the catheter within a 360-degree arc. The perception to the physician is that there is an empty space through which the catheter is now passing. The tactile sense is distinctly different than when the catheter was first placed or during the first few coblation passes. Upon appreciation of that sensation, the catheter is withdrawn into the introducer needle, and both are removed simultaneously.

Cervical coblation requires the same preliminary steps leading to patient positioning, except that light sedation should be used for all patients. With the patient

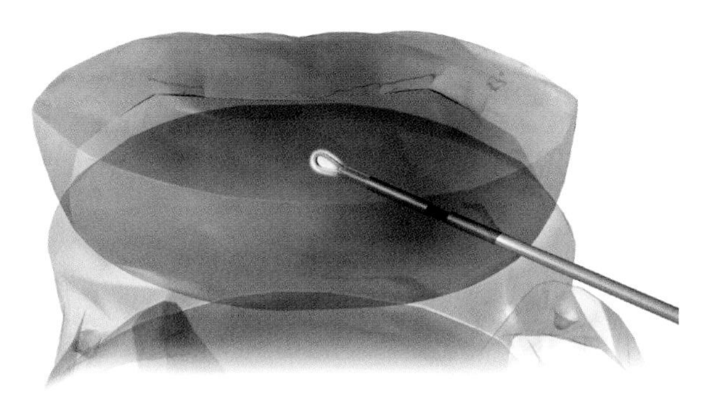

FIGURE 32–7 Illustration of proper introducer needle and catheter placement.

in the supine position, the x-ray gantry angle is rotated in a counterclockwise manner if a right-sided approach is used. While this is being done, the surgeon is visualizing the region of the ipsilateral neural foramen. Rotation should cease just as it comes into view. Cephalocaudal tilting of the gantry angle is performed until the end plates are parallel. Placement of the introducer needle into the central portion of the disk without encroaching upon the end plates is now feasible (Figs. 32–7, 32–8). The catheter is then gently advanced through the introducer needle and locked in place by the Luer-lock mechanism. When correct placement of the coblation catheter has been confirmed by reviewing the anteroposterior and lateral fluoroscopic images, a 0.5 second burst of coagulation is provided. If there is any involuntary extremity motion or pain perceived, catheter positioning must be reconfirmed. If neither of these symptoms occurs, ablation can be safely performed. To accomplish this, the catheter is rotated in a continuous 360-degree arc over a 6- to 10-second interval. Our preference is to perform the initial ablation just beyond the central portion of the disk. Upon completion one or two successive ablations are conducted in slightly different locations. The introducer needle is slightly withdrawn, with the catheter still locked in position such that it rests in the midline. The same technique is followed to accomplish one final ablation just proximal to the midline position of the disk. Prior to each ablation a short coagulation stimulus is provided. Following these two or three ablations, the catheter is withdrawn into the introducer needle, and both are simultaneously removed.

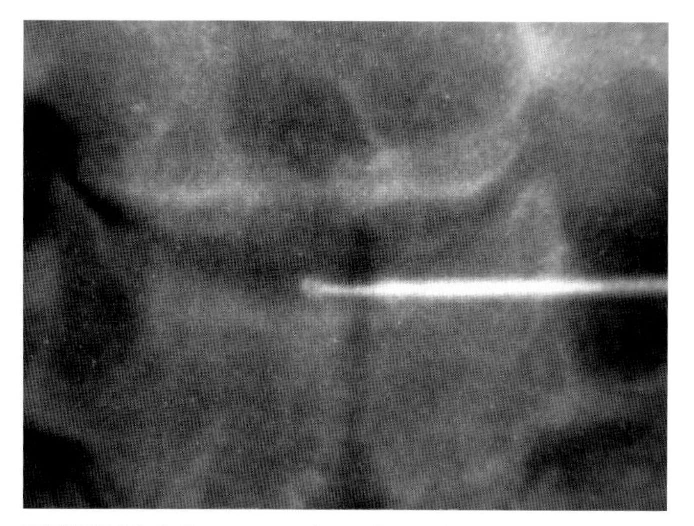

FIGURE 32–8 Anteroposterior radiograph of introducer needle and catheter in central region of the C4–C5 disk.

Complications

As with any percutaneous spinal procedure, potential complications can arise. Complications can relate to the needle and procedural technique, or they can be related to periprocedural factors. Technique-related complications include nerve root injury, diskitis, osteomyelitis, cellulitis, uncontrolled bleeding, dural puncture, annular injury, and vertebral end-plate injury. Vertebral end-plate osteonecrosis and subchondral marrow changes have been described in the laser diskectomy literature.[24] Although this has not been described as a complication of nucleoplasty, it is a theoretical complication. This can be avoided by entering the disk space with the introducer needle and catheter parallel to the end plates. Periprocedural complications may involve adverse reactions to anesthetic, sedative/analgesic medications, perioperative antibiotic prophylaxis, or intravenous fluid management. Preliminary data on complications and side effects of lumbar nucleoplasty reported soreness at the injection site as the most common side effect, which dropped rapidly after the first 72 hours postprocedure. Numbness and tingling were the next most commonly reported side effects. No major complications were observed in this small preliminary study of 19 patients. Although not yet published, we reported similar findings in a cohort of 53 patients undergoing 54 coblation procedures. In this group, 4% described increased back pain, 4% new leg pain, and 10% new numbness/tingling that persisted through the 2-week study interval. All occurrences of increased back pain resolved within 3 months. No patient considered the new leg pain, numbness, or tingling to be functionally limiting. Because the extremity symptoms presented in a nondermatomal manner for each subject, we have yet to develop a definitive explanation for those symptoms.

The potential complications following cervical coblation include laceration of the ipsilateral internal carotid artery, vertebral artery, or jugular vein. The spinal cord can be impaled, or the trachea or esophagus can be pierced. If the esophageal wall is breached, there is a dramatic increase in the risk of diskitis unless a new introducer needle is used. A common event is passage through the thyroid and the development of a hematoma. This side effect is invariably transient provided repeated prodding of the thyroid did not occur. Firm external compression for 5 minutes following the completion of the coblation procedure is recommended if concern about thyroid injury arises. One of the simplest ways to minimize these potential complications is to perform this technique only from the right side because the esophagus and trachea tend to rest slightly left of the midline. Using a sterile marking pen to outline the internal carotid may be helpful; however, we do not routinely do this. At the C2–C3 and less commonly the C3–C4 level, the esophagus may overlie or rest very close to the anticipated path for the introducer needle. We have our patients swallow a barium paste to outline the margins of the esophagus, thereby allowing us to avoid this bacterial reservoir. There are instances in which the introducer needle will back up after proper positioning has been accomplished. It is therefore strongly recommended that the introducer needle and catheter position be checked prior to stimulating with coagulation. Finally, it cannot be overemphasized that the most important issue to avoid serious postprocedure sequelae is physician experience. Cervical coblation is not for novices or those who have not performed numerous cervical diskograms.

Case Illustration

A 30-year-old athletic district manager for a pharmaceutical firm presented with the spontaneous development and 6-week history of posterior thigh and calf pain greater than low-back pain (90% extremity). Examination revealed an absent ankle jerk in the involved extremity, positive straight leg raise at 60 degrees, and 4+/5 strength of the gluteus maximus and gastrocnemius. Given his definitively articulated desire to avoid any invasive procedure, despite a pain intensity of 75 out of 100 on the visual analogue scale, a comprehensive rehabilitation program consisting of a Cox-2 specific nonsteroidal anti-inflammatory agent, active physical therapy, and avoidance of provocative factors was prescribed. His symptoms gradually abated over a 4-month period, such that the patient rated them a 10 to 20 out of 100. He was able to return to his usual athletic endeavors, lifting weights and running, with some minimal limitation. Two months later, the same presenting symptoms and intensity level recurred. Two weeks after this flare-up, he requested that surgery be performed. He did not want to take the time to undergo selective nerve root blocks in conjunction with physical therapy. An MRI was ordered, confirming the diagnosis of an S1 radiculopathy consequent to an L5–S1 focal protrusion (Figs. 32–9, 32–10). Lumbar nucleoplasty using coblation was suggested because the protrusion was contained, and there was adequate disk height (Fig. 32–11). He

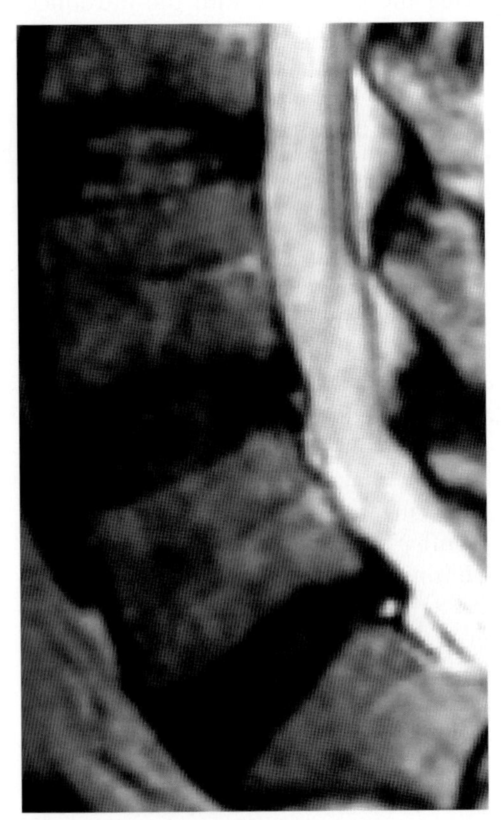

FIGURE 32–9 Sagittal T2-weighted image demonstrating a contained focal protrusion at L5–S1.

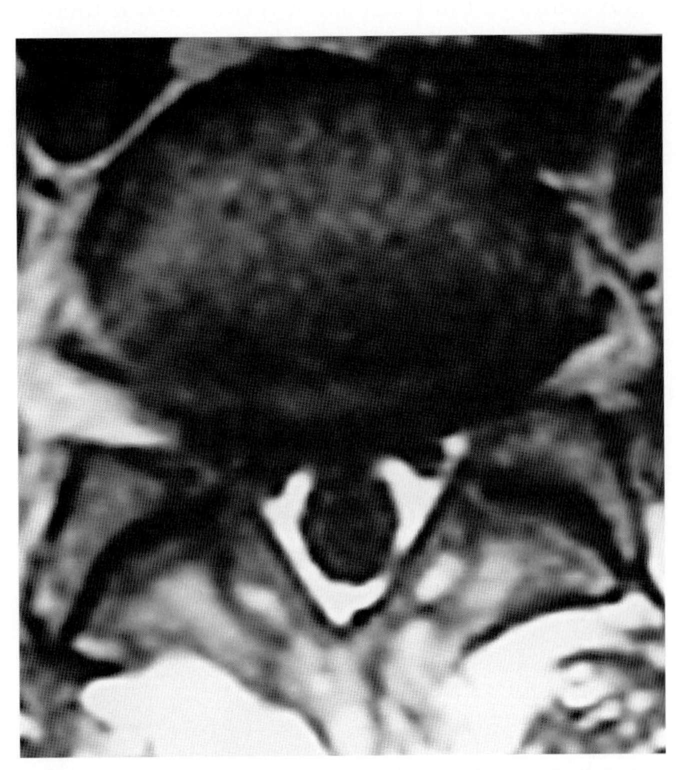

FIGURE 32–10 Axial T2-weighted image demonstrating dorsal displacement of the right S1 nerve root.

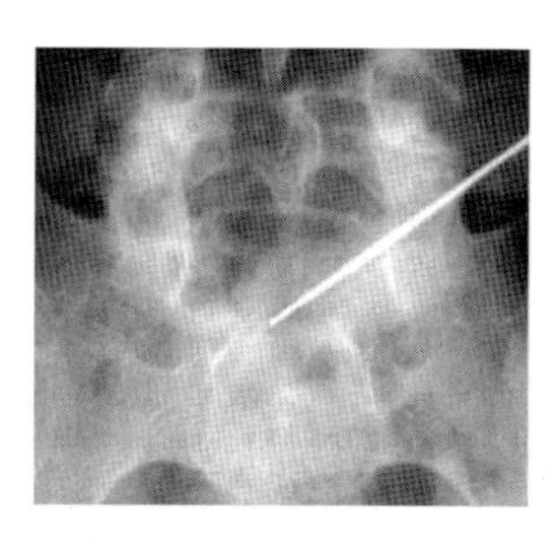
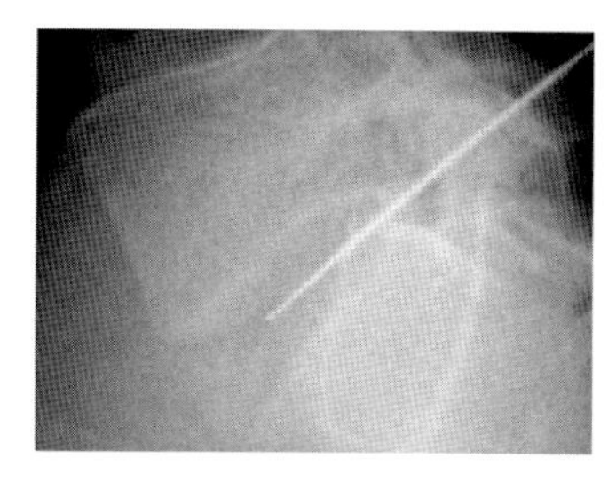

FIGURE 32–11 (A) Posteroanterior and **(B)** lateral views of the coblation catheter within the central portion of the disk.

experienced complete pain relief (0/100) the morning following the performance of nucleoplasty. There was no myotomal deficit at 2-week follow up. The patient was released to participate in his usual activities without any limitations. At each of his follow-up visits over the course of 1 year, the result had not deteriorated along any dimension.

Nucleoplasty presents a new minimally invasive treatment for herniated disks utilizing radiofrequency energy for partial removal of the nucleus pulposus. It is safe over other minimally invasive techniques because the temperature is kept low during ablation, avoiding the chances of any neural injury. It has the potential to provide a viable, safe, and effective treatment of low-back pain or radicular pain associated with a contained lumbar disk herniation. Because present clinical experience is limited, prospective controlled, randomized trials are required to determine the efficacy of this procedure over other less invasive techniques.

REFERENCES

1. Mixter WJ, Barr JS. Rupture of the intervertebral disc with involvement of the spinal canal. *N Engl J Med*. 1934;211:210–215.
2. Lutz GE, Vad V, Wisneski R. Fluoroscopic transforaminal lumbar epidural steroids: an outcome study. *Arch Phys Med Rehabil*. 1998;79:1362–1366.
3. Riew KD, Yin Y. The effect of nerve root injections on the need for operative treatment of lumbar radicular pain. *J Bone Joint Surg Am*. 2000;82:1589–1593.
4. Weiner B, Fraser R. Foraminal injection for lateral lumbar disc herniations. *J Bone Joint Surg (Br)*. 1997;79:804–807.
5. Kraemer J, Ludwig J, Bickert U, Owzcarek V, Traupe M. Lumbar epidural perineural injection: a new technique. *Eur Spine J*. 1997;6:357–361.
6. Smith L, Brown JE. Treatment of lumbar intervertebral disc lesions by direct injection of chymopapain. *J Bone Joint Surg (Br)*. 1967;49:502–519.
7. Pfirrmann CWA, Oberholzer PA, Zanetti M, et al. Selective nerve root blocks for the treatment of sciatica: evaluation of injection site and effectiveness—a study with patients and cadavers. *Radiology*. 2001;221:704–711.
8. Poynton AR, O'Farrell DA, Mulcahy D. Chymopapain chemonucleolysis: a review of 105 cases. *J R Coll Surg Edinb*. 1998;43:407–409.
9. Scwetschenau PR, Ramirez A, Johnson J. Double blind evaluations of intradiscal chymopapain for herniated lumbar discs: early results. *J Neurosurg*. 1976;45:622–627.
10. Javid MJ, Nordby EJ, Ford LT. Safety and efficacy of chymopapain (chymodiactin) in herniated nucleus pulposus with sciatica. *JAMA*. 1983;249:2489–2494.
11. Fraser RD. Chymopapain for the treatment of intervertebral disc herniation: the final report of a double-blind study. *Spine*. 1984;9:815–817.
12. Gogan WJ, Frazer RD. Chymopapain: a 10 year double blind study. *Spine*. 1992;17:388–394.
13. Wittenberg RH, Oppel S, Rubenthaler FA, Steffen R. Five-year results from chemonucleolysis with chymopapain or collagenase: a prospective randomized study. *Spine*. 2001;26:1835–1841.
14. Kambin P. Arthroscopic microdiskectomy. *Mt Sinai J Med*. 1991;58:159–164.
15. Onik G, Maroon J, Helms C, et al. Automated percutaneous diskectomy: initial patient experience, work in progress. *Radiology*. 1987;162:129–132.
16. Revel M, Payan C, Vallee C, et al. Automated percutaneous lumbar discectomy versus chemonucleolysis in the treatment of sciatica. a multicenter trial. *Spine*. 1993;18:1–7.
17. Mayer HM, Brock M. Percutaneous endoscopic discectomy: surgical technique and preliminary results compared to microsurgical discectomy. *J Neurosurg*. 1993;78:216–225.
18. Choy DS, Altman P. Fall of intradiscal pressure with laser ablation. *J Clin Laser Med Surg*. 1995;13:149–151.
19. Sharps L, Isaac Z. Percutaneous disc decompression using nucleoplasty. *Pain Physician*. 2002;5:121–126.
20. Singh V, Slipman CW. Discogenic pain and intradiscal therapies. In: Manchikanti L, Slipman CW, Fellows B, eds. *Low Back Pain: An Interventional Approach to Diagnosis and Treatment*. Paducah, KY: ASIPP Publishers; 2002:411–420.
21. Chatterjee S, Foy PM, Findlay GF. Report of a controlled clinical trial comparing automated percutaneous lumbar discectomy and microdiscectomy in the treatment of contained lumbar disc herniation. *Spine*. 1995;20:734–738.
22. Carragee EJ, Kim DH. A prospective analysis of magnetic resonance imaging findings in patients with sciatica and lumbar disc herniation: correlation of outcomes with disc fragment and canal morphology. *Spine*. 1997;22:1650–1660.
23. Slipman CW, Palmitier RA, DeDianous DK. Injection techniques. In: Grabois M, Hart H, Garrison J, Lehmhuhl D, eds. *Physical Medicine and Rehabilitation: The Complete Approach*. Boston: Blackwood Science Publishers; 1999:458–486.
24. Tonami H, Kuginuki M, Kuginuki Y, et al. MR imaging of subchondral osteonecrosis of the vertebral body after percutaneous laser diskectomy. *Am J Roentgenol*. 1999;173:1383–1386.

■ SECTION SIX ■

Image-Guided Endoscopic Spine Surgery

33

Fluoroscopic Image-Guided Spine Surgery

KEVIN T. FOLEY, MICHAEL A. LEFKOWITZ, AND Y. RAJA RAMPERSAUD

Fluoroscopy is an imaging technique that is familiar to spinal surgeons. It is routinely employed to improve intraoperative visualization of bony anatomy. By replacing direct visualization with radiographic visualization, it has enabled a reduction in surgical exposure, duration, and blood loss. Its use has facilitated a variety of complex spinal procedures, including pedicle screw insertion, interbody cage placement, odontoid screw insertion, and atlantoaxial transarticular screw fixation. Despite its widespread acceptance and utility, however, fluoroscopy has disadvantages. The most notable is occupational radiation exposure, particularly to the surgeon's hands.[1–3] Data have suggested that spinal surgeons, in particular, are at significant risk for fluoroscopy-related radiation exposure.[4] Furthermore, the C-arm can be cumbersome to maneuver around a sterile operative field. Because only a single projection can be visualized at one time (without a second fluoroscope), it is necessary to reposition the C-arm during procedures that require multiple planes of visualization. This process is often tedious, time consuming, and frustrating.

A desire to improve intraoperative visualization led to the development of image-guided surgery systems for spinal surgery. The first such systems were CT based and were an extension of systems used for cranial neurosurgery. Further development of image-guided technology has resulted in a second class of systems that differ in terms of the type of imaging that is used to provide the image guidance. These systems are based on fluoroscopy itself. By combining current C-arm fluoroscopy with computer-aided surgical technology, many advantages of fluoroscopy can be enhanced and its disadvantages minimized or eliminated.

A fluoroscopy-based system employs commonly available C-arms augmented with accessories that allow accurate measurement of the relationship between the C-arm and the patient. The system takes patient and C-arm position data for a given projection and relates the data to the fluoroscopic image from that projection. After calibrating the system with positional and fluoroscopic data from one or more projections, the computer generates a mathematical model of the fluoroscopic image that enables the superimposition of tracked surgical instruments onto the saved fluoroscopic images. Thus, the real-time position of these instruments is displayed as it relates to one or more previously acquired fluoroscopic images, even in multiple planes, simultaneously. We term this process *virtual fluoroscopy* (Fig. 33–1). The advantages of virtual fluoroscopy are that no special preoperative study is required, intraoperative patient registration is automated, and the images may be updated as necessary in the operating room. Fluoroscopy-based systems are available that are either integrated with conventional image-guided surgery systems (FluoroNav Virtual Fluoroscopy System and StealthStation, Medtronic Surgical Navigation Systems, Louisville, CO) or exist as stand-alone devices (StealthStation Ion Fluoroscopic Navigation System, Medtronic Surgical Navigation Systems, Broomfield, CO).

Materials and Methods

A typical virtual fluoroscopy system consists of an image-guidance computer system, a commercially available fluoroscopic C-arm, a calibration device that

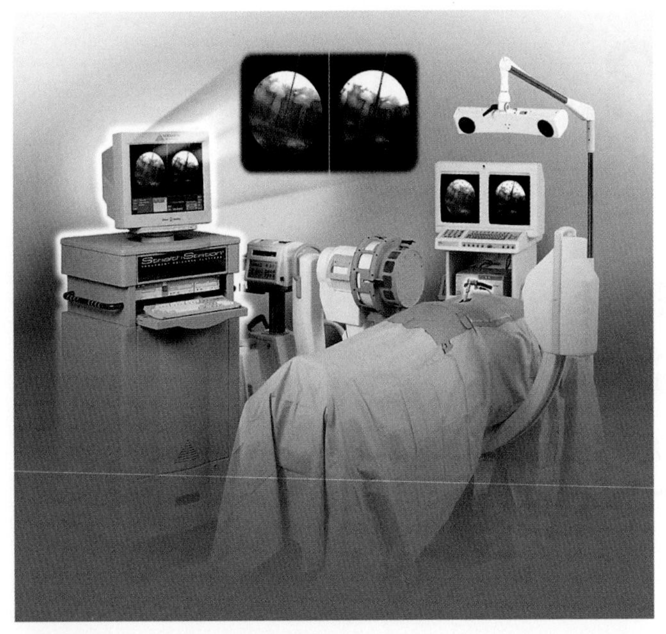

FIGURE 33–1 Virtual fluoroscopy. Operating room setup integrating fluoroscopic images with previously acquired images.

attaches to the C-arm, and specially modified surgical instruments that are capable of being tracked by the image-guidance system. The system may be operated by the surgeon through a sterile interface, or it may be operated by an assistant. The operation of a virtual fluoroscopy system may be divided into four basic steps (Fig. 33–2):

Step 1: fluoroscopic image acquisition

- Conventional fluoroscopic images are automatically transferred to the computer for image processing.

Step 2: C-arm and patient position measurement

- Information about the relative position of the C-arm and the patient is acquired.
- Measurement is done by cameras that detect the location of light-emitting diodes or passive reflectors that have been attached to the C-arm and the patient.
- The markers that are attached to the patient are in the form of a dynamic reference array (DRA), which rigidly attaches to the portion of the patient's anatomy that is to be imaged. Other means of position sensing (e.g., electromagnetic, sonic, mechanical, etc.) can also be used.

Step 3: merging of the fluoroscopic images with their unique C-arm and patient positions to create a mathematical model (mapping) of the image formation process

- The computer calibrates the acquired fluoroscopic image by taking into account the positional data acquired in the second step.
- Based on the inputted images, a mathematical mapping function is generated that allows a virtual fluoroscopic image to be produced for a unique combination of C-arm and patient position.
- The calibration process compensates for such factors as gravity-dependent changes in the C-arm image center, the effect of external electromagnetic fields generated by electrical equipment in the operating room, and the effect of changes in the C-arm's position with respect to the earth's magnetic field.
- Because of these compensation factors, which are unique to every C-arm position, it is necessary that every acquired image be independently calibrated. This can be accomplished quickly and efficiently through the use of a computerized algorithm.

Step 4: measurement of the position of surgical instruments in the operative field so that their likeness may be superimposed on the virtual fluoroscopic images

- The computer determines the position of one or more trackable surgical instruments using a position-measuring camera, then superimposes an image of the instrument(s) in the virtual fluoroscopic display.
- Dedicated tracked awls, probes, taps, and screwdrivers are available, and any rigid surgical instrument may be tracked with the assistance of a universal tool array.
- The system is capable of correctly displaying the position of the surgical instrument(s) in any of the previously acquired fluoroscopic images, in multiple planes, simultaneously. The system also allows the actual projection of a surgical instrument (in one color) and the simultaneous projection of the linear extension of that instrument's proposed trajectory (in a second color).

System Accuracy

The accuracy of various virtual fluoroscopy systems has been tested experimentally. Foley et al[5] performed a cadaver study comparing live and virtual fluoroscopic images in which a tracked probe was inserted into pedicles from L1 to S1. Differences in positioning the probe tip and probe trajectory angle were measured for the live and virtual images. The mean error in probe tip localization was 0.97 ± 0.40 mm (99% confidence interval = 2.2 mm, maximum probe tip error = 3 mm). The mean trajectory angle difference between the virtual and actual probe images was 2.7 degrees ± 0.6 degrees (99% confidence interval = 4.6 degrees, maximum trajectory angle difference = 5 degrees). (Fig. 33–3)

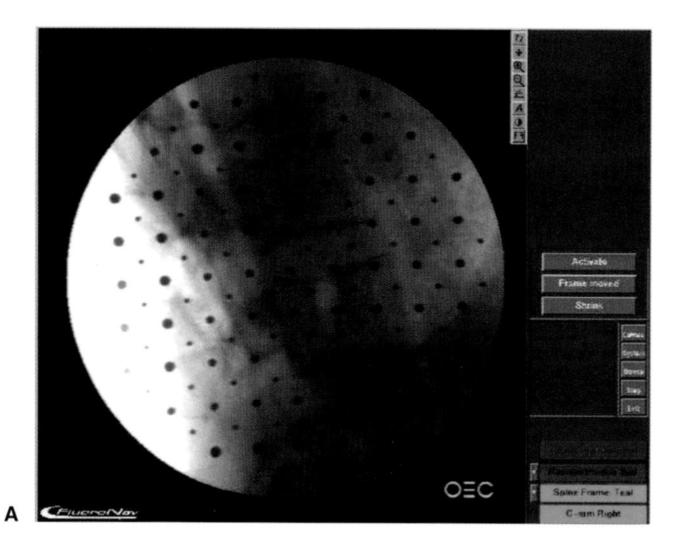

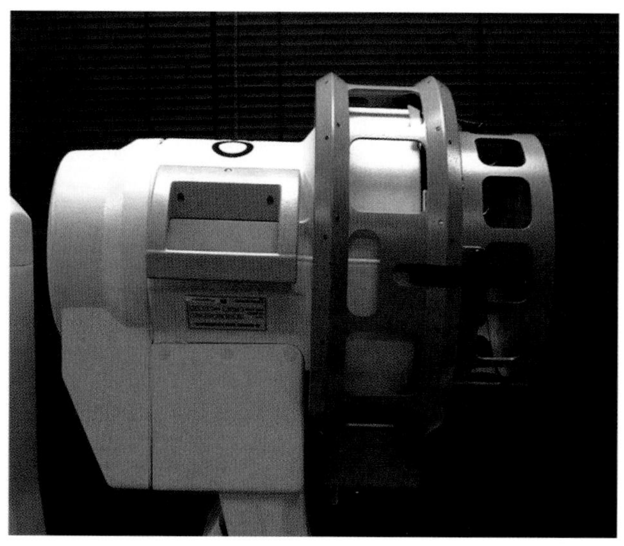

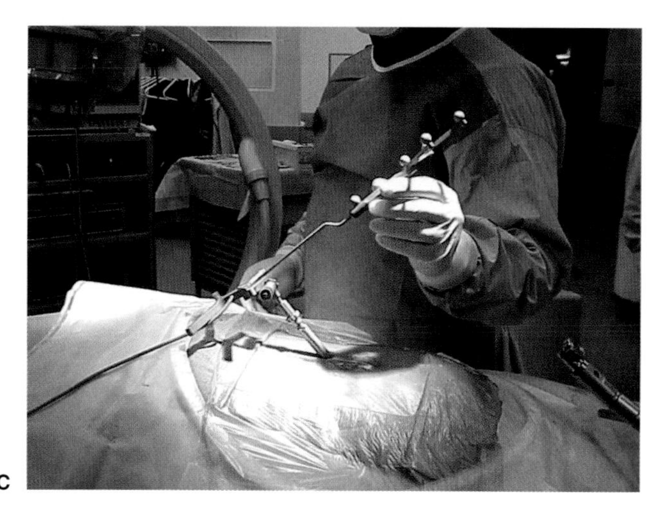

FIGURE 33–2 Fluoroscopic image-guided spine surgery. **(A)** Fluoroscopic images are acquired and calibrated (anteroposterior, lateral, oblique, etc.). **(B)** Calibration target with affixed light-emitting diodes attached to an OEC Model 9600 C-arm fluoroscope. **(C)** The reference arc is applied to the anatomy; any rigid surgical instrument can now be tracked simultaneously on all views.

Operative Techniques

Open Pedicle Screw Insertion

The steps for open pedicle screw insertion are:

- The DRA is rigidly affixed to the spinous process of the vertebra in which pedicle screws are to be placed.
- Fluoroscopic views normally obtained by the surgeon are then acquired. These may include lateral views, anteroposterior views, or oblique ("owl's-eye") views down the length of the pedicle.
- By positioning the tracked instruments over the pedicle, the anticipated entry point and trajectory of the instruments may be displayed prior to probing the pedicle.
- The system will also allow the virtual projection of pedicle screws of a selected length and diameter onto the chosen trajectory.
- The use of tracked awls, probes, and taps permits continuous visualization of the instruments along their course through the pedicle and into the vertebral body.
- The fluoroscope may be used in the live mode at any time during the procedure for visualization of instrument or screw position.

Percutaneous Pedicle Screw Insertion

Because the virtual fluoroscopy system does not rely on direct exposure of the spine for registration, percutaneous screws may be inserted.

- A small incision is made over the spinous process of one of the levels to be instrumented. The DRA is rigidly attached to the spinous process.
- The desired fluoroscopic projections (i.e., AP, lateral, and oblique) are obtained and calibrated.

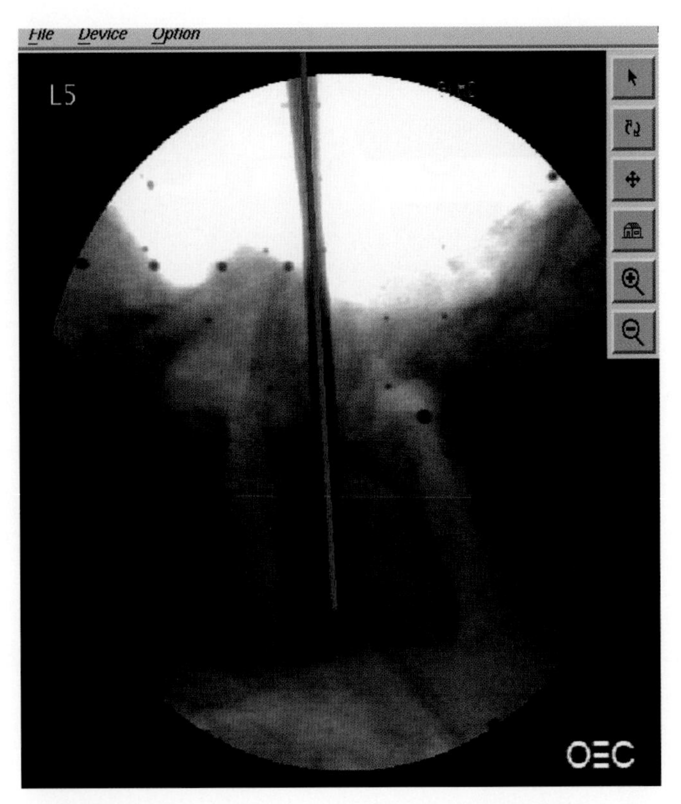

FIGURE 33–3 Trajectory angle difference between the virtual and actual probe images. The virtual angle is in red over the actual value.

- A tracked, sharp-tip probe is placed on the skin surface over the pedicle. The trajectory of the probe may be virtually extended through the pedicle to visualize the anticipated course of the pedicle screw (Fig. 33–4A).
- A stab incision is made at the skin entry point, and a K-wire and dilators are used to dissect through the paraspinous muscles to the pedicle surface. The dilators are withdrawn, and a tracked awl and probe are used to form a pilot hole in the pedicle under virtual fluoroscopic guidance.
- As described in the conventional pedicle screw insertion section, the trajectory of the instruments may be virtually extended to visualize the pathway of the screw prior to probing the pedicle (Fig. 33–4B).

Atlantoaxial Transarticular Screw Fixation

The steps for atlantoaxial transarticular screw fixation are:

- The patient is put in the prone position with the head affixed in a Mayfield headrest. It is important to have the headrest positioned in such a fashion as to allow anteroposterior views of the atlantoaxial complex to be obtained.
- Under lateral fluoroscopic guidance, the atlantoaxial subluxation is gently reduced, and the head is fixed in place.
- A conventional midline occiput to C3 exposure is performed so that the C1 and C2 lateral masses and the C1–C2 and C2–C3 facet joints are revealed.
- The DRA is attached to the C2 spinous process. At this point, anteroposterior and lateral fluoroscopic images are obtained and calibrated.
- The preoperative CT and MRI scans are reviewed for information on the optimal screw entry point and trajectory. A typical entry point is ~2 to 3 mm above the C2–C3 facet joint line and 2 to 3 mm lateral to the junction of the C2 lamina and lateral mass.

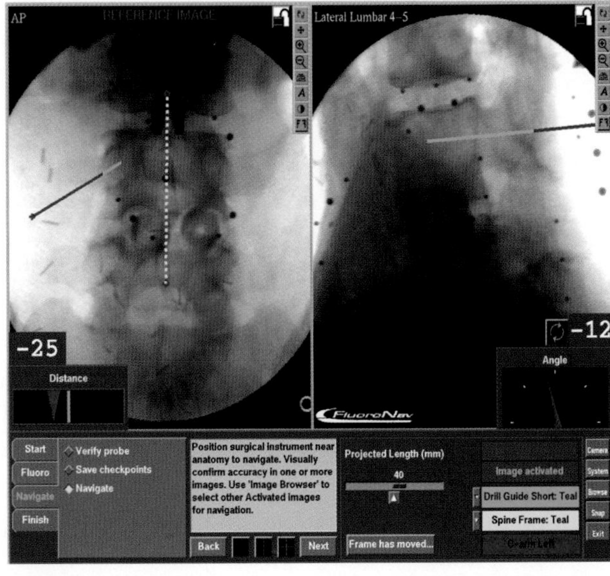

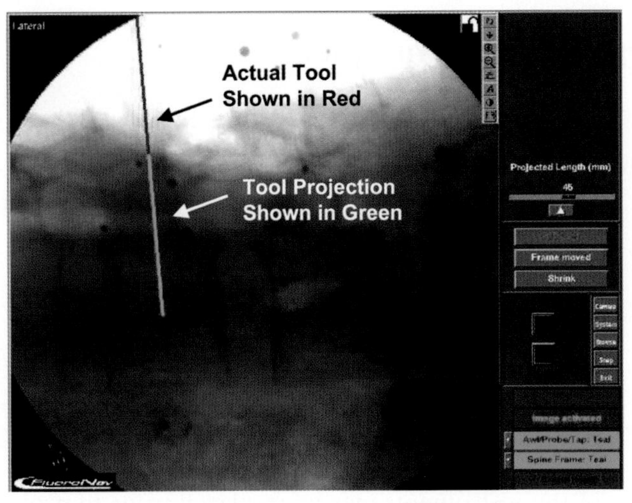

FIGURE 33–4 (A,B) Trajectory of the probe may be virtually extended through the pedicle to visualize the anticipated course of the pedicle screw.

- A tracked probe is placed on the skin surface at the cervicothoracic junction, 1.5 to 2 cm lateral to the midline. The trajectory of the probe is virtually extended through the C2 inferior facet, the C2 pars, across the C1–C2 joint, into the Cl lateral mass, to the posterior cortex of the Cl anterior arch. The position of the probe is adjusted until a proper trajectory is observed.
- A paramedian stab incision is then made where the probe contacts the skin, and a tracked drill guide is inserted through this incision and the underlying paraspinous tissues to the C2–C3 facet. The entry point is decorticated. A drill is then passed through the tracked guide and is used to create a pilot hole along the C1–C2 transarticular pathway.
- The trajectory of the drill and guide is followed using virtual fluoroscopy, simultaneously visualizing this trajectory in the anteroposterior and lateral views. Progress of the actual drill tip is followed using live lateral fluoroscopy. An appropriate-length screw is inserted once the pilot hole has been tapped. The process is repeated on the contralateral side.

Odontoid Screw Insertion

The steps for odontoid screw insertion are:

- The patient is positioned supine with the neck extended. The odontoid fracture is reduced under live fluoroscopy. The proper position is maintained using a Mayfield apparatus.
- The DRA is attached to the Mayfield apparatus. Open-mouth and lateral fluoroscopic images of C2 are obtained, calibrated, and saved using a single fluoroscope. The C-arm is returned to the lateral position.
- An incision is made at the level of the C5–C6 interspace, and dissection proceeds down to the ventral surface of the cervical spine, as far rostral as the C2–C3 interspace.
- A shallow, midline trough is created in the ventral surface of the C3 vertebral body and the C2–C3 anulus to facilitate a steep trajectory for the screw.
- A tracked drill guide is positioned against the anterior, inferior aspect of the C2 vertebral body in the midline. Proper position is confirmed with the open-mouth and lateral virtual fluoroscopic views (Fig. 33–5).
- A K-wire is then inserted through this drill guide to penetrate the anterior aspect of the inferior C2 end plate and directed through the middle of the dens to a point just proximal to its tip.
- Progress of the K-wire is monitored with live lateral fluoroscopy. After the K-wire has been appropriately positioned, the screw length is measured using a gauge, and a self-tapping, cannulated lag screw is inserted over the K-wire.
- The K-wire remains in place while the screw is being inserted to maintain the proper alignment of the dens with the C2 body. The K-wire is removed after the screw has been fully inserted. To achieve the proper lag effect, the lag screw threads must lie distal to the fracture line.

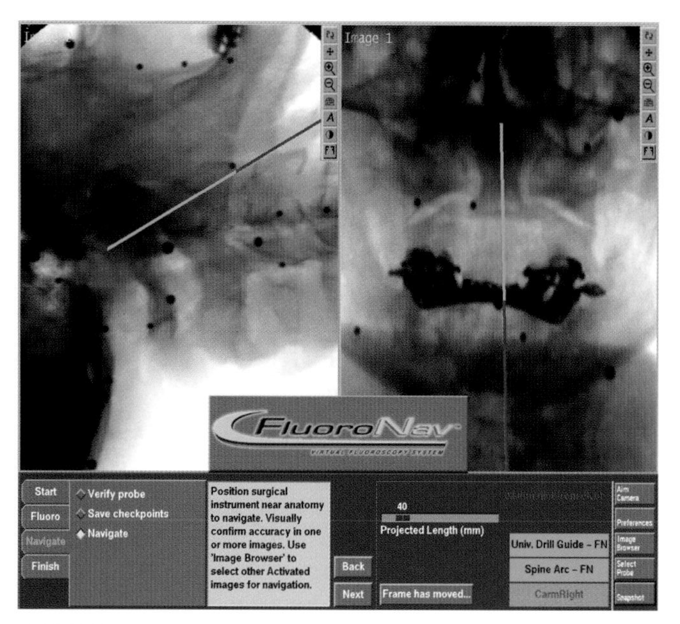

FIGURE 33–5 Open-mouth (right) and lateral (left) virtual fluoroscopic views during odontoid screw insertion.

A virtual fluoroscopy system for spinal and musculoskeletal procedures offers several distinct advantages over conventional C-arm fluoroscopy. First, radiation exposure to the patient and surgical team is reduced. The system eliminates the need to obtain multiple images to update instrument position. Rather, the instrument is tracked by the digitizer, and its real-time position is overlaid onto the previously acquired fluoroscopic view(s). In addition, bilateral localization at any given spinal level(s) can be performed using a single image, further reducing fluoroscopy time. Furthermore, because preacquired fluoroscopic images are used for navigation, the surgical team can stand at a safe distance during "live" fluoroscopy, minimizing or eliminating the need for wearing lead shielding. Second, a single C-arm unit is turned into a multiplanar device. The surgeon can preacquire several images in several planes and use them for navigation. The system overlays a tracked tool's position onto all of the preacquired views simultaneously (up to four views). Thus, virtual fluoroscopy eliminates the need to repeatedly reposition the C-arm and enables the surgeon to achieve a desired trajectory in a much more efficient manner. Third, after acquiring the desired images, the surgeon can move the C-arm out of the operative field, minimizing or eliminating the ergonomic challenges of C-arm use, particularly in spinal procedures. Fourth, the computational power of the image-guided computer allows further enhancement of standard fluoroscopy by providing real-time quantitative information to the surgeon. For example, in planning pedicle screw insertion, the distance of the screw insertion point from the midline and the desired axial trajectory can be obtained from the patient's preoperative CT or MRI scan (e.g., the diagnostic study, not a specially formatted image-guided study). After obtaining a true anteroposterior fluoroscopic view and defining the midline with the virtual fluoroscopy system software, the surgeon can see a real-time numerical display of the angular trajectory of an instrument relative to the midsagittal plane (in degrees) and the distance of its tip from the midline (in millimeters).

Foley et al[6] performed a study of lumbar pedicle screw fixation using a novel percutaneous technique. A virtual fluoroscopy system (FluoroNav) was used as the imaging modality. Twelve patients were successfully treated using this technique. The versatility of the imaging system allowed registration of unexposed spine elements for the percutaneous procedure. Registration was completely automated, requiring no surgeon input, and occurred in seconds. All percutaneous pedicle screws were successfuly placed.

Technology is currently being developed that may ultimately allow intraoperative registration of the spine with fluoroscopic imaging. This may eliminate the need for time-consuming tactile anatomical registration. Two-dimensional fluoroscopic registration could then be used as an adjunct to CT or MRI to allow for three-dimensional real-time navigation. In fact, the development of isocentric C-arm fluoroscopy, which generates CT images using an intraoperative fluoroscope, may offer another means of three-dimensional navigation using a two-dimensional intraoperative imaging source. Finally, it is quite likely that virtual fluoroscopy technology will be routinely integrated into C-arm fluoroscopes, allowing the surgeon to use a single device in either a "live" or virtual mode, as navigational needs dictate.

REFERENCES

1. International Commission on Radiological Protection. Publication 60: recommendations of the International Commission on Radiological Protection. *Ann ICRP.* 1991;21:1–3.
2. Mehlman CT, DiPasquale TG. Radiation exposure to the orthopaedic surgical team during fluoroscopy: how far away is far enough? *J Orthop Trauma.* 1997;11:392–398.
3. Sanders R, Koval KJ, DiPasquale T, et al. Exposure of the orthopaedic surgeon to radiation. *J Bone Joint Surg Am.* 1993;75:326–330.
4. Rampersaud YR, Foley KT, Shen AC, et al. Radiation exposure to the spine surgeon during fluoroscopically assisted pedicle screw insertion. *Spine.* 2000;25:2637–2645.
5. Foley KT, Rampersaud YR, Simon DA. Virtual fluoroscopy: multiplanar x-ray guidance with minimal radiation exposure. *Eur Spine J.* 1999;8(suppl 1):S36.
6. Foley KT, Gupta SK, Justis JR, Sherman MC. Percutaneous pedicle screw fixation of the lumbar spine. *Neurosurgical Focus.* 2001;10:1–8.

34

Image-Guided Endoscopic and Minimally Invasive Spine Surgery

CALVIN R. MAURER JR., RAMIN SHAHIDI, JAY B. WEST, AND DANIEL H. KIM

Electronic videoendoscopy is commonly performed for a wide variety of diagnostic and therapeutic procedures due to the advent of miniature charge–coupled device (CCD) cameras and associated microelectronics. An *endoscope* is basically a long tube through which an image of the surgical space inside the body is transmitted to the surgeon. This tube may be rigid for areas easily accessible through an incision, or flexible to extend through twisting paths, as in pulmonary airways or the gastrointestinal tract. In current systems, the image is presented on a video monitor. The image is passed through the tube, either by lens optics in a rigid endoscope or by fiberoptics in a flexible endoscope, to a CCD video camera at the surgeon's end.[1] Improvements in CCD technology have alternatively made it possible to locate the CCD array at the endoscope tip. A light source is transmitted to the endoscope tip through fiberoptics in all endoscopes. This technology is packed into a tube ranging from a few millimeters to a centimeter in diameter. For some operations, typically those that require flexible endoscopes, instruments are passed through a working channel in the endoscope. In operations where the surgical space is more easily accessible, a rigid endoscope and multiple instruments are inserted through separate incisions.

Open spine surgery requires extensive soft tissue dissection. Muscle retraction during surgery has been shown to cause short-term damage and long-term, degenerative changes.[2–5] Most of the recovery involved in open spinal procedures is due to the soft tissue dissection and muscle trauma.[6] This trauma necessitates long recovery time and extended loss of work.[7,8] Recovery from open spinal surgery exposes the patient to prolonged opiate analgesia. Pain management researchers agree that such analgesia poses a nontrivial risk of initiating, or exacerbating, addiction in the recovering patient.[9,10]

In minimally invasive surgical procedures, endoscopes are inserted through natural orifices of the body or small (typically 5–10 mm) incisions. The endoscope illuminates the surgical region of interest and transmits camera images to a video monitor. Such minimally invasive procedures as endoscopic/percutaneous laminotomy, diskectomy, pedicle screw fixation, and vertebroplasty can reduce morbidity relative to traditional open procedures. Surgery performed through small incisions is often much less traumatic than the same surgery done through large incisions. Minimally invasive procedures have proven to be effective, reduce postoperative pain, shorten the hospital stay, help the patient resume normal activity, and reduce the surgical complication rate.[11–19]

These advantages unfortunately do not come without costs. What is better for the patient is often awkward for the surgeon, who has typically relied heavily on dexterity, tactile feedback, and excellent hand–eye coordination, and who now must operate while looking at a video monitor displaying endoscopic images. Dexterity limitations[20] and tactile limitations[21] are obvious and well known. There are also several fundamental vision problems. The surgeon's natural hand–eye coordination is severely degraded, and there are difficulties with depth perception and spatial orientation.[22] These visualization problems (compared with open surgery) are due to a variety of factors, including monocular vision (although stereoscopic systems are possible), a limited field of view, peripheral image distortions, and the projection of a natural three-dimensional (3D) surgical scene on a two-dimensional (2D) display. Also, endoscopes can display only visible surfaces, and it is therefore generally difficult to visualize tumors, nerves, vessels, and other anatomic structures that lie beneath opaque tissue.

Image-guided surgery (IGS) systems are widely used in a variety of cranial and open spinal procedures.[23–26] Such systems have the promise of addressing some of the visualization problems inherent with endoscopic and minimally invasive spine surgery. This chapter will describe currently available fluoroscopy-based and CT-based IGS systems, review some of the key issues and challenges for the application of these systems to image-guided endoscopic and minimally invasive spine surgery, discuss the relevance of IGS for pedicle screw placement, and describe a promising new approach called *image-enhanced endoscopy.*

Fluoroscopy-Based Image-Guided Surgery

Fluoroscopy is an imaging method that is useful and familiar to musculoskeletal surgeons. It is routinely employed for intraoperative visualization of patient anatomy, particularly bony anatomy, and surgical instrument position. Such radiographic visualization facilitates reduced surgical exposure and improved accuracy for a wide variety of spine procedures.

Despite its widespread acceptance and utility, fluoroscopy has limitations and disadvantages. Perhaps the most important disadvantage is occupational radiation exposure, particularly to the surgeon's hands.[27–29] Data have suggested that spinal surgeons, in particular, are at significant risk for fluoroscopy-related radiation exposure.[30] Another limitation associated with conventional use of a C-arm fluoroscope is that only one x-ray projection image can be acquired and visualized at a time (without using a second fluoroscope). Thus, for procedures that require the use of images obtained from multiple orientations, it is necessary to reposition the C-arm repeatedly throughout the procedure. Frequent repositioning of a C-arm fluoroscope in a crowded operative field is often ergonomically challenging. Furthermore, it is generally difficult to position and orient a surgical probe or instrument properly when it can be seen in only one projection image at a time.

Fluoroscopy-based IGS systems have been developed to overcome these limitations and disadvantages. Such systems track surgical probes and instruments and display their positions in real time on one or more previously acquired fluoroscopic images. Some authors refer to this process as *virtual fluoroscopy*[31–33] (see note "a"). The fundamental ideas of fluoroscopy-based IGS were first presented by Potamianos et al[34,35] and subsequently developed by other investigators.[31,36–40] The original work used a robotic manipulator. Most current systems use an optical tracking system.[31] Several systems are available (e.g., the FluoroNav Virtual Fluoroscopy System, which is integrated in the StealthStation Treatment Guidance System, Medtronic, Surgical Navigation System, Louisville, CO).

The main components of a typical fluoroscopy-based IGS system are a computer workstation and monitor, a tracking system, a conventional C-arm fluoroscope, a calibration device that attaches to the imaging head of the fluoroscope, a spine clamp with a dynamic reference frame (DRF), and a variety of optically tracked instruments (Fig. 34–1). The calibration device basically consists of two parallel plates that contain radiopaque metal spheres. Although various kinds of tracking systems can be used, including electromagnetic, magnetic, and ultrasonic, most current systems use an optical tracking system. Such a system generally consists of two or more optical sensors or cameras that detect infrared light emitting diodes (IREDs) or photoreflective spheres or disks that are mounted on the calibration device, the DRF attached to the spine clamp, and the surgical instruments. Using mathematical principles of localization by triangulation, the system determines the spatial position and orientation of the instruments (and DRF and calibration device) to provide real-time navigation. Multiple instruments can be tracked simultaneously during a procedure. In the case of actively tracked instruments using IREDs, each instrument IRED array is strobed individually by the tracking system. In the case of passively tracked instruments using photoreflective spheres or disks, the tracking system can identify different instruments if they have distinct marker configurations.

At the beginning of surgery, the fluoroscope is positioned in the usual fashion, the calibration device is attached to the imaging head (image intensifier), and the fluoroscope is sterilely draped. The DRF is attached to the spinous process of the spine segment of interest, or an adjacent segment, with a clamp or a modified screw.[41,42] The DRF allows patient movement to be tracked. One or more fluoroscopic images are obtained with the vertebral segments of interest centered in the field of view to minimize the effects of parallax. Each fluoroscopic image is transferred at the time of acquisition from the fluoroscope to the computer workstation through a standard video cable (or a digital link). The optical tracking system simultaneously determines the position of the calibration device and the DRF and thereby determines the position of the C-arm relative to the patient at the time of image acquisition. The computer digitizes the acquired fluoroscopic image and calibrates the image using the positions of the

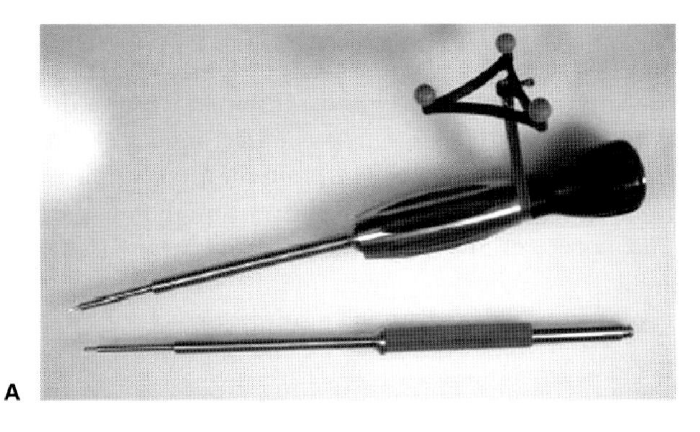

A

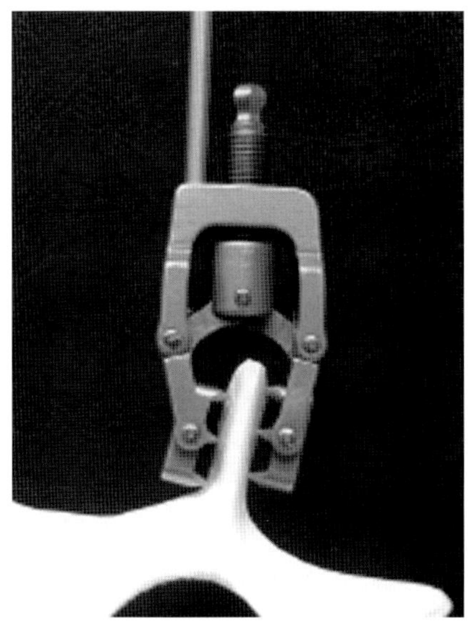

B

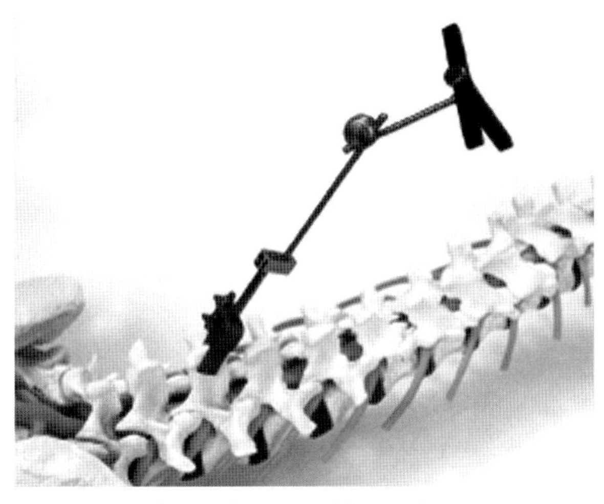

C

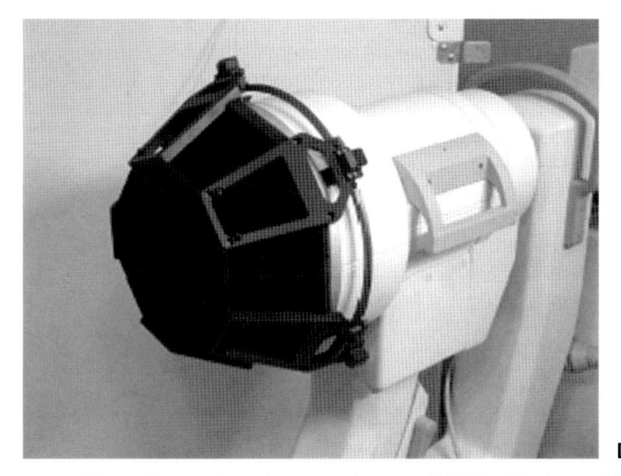

D

FIGURE 34–1 Some image-guided spine surgery system components. **(A)** An awl with an array of photoreflective spheres. Other surgical tools that can be tracked and used with an image-guided surgery (IGS) system include a bone tap, pedicle probe, drill guide, drill, and screwdriver. **(B)** A spine clamp attached to a spinous process. **(C)** A spine clamp with a dynamic reference frame (DRF) of infrared light emitting diodes (IREDs). **(D)** A calibration device attached to the imaging head of a C-arm fluoroscope. The calibration device basically consists of two parallel plates containing radiopaque metal spheres and has many IREDs mounted around its circumference.

radiopaque calibration markers that appear in the fluoroscopic image (Fig. 34–2) and the position of the C-arm relative to the patient. During the calibration process, the computer constructs a mathematical model of the fluoroscopic image formation process, which describes where a given position relative to the patient projects onto the fluoroscopic image. The mathematical model can be different for every acquired image for a variety of reasons (e.g., mechanical deformation of the C-arm, geometric distortion in the image intensifier image due to a change in position of the image intensifier relative to the earth's magnetic field and electromagnetic fields near the C-arm generated by electrical devices in the operating room). Because of this, the calibration device is left on the imaging head, and calibration is performed independently for every acquired fluoroscopic image. After the fluoroscopic images are acquired and calibrated, the optical tracking system determines the positions of instruments and the DRF and uses the relative instrument positions plus the image formation model to overlay in real-time graphic representations of the tracked instruments on all preacquired fluoroscopic images (Fig. 34–2). The graphic overlays appear where the instruments would appear if new fluoroscopic images were acquired. Additional information can also be displayed, such as the trajectory (linear extension) of the instrument.

Fluoroscopy-based IGS has several distinct advantages over conventional C-arm fluoroscopy.[31] First, radiation

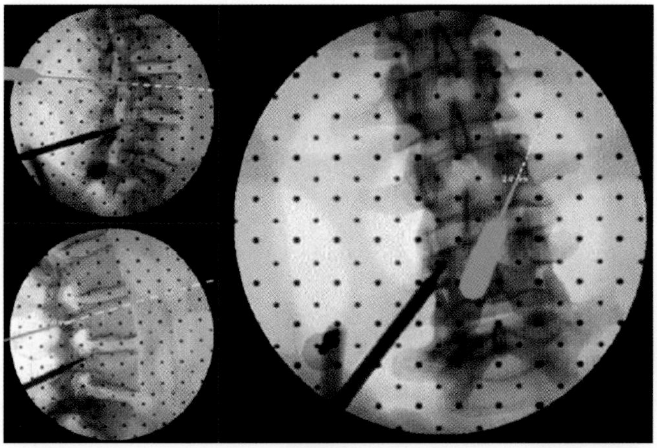

FIGURE 34–2 Fluoroscopy-based surgical navigation. In a fluoroscopy-based image-guided surgery (IGS) system, surgical probes and instruments are tracked and their changing positions overlaid in real time on previously acquired fluoroscopic images. The surgeon can acquire several images from different orientations and use all or some of them simultaneously for multiplanar navigation. This eliminates the need to reposition the C-arm repeatedly, as is necessary during conventional fluoroscopy. In this example, a probe (green) and its linear extension (yellow dotted line) are displayed on anteroposterior (right panel) and lateral (two left panels) fluoroscopic images. The original position of the probe can be seen as a dark structure in the previously acquired images. The black dots in the fluoroscopic images are radiopaque markers contained in the calibration device that attaches to the C-arm and are used for image calibration.

exposure to the patient and the surgical team is substantially reduced. Surgical probes and instruments are tracked and their positions overlaid on previously acquired fluoroscopic images. Thus, unlike conventional fluoroscopy, it is not necessary to acquire a temporal sequence of images to follow a probe or instrument. Because the fluoroscopic images used for surgical navigation are acquired once, or at most a few times, during the procedure, the surgical team can stand at a safe distance during image acquisition, thereby minimizing if not eliminating the need to wear heavy lead shielding. Second, the surgeon can acquire several images from different orientations and use all or some of them simultaneously for multiplanar navigation; the positions of tracked surgical probes and instruments are overlaid in real time on all preacquired fluoroscopic images. This eliminates the need to reposition the C-arm repeatedly, as is necessary during conventional fluoroscopy. Third, the C-arm fluoroscope may be removed from the operative field after image acquisition, which improves the ergonomics in a crowded surgical environment. Fourth, a fluoroscopy-based IGS system can enhance conventional fluoroscopy images by providing additional quantitative information to the surgeon. For example, the trajectory of the instrument can be displayed (e.g., the instrument can be displayed in one color and its linear extension in another color), and such measurements as distances (e.g., pedicle screw length or probe tip distance from midline) and angles (e.g., instrument trajectory angle relative to the midsagittal plane) can be obtained. Finally, there are several advantages relative to conventional IGS systems that use preoperative computed tomography (CT) or magnetic resonance imaging (MRI). No specially acquired preoperative image is required, which eliminates the associated time, cost, and logistical difficulties. Also, the challenging and time-consuming task of preoperative image-to-physical registration is not necessary. Because fluoroscopy is an intraoperative imaging technique, intraoperative image, updating is achieved simply by acquiring a new fluoroscopic image; for example, after patient movement or a change in intersegmental relationships caused by a surgical intervention (distraction of an interspace, reduction of a deformity). Validation of the virtual instrument overlays is achieved simply by acquiring a fluoroscopic image and visually comparing the position of the instrument in the image with the virtual overlay.

The most important limitation of fluoroscopy-based IGS is that navigation is based on 2D x-ray projection images rather than 3D CT images. The 3D anatomy must be inferred from the 2D projection information. The clinical interpretation of 2D images is highly dependent on the skill and experience of the surgeon. The other main limitation is the nature of fluoroscopic images. For example, it is often difficult to obtain clinically adequate fluoroscopic images in an obese patient. Such radiopaque surgical tools as retractors obscure patient anatomy. It is important to use good fluoroscopic technique. In particular, the surgical region of interest should be centered in the fluoroscopic image field of view to minimize the effects of parallax.

CT-Based Image-Guided Surgery

Spinal IGS applications are a relatively recent addition to neurosurgery and were adapted from well-established cranial IGS technology.[23–26] The purpose of applying stereotactic principles to spine surgery is to improve the surgeon's orientation to the unexposed anatomy. The 3D anatomy of the spinal column can present difficulties for even the most experienced surgeon. This is especially true for percutaneous and endoscopic approaches. The ability to conceptualize the 3D anatomy of the spinal column from any particular approach varies among surgeons. It is highly dependent on the correct interpretation of both preoperative and intraoperative images. As mentioned previously, the most important limitation of fluoroscopy-based IGS is that navigation is based on 2D x-ray projection images. This can provide only a 2D projection view of complex 3D anatomy. The surgeon must estimate the position of unexposed spinal structures based on an interpretation of these 2D projection images and a knowledge of pertinent anatomy. Such inference can result in varying degrees of inaccuracy (e.g., when placing screws in the spinal column). A CT-based IGS system facilitates this image interpretation process by providing a variety of 2D reformatted image slices and 3D renderings and displaying in real time the position and orientation of tracked instruments on these images. The primary advantage of CT-based IGS is that navigation is based on 3D preoperative CT images, which fundamentally allows a CT-based system to reveal better 3D anatomical information to the surgeon than a fluoroscopy-based system.

The general steps required to perform CT-based IGS for spinal procedures are relatively similar for all systems. Prior to surgery, a CT image of the appropriate spinal segments is obtained using a specific protocol. The CT image consists of a 3D volume of contiguous axial CT image slices. The scan protocol is often recommended by the IGS vendor to ensure correct image parameters. The spatial resolution of the image is limited by the voxel dimensions: spatial sampling (discretization) of the underlying continuous image constitutes loss of information by partial volume averaging, so structural information on the scale of the voxel dimension and smaller is lost. Thus, it is helpful to acquire images for IGS that have small voxel dimensions. We believe that CT images for IGS should be acquired with ~1 mm slice thickness or smaller.

Once the patient has been scanned, the image is transferred to the IGS computer workstation (e.g., via a network or optical media). Preoperative planning is performed at the IGS computer workstation at the surgeon's convenience. The software is used to reconstruct the images. A wide variety of 2D reformatted image slices and 3D renderings based on the preoperative CT image are possible (Fig. 34–3). The 2D reformatted image slices can be standard triplanar (i.e., axial, sagittal, and coronal) views as well as views parallel and orthogonal to a planned trajectory or axis of a planned pedicle screw. The 3D rendering can be rotated, and in some systems the color and transparency of various tissues and segmented volumes of interest can be interactively adjusted. The combination of zoom, pan, slice scrolling, a distance measurement tool, multiple 2D reformatted image slices, and a rotatable 3D rendering allows the surgeon to understand the anatomical relationships, which is especially important in the presence of diseased and distorted anatomy. For pedicle screw placement, the position (entry point), trajectory, and screw dimensions (length and width) can be interactively manipulated and evaluated to obtain an appropriate fit. The plan can be stored and used intraoperatively to select the appropriate screw, to find the entry point, and to follow the selected trajectory. Most systems provide some type of targeting view during placement, which is generally more useful than other views during actual placement and minimizes the number of images displayed on the computer screen. Some authors report that for pedicle screw placement, the ability of the planning software to help the surgeon understand complex anatomical relationships and determine an appropriate pedicle screw entry point, trajectory, and dimensions improves surgical planning and is of equal or greater importance than the use of the IGS system for intraoperative navigation.[43–45]

The main components of a CT-based IGS system are basically the same as those of a fluoroscopy-based IGS system, except that there is not a C-arm fluoroscope or calibration device that attaches to the fluoroscope: a computer workstation and monitor, a tracking system, a spine clamp with a DRF, and a variety of optically tracked instruments. The patient is positioned on the operating room table as for a conventional spinal procedure. The computer monitor is placed so that the surgeon has a clear view. Some systems have a lightweight, flat-panel monitor mounted on a boom that can be positioned over the operative field. These displays, which are covered by a clear, sterile drape during surgery, sometimes have a touch-sensitive screen so that the surgeon can easily interact with the software during the procedure. The optical position sensor (camera array) is placed such that it will have an unobstructed view of the surgical field. The best location is generally near the foot or head of the table. The line of sight between the camera and the tracked instruments should be maintained during the procedure. The use of a DRF attached to the spinous process of the spine segment of interest allows the optical position sensor to be repositioned as necessary.

A standard exposure of the spinal levels is performed for an open IGS procedure. The DRF is securely fixed to the spinous process at the level, or adjacent to the level, on which to be operated (Fig. 34–1). The registration process is then performed, as will be described in detail later. Intraoperative navigation begins after registration is finished. We believe that it is extremely important that the surgeon identify and locate several anatomical landmarks to visually assess and verify that the IGS system is working properly and that the registration is sufficiently accurate for the surgical procedure before using the system for surgical navigation. The optical tracking system determines the positions of instruments and the DRF, and uses the relative instrument positions to overlay in real time graphic representations of the tracked instruments on a variety of 2D reformatted image slices and 3D renderings based on the preoperative CT image (Fig. 34–3). A variety of surgical instruments can be tracked,

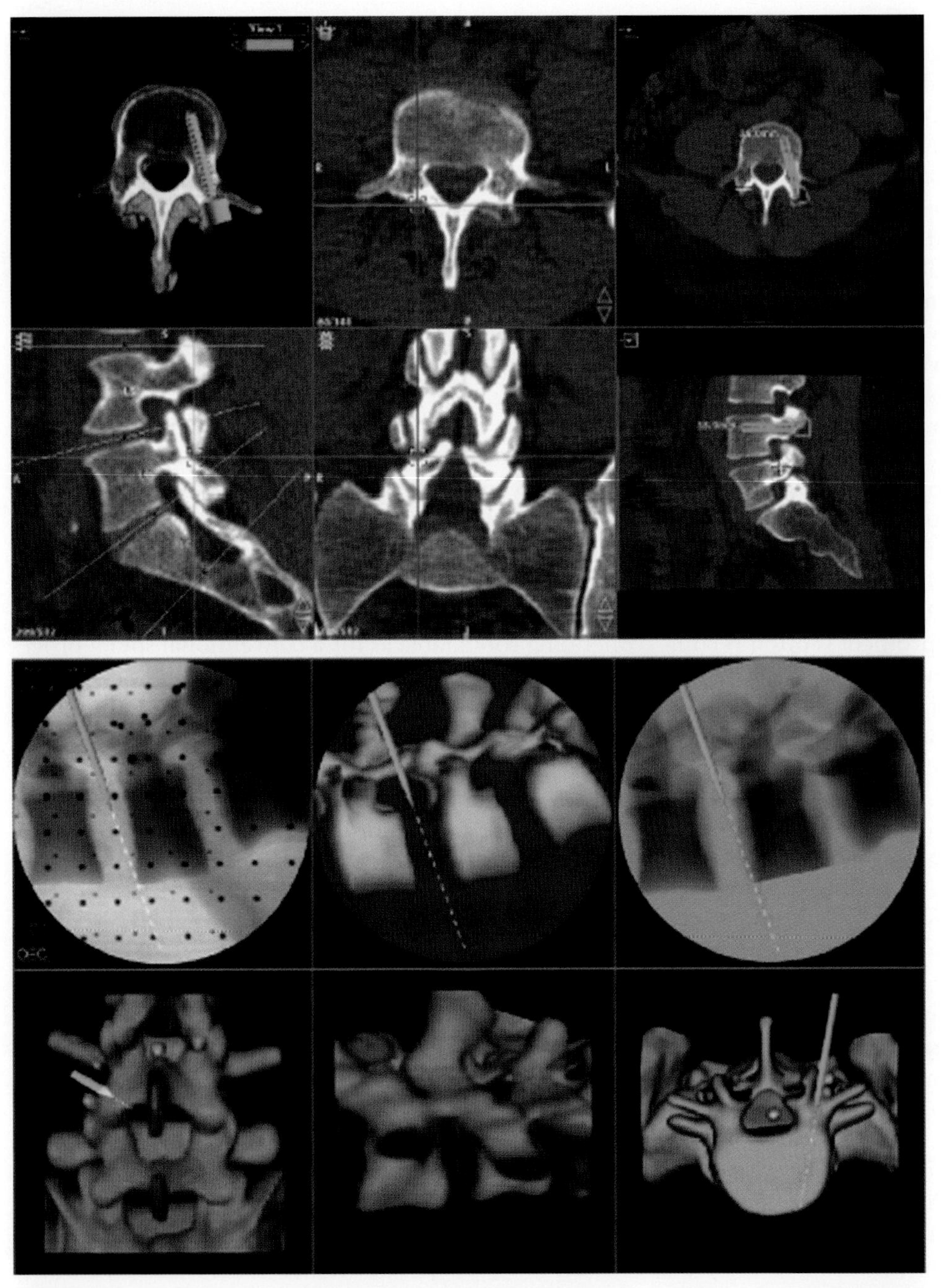

FIGURE 34–3 Illustration of CT-based surgical planning (top) and guidance (bottom). A wide variety of 2D reformatted image slices and three-dimensional renderings based on the preoperative CT image is possible for both planning and guidance. *Top:* Preoperative planning for pedicle screw placement in a clinical case. The middle two and bottom left panels are standard triplanar (i.e., axial, sagittal, and coronal) reformatted image slices through a user-defined cursor position. Similar views though the tip of a tracked instrument are possible during navigation. The right two panels are orthogonal reformatted image slices through the axis of the planned pedicle screw. Similar views through the trajectory of a tracked instrument are possible during navigation. The top left panel is a volume rendering of the vertebra below a plane through the axis of the planned pedicle screw. *Bottom:* Intraoperative navigation in a phantom experiment. The top middle and bottom three panels illustrate a variety of 3D renderings during navigation. Image-to-physical registration for this experiment was accomplished by matching the positions of bone-implanted markers visible in the CT with the positions of the markers visible in a pair of fluoroscopic images (one is shown in the upper left panel). This is fiducial-based 2D–3D registration. Regardless of how registration is accomplished, synthetic x-ray projection images called digitally reconstructed radiographs (DRRs) can be generated from the preoperative CT image (top right panel).

including a standard pointer, bone tap, pedicle probe, drill guide, drill, screwdriver, and awl.

Image-to-Physical Registration

Registration is the determination of a mapping or transformation between the coordinates in one space and those in another, such that points in the two spaces that correspond to the same anatomical point are mapped to each other. To use preoperatively acquired 3D images for intraoperative therapy guidance, the images must be registered to a patient coordinate system defined in the operating room. Image-to-physical registration is one of the fundamental steps in all image-guided interventions. Surgical navigation systems use the image-to-physical registration transformation to track in real time the changing position of a surgical probe on a display of the preoperative images or to direct a needle to a surgical target visible in the images. Rapid and accurate registration remains one of the major technical difficulties of CT-based spinal IGS procedures.

Image-to-physical registration is commonly performed using geometric features, which include anatomical landmarks, surfaces, fiducials, and frames. Unlike cranial surgery, a stereotactic frame system is not practical for spine surgery.[b] The use of the skin surface or skin-affixed fiducials, which are commonly used in cranial IGS, produces unacceptably high registration error in spinal applications because of very substantial skin movement with respect to bony structures.[49,50] In open spinal IGS procedures, point-based registration is popular. This involves finding the coordinates of corresponding points in the preoperative CT image and the physical space of the patient. Such bony anatomical landmarks as the tip of the spinous or transverse process or a prominent facet or osteophyte are identified in the preoperative CT image on the IGS computer workstation display and localized in the physical space of the patient by touching the landmarks with a tracked probe. The corresponding landmark positions are then aligned in a least-squares sense by the IGS computer workstation. In our experience, manual localization of anatomical landmarks is easier and more accurate when multiple orthogonal views are used simultaneously during the interactive visual identification process. For localization of anatomical landmarks, intraobserver precision is better than interobserver precision[51]; thus, manual localization of landmarks is typically more accurate if the same person localizes the landmarks in both the image and the physical space. The registration procedure is typically faster if the surgeon localizes the points in CT before the procedure. To maximize accuracy, the points should be picked according to a few simple guidelines[52,53]: use as many markers as is feasible (i.e., at least three noncollinear markers are required mathematically; we generally use six), place markers so that the centroid of their configuration is near the regions that are most critical during surgery, keep the markers as far apart as possible, and avoid linear and near-linear fiducial configurations. Bone-implanted fiducial markers, which have been shown to have high registration accuracy in cranial IGS,[54] have also been used to improve accuracy in spinal IGS.[55,56] Another image-to-physical registration method is surface-based registration. In this case, the probe is moved along the surface of the vertebra, and the recorded surface points are matched to a vertebral bone surface model extracted from the CT image. Registration accuracy is largely dependent on the surgeon carefully performing the surface mapping process; a casual approach to this step can easily create substantial registration errors. The surface-based registration requires an accurate segmentation, takes substantially more time to collect the surface information, and requires a thorough soft tissue debridement of the exposed spinal surface. The point and surface information can be used together to improve accuracy.[57,58]

These point- and surface-based registration approaches are unfortunately applicable only for open IGS procedures. They are not useful for such new minimally invasive techniques as percutaneous and endoscopic spinal surgery. Assaker et al[41,42] proposed a registration method for endoscopic spine surgery that involves mounting a reference frame on a long percutaneous shaft that is screwed into a pedicle and acquiring the preoperative CT after frame implantation. The frame functions both as a fiducial reference system for registration and as a DRF that tracks patient motion intraoperatively. The technique was shown experimentally[41] and clinically[42] to be accurate and useful for guiding a surgical tool through an endoscope. Nonetheless, frame insertion is a lengthy procedure (the authors reported 90 minutes), and patient transfer is logistically difficult because of the frame implant protruding out of the back. Thus, it is unlikely that this approach will achieve widespread acceptance or use. Another more promising approach is to use a tracked ultrasound probe to measure points on the vertebral bone surface noninvasively.[59–63] Because the intensity reflection coefficient, which is the ratio of the pressure reflected to the pressure incident, is quite high for bone–tissue interfaces, ultrasound echoes corresponding to bone–tissue interfaces have high signal amplitude and are easily identified. These bone surface points can then be matched to a vertebral bone surface model extracted from the CT image. Excellent results have been obtained in the laboratory, but we are unaware of any commercially available product using this approach.

The preoperative 3D image can be registered to an intraoperative 2D image as an alternative. The 2D–3D

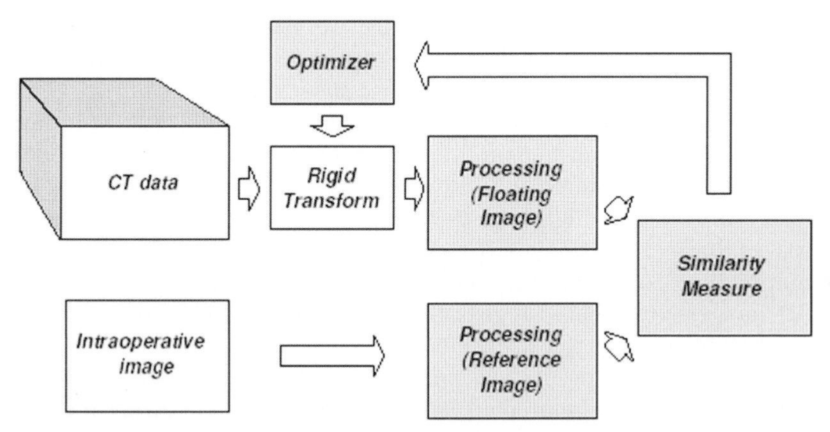

FIGURE 34–4 Schematic overview of the 2D–3D registration process. For intensity-based 2D–3D registration, the reference image is an intraoperative x-ray projection (2D) image. It is used as is with little or no processing. The floating image is a CT (3D) image. It is processed by generating DRRs (synthetic x-ray projection images) for various orientations of the CT image relative to the x-ray imaging system. The optimizer searches for the rigid transformation that produces the DRR that is most similar to the real x-ray projection image. The optimal transformation is used to align the CT coordinate system with that of the operating room (patient).

problem involves taking one or more (in practice, generally two or more) x-ray projection (2D) images of the patient's anatomy and using these projection images to determine the rigid transformation that best aligns the coordinate system of the CT (3D) image with that of the x-ray projection images and the operating room. For spinal IGS, the x-ray projection images would typically be C-arm fluoroscopic images, although such digital flat-panel x-ray cameras as amorphous silicon detectors should start becoming widely available during the next 5 years. Figure 34–4 shows a schematic representation of the 2D–3D process. In general, most of the proposed solutions to this problem fit in this general framework.

One general approach is feature-based 2D–3D. The first reported method is based on image contours.[64] It requires segmentation of the object surface in preoperative CT images and the object contour in intraoperative projection x-ray images. The registration is performed by minimizing a distance-based cost function between the 3D surface model and the back-projection lines stemming from the 2D contour points. A variation of this approach minimizes a 2D distance instead of a 3D distance (by forward projecting the 3D surface model onto the x-ray image). Algorithms based on contours have adequate execution speed for use in a clinical context, but the interactive selection of object contours on the x-ray images is difficult and time consuming, and the accuracy of the registration is highly dependent on the contour segmentation. The best currently available feature-based 2D–3D approach uses metal fiducials implanted in the spine for point-based alignment. There are several fiducial-based 2D–3D systems in use[65] and under development[66] for intraoperative image-guided radiotherapy of spinal lesions. The implanted fiducial 2D–3D approach is relatively quick, quite accurate, and clinically robust.[67] Artificial fiducial markers, however, although less invasive than a rigid frame, still require a surgical implantation procedure. This entails risk, especially in the cervical spine, where the vertebral structures are small and fragile. There is also the issue of whether or not it is acceptable to leave fiducials permanently implanted. One report proposes attaching a metal wire to the fiducial to facilitate removal of the marker after the procedure.[56]

Perhaps the most promising approach for spinal IGS applications is intensity-based 2D–3D.[33,68–71] In this case, the reference image is one or more x-ray projection images, and the floating image is a CT image. The method involves computing synthetic x-ray images, which are called digitally reconstructed radiographs (DRRs), by casting rays using a known camera geometry through the CT image. The DRR pixel values are simply the summations of the CT values encountered along each projection ray. The pose (position and orientation) of the CT image is adjusted iteratively until the DRR it produces is most similar to the x-ray projection image. The accuracy of intensity-based 2D–3D image registration has been well validated for the head and is ~1 mm.[72] It is inherently more difficult to register the spine than the head because vertebrae are substantially smaller than the cranium. Nonetheless, although these methods are basically untested on clinical spine image data, very preliminary results in a report based on data from four patients suggests that a registration accuracy of 1 to 2 mm can be achieved in the spine.[73]

In summary, image-to-physical registration methods currently incorporated in commercially available CT-based IGS systems require open exposure of bony anatomy to perform registration. Several commercial vendors are currently developing 2D–3D registration techniques that use intraoperative C-arm fluoroscopy for their spinal IGS applications, and at least one is performing preliminary clinical evaluation. It is possible, even likely, that in the next few years one or more commercial products that are fast, accurate, and robust will become available. Such fluoroscopic image-based registration methods will not require open exposure of bony anatomy, and the availability of such products will advance the use of CT-based IGS for percutaneous and endoscopic spine procedures.

Example Application: Pedicle Screw Insertion

There are several types of spine procedures for which the use of IGS promises to improve patient health outcomes, including instrumentation and percutaneous procedures, resection of tumors and arteriovenous malformations, treatment of spinal instability, and treatment of disk disease.[74] For example, image guidance has been reported to help the surgeon to perform such complex spine procedures as pedicle screw insertion,[75–78] atlantoaxial transarticular screw fixation,[45,79,80] transoral cervicomedullary junction decompression,[45,81] anterior cervical corpectomy,[82,83] and posterior lumbar interbody fusion.[84] We will focus here on one application: pedicle screw insertion.

It is well accepted that pedicle screws and rods provide superior stability in comparison to other posterior spinal fixation techniques. Biomechanical studies have shown that pedicle screw fixation provides increased rigidity and construct stiffness.[85–87] Pedicle fixation of the spinal column has gained greater acceptance as improved instrumentation and clinical effectiveness have become apparent.[88,89] Several complex spinal abnormalities, including degenerative diseases, trauma, neoplasms, and infections, are commonly treated with instrumentation to promote fusion via stabilization.

Transpedicular screw placement can be challenging, however, and there has been considerable debate over the safety of pedicle screw placement in the thoracic spine.[86,90–92] There is considerable variation among vertebrae in both the relationship of the transverse process to the axis of the pedicle and the angle of the pedicle to the vertebral body. This is especially true in the thoracic vertebrae.[93] Unlike the ovoid-shaped lumbar pedicle, the cross-sectional morphology of an individual thoracic pedicle is widely variable.[94] Freehand placement of pedicle screws using anatomical landmarks may be imprecise, especially when the anatomical features of the diseased segments and the adjacent neural structures are distorted. Serious complications that result from screw misplacement or pedicle cortex perforation can lead to devastating neurologic or vascular damage. Cadaveric and clinical studies in which conventional surgical techniques (i.e., freehand placement using anatomical landmarks and fluoroscopy) were used have reported alarmingly high pedicle screw misplacement (cortical violation) rates, from 3 to 55% for thoracic screws and 5 to 41% for lumbar screws.[86,90–92,95–105]

The use of IGS systems for pedicle screw placement can improve the accuracy of placement. Studies on pedicle screw placement using image guidance have reported a substantially lower misplacement rate (0–14%) for thoracic and lumbar screws.[43,75–77,95,100,106–112] In a study in which 48 thoracic screws were placed from T1 to T12 in two cadavers, half using anatomical landmarks and fluoroscopy and the other half using an IGS system, almost 50% of the screws placed conventionally perforated the pedicle cortex, whereas only one (4%) of the screws placed using image guidance disrupted the cortex.[95] In a randomized clinical study of thoracolumbar or lumbosacral pedicle screw instrumentation, the pedicle perforation rate was 13.4% in the conventional group and 4.6% in the image-guided group.[100] It is important that whereas reported neurologic sequelae from conventional pedicle screw placement are typically ~5%, no such complications have been reported in clinical studies in which an IGS system has been used for screw placement.

Because fluoroscopy-based IGS uses only the position of the tracked fluoroscope and the positions of the radiopaque markers (contained in the calibration device) in the fluoroscopic image, registration is automatic and independent of exposed anatomy. Thus, fluoroscopy-based IGS, unlike CT-based IGS (until registration methods become available that do not require exposure of bone anatomy), can be used for percutaneous pedicle screw placement. Foley et al[113] described the following procedure for percutaneous placement of lumbar pedicle screws using fluoroscopy-based IGS. After visualizing the spine segments of interest with anteroposterior and lateral conventional C-arm fluoroscopy, a small incision is made over the spinous process at one of the segment levels being fused, and a DRF is rigidly attached to the process. Fluoroscopic images are obtained for anteroposterior, lateral, and optionally oblique views, transferred to the computer workstation, calibrated, and stored. A tracked probe is placed on the skin surface. Graphic representations of the probe position and its trajectory (virtual extension) are overlaid in real time on the preacquired fluoroscopic images. The virtual extension of the probe allows the surgeon to choose a trajectory that traverses the pedicle of interest. After making a stab incision at the skin entry point, a K-wire is used to perforate the fascia, and sequential dilators are used to dilate the fascia and bluntly separate the paraspinous muscles down to the vertebral surface.[114] The dilators are removed, and a tracked awl and a tracked pedicle probe are used to create a pilot hole in the pedicle while monitoring the positions and trajectories of these tracked instruments on the preacquired fluoroscopic images. Although it is not currently possible to use CT-based IGS for intraoperative guidance during percutaneous pedicle screw placement, the planning software that is part of most CT-based IGS systems can be used, if a preoperative CT image is available, to help the surgeon understand complex anatomical relationships and determine an appropriate pedicle screw entry point, trajectory, and dimensions. As an alternative, the pedicle screw dimensions can be chosen using measurement tools available in the fluoroscopy-based IGS system.

Although the accuracy of IGS systems is quite good, one must be aware that the margins of error are small in many areas of the spine for common procedures. Rampersaud et al[115] reported an interesting study regarding the accuracy requirements for image-guided pedicle screw placement. The authors developed a geometric model of the pedicle and pedicle screw and used this model to compute maximum permissible rotational and translational errors for pedicle screw placement when using clinically relevant screw diameters in the cervical, thoracic, and thoracolumbar spine that would avoid pedicle wall perforation. They concluded from their mathematical analysis that extremely high accuracy is necessary to place pedicle screws at many levels of the spine (especially midcervical, midthoracic, and thoracolumbar) without perforating the pedicle wall, and that these accuracy requirements exceed the overall accuracy of current commercially available IGS systems, based on clinical utility errors reported in the literature.[c] In view of the findings of the numerous reports in the literature (cited ealier) that show that the use of IGS systems improves the accuracy of pedicle screw placement, the authors hypothesized that IGS systems help bring the surgeon close to the optimal screw entry point and trajectory, and that further refinements to the screw path result from haptic feedback and the self-centering, mechanical constraint provided by the pedicle wall. These findings suggest that surgeons should consider the use of a manual pedicle probe rather than a drill, and that robotic pedicle screw placement should be viewed with caution. The findings also emphasize that an IGS system is a tool; the system can be of great assistance to the surgeon, but it cannot replace a thorough understanding of the pertinent spinal anatomy and the proper spinal stabilization techniques, and it is not a substitute for surgical skill and vigilance.

Image-Enhanced Endoscopy

A fundamental limitation of endoscopes is that they can display only visible surfaces; it is therefore generally difficult to visualize tumors, nerves, vessels, and other anatomical structures that lie beneath opaque tissue. Virtual endoscopy systems have been widely used for visualizing internal anatomy.[32,118–120] Such systems generate virtual endoscopic images by locating a viewpoint inside an organ and visualizing 3D medical images (generally CT images, but sometimes MR or ultrasound images) with an appropriate rendering technique. An important advantage of virtual endoscopy compared with real endoscopy is that anatomical structures that lie beyond the surface of the structure being observed can be visualized.

A relatively new method for IGS called *image-enhanced endoscopy* has been developed to overcome the visibility limitation of endoscopes.[121] Registered real and virtual endoscopic images are displayed simultaneously. The virtual endoscopic images are perspective volume renderings generated from the same view as the endoscope camera using a preoperative image (e.g., CT or MRI). The simultaneous display of real and virtual endoscopic images combined with the ability to vary tissue transparency in the virtual images (which is easily accomplished with volume rendering) provides surgeons with the ability to see beyond visible surfaces and thus provides additional exposure during surgery. Image-enhanced endoscopy is a potentially useful addition to conventional IGS systems, which generally show only the position of the tip (and sometimes the orientation) of a surgical instrument or probe on reformatted image slices.

The pose (position and orientation) of the endoscope is tracked using an optical tracking system by rigidly attaching a universal tracker (Fig. 34–5). Generation of virtual images that are accurately registered to the real endoscopic images requires calibration of the tracked

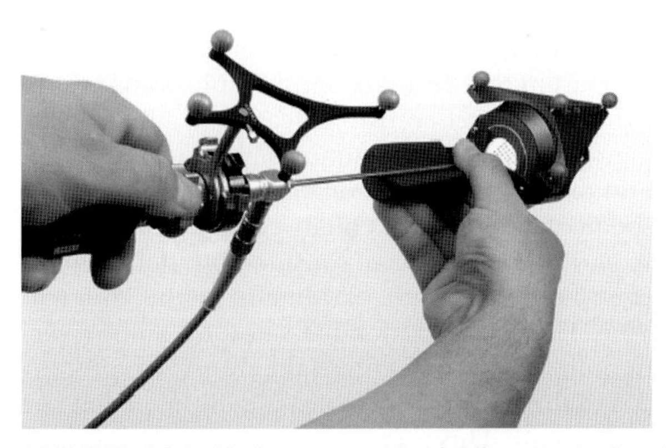

FIGURE 34–5 Endoscope with rigidly attached universal tracker placed in the endoscope calibration unit. The endoscope is placed in the calibration unit with the tip of its lens ~15 mm away from a calibration grid. The sets of known physical and localized image coordinates for the identified dots (calibration grid target features) are used to determine the calibration parameters of the endoscope camera. (With permission from Shahidi R, Bax MR, Maurer CR Jr, et al. Implementation, calibration and accuracy testing of an image-enhanced endoscopy system. *IEEE Trans Med Imaging.* 2002;21:1524–1535.)

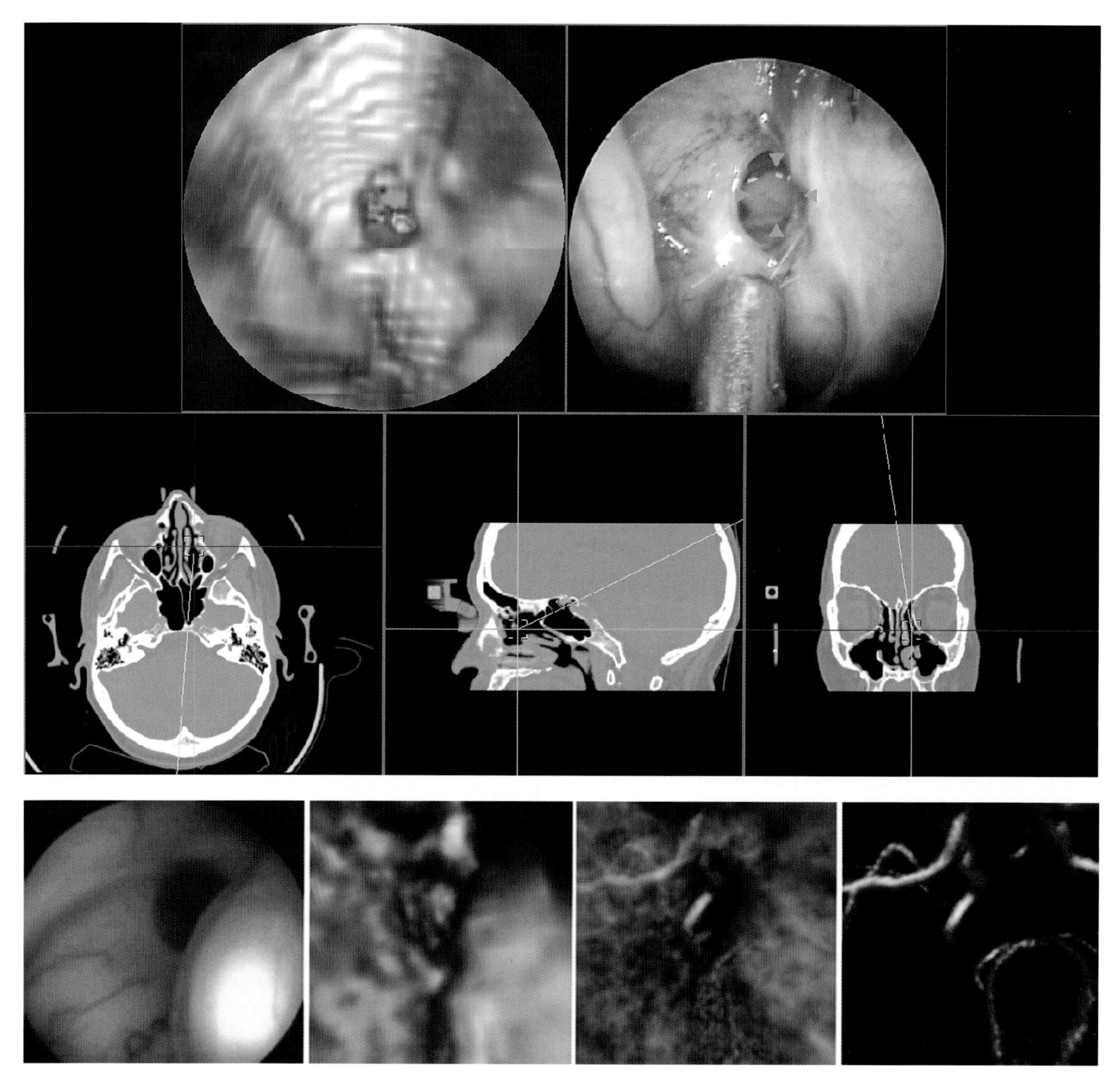

FIGURE 34–6 Two examples of cranial image-guided surgery (IGS) applications that illustrate the potential usefulness of image-enhanced endoscopy. *Top:* The bottom three panels show the position and orientation of an optically tracked instrument during surgery for treatment of recurrent acute rhinosinusitis displayed on triplanar (axial, sagittal, and coronal) reformatted preoperative CT image slices. The top right panel shows a real endoscopic video image. The top left panel shows a synthetic (virtual) 3D perspective rendering generated from the same view as the endoscope using the CT image. During a preoperative review of the CT image, it was noted that the sphenoid sinus had pneumatized around the left optic nerve. Intraoperatively, the real endoscopic video image and the virtual endoscopic image were used to guide surgical dissection without entering the sphenoid sinus or hitting the optic nerve (antitargeting). The optic nerve is shown in green (top left panel). *Bottom:* The left image is a real endoscopic video image from a patient undergoing third ventriculostomy for treatment of myelomeningocele-related hydrocephalus. The remaining three images show synthetic (virtual) 3D perspective renderings generated from the same view as the endoscope using a preoperative MRI. These three renderings were generated by making the ventricular wall increasingly transparent (from left to right). The circle of Willis observed in isolation of the soft tissue allowed the surgeon to appreciate anomalous third ventricle floor anatomy and select an optimal location, away from the basilar artery, for fenestration of the floor of the third ventricle. (Modified with permission from Shahidi R, Bax MR, Maurer CR Jr, et al. Implementation, calibration and accuracy testing of an image-enhanced endoscopy system. *IEEE Trans Med Imaging.* 2002;21:1524–1535.)

endoscope. The endoscope is placed in the calibration unit with the tip of its lens ~15 mm away from a calibration grid. The sets of known physical and localized image coordinates for the identified dots (calibration grid target features) are used to determine the calibration parameters of the endoscope camera. During the calibration process, the computer constructs a mathematical model of the endoscope image formation process, which describes where a given position relative to the patient projects onto the endoscopic images.

Image-enhanced endoscopy has not yet been applied to spine surgery. Figure 34–6 shows two examples of cranial IGS applications that illustrate the potential usefulness of image-enhanced endoscopy. It is currently relatively easy to generate virtual endoscopic images for visualizing vertebrae, disks, and tumors using CT images for spinal IGS applications. It should also be possible to visualize nerves and vessels using special MR image protocols. We believe that image-enhanced endoscopy may play an important role in the development of image-guided endoscopic surgery.

Conclusions

Current technical developments in modern endoscopic surgery are fascinating, and the developmental potential is very promising. Endoscopic and percutaneous spinal procedures have proved to be safe, effective, and minimally invasive. Despite the attractive character of such approaches, most surgeons still have limited experience with them. One of the reasons is their long learning curve. The absence of a 3D direct view of the surgical field and the lack of convenient guidance methods in endoscopic procedures make them frustrating, increase the operating time, and do not encourage new surgeons to adopt these techniques. We believe that surgical navigation technology will play an important role in helping to guide the surgeon in real time through an endoscopic approach, which can substantially decrease the time of the learning curve, making the surgery safer and less frustrating. It may also be a useful educational assistance to spine surgeons in training. Moreover, even for experienced surgeons, guidance can potentially decrease the operating time and optimize implant placement and resection of small and difficult to find spinal lesions. Nonetheless, it should be stressed that traditional knowledge of the anatomical relationships of the spine must never be replaced by reliance on IGS technology.

REFERENCES

1. Knyrim K, Seidlitz H, Vakil N, Classen M. Perspectives in electronic endoscopy: past, present and future of fibers and CCDs in medical endoscopes. *Endoscopy.* 1990;22(suppl 1):2–8.
2. Gejo R, Matsui H, Kawaguchi Y, Ishihara H, Tsuji H. Serial changes in trunk muscle performance after posterior lumbar surgery *Spine.* 1999;24:1023–1028.
3. Kawaguchi Y, Matsui H, Tsuji H. Back muscle injury after posterior lumbar spine surgery, I: Histologic and histochemical analyses in rats. *Spine.* 1994;19:2590–2597.
4. Kawaguchi Y, Matsui H, Tsuji H. Back muscle injury after posterior lumbar spine surgery, II: Histologic and histochemical analyses in humans. *Spine.* 1994;19:2598–2602.
5. Kawaguchi Y, Matsui H, Tsuji H. Back muscle injury after posterior lumbar spine surgery: a histologic and enzymatic analysis. *Spine.* 1996;21:941–944.
6. Mathews HH, Mathern BE. Percutaneous procedures in the lumbar spine. In: An HS, ed. *Principles and Techniques of Spinal Surgery.* Baltimore: Williams & Wilkins; 1997:731–745.
7. Deyo RA, Cherkin DC, Conrad D, Volinn E. Cost, controversy, crisis: low back pain and the health of the public. *Annu Rev Public Health.* 1991;12:141–156.
8. Deyo RA, Cherkin DC, Loeser JD, Bigos SJ, Ciol MA. Morbidity and mortality in association with operations on the lumbar spine: the influence of age, diagnosis, and procedure. *J Bone Joint Surg Am.* 1992;74:536–543.
9. Portenoy RK. Opioid therapy for chronic nonmalignant pain: a review of the critical issues. *J Pain Symptom Manage.* 1996;11:203–217.
10. Portenoy RK. Opioid therapy for chronic nonmalignant pain: clinician's perspective. *J Law Med Ethics.* 1996;24:296–309.
11. Coltharp WH, Arnold JH, Alford WC Jr, et al. Videothoracoscopy: improved technique and expanded indications. *Ann Thorac Surg.* 1992;53:776–779.
12. Huang TJ, Hsu RWW, Liu HP, et al. Video-assisted thoracoscopic treatment of spinal lesions in the thoracolumbar junction. *Surg Endosc.* 1997;11:1189–1193.
13. Huang TJ, Hsu RWW, Liu HP, Liao YS, Shih HN. Technique of video-assisted thoracoscopic surgery for the spine: new approach. *World J Surg.* 1997;21:358–362.
14. Kaiser LR. Video-assisted thoracic surgery: current state of the art. *Ann Surg.* 1994;220:720–734.
15. Mack MJ, Aronoff RJ, Acuff TE, et al. Present role of thoracoscopy in the diagnosis and treatment of diseases of the chest. *Ann Thorac Surg.* 1992;54:403–409.
16. McAfee PC, Regan JR, Fedder IL, Mack MJ, Geis WP. Anterior thoracic corpectomy for spinal cord decompression performed endoscopically. *Surg Laparosc Endosc.* 1995;5:339–348.
17. McAfee PC, Regan JR, Zdeblick T, et al. The incidence of complications in endoscopic anterior thoracolumbar spinal reconstructive surgery: a prospective multicenter study comprising the first 100 consecutive cases. *Spine.* 1995;20:1624–1632.
18. McLain RF. Endoscopically assisted decompression for metastatic thoracic neoplasms. *Spine.* 1998;23:1130–1135.
19. Regan JJ, Guyer RD. Endoscopic techniques in spinal surgery. *Clin Orthop.* 1997;335:122–139.
20. Treat MR. A surgeon's perspective on the difficulties of laparoscopic surgery. In: Taylor RH, Lavallee S, Burdea G, Mösges R, eds. *Computer-Integrated Surgery: Technology and Clinical Applications.* Cambridge, MA: MIT Press; 1996:559–560.
21. Schippers E, Schumpelick V. Requirements and possibilities of computer-assisted endoscopic surgery. In: Taylor RH, Lavallee S, Burdea G, Mösges R, eds. *Computer-Integrated Surgery: Technology and Clinical Applications.* Cambridge, MA: MIT Press; 1996:561– 565.
22. Tendick F, Jennings RW, Tharp G, Stark L. Perception and manipulation problems in endoscopic surgery. In: Taylor RH, Lavallee S, Burdea G, Mösges R, eds. *Computer-Integrated Surgery: Technology and Clinical Applications.* Cambridge, MA: MIT Press; 1996:567–575.
23. Alexander E III, Maciunas RJ. eds. *Advanced Neurosurgical Navigation.* New York: Thieme Medical Publishers; 1999.
24. Barnett GH, Roberts DW, Maciunas RJ, eds. *Image-Guided Neurosurgery: Clinical Applications of Surgical Navigation.* St. Louis, MO: Quality Medical Publishing; 1998.

25. Germano IM, ed. *Advanced Techniques in Image-Guided Brain and Spine Surgery.* New York: Thieme Medical Publishers; 2002.
26. Gildenberg PL, Tasker RR, eds. *Textbook of Stereotactic and Functional Neurosurgery.* New York: McGraw-Hill; 1998.
27. International Commission on Radiological Protection (ICRP). Recommendations of the International Commission on Radiological Protection, ICRP Publication 60. *Ann ICRP.* 1991;21: 1–201.
28. Mehlman CT, DiPasquale TG. Radiation exposure to the orthopaedic surgical team during fluoroscopy: how far away is far enough? *J Orthop Trauma.* 1997;11:392–398.
29. Sanders R, Koval LK, DiPasquale TG, Schmelling G, Stenzler S, Ross E. Exposure of the orthopaedic surgeon to radiation. *J Bone Joint Surg Am.* 1993;75:326–330.
30. Rampersaud YR, Foley KT, Shen AC, Williams S, Solomito M. Radiation exposure to the spine surgeon during fluoroscopically assisted pedicle screw insertion. *Spine.* 2000;25:2637–2645.
31. Foley KT, Simon DA, Rampersaud YR. Virtual fluoroscopy: computer-assisted fluoroscopic navigation. *Spine* 2001;26:347–351.
32. Vining DJ, Liu K, Choplin RH, Haponik EF. Virtual bronchoscopy: relationships of virtual reality endobronchial simulations to actual bronchoscopic findings. *Chest.* 1996;109:549–553.
33. Lemieux L, Jagoe R, Fish DR, Kitchen ND, Thomas DGT. A patient-to-computed-tomography image registration method based on digitally reconstructed radiographs. *Med Phys.* 1994;21:1749–1760.
34. Potamianos P, Davies BL, Hibberd RD. Intra-operative imaging guidance for keyhole surgery: methodology and calibration. Proc *First Int Symp Medical Robotics and Computer Assisted Surgery.* 1994;98– 104.
35. Potamianos P, Davies BL, Hibberd RD. Intra-operative registration for percutaneous surgery. Proc *Second Annu Int Symp Medical Robotics and Computer Assisted Surgery.* 1995;156–164.
36. Brack C, Burgkart R, Czopf A, et al. Accurate x-ray-based navigation in computer-assisted orthopedic surgery. In: Lemke HU, Vannier MW, Inamura K, Farman AG, eds. *Computer Assisted Radiology and Surgery.* Amsterdam: Elsevier Science; 1998:716–722.
37. Hofstetter R, Slomczykowski M, Bourquin I, Nolte L-P. Fluoroscopy based surgical navigation: concept and clinical applications. In: Lemke HU, Vannier MW, Inamura K, eds. *Computer Assisted Radiology and Surgery.* Amsterdam: Elsevier Science; 1997:956–960.
38. Hofstetter R, Slomczykowski M, Sati M, Nolte L-P. Fluoroscopy as an imaging means for computer-assisted surgical navigation. *Comput Aided Surg.* 1999;4:65–76.
39. Phillips R, Viant WJ, Mohsen AMMA, et al. Image guided orthopaedic surgery: design and analysis. *Trans Inst Meas Contr.* 1995;17:251–264.
40. Yaniv Z. *Fluoroscopic Image Processing and Registration for Computer-Aided Orthopaedic Surgery* [master's thesis]. Jerusalem: Hebrew University; 1998.
41. Assaker R, Cinquin P, Cotten A, Lejeune JP. Image-guided endoscopic spine surgery, I: A feasibility study. *Spine.* 2001;26:1705– 1710.
42. Assaker R, Reyns N, Pertruzon B, Lejeune JP. Image-guided endoscopic spine surgery, II: Clinical applications. *Spine.* 2001;26: 1711–1718.
43. Berlemann U, Monin D, Arm E, Nolte L-P, Ozdoba C. Planning and insertion of pedicle screws with computer assistance. *J Spinal Disord.* 1997;10:117–124.
44. Ondra SL, Karahalios D. Image guidance for scoliosis. In: Germano IM, ed. *Advanced Techniques in Image-Guided Brain and Spine Surgery.* New York: Thieme Medical Publishers; 2002:191–196.
45. Welch WC, Subach BR, Pollack IF, Jacobs GB. Frameless stereotactic guidance for surgery of the upper cervical spine. *Neurosurgery.* 1997;40:958–963.
46. Hamilton AJ. Radiosurgical treatment of spinal metastases. In: Maciunas RJ, ed. *Advanced Techniques in Central Nervous System Metastases.* Park Ridge, IL: American Association of Neurological Surgeons; 1998:255–268.
47. Hamilton AJ, Lulu BA, Fosmire H, Stea B, Cassady JR. Preliminary clinical experience with linear accelerator-based spinal stereotaxic radiosurgery. *Neurosurgery.* 1995;36:311–319.
48. Lax I, Blomgren H, Naslund I, Svanstrom R. Stereotactic radiotherapy of malignancies in the abdomen: methodological aspects. *Acta Oncol.* 1994;33:677–683.
49. Brodwater BK, Roberts DW, Nakajima T, Friets EM, Strohbehn JW. Extracranial application of the frameless stereotactic operating microscope: experience with the lumbar spine. *Neurosurgery.* 1993;32:209–213.
50. Bryant JT, Reid JG, Smith BL, Stevenson JM. A method for determining vertebral body positions in the sagittal plane using skin markers. *Spine.* 1989;14:258–265.
51. Dean D, Palomo M, Subramanyan K, et al. Accuracy and precision of 3D cephalometric landmarks from biorthogonal plain-film x-rays. *Proc SPIE.* 1998;3335:50–58.
52. Maurer CR Jr, Rohlfing T, Dean D, et al. Sources of error in image registration for cranial image-guided surgery. In: Germano IM, ed. *Advanced Techniques in Image-Guided Brain and Spine Surgery.* New York: Thieme Medical Publishers; 2002:10–36.
53. West JB, Fitzpatrick JM, Toms SA, Maurer CR Jr, Maciunas RJ. Fiducial point placement and the accuracy of point-based, rigid-body registration. *Neurosurgery.* 2001;48:810–817.
54. Maurer CR Jr, Fitzpatrick JM, Wang MY, Galloway RL Jr, Maciunas RJ, Allen GS. Registration of head volume images using implantable fiducial markers. *IEEE Trans Med Imaging.* 1997;16:447– 462.
55. Salehi SA, Ondra SL. Use of internal fiducial markers in frameless stereotactic navigational systems during spinal surgery: technical note. *Neurosurgery.* 2000;47:1460–1462.
56. Winkler D, Vitzthum H-E, Seifert V. Spinal markers: a new method for increasing accuracy in spinal navigation. *Comput Aided Surg.* 1999;4:101–104.
57. Maurer CR Jr, Aboutanos GB, Dawant BM, Maciunas RJ, Fitzpatrick JM. Registration of 3-D images using weighted geometrical features. *IEEE Trans Med Imaging.* 1996;15:836–849.
58. Maurer CR Jr, Maciunas RJ, Fitzpatrick JM. Registration of head CT images to physical space using a weighted combination of points and surfaces. *IEEE Trans Med Imaging.* 1998;17: 753–761.
59. Brendel B, Winter S, Rick A, Stockheim M, Ermert H. Registration of 3D CT and ultrasound datasets of the spine using bone structures. *Comput Aided Surg.* 2002;7:146–155.
60. Herring JL, Dawant BM, Maurer CR Jr, Muratore DM, Galloway RL Jr, Fitzpatrick JM. Surface-based registration of CT images to physical space for image-guided surgery of the spine: a sensitivity study. *IEEE Trans Med Imaging.* 1998;17:743–752.
61. Lavallee S, Troccaz J, Sautot P, et al. Computer-assisted spinal surgery using anatomy-based registration. In: Taylor RH, Lavallee S, Burdea G, Mösges R, eds. *Computer-Integrated Surgery: Technology and Clinical Applications.* Cambridge, MA: MIT Press; 1996: 425–449.
62. Maurer CR Jr, Gaston RP, Hill DLG, et al. AcouStick: a tracked A-mode ultrasonography system for registration in image-guided surgery. In: Taylor CJ, Colchester ACF, eds. *Proceedings of the Second International Conference on Medical Imaging Computing and Computer-Assisted Intervention.* Berlin: Springer-Verlag; 1999: 953–962.
63. Trobaugh JW, Richard WD, Smith KR, Bucholz RD. Frameless stereotactic ultrasonography: method and applications. *Comput Med Imaging Graph.* 1994;18:235–246.
64. Lavallee S, Szeliski R. Recovering the position and orientation of free-form objects from image contours using 3D distance maps. *IEEE Trans Pattern Anal Mach Intell.* 1995;17:378–390
65. Murphy MJ, Adler JR Jr, Bodduluri M, et al. Image-guided radiosurgery for the spine and pancreas. *Comput Aided Surg.* 2000;5: 278–288.

66. Medin PM, Solberg TD, De Salles AAF, et al. Investigations of a minimally invasive method for treatment of spinal malignancies with LINAC stereotactic radiation therapy: accuracy and animal studies. *Int J Radiat Oncol Biol Phys.* 2002;52:1111–1122.
67. Murphy MJ. Fiducial-based targeting accuracy for external-beam radiotherapy. *Med Phys.* 2002;29:334–344.
68. Brown LMG, Boult TE. Registration of planar film radiographs with computed tomography. *Proc IEEE Workshop Math Meth Biomed Image Anal.* 1996;42–51.
69. Penney GP, Batchelor PG, Hill DLG, Hawkes DJ. Validation of a two- to three-dimensional registration algorithm for aligning preoperative CT images and intraoperative fluoroscopy images. *Med Phys.* 2001;28:1024–1032.
70. Penney GP, Weese J, Little JA, Desmedt P, Hill DLG, Hawkes DJ. A comparison of similarity measures for use in 2D–3D medical image registration. *IEEE Trans Med Imaging.* 1998;17:586–595.
71. Weese J, Penney GP, Buzug TM, Hill DLG, Hawkes DJ. Voxel-based 2-D/3-D registration of fluoroscopy images and CT scans for image-guided surgery. *IEEE Trans Inf Technol Biomed.* 1997;1: 284–293.
72. Chang SD, Main W, Martin DP, Gibbs IC, Heilbrun MP. An analysis of the accuracy of the CyberKnife: a robotic frameless stereotactic radiosurgical system. *Neurosurgery.* 2003;52:140–147.
73. Russakoff DB, Rohlfing T, Ho A, et al. Evaluation of intensity-based 2D–3D spine image registration using clinical gold-standard data. Second International Workshop on Biomedical Image Registration. Berlin: Springer-Verlag; 2003:151–160.
74. Cleary K, Anderson J, Brazaitis M, et al. Final report of the Technical Requirements for Image-Guided Spine Procedures Workshop. *Comput Aided Surg.* 2000;5:180–215.
75. Glossop ND, Hu RW, Randle JA. Computer-aided pedicle screw placement using frameless stereotaxis. *Spine.* 1996;21:2026–2034.
76. Kalfas IH, Kormos DW, Murphy MA, et al. Application of frameless stereotaxy to pedicle screw fixation of the spine. *J Neurosurg.* 1995;83:641–647.
77. Laine T, Schlenzka D, Makitalo K, Tallroth K, Nolte L-P, Visarius H. Improved accuracy of pedicle screw insertion with computer-assisted surgery: a prospective clinical trial of 30 patients. *Spine.* 1997;22:1254–1258.
78. Lavallee S, Sautot P, Troccaz J, Cinquin P, Merloz P. Computer-assisted spine surgery: a technique for accurate transpedicular screw fixation using CT data and a 3-D optical localizer. *J Image Guid Surg.* 1995;1:65–73.
79. Silveri CP, Vaccaro AR. Posterior atlantoaxial fixation: the Magerl screw technique. *Orthopedics.* 1998;21:455–459.
80. Weidner A, Wahler M, Chiu ST, Ullrich CT. Modification of C1–C2 transarticular screw fixation by image-guided surgery. *Spine.* 2000;25:2668–2674.
81. Pollack IF, Welch WC, Jacobs GB, Janecka IP. Frameless stereotaxic guidance: an intraoperative adjunct in the transoral approach for ventral cervicomedullary junction decompression. *Spine.* 1995;20:216–220.
82. Albert TJ, Klein GR, Vaccaro AR. Image-guided anterior cervical corpectomy: a feasibility study. *Spine.* 1999;24:826–830.
83. Bolger C, Wigfield C. Image-guided surgery: applications to the cervical and thoracic spine and a review of the first 120 procedures. *J Neurosurg.* 2000;92:175–180.
84. Lefkowitz MA, Foley KT. Computer-assisted image-guided fluoroscopy (virtual fluoroscopy). In: Germano IM, ed. *Advanced Techniques in Image-Guided Brain and Spine Surgery.* New York: Thieme Medical Publishers; 2002:207–217.
85. Ferguson RL, Tencer AF, Woodard P, Allen B Jr. Biomechanical comparisons of spinal fracture models and the stabilizing effects of posterior instrumentation. *Spine.* 1988;13:453–460.
86. Vaccaro AR, Rizzolo SJ, Allardyce TJ, et al. Placement of pedicle screws in the thoracic spine, I: Morphometric analysis of the thoracic vertebrae. *J Bone Joint Surg Am.* 1995;77:1193–1199.
87. Wood KB, Wentorf FA, Ogilvie JW, Kim KT. Torsional rigidity of scoliosis constructs. *Spine.* 2000;25:1893–1898.
88. Gaines RW Jr. The use of pedicle-screw internal fixation for the operative treatment of spinal disorders. *J Bone Joint Surg Am.* 2000; 82:1458–1476.
89. Yuan HA, Garfin SR, Dickman CA. A historical cohort study of pedicle screw fixation in thoracic, lumbar, and sacral spine fusions. *Spine.* 1994;19(suppl 20):2279S–2296S.
90. Cinotti G, Gumina S, Ripani M, Postacchini F. Pedicle instrumentation in the thoracic spine: a morphometric and cadaveric study for placement of screws. *Spine.* 1999;24:114–119.
91. Vaccaro AR, Rizzolo SJ, Balderston RA, et al. Placement of pedicle screws in the thoracic spine, II: An anatomical and radiographic assessment. *J Bone Joint Surg Am.* 1995;77:1200–1206.
92. Weinstein JN, Spratt KF, Spengler D, Brick C, Reid S. Spinal pedicle fixation: reliability and validity of roentgenogram-based assessment and surgical factors on successful screw placement. *Spine.* 1988;13:1012–1018.
93. McCormack BM, Benzel EC, Adams MS, Baldwin NG, Rupp FW, Maher DJ. Anatomy of the thoracic pedicle. *Neurosurgery.* 1995; 37:303–308.
94. Kothe R, O'Holleran JD, Liu W, Panjabi MM. Internal architecture of the thoracic pedicle: an anatomic study. *Spine.* 1996;21: 264–270.
95. Abitbol JJ, Smith MM, Foley KT. Thoracic pedicle screw placement accuracy: image-interactive guidance versus conventional techniques. Paper presented at: Annual Meeting of the Congress of Neurological Surgeons; 1996; Montreal.
96. Castro WHM, Halm H, Jerosch J, Malms J, Steinbeck J, Blasius S. Accuracy of pedicle screw placement in lumbar vertebrae. *Spine.* 1996;21:1320–1324.
97. Esses SI, Sachs BL, Dreyzin V. Complications associated with the technique of pedicle screw fixation: a selected survey of ABS members. *Spine.* 1993;18:2231–2239.
98. Farber GL, Place HM, Mazur RA, Jones DEC, Damiano TR. Accuracy of pedicle screw placement in lumbar fusion by plain radiographs and computed tomography. *Spine.* 1995;20:1494–1499.
99. Hsu KY, Zucherman JF, White AH, Wynne G. Internal fixation with pedicle screws. In: White AH, Rothman RH, Roy CD, eds. *Lumbar Spinal Surgery.* St. Louis, MO: CV Mosby; 1987:322–338.
100. Laine T, Lund T, Ylikoski M, Lohikoski J, Schlenzka D. Accuracy of pedicle screw insertion with and without computer assistance: a randomized controlled clinical study in 100 consecutive patients. *Eur Spine J.* 2000;9:235–240.
101. Liljenqvist UR, Halm HF, Link TM. Pedicle screw instrumentation of the thoracic spine in idiopathic scoliosis. *Spine.* 1997; 22: 2239–2245.
102. Odgers CJ, Vaccaro AR, Pollack ME, Cotler JM. Accuracy of pedicle screw placement with the assistance of lateral plain radiography. *J Spinal Disord.* 1996;9:334–338.
103. Schulze CJ, Munzinger E, Weber U. Clinical relevance of accuracy for pedicle screw placement: a computed tomographic-supported analysis. *Spine.* 1998;23:2215–2220.
104. Suk SI, Lee CK, Kim WJ, Chung YJ, Park YB. Segmental pedicle screw fixation in the treatment of thoracic idiopathic scoliosis. *Spine.* 1995;20:1399–1405.
105. Xu R, Ebraheim NA, Ou Y, Yeasting RA. Anatomic considerations of pedicle screw placement in the thoracic spine: Roy-Camille technique versus open-lamina technique. *Spine.* 1998;23:1065–1068.
106. Amiot LP, Lang K, Putzier M, Zippel H, Labelle H. Comparative results between conventional and computer-assisted pedicle screw installation in the thoracic, lumbar, and sacral spine. *Spine.* 2000;25:606–614.
107. Carl AL, Khanuja HS, Sachs BL, et al. In-vitro simulation: early results of stereotaxy for pedicle screw placement. *Spine.* 1997;22: 1160–1164.

108. Choi WW, Green BA, Levi AD. Computer-assisted fluoroscopic targeting system for pedicle screw insertion. *Neurosurgery*. 2000; 47:872–878.
109. Foley KT, Smith MM. Image-guided spine surgery. *Neurosurg Clin N Am*. 1996;7:171–186.
110. Merloz P, Tonetti J, Pittet M, Coulomb L, Lavallee S, Sautot P. Pedicle screw placement using image-guided techniques. *Clin Orthop*. 1998;354:39–48.
111. Schwarzenbach O, Berlemann U, Jost B, et al. Accuracy of computer-assisted pedicle screw placement: an in-vivo computed tomography analysis. *Spine*. 1997;22:452–458.
112. Youkilis AS, Papadopoulos SM. Thoracic instrumentation: stereotactic navigation for placement of pedicle screws in the thoracic spine. In: Germano IM, ed. *Advanced Techniques in Image-guided Brain and Spine Surgery*. New York: Thieme Medical Publishers; 2002:182–190.
113. Foley KT, Gupta SK, Justis JR, Sherman MC. Percutaneous pedicle screw fixation of the lumbar spine. *Neurosurg Focus*. 2001;10:1–8.
114. Foley KT, Smith MM. Microendoscopic discectomy. *Tech Neurosurg*. 1997;3:301–307.
115. Rampersaud YR, Simon DA, Foley KT. Accuracy requirements for image-guided spinal pedicle screw placement. *Spine*. 2001;26:352–359.
116. Glossop ND, Hu RW. Practical accuracy assessment of image-guided spine surgery. Paper presented at: Second Annual North American Program on Computer Assisted Orthopedic Surgery; 1998; Pittsburgh, PA.
117. Foley KT, Rampersaud YR, Simon DA. Virtual fluoroscopy: multiplanar x-ray guidance with minimal radiation exposure. *Eur Spine J*. 1999;8(suppl 1):S36.
118. Haponik EF, Aquino SL, Vining DJ. Virtual bronchoscopy. *Clin Chest Med*. 1999;20:201–217.
119. Higgins WE, Ramaswamy K, Swift RD, McLennan G, Hoffman EA. Virtual bronchoscopy for three-dimensional pulmonary image assessment: state of the art and future needs. *Radiographics*. 1998;18:761–778.
120. Rubin GD, Beaulieu CF, Argiro V, et al. Perspective volume rendering of CT and MR images: applications for endoscopic imaging. *Radiology*. 1996;199:321–330.
121. Shahidi R, Bax MR, Maurer CR Jr, et al. Implementation, calibration and accuracy testing of an image-enhanced endoscopy system. *IEEE Trans Med Imaging*. 2002;21:1524–1535.

---

[a] *A virtual image is a synthetic (e.g., computer-generated) image. For example,* virtual endoscopy *refers to a process in which synthetic endoscopic images are generated from CT or MR images.*[32] *It is well known that synthetic x-ray projection images can be generated from CT images; such virtual images are called digitally reconstructed radiographs.*[33] *Such images are virtual fluoroscopy images in the normal use of the word* virtual *in the context of imaging. In fluoroscopy-based IGS systems, a representation of a tracked probe or instrument is overlaid on a previously acquired real fluoroscopic image. Thus, we feel that the phrase* virtual fluoroscopy *as used in Reference 31 is potentially misleading. We use the generic description* fluoroscopy-based image-guided surgery *in this chapter.*

[b] *Spinal lesions have a fixed relationship to the spine, but fixing the spine in a stereotactic frame is technically challenging and cumbersome. A frame that attaches to the vertebral bodies has been developed for radiosurgery of spinal tumors.*[46,47] *This, however, requires multiple incisions under general anesthesia, risks surgical complications, and, in combination with the radiosurgery treatment, results in a long procedure. An alternative system that can be used for spine radiosurgery is an external stereotactic frame that encloses the body from head to midthigh and stabilizes the patient via a foam pad within.*[48] *Because there is no rigid fixation, however, this system allows for some residual patient movement. Hamilton*[46] *estimates that the invasive frame spinal targeting error is approximately 2.5 mm, and the error of the Lax body frame is up to 10 mm.*

[c] *For example, Glossop and Hu*[116] *reported an average of 2 to 3 mm translational error and 4 to 7 degrees of rotational error for pedicle screw placement using a CT-based IGS system. The translational error is consistent with theoretical predictions (see Figure 3 in reference 53), and is similar to error values reported for cranial applications using CT-based IGS systems.*[52] *Foley et al*[117] *observed a mean probe tip position error of 0.97 ± 0.40 mm and a mean trajectory angle error of 2.7 ± 0.6 degree by measuring the difference between the graphic representation of a tracked instrument and its real position in a newly acquired fluoroscopic image during pedicle screw placement using a fluoroscopic-based IGS system. The fluoroscopy–based IGS system errors are 2D errors, which are less than more clinically relevant 3D errors. Rampersaud et al*[115] *found a maximum permissible translational error of less than 1 mm and rotational error of less than 5 degrees at the midcervical spine, midthoracic spine, and thoracolumbar junction.*

SECTION SEVEN

Robotic Spine Surgery

35

Robotic Endoscopic Spine Surgery

DAVID LE, RUSSELL WOO, AND DANIEL H. KIM

Innovations in endoscopic technique and equipment continue to broaden the range of applications in spine surgery; however, these procedures have yet to gain widespread adoption due to the challenges of mastering endoscopic technique. Difficulties remain in achieving dexterity and precision of instrument control within the confines of a limited operating space, further compounded by the need to operate from a video image. The application of robotic technology has the potential of contributing significantly to the advancement of endoscopic spine surgery.

History of Minimally Invasive Surgery

The introduction of computer guidance and robotics into surgical procedures has been driven by the desire to make operations both less invasive and more precise. Minimally invasive surgical (MIS) techniques have become increasingly widespread in multiple surgical disciplines; specifically, the fields of general surgery, gynecology, orthopedics, thoracic surgery, and urology have all seen the adoption of minimally invasive techniques in the treatment of a variety of surgical conditions. The goal of MIS is to reduce a patient's pain and recovery time by decreasing the trauma of large incisions required by conventional open surgery. Additional benefits include improved cosmesis, reduced convalescence and hospital costs, and less time away from productive work.[1]

The basic arrangement of an MIS procedure involves the introduction of cannulas into the abdominal or thoracic cavity through small incisions generally no larger than 1 cm. A video endoscope for imaging and an array of endoscopic operative instruments are then introduced through these cannulas. Although the adoption of minimally invasive techniques has occurred primarily since the 1990s, we can trace their origin to the earliest eras of Western medicine.

As early as 400 BC, Hippocrates detailed the use of a speculum for examining the anorectum. Although endoscopy can trace its roots to the ancient Greeks, the first significant procedures were not performed until the past century. In 1901, the German surgeon George Kelling used a cystoscope to examine the abdomen of a dog after air insufflation.[2] Several years later, Hans Christian Jacobaeus of Stockholm, Sweden, first reported a clinically significant laparoscopy procedure in which he used a simple laparoscope with a light source at the end, with air insufflation through the scope.[2] Dr. Jacobaeus coined the term *laparothorakoskopie.*

Over the next century, the techniques of laparoscopic surgery began to slowly mature. In 1920, Zollikofer of Switzerland advocated the use of carbon dioxide gas for insufflation instead of filtered air or nitrogen.[2] In 1929, Kalk described several diagnostic and therapeutic laparoscopic procedures and advocated the use of a second puncture site to establish pneumoperitoneum. In addition, Janos Veress of Hungary and O. Goetz of Germany developed needles capable of establishing pneumoperitoneum.[2] Today, the Veress needle continues to be used widely in laparoscopic techniques.

The Modern Era of Minimally Invasive Surgery

Following the pioneering advances of the early twentieth century, the last few decades have been marked by the progressive acceptance and adoption of minimally invasive techniques to multiple surgical disciplines. By the 1970s, gynecologists worldwide began to embrace laparoscopy for diagnostic and simple therapeutic uses. The adoption of laparoscopic techniques in the field of general surgery followed a decade later. The first laparoscopic appendectomy was performed by Semm in 1983, and the first laparoscopic cholecystectomy was performed by Philip Mouret of France in 1987.[2]

Since then, minimally invasive techniques have been applied to almost all surgical fields. With many recognized benefits, including smaller incisions, reduced postoperative pain, rapid recovery, and shorter hospital stay, such techniques have now become the standard of care for a variety of operations.

Limitations of MIS

Although MIS techniques have revolutionized many surgical procedures, the introduction of MIS has also brought with it certain unique complexities that are not present with conventional open surgery.

Movement Limitations

First, MIS instruments work through cannulas, or ports, in the body wall. These ports act as pivot points that consequently reverse the direction of motion of the instrument tip in relation to the motion of the instrument handle. For instance, to move the tip to the left inside the body cavity requires the surgeon to move his or her hands to the right outside the body, and so on. This reversal of motion creates nonintuitive control of the instruments that is mentally taxing, especially as the complexity of the surgical task increases.

Second, the majority of MIS instruments consist of an end effector mounted to the tip of a long, rigid shaft. The endoscopic cannula allows these instruments to pivot around the fixed point within the body wall, but it restricts motion laterally. The six degrees of freedom of position and orientation (defined as motion along the *x*, *y*, and *z* axes and rotation about each of these axes) of open instruments is therefore reduced to 4 degrees of motion (i.e., pitch, yaw, roll, and insertion) for MIS procedures (Fig. 35–1). An additional two degrees of freedom could be restored to MIS instruments by constructing articulations at the distal end, past the location of the cannula pivot point (Fig. 35–2); however, the precise and dynamic control of these distal articulations would be difficult to coordinate without the assistance of computer control.

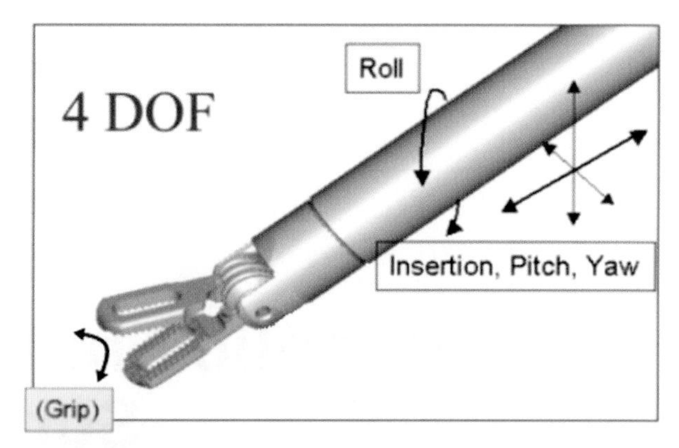

FIGURE 35–1 Traditional 4-degrees-of-freedom endoscopic instrument.

Haptic Limitations

The long shafts of MIS instruments force a separation of the surgeon's hands from the operative anatomy, which significantly decreases the amount of tactile sensation and force reflection available. The extended length of the instruments also significantly magnifies any existing hand tremor. Furthermore, the excursion of an instrument tip is highly dependent on its depth of insertion. For instance, an instrument that is shallowly inserted requires comparatively large hand movements to accomplish a given instrument movement inside the body; a deeply inserted instrument requires much less hand movement to sweep the instrument tip around. As a result, the dynamics of the instrument change constantly as it is inserted and retracted throughout a procedure. Overall, all these factors can lead to less precise and less predictable movements when compared with standard, open surgical instruments.

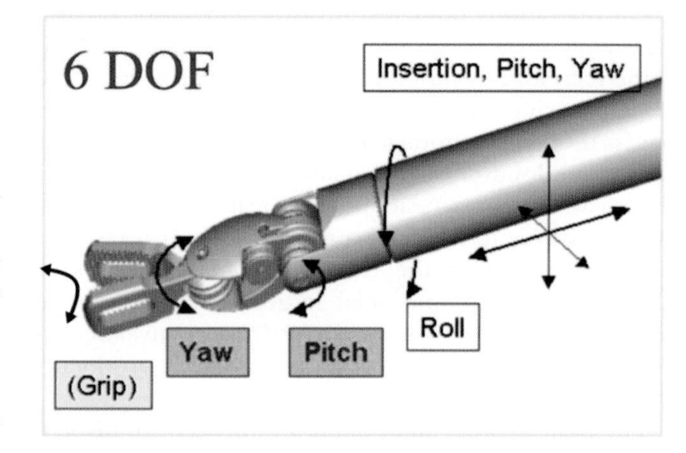

FIGURE 35–2 Fully articulated 6-degrees-of-freedom robotic instrument.

Visual Limitations

The introduction of an endoscope forces a surgeon to be visually guided by a video image instead of direct vision. The video monitor is often located on the far side of the patient, and the differences in orientation between the endoscope, instruments, and monitor require the surgeon to perform a difficult mental transformation between the visual and motor coordinate frame.[3] This problem is further exacerbated whenever an angled endoscope is used.

The majority of conventional endoscopes are built around a single lens train that is only capable of displaying images in a flat two-dimensional format. This removes much of the depth cues of normal binocular vision, complicating such tasks as dissection between tissue planes. Some stereoscopic vision systems exist, but their performance is limited in resolution and contrast due to the endoscope itself as well as the display technology.

In addition to these limitations, conventional endoscopes often require a dedicated assistant to hold and manipulate them. The natural tremors and movements of the handling assistant are exacerbated by the magnified image.

Robotics in Surgery

The first reference to the word *robot* is thought to have appeared in the play *Rossum's Universal Robots* by the Czechoslovakian playwright Karel Capek, which debuted in London in 1921. The word *robot* was derived from the Czech word *robota,* which refers to a serf or a person whose role is to perform forced labor.[4] Since then, the term *robot* has been used to refer to a variety of electromechanical devices designed to perform specific tasks. The Robotics Industries Association has more recently defined an industrial robot as a "reprogrammable, multifunctional manipulator designed to move material, parts, tools, or other specialized devices through various programmed motions for the performance of a variety of tasks." In contrast, *Webster's* dictionary defines a robot as "a machine that looks like a human being and performs various complex acts (as walking or talking) of a human being."[5]

For several decades robots have served in numerous and varied applications (e.g., manufacturing, deep-sea exploration, detonation of munitions, military surveillance, and entertainment). In contrast, the use of robotic technology in surgery is still a relatively young field. Surgical procedures have advanced rapidly since the 1980s because of the large technology base that has been developed in robotics research. Improvements in mechanical design, kinematics, and control algorithms that were originally created for industrial robots are directly applicable to many surgical applications.

TABLE 35–1 Classification of robotic surgical systems

Type of System	*Definition*	*Example*
Autonomous	System carries out treatment without immediate input from the surgeon	Cyberknife ROBODOC
Surgical assist	Surgeon and robot share control	Aesop
Teleoperators	Input from the surgeon directs movement of instruments	Intuitive Surgical da Vinci system Computer Motion Zeus system

The first recorded application of robotics in a surgical procedure was for computed tomography (CT)-guided stereotactic brain biopsy in 1987.[6] Since then, technological advances have led to the development of several different robotic systems. These systems vary significantly in complexity and function.

Classification of Robotic Surgery Systems

Robots can interact with surgeons in many ways. One classification of robots is in terms of the level of autonomy exercised by the robot (Table 35–1). One class operates autonomously in that the robots carry out a preoperative plan without any immediate control from the surgeon. The tasks performed are typically focused or repetitive, but they require a degree of precision not attainable by human hands. The second class of robots operates as surgical assist devices, meaning that the surgeon and robot share control. In the final class of robots, every function is explicitly controlled by the surgeon. The hand motions of the surgeon at the control console are tracked by the electronic controller, then relayed to the slave robot in such a manner that the instrument tips perfectly mirror every movement of the surgeon. Because the control console is physically separated from the slave robot, these systems are referred to as *teleoperators.*

Autonomous Systems

ROBODOC

Orthopedic surgery was one of the first areas of surgery to adopt the use of robotics. In comparison with soft tissue, bones deform minimally during cutting and are more amenable to image-guided technology. The result is that robotic procedures can result in far better agreement with a preoperative plan than the analogous manual procedure.

The ROBODOC system began development in 1986[7] to address potential human errors in performing cementless total hip replacement. In this procedure, the hip joint is disarticulated, and the femoral head and acetabular cup are resected. The acetabular cup is replaced by a metal and polymer prosthetic. The femoral implant consists of a long metal shaft that is inserted into a deep cavity that must be milled along the longitudinal axis of the femur. These femoral implants were originally cemented in place; however, long-term data showed that the cement was prone to cracking, loosening, or causing osteolysis that would ultimately lead to failure of the implant. Newer cementless implants have a porous metal surface and rely on natural bone ingrowth for fixation. This ingrowth requires close proximity between the implant and the bone surface, so long-term success is highly dependent on a tight fit between the two.

The ROBODOC system provides two advantages over the manual procedure. First, several clinical trials have confirmed that the robotically milled femoral pockets are more accurately formed.[7,8] Second, the preoperative CT images that are used to plan the bone-milling procedure allow the surgeon to optimize the implant size and placement for each patient.

Cyberknife

Another excellent example of an autonomous robotic system is the Cyberknife (Accuracy, Inc., Sunnyvale, CA). The system was first developed in 1994 as a noninvasive means to align treatment beams precisely for frameless stereotactic radiosurgery of brain tumors.[9] There are three fundamental differences from conventional frame-based radiosurgery.[10] First, the treatment site is referenced to such internal radiographic features as skeletal anatomy or implanted fiducials rather than a stereotactic frame. Second, it uses real-time radiography to establish the position of the lesion during treatment, then dynamically brings the treatment beam into alignment with the observed position of the treatment site. Third, treatment beams may be aimed independently without a fixed isocenter, and changes in patient position are compensated for by adaptive beam pointing.

In practice, treatment begins with a contrast CT scan of the region of interest for preoperative planning and also for reference in the targeting process. Magnetic resonance imaging (MRI) scans can further be obtained and fused with the CT images to provide a composite study. Radiotherapy treatment plans are then formulated by a team of neurosurgeons, radiation physicists, and radiation oncologists.

The delivery of an image-guided radiosurgery treatment follows a "step-and-shoot" sequence. Once the patient is placed in a position approximating the preoperative CT scan, the imaging system acquires a pair of alignment radiographs to determine the initial treatment site in the robot coordinate system. The robotic arm then moves the x-ray linear accelerator through a series of predetermined positions, or nodes, surrounding the patient. At each node, the robotic arm stops and reacquires a new pair of images from which the target position is redetermined. After the position of the target is confirmed, the arm adapts beam pointing to compensate for any movement, and the linear accelerator delivers the preplanned radiation dose for that direction. The complete process is repeated for each node. In the typical case, the system will deliver 6 to 30 Gy at the tumor margin, distributed among 100 intersecting beams. Remeasurement intervals between delivery doses are between 20 and 40 seconds.[9]

The Cyberknife system is completely autonomous in that once the treatment plan is formulated, it carries out its travel path from beginning to end without human input. Corrections to beam point are calculated entirely "on the fly" based on its imbedded computer algorithm. Although an attendant physician is always present to supervise the treatment session, the computer algorithm rarely requires intervention.

Since 1994, the system has been used to treat more than 1000 patients with benign and malignant intracranial tumors[11] as well as 16 patients with spinal cord lesions.[10] Studies using a dosimetric phantom have shown the system to be highly accurate in its targeting, with an observed root mean squared radial error of 1.8 mm, comparable to a typical stereotactic frame–based radiosurgical system.[9,12]

Surgical Assist Devices

The second classification of surgical robotic systems currently in use is the surgical assist device. One example is a robotic system for bone cutting in knee joint replacement procedures.[13] The surgeon grasps the cutting tool at the end of a low-impedance robot manipulator and moves the tool to reshape the bone to fit the prosthetic joint. The robot monitors the surgeon's actions and permits free motion in the appropriate cutting region, but applies forces to prevent motion into regions where bone should not be removed. This allows the surgeon to supervise and control the robot, using human sensing and judgment, while it also provides active constraints that increase safety and accuracy of the cutting process.

AESOP

The most widely used example of this type of robot is AESOP (Automatic Endoscopic System for Optimal Positioning; Computer Motion, Inc., Goleta, CA) (Fig. 35–3). In essence, AESOP is a voice-activated robotic endoscope holder and manipulator. It allows a surgeon to attach a scope to a robotic arm that provides a steady image by eliminating the natural movements inherent in a live camera holder. The surgeon is then able to reposition the camera by voice commands. In addition, the surgeon has the ability to preset camera positions, enabling rapid repositioning of the image to different areas of the operative field. Today, AESOP is used in many different surgical disciplines, including general surgery, gynecological surgery, cardiothoracic surgery, and urology.[14,15]

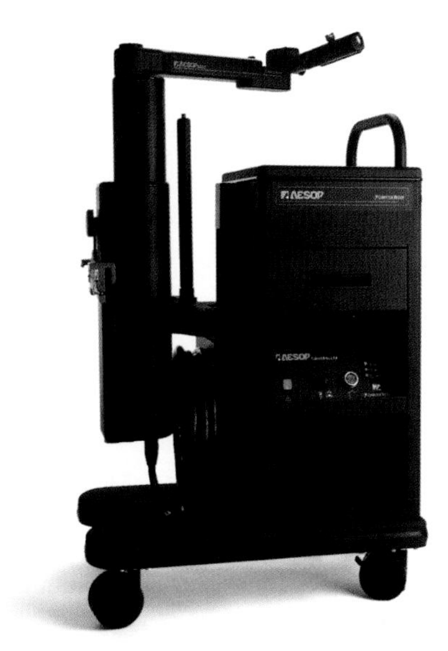

FIGURE 35–3 AESOP Robotic Endoscope Holder (courtesy of Computer Motion, Goleta, CA).

To date, several studies have evaluated the effects of such robotic surgical assist devices as the AESOP system on such specific parameters as operative time and operative outcomes. Overall, these studies appear to conclude that although such camera manipulating assist systems do not significantly alter operative times, patient length of stay, or operative morbidity, they do provide the subjective sense that there is less inadvertent movement of the laparoscope.[16] In addition, the studies conclude that such systems may be beneficial in that they decrease the need for an operative assistant assigned to hold the laparoscope, thereby enabling "solo" laparoscopic surgery in some cases.

Teleoperators

In the realm of true operative procedures, there currently are only two systems commercially available: the da Vinci Surgical System by Intuitive Surgical, Inc. (Sunnyvale, CA) and the Zeus system by Computer Motion (Goleta, CA).

Although these systems are popularly referred to as surgical "robots," this is a misnomer, because the term *robot* implies autonomous movement. In neither da Vinci nor Zeus does the system operate without the immediate control of a surgeon. A better term may be *computer-enhanced telemanipulators*. For the sake of consistency with published literature, however, this chapter will continue to refer to such systems as robots.

The integration of computer technology into both the da Vinci and Zeus systems helps to resolve many of the limitations of MIS. By scanning the surgeon's hand motions, information is relayed to the instruments to move them in the corresponding direction and orientation. Intuitive nonreversed instrument control is therefore restored, while also preserving the noninvasive nature of the MIS approach.

The presence of a computer control system allows one to filter out inherent hand tremor, thus making the motion of the instrument tips steadier than it is with the unassisted hand. In addition, the system allows for variable motion scaling from the surgeon's hand to the instrument tips. For instance, a 3:1 scale factor maps 3 cm of movement of the surgeon's hand into 1 cm of motion at the instrument tip. In combination with image magnification from the video endoscope, motion scaling makes delicate motions easier and more precise.[17]

In both systems, the instruments are also engineered with articulations at the "wrist" distally that increases their dexterity compared with simpler MIS tools. The da Vinci system alone possesses instruments capable of the full 6 degrees of freedom of the human wrist.

The da Vinci System

The da Vinc system is made up of two major components[18] (Figs. 35–4, 35–5, 35–6, 35–7). The first is the surgeon's console, which houses the visual display system, the surgeon's control handles, the user interface buttons, and the electronic controller. The second component is the patient side cart, which consists of two arms that control the operative instruments, and a third arm, which controls the video endoscope.

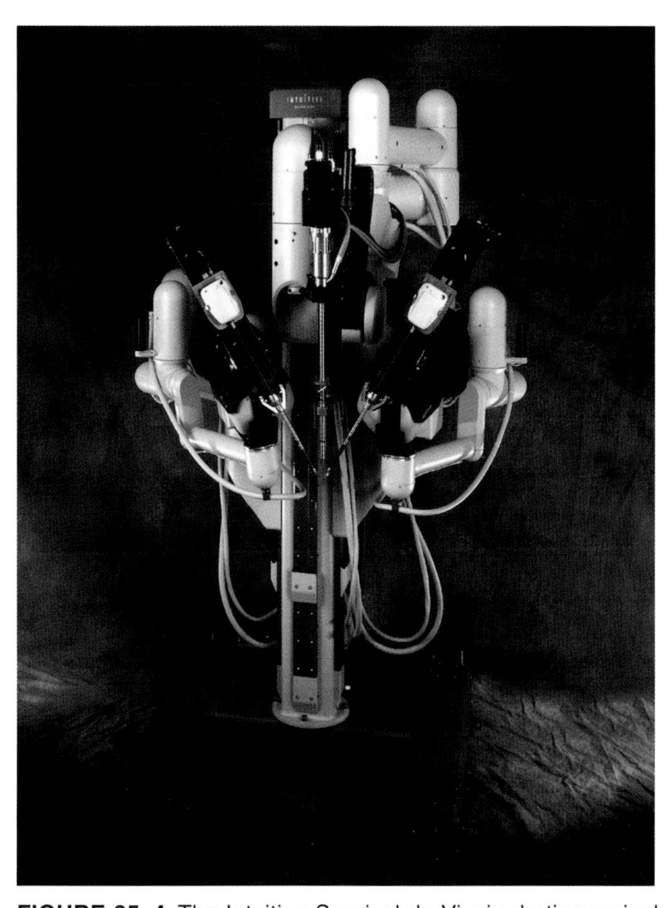

FIGURE 35–4 The Intuitive Surgical da Vinci robotic surgical system (courtesy of Intuitive Surgical, Sunnyvale, CA).

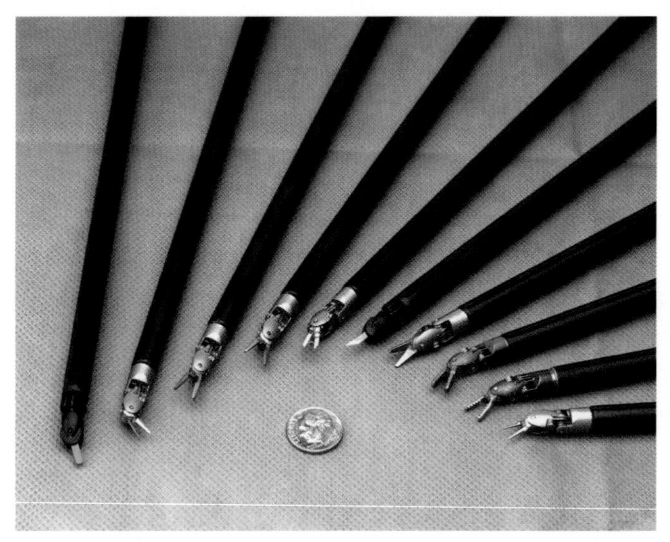

FIGURE 35–5 An array of fully articulated, six-degrees-of-freedom robotic endoscopic instruments (courtesy of Intuitive Surgical, Sunnyvale, CA).

The operative surgeon is seated at the surgeon's console, which can be located up to 10 m away from the operating table. Within the console are located the surgeon's control handles, or masters, which act as high-resolution input devices that read the position, orientation, and grip commands from the surgeon's fingertips. They also act as haptic displays that transmit forces and torques back to the surgeon's hand in response to various measured and synthetic force cues. This control system also allows for computer enhancement, enabling motion scaling and tremor reduction.

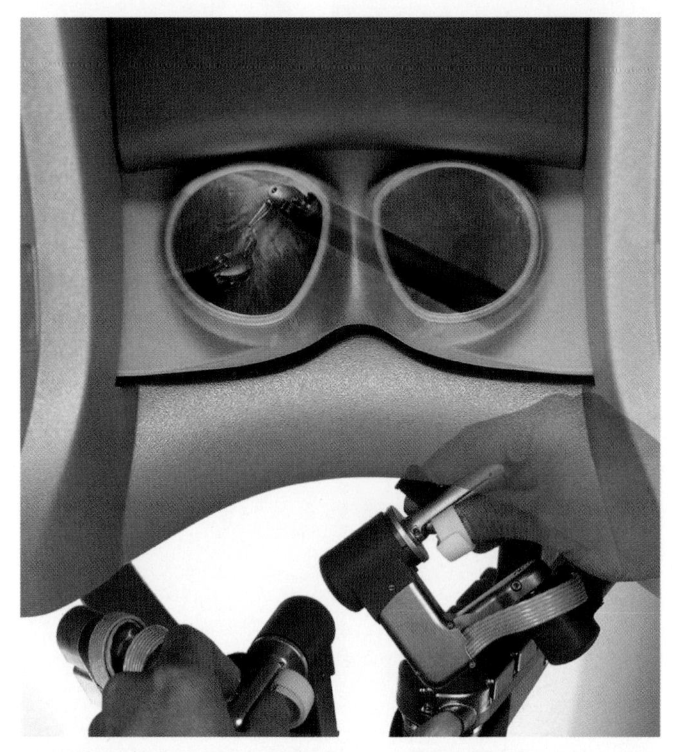

FIGURE 35–6 At the surgeon's console, alignment of the visual axis to the master controls creates the illusion that the surgeon's hands are operating virtually within the patient (courtesy of Intuitive Surgical, Sunnyvale, CA).

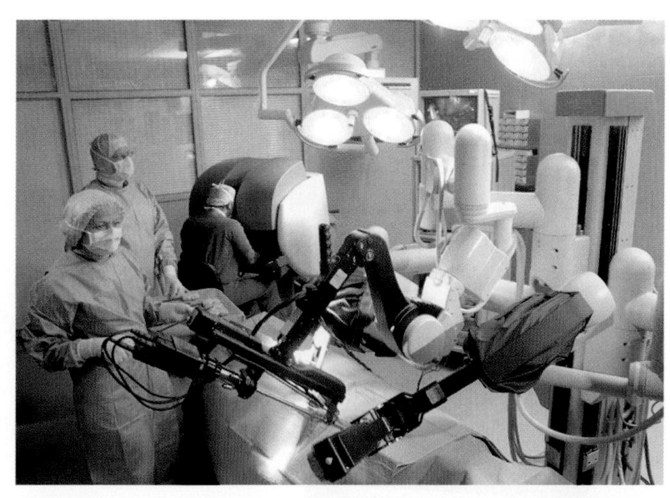

FIGURE 35–7 Arrangement of the da Vinci system within an operating room (courtesy of Intuitive Surgical, Sunnyvale, CA).

The image of the operative site is projected to the surgeon through a high-resolution stereo display system that uses two medical-grade cathode ray tube (CRT) monitors to display a separate image to each of the surgeon's eyes. The surgeon's brain then fuses the two separate images into a virtual three-dimensional construct. The image plane of the stereo viewer is superimposed over the range of motion of the masters, which restores visual alignment and hand–eye coordination. In addition, because the image of the endoscopic instrument tip is overlaid on top of where the surgeon senses his or her hands, the end effect is that the surgeon feels that his or her hands are virtually inside the patient's body.

Since its inception in 1995, the da Vinci system has received generalized clearance for surgery under European CE guidelines; in the United States it has received clearance for general, thoracic surgery, and urologic procedures such as the radical prostatectomy. In addition, the da Vinci system recently received FDA clearance for cardiac procedures involving a cardiotomy. To date, thousands of surgical procedures in multiple disciplines have been performed using the da Vinci system.[19–21]

The Zeus System

The Zeus system (Computer Motion, Goleta, CA) is a telemanipulator system that consists of a surgeon's console and three robotic arms (Figs. 35–8, 35–9, 35–10). The surgeon operates from a console several feet away from the operating table. There the surgeon uses hand-held manipulators to control the two robotic arms and

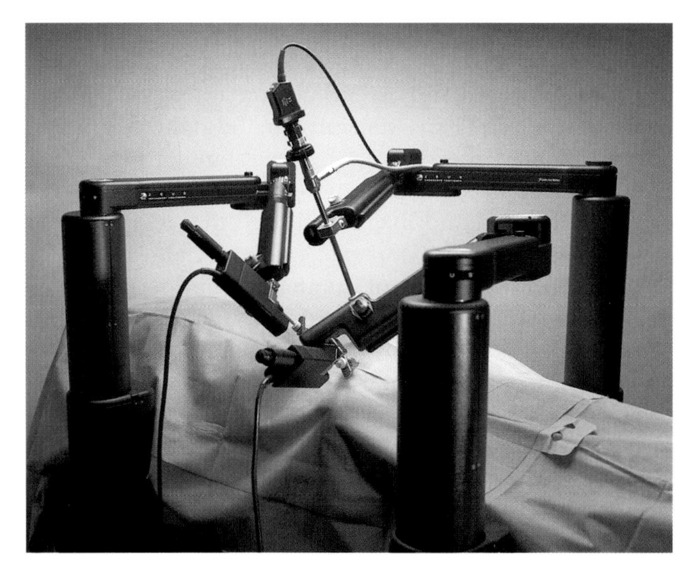

FIGURE 35–8 The Computer Motion Zeus robotic surgical system (courtesy of Computer Motion, Goleta, CA).

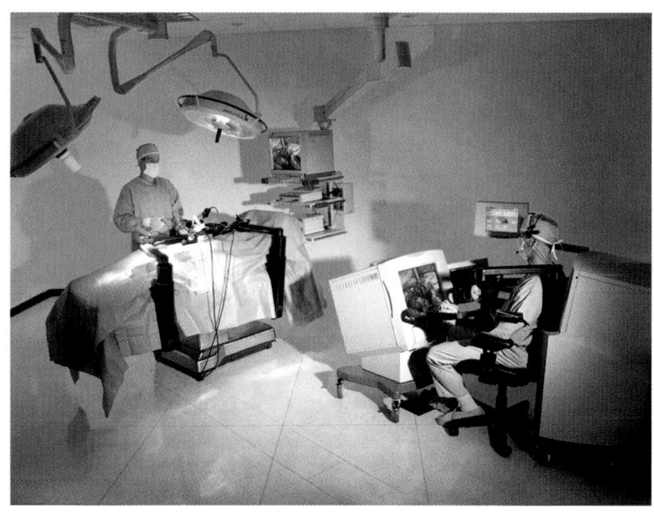

FIGURE 35–10 The Zeus system as arranged in an operating room (courtesy of Computer Motion, Goleta, CA).

surgical instruments, a foot pedal to activate the computer driven system, and voice commands to direct a camera controlled by an AESOP arm.[22] Like the da Vinci system, the Zeus system offers tremor reduction and motion scaling.

The Zeus system consists of three modular, freestanding robotic arms that are attached to the operating table. This design allows the system to be oriented to many different configurations. The Zeus system also features 3.5 to 5.0 mm instruments, several of which are capable of increased articulation through the Zeus Microwrist. This joint provides the instrument with an additional degree of freedom at the wrist, giving a total of 5 degrees of freedom. The Zeus system also features the ability to accommodate a variety of visualization options (3D and 2D) and scope sizes. Although these options are available, 3D visualization does not appear to be a core feature of this system. The Zeus system is similarly compatible with a variety of instruments from several off-the-shelf manufacturers.

The Zeus system has also received generalized clearance for surgery under European CE guidelines. In the United States, the Zeus system has received FDA clearance for general laparoscopy and is currently undergoing FDA trials for thoracic and cardiac procedures. To date, the Zeus system has been used to perform multiple operations in many surgical disciplines throughout the world.[22–24]

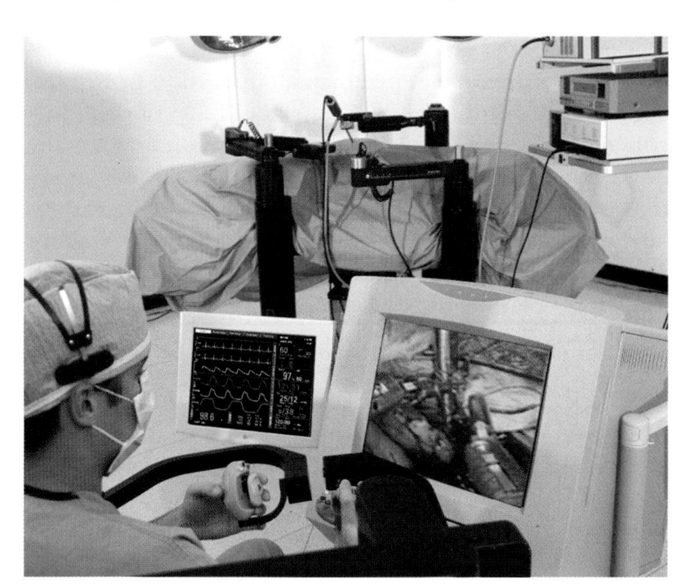

FIGURE 35–9 The surgeon's console with its video display and master controls (courtesy of Computer Motion, Goleta, CA).

Application to Endoscopic Spine Surgery

Procedures such as thoracoscopic diskectomy, vertebrectomy, and interbody fusion can all be performed using existing endoscopic equipment; however, mastery of these techniques in an endoscopic environment is challenging. Compared with open surgery, few would argue with the assertion that significant sacrifices are made in terms of the maneuverability and dexterity of the instrument tips, the precision and delicacy of dissection, and the sheer ease with which procedures may be accomplished.

There are several distinct and compelling advantages associated with the use of the surgical robot, which suggests that this particular technology is capable of significantly enhancing current operative technique. Unlike conventional instrumentation, which requires manipulation in reverse, the proportional movement of the robotic device allows the instruments to follow the movement of the surgeon's hands directly. The intuitive control of the instruments is particularly advantageous for the novice endoscopist. In addition to mimicking the surgeon's movements in an intuitive manner, the robotic instruments offer six degrees of freedom plus grip, two more than conventional instruments. This technology permits a large range of motion and rotation that follows the natural range of articulation of the human wrist, and may be particularly helpful when working space is limited. The electronic control system is capable of filtering out hand tremors as well as motion scaling, whereby gross hand movements at the surgeon's console may be translated to much finer movement of the instrument tips at the operative site. The 3D vision system adds a measure of safety and surgical control beyond what is available with the traditional endoscope. The 3D display improves depth perception, and the ability to magnify images by a factor of 10 allows extremely sensitive and accurate surgical manipulation. The alignment of the visual axis with the surgeon's hands in the console further enhances hand–eye coordination to a degree uncommon in traditional endoscopic surgery.

Future Directions

Although the current robotic systems represent great strides in technology, the possibilities for innovation are virtually endless.

The use of a video image that is processed through a computer system rather than direct vision allows for the overlay of any number of images or information. For instance, vital signs and other patient data may be projected directly in front of the surgeon's eyes while he or she is operating. A 3D image of a tumor may be directly overlaid on top of the operative field as the dissection is performed. Virtual models of heart valves, orthopedic implants, or vascular conduits may be test fitted before the costly objects are requisitioned.

Because the computer systems may be made aware of both the patient's anatomy and the position of the operative instruments, a virtual "safety envelope" may be defined. The system can then track the surgeon's hand movements and prevent inadvertent damage to collateral tissue.

One of the "holy grails" of robotic surgery is to endow the systems with true force reflection and haptic feedback; however, the presence of the numerous mechanical joints inherently imparts additional friction to the entire kinematic chain. It is therefore difficult to distinguish friction that originates from the robotic system and forces from living tissue. This limitation will be overcome with the development of newer computer algorithms and microsensors that can be positioned at the tips of the instruments.

The control handles of such a system as the da Vinci both sense a surgeon's hand movements and are electronically powered and can relay force information back to the surgeon. Tissue tension can be delivered, as in conventional surgery, as can any range of biological data. For instance, the pulsations of a diminutive artery can be enhanced and magnified such that it is palpable to the surgeon at the console. Other variables that are not in the average realm of human perception (e.g., oxygen tension, temperature, and density) may also be conveyed, as demonstrated by the National Aeronautics and Space Administration Smart Probe project.[25]

The fact that robotic systems can track a surgeon's hand movements brings with it the ability to record that wealth of data. Thus, every nuance of a master surgeon's performance, as well as the visual information from the operation, may be preserved. All that information may then be replayed in its entirety for those in training. Rather than stumble through an operation step by step, a novice may be able first to mimic, then to perform, an operation as it was meant to be. This "player piano" model may be invaluable in surgical education and could change the manner in which future generations learn to operate.

Computer systems are also much more facile than the human mind at processing complex coordinate frames of reference. For example, the operative instruments can be programmed to always align with the axis of view of the endoscope. Thus, wherever the endoscope is angled, it would appear to the surgeon that he or she is positioned at the end of the endoscope. For instance, an angled endoscope inserted into the mouth and directed back toward the nasopharynx could establish a vantage point for the operative instruments such that one could seem to operate through the back of the patient's head.

A much-popularized idea is the concept of telesurgery, whereby a surgeon can perform an operation from a distance by means of a remote interface. This concept, first conceived for military applications, would allow for the delivery of surgical care to remote or inhospitable areas. It also allows a surgeon the ability to perform operations far beyond his or her immediate geographical vicinity. The world's first transatlantic laparoscopic cholecystectomy has been performed remotely, in which a surgeon located in New York operated on a patient in Strasbourg, France.[26] This concept, however, is still severely limited by the capability of current bandwidth as well as the speed of light. A less ambitious application is telementoring, whereby an experienced specialist can observe and advise a surgical team operating in a remote location. A growing number of procedures have already been accomplished using this technology.[27]

The advent of minimally invasive surgery has brought with it a wealth of potential benefits for patients and the health care system; however, the inherent limitations of operating in an endoscopic setting pose significant challenges for the surgeon, and this is only magnified as procedures become more complex (e.g., those encountered in spine surgery). The incorporation of robotic and computer technology has the potential to contribute significantly to the advancement of this area. As the technology continues to be refined, its ultimate acceptance will demand that issues of cost, training, safety, efficacy, and clinical utility all be addressed. There remains much work to be done, yet also much good to be gained.

REFERENCES

1. Hunerbein M, Gretschel S, Rau B, Schlag PM. Reducing trauma with minimally invasive surgery: evidence and new strategies. *Chirurg.* 2003;74:282–289.
2. Filipi CJ. A history of endoscopic surgery. In: Arregui ME, Jr., Katkhouda N, McKernan JB, Reich H, eds. *Principles of Laparoscopic Surgery: Basic and Advanced Techniques.* New York: Springer-Verlag;1995:3–20.
3. Tendick F Jr, Tharp G, Stark L. Sensing and manipulatin problems in endoscopic surgery: experiment, analysis, and observation. *Presence.* 1993;2:66–81.
4. Alok Shrivastava MM. Surgical robots: the “genie” is out. In: Hemal A, ed. *Contemporary Trends in Laparoscopic Urologic Surgery.* New Delhi: BI Churchill Livingston; 2002:289–297.
5. Webster M. Online dictionary, Merriam Webster. Available at: http://www.m-w.com/netdict.htm. Accessed June 9, 2003.
6. Young RF. Application of robotics to stereotactic neurosurgery. *Neurol Res.* 1987;9:123–128.
7. Bargar WL, Bauer A, Borner M. Primary and revision total hip replacement using the Robodoc system. *Clin Orthop.* 1998;354:82–91.
8. Jerosch J, von Hasselbach C, Filler T, Peuker E, Rahgozar M, Lahmer A. Increasing the quality of preoperative planning and intraoperative application of computer-assisted systems and surgical robots-an experimental study. *Chirurg.* 1998;69:973–976.
9. Adler JR Jr, Murphy MJ, Chang SD, Hancock SL. Image-guided robotic radiosurgery. *Neurosurgery.* 1999;44:1299–1306; discussion 306–307.
10. Ryu SI, Chang SD, Kim DH, et al. Image-guided hypo-fractionated stereotactic radiosurgery to spinal lesions. *Neurosurgery.* 2001;49:838–846.
11. Chang SD, Main W, Martin DP, Gibbs IC, Heilbrun MP. An analysis of the accuracy of the CyberKnife: a robotic frameless stereotactic radiosurgical system. *Neurosurgery.* 2003;52:140–146; discussion 146–147.
12. Schell MC, Larson DA, Keavitt DD, Lutz WR, Padgarsak EB, Wu A. Stereotactic radiosurgery. In: *AAPM Task Group 42 Report.* Boston: American Association of Physicists in Medicine; 1995: 6–8.
13. Jakopec M, Harris SJ, Rodriguez y Baena F, Gomes P, Cobb J, Davies BL. The first clinical application of a “hands-on” robotic knee surgery system. *Comput Aided Surg.* 2001;6:329–339.
14. Mettler L, Ibrahim M, Jonat W. One year of experience working with the aid of a robotic assistant (the voice-controlled optic holder AESOP) in gynaecological endoscopic surgery. *Hum Reprod.* 1998;13:2748–2750.
15. Okada S, Tanaba Y, Yaegashi S, et al. Initial use of the newly developed voice-controlled robot system for a solitary pulmonary arterio-venous malformation. *Kyobu Geka.* 2002;55:871–875.
16. Merola S, Weber P, Wasielewski A, Ballantyne GH. Comparison of laparoscopic colectomy with and without the aid of a robotic camera holder. *Surg Laparosc Endosc Percutan Tech.* 2002;12:46–51.
17. Falk V, Guthart G, Salisbury JK, Wather T, Gummert J, Mohr F. Dexterity enhancement in endoscopic surgery by a computer controlled mechanical wrist. *Min Inv Therapy Allied Technol.* 1999;8: 235–242.
18. Guthart GS. The intuitive telesurgery system: overview and application. Paper presented at: IEEE International Conference on Robotics and Automation; April 10, 2000; San Francisco.
19. Chitwood WR Jr, Nifong LW, Elbeery JE, et al. Robotic mitral valve repair: trapezoidal resection and prosthetic annuloplasty with the da Vinci surgical system. *J Thorac Cardiovasc Surg.* 2000; 120:1171–1172.
20. Menon M, Tewari A, Baize B, Guillonneau B, Vallancien G. Prospective comparison of radical retropubic prostatectomy and robot-assisted anatomic prostatectomy: the Vattikuti Urology Institute experience. *Urology.* 2002;60:864–868.
21. Talamini M, Campbell K, Stanfield C. Robotic gastrointestinal surgery: early experience and system description. *J Laparoendosc Adv Surg Tech A.* 2002;12:225–232.
22. Hollands CM, Dixey LN. Applications of robotic surgery in pediatric patients. *Surg Laparosc Endosc Percutan Tech.* 2002;12:71–76.
23. Goh PM, Lomanto D, So JB. Robotic-assisted laparoscopic cholecystectomy. *Surg Endosc.* 2002;16:216–217.
24. Margossian H, Falcone T. Robotically assisted laparoscopic hysterectomy and adnexal surgery. *J Laparoendosc Adv Surg Tech A.* 2001;11:161–165.
25. Soller BR, Cabrera M, Smith SM, Sutton JP. Smart medical systems with application to nutrition and fitness in space. *Nutrition.* 2002; 18:930–936.
26. Marescaux J, Leroy J, Rubino F, et al. Transcontinental robot-assisted remote telesurgery: feasibility and potential applications. *Ann Surg.* 2002;235:487–492.
27. Marescaux J, Rubino F. Telesurgery, telementoring, virtual surgery, and telerobotics. *Curr Urol Rep.* 2003;4:109–113.

Index

Page numbers in italics indicate figures and tables.